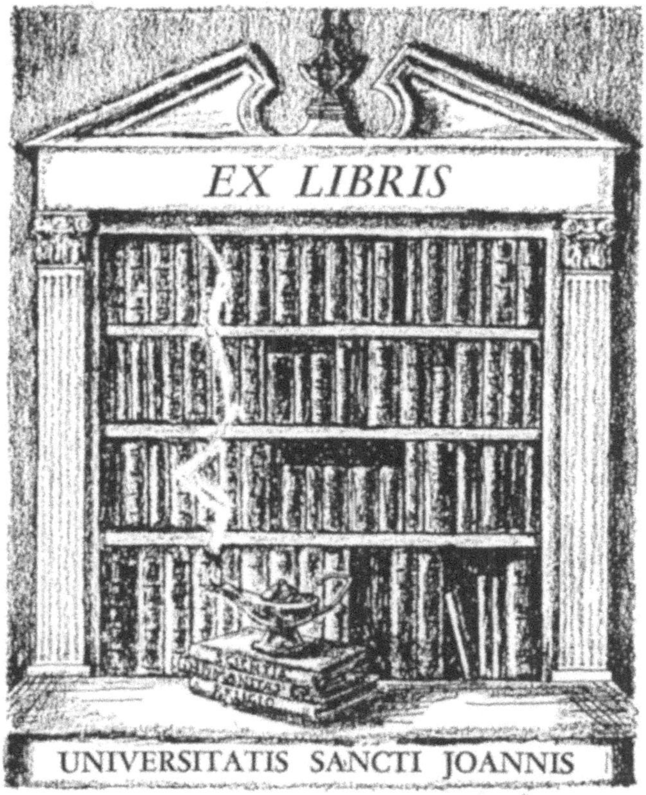
EX LIBRIS
UNIVERSITATIS SANCTI JOANNIS

OXYGEN TRANSPORT TO TISSUE – II

ADVANCES IN EXPERIMENTAL MEDICINE AND BIOLOGY

Recent Volumes in this Series

Volume 67
ATHEROSCLEROSIS DRUG DISCOVERY
Edited by Charles E. Day • 1976

Volume 68
CURRENT TRENDS IN SPHINGOLIPIDOSES AND ALLIED DISORDERS
Edited by Bruno W. Volk and Larry Schneck • 1976

Volume 69
TRANSPORT PHENOMENA IN THE NERVOUS SYSTEM: Physiological and Pathological Aspects
Edited by Giulio Levi, Leontino Battistin, and Abel Lajtha • 1976

Volume 70
KININS: Pharmacodynamics and Biological Roles
Edited by F. Sicuteri, Nathan Back, and G. L. Haberland • 1976

Volume 71
GANGLIOSIDE FUNCTION: Biochemical and Pharmacological Implications
Edited by Giuseppe Porcellati, Bruno Ceccarelli, and Guido Tettamanti • 1976

Volume 72
FUNCTIONS AND METABOLISM OF PHOSPHOLIPIDS IN THE CENTRAL AND PERIPHERAL NERVOUS SYSTEMS
Edited by Giuseppe Porcellati, Luigi Amaducci, and Claudio Galli • 1976

Volume 73A
THE RETICULOENDOTHELIAL SYSTEM IN HEALTH AND DISEASE: Functions and Characteristics
Edited by Sherwood M. Reichard, Mario R. Escobar, and Herman Friedman • 1976

Volume 73B
THE RETICULOENDOTHELIAL SYSTEM IN HEALTH AND DISEASE: Immunologic and Pathologic Aspects
Edited by Herman Friedman, Mario R. Escobar, and Sherwood M. Reichard • 1976

Volume 74
IRON AND COPPER PROTEINS
Edited by Kerry T. Yasunobu, Howard F. Mower, and Osamu Hayaishi • 1976

Volume 75
OXYGEN TRANSPORT TO TISSUE–II
Edited by Jürgen Grote, Daniel Reneau, and Gerhard Thews • 1976

OXYGEN TRANSPORT TO TISSUE – II

Edited by
Jürgen Grote
University of Mainz
Mainz, West Germany

Daniel Reneau
Louisiana Tech University
Ruston, Louisiana

and

Gerhard Thews
University of Mainz
Mainz, West Germany

PLENUM PRESS • NEW YORK AND LONDON

Library of Congress Cataloging in Publication Data

International Symposium on Oxygen Transport to Tissue, 2d, Mainz, 1975.
Oxygen transport to tissue, II.

(Advances in experimental medicine and biology; 75)
Includes index.
1. Blood gases–Congresses. 2. Oxygen transport (Physiology)–Congresses. 3. Oxygen in the body–Congresses. 4. Tissue respiration–Congresses. I. Grote, Jürgen. II. Reneau, Daniel, D. III. Thews, Gerhard, 1926- IV. Title. V. Series.
QP99.3.09I54 1975 599'.01'24 75-25951

DOI 10.1007/978-1-4684-3273-2

Proceedings of the Second International Symposium on Oxygen Transport to Tissue held in Mainz, West Germany, March 12-14, 1975

A Division of Plenum Publishing Corporation
227 West 17th Street, New York, N.Y. 10011

International Society of Oxygen Transport to Tissue

Preface

This volume contains those papers which were presented at the Second International Symposium on Oxygen Transport to Tissue, together with the discussions which followed. These discussions were generously summarized by the chairmen of the various sessions.

This symposium in Mainz was the third international meeting, after those held in Dortmund in 1971 and Charleston-Clemson in 1973, which dealt primarily with problems relating to oxygen transport to tissue under physiological and pathophysiological conditions. It was the second symposium conducted by the International Society on Oxygen Transport to Tissue which was founded in 1973.

We dedicate this volume to the memory of the first president of the International Society on Oxygen Transport to Tissue, Dr. Melvin H. Knisely.

July, 1975

Jürgen Grote

Daniel D. Reneau

Gerhard Thews

Contents

Session IV - OXYGEN DIFFUSION IN BLOOD AND TISSUE

Session V - MATHEMATICAL MODELS TO DESCRIBE

OXYGEN TRANSPORT IN BLOOD AND TISSUE

Session VII - OXYGEN SUPPLY OF THE CENTRAL NERVOUS SYSTEM II

Session VIII - OXYGEN SUPPLY OF DIFFERENT ORGANS

Session IX - COMMON ASPECTS OF OXYGEN SUPPLY

Session XI - RESPIRATORY GAS EXCHANGE AND METABOLISM IN TUMOR TISSUE II

WELCOME

Ladies and Gentlemen, dear Colleagues:

May I heartly welcome you to Mainz and express my appreciation for your participation in our 1975 conference. The numerous papers submitted have shown that the members of the International Society of Oxygen Transport to Tissue were again in the past year very successful in their scientfic research.

In spite of the large participation this year, we have attempted to keep the conference here in Mainz within the scope of a symposium so as to provide wide room for discussion. It seems to me that such a working conference provides the best opportunity for the exchange of personal experiences.

In this vein, I would propose that in the future a large congress based on the highly successful models of Charleston and Clemson be scheduled alternately with a smaller symposium. You will notice that we have reduced the social program to fit the scope of a symposium. We hope that the informal evening activities will provide you maximum opportunities for personal discussions.

The last conference began with Dr. Knisely's excellent survey of the historical development of our field of research. Little can be added to this. Therefore, I would like in utmust brevity, to say a few words about future trends in our work. The developments of the theoretical analysis and of techniques for measurement of Oxygen Transport to Organs have, in recent years, made remarkable progress. Although we are as yet far from a complete understanding of the processes of Oxygen Transport, we have reached that point where we can expect an increasing completeness of our knowledge but at the same time can anticipate no basically new knowledge. It is at this point, therefore, that we must ask ourselves, "What uses have such limited results for the general population?"

On the other hand, there is a multitude of problems in medicine to whose solutions our methods could contribute. I am of the conviction that in planning our future work we should actively consider the possibilities of practical application. This deals with that not exactly new question of the relationship between basic research and applied research.

If I perceive developments correctly, the previously existing boundaries between these two directions of research will soom disappear. I am also convinced that this division is no longer justified in view of the public's expectations. Research is generally financed publicly and it is therefore legitimate that an improvement in the quality of life be expected from these investments.

In view of this, we have included in this year's program two special topics wherein the relationship between basic research and application in medicine is particularly close: Gas Exchange and Metabolism in Tumor Tissue and Perinatal Oxygen Supply.

Before we begin with the papers and discussions, I have one last item: Past President Dr. Knisely is unfortunately not able to be with us because of ill health. I ask your permission to send him the following telegram in your name:

"Dear Dr. Knisely,
The participants of the 2nd Symposium on Oxygen Transport to Tissue send their warmest greetings and sincere wishes for your recovery. We thank you for your valuable work in the service of science and particularly for our Society OTT."

In conclusion, I wish to thank all those who have helped in the preparation of this Symposium. To the Akademie der Wissenschaften und der Literatur zu Mainz, in particular to its President, Professor Bredt, and its General Secretary, Dr. Brenner, I offer special thanks for their generosity in making available to us their facilities.

Likewise, I wish to thank the members of the Physiologisches Institut der Universität Mainz who have helped with the organization. Unfortunately it is not possible for me to mention the names of all those who helped. However, we are particularly indebted to two colleagues, the meeting coordinators, Dr. Grote and Dr. Reneau, and we thank them sincerely.

I hope that your stay in Mainz will be a most pleasant one and I now open the 2nd Symposium on Oxygen Transport to Tissues with the wish for success in the course and results of the next days.

Professor Dr. Gerhard THEWS

Oxygen Measurements in Blood and Tissue

A METHOD FOR SIMULTANEOUS MEASUREMENTS OF BIOELECTRIC ACTIVITY AND LOCAL TISSUE PO_2 IN THE CNS

A.Lehmenkühler, H.Caspers, E.-J.Speckmann

Institute of Physiology, Univ. of Münster

44 Münster, FR Germany

Previous investigations have shown that recordings of tissue PO_2 in central nervous structures by means of the polarographic method may be considerably distorted, if Pt-microelectrodes are used in connection with a remote reference point (4). Such distortions are due to DC potentials generated by neural networks of the CNS in a variety of physiological and pathological conditions (c.f. 2). The bioelectric DC potentials interfere with the polarizing voltage in the polarographic circuit and can simulate changes in PO_2, since a sufficient polarographic step in the current-voltage curves of Pt-microelectrodes is often missing. To avoid this source of error, a recording device has to be used which allows either to reduce the pick up of DC potentials to a minimum or to compensate for them. These requirements are fulfilled by concentric or double microelectrodes in which the AgAgCl-reference is coupled to the active Pt-tip at a distance of a few microns (c.f. 4). Meanwhile various technical versions of such electrode arrangements have proved their reliability (s. also 1).

Concentric or double microelectrodes may be applied, whenever changes of the PO_2 within a physiological range of fluctuations are to be measured. With higher oxygen pressures, however, the use of such electrode arrangements becomes complicated. This fact is due to a non-linearity of the current/O_2-pressure characteristic which develops with increasing PO_2

levels. A typical finding is illustrated in Fig. 1A,C. In this experiment a compound Pt-AgAgCl microelectrode with a total tip diameter of a few microns was tested in a Ringer's solution equilibrated with different PO_2 values in a hyperbaric chamber. A stabilized polarographic voltage of, most often, 550 mV was applied. The effective polarizing voltage between the Pt-tip and a gross AgAgCl bath electrode was continuously monitored by means of a high impedance preamplifier. Fig. 1A shows the simultaneous recording of the effective polarizing voltage (V_p) and of the polarographic current ($I\ O_2$) during the first stepwise variation of the PO_2 from 0-1 ata achieved by changing the equilibrating gases from nitrogen to oxygen. This PO_2 shift induced a considerable transient fall of the effective polarizing voltage. In Fig. 1C the results of further stepwise increases in PO_2 are summarized graphically.

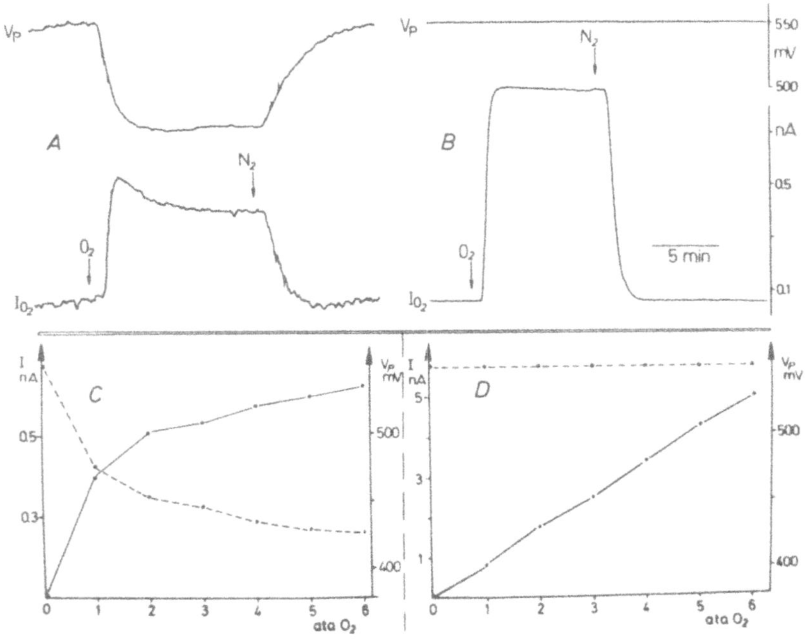

Fig. 1
Polarizing voltage (V_p) and O_2-current ($I\ O_2$) during replacement of N_2- by O_2-equilibrated test solution with unclamped (A) and clamped V_p (B). The relation between $I\ O_2$ and O_2-pressure in both cases are displayed in C and D. The graph in C corresponds to measurements as in A, the graph in D to those in B. $I\ O_2$ = continuous line; V_p = broken line.

Steady state values of the polarographic current and of the effective polarizing voltage are plotted versus the PO_2 displayed on the abscissa. The graph reveals that the polarographic current rises in a non-proportional relation with increasing PO_2. This curve is nearly mirrored by the relationship between the effective polarizing voltage and the PO_2. The finding suggests that the progressive flattening of the current curve is due mainly to the decrease of the polarizing voltage which obviously results from the high impedance (10-100 MΩ) of the AgAgCl micro-reference electrode. The drop in voltage with increasing PO_2 is practically missing if low resistance gross reference electrodes are used.

Within a physiological range of PO_2 fluctuations the non-linearity of the current-PO_2 curve can be neglected. However, at higher oxygen pressures, especially at hyperbaric values, considerable errors of PO_2 measurements can occur. Therefore a method had to be developed which prevents non-linearity of the current-PO_2 curve as well as interferences of the polarizing voltage with bioelectric DC potentials. This was realized by dividing the PO_2 reference system into a current-free microelectrode and a current-carrying macroelectrode. A low resistance electrode located at a remote inactive point is used as current reference in the polarographic circuit. A microelectrode in the immediate vicinity of the Pt-tip monitors the tissue potential, which is used to clamp the polarizing voltage between tissue and Pt-tip by means of an electronic circuit. The voltage-reference microelectrode consists of a bent micropipette with a tip diameter of about 1 µ filled with 0.9% NaCl solution. This electrode is fixed to the Pt-electrode over a length of 2 mm with the intertip distance amounting to a few microns. As a current reference electrode a remote AgAgCl macroelectrode with a tip diameter of about 2 mm is used. Pt-microneedles serve as polarographic electrodes according to the technique described by Baumgärtl and Lübbers (1).

A block diagram of the electric circuit is shown in Fig. 2. Local bioelectric potentials at the site of the Pt-electrode are recorded by a microelectrode (ME) via a "neutralized capacitance" DC preamplifier. The tissue potential (V_T) and the polarizing voltage (V_P) are added by the operational amplifier 1. The output signal (V_P + V_T) is led to the (+) inputs of the opera-

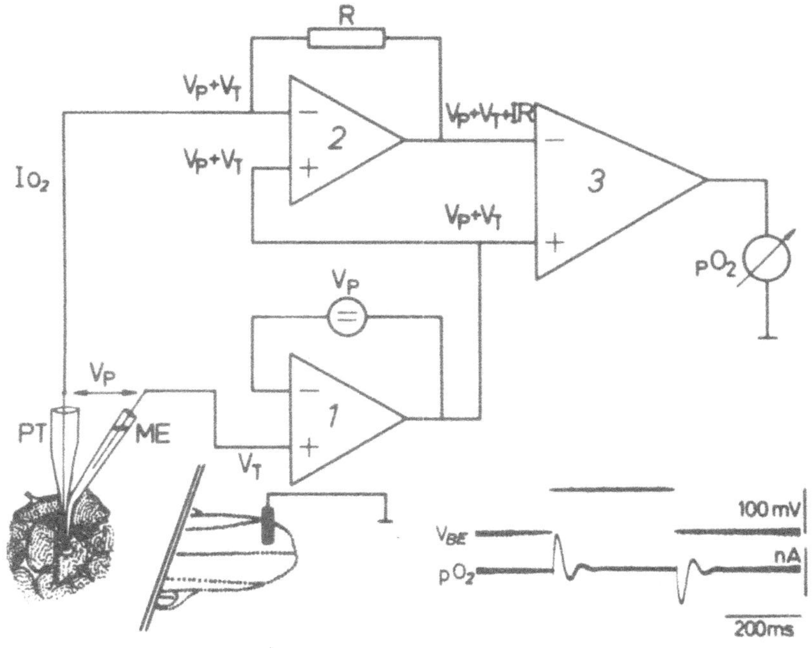

Fig. 2
Equivalent circuit for clamping the polarizing voltage between the tip of a platinum needle electrode and the tip of a micropipette. Pt = platinum needle electrode; ME = micropipette filled with 0.9% NaCl solution; V_P = polarizing voltage; V_T = bioelectric voltage of the tissue; $I\ O_2 = O_2$ current; R = resistor; 1, 2, 3 = operational amplifiers. Inserted tracings: Simultaneous recording of potential between an AgAgCl bath electrode and circuit ground (V_{BE}) and of the PO_2 signal during a rectangular pulse of 100 mV.

tional amplifiers 2 and 3. Amplifier 2 is designed as current to voltage converter. By feeding back the amplified signal through the resistor (R) to the corresponding (-) input, the difference between the potentials of the Pt-tip and the tissue is adjusted to the polarizing voltage (V_P). The operational amplifier 3 measures the difference between the output signals of the amplifiers 1 and 2 which is proportional to the O_2 current ($I\ O_2$). The properties of the V_P control circuit were tested in air-equilibrated Ringer's solution. The inserted tracings in Fig. 2 demonstrate that transient changes of the oxygen current evoked by a 100 mV rectangular variation of the bath potential returned to the initial value within 100 msec. The curves in Fig. 1B show that the polarizing voltage V_p remains stable during a stepwise increase of the oxygen pressure in the test fluid, if the described clamping circuit is applied. Correspondingly the relation between O_2-current and PO_2 becomes linear over the entire O_2-pressure range (Fig. 1D).

As compared with other methods (3) the described electronic arrangement has some further advantages. The microelectrode controlling the effective polarizing voltage can be used for simultaneous recordings of DC potentials at the immediate recording site of the PO_2. Moreover, this electrode may serve as a voltage reference also for additional measurements, e.g. of ion activities. In this way the total diameter of multiple electrode arrangements can be reduced.

Literature

1. BAUMGÄRTL, H. and LÜBBERS, D.W. Platinum needle electrode for polarographic measurement of oxygen and hydrogen. In: M. KESSLER et al. (Eds.) Oxygen supply. Theoretical and practical aspects of oxygen supply and microcirculation of tissue. pp. 130-136. Urban und Schwarzenberg, München-Berlin-Wien, 1973

2. CASPERS,H. and SPECKMANN, E.-J. Cortical DC shifts associated with changes of gas tensions in blood and tissue. In: A. REMOND (Ed.-in-chief) Handbook of Electroencephalography and Clinical Neurophysiology, Vol. 10 Part A, pp. 41-65. Elsevier, Amsterdam, 1974

3. KUNKE, S., ERDMANN, W., and METZGER, H. A new method for simultaneous PO_2 and action potential measurement in microareas of tissue. J.appl.Physiol., 1972, 32: 436-438

4. SPECKMANN, E.-J. und CASPERS, H. Messung des Sauerstoffdrucks mit Platinmikroelektroden im Zentralnervensystem. Pflügers Arch., 1970, 318: 78-81

OXYGEN FIELDS INDUCED BY RECESSED AND NEEDLE OXYGEN MICROELECTRODES IN HOMOGENEOUS MEDIA

Gary Schneiderman and Thomas K. Goldstick

Chemical Engineering Department
Northwestern University
Evanston, Illinois 60201 USA

Accurate interpretation of the experimental results obtained with oxygen microelectrodes requires a knowledge of the extent to which the PO_2 disturbance generated by the electrode extends into the medium under study. We have developed computer simulations (1) of the PO_2 fields surrounding the two most common types of microelectrodes, recessed and needle. The simulations allow us to characterize a probe from its approximate shape and its electrical current before and after membrane application. It also allows us to decide, on theoretical grounds, which microelectrode design would be best for a particular experiment. The theoretical model described here is for a cathode in a homogeneous, non-consuming medium. It would, however, be equally valid in a medium consuming O_2 at a constant rate (2) and the results found here would be similar to those in a real tissue.

Previous mathematical simulations of O_2 microelectrode operation have not properly portrayed the actual geometry. For analytical facility, previous studies (2-5) have employed a spherosymmetric geometry to model the microelectrode. Although certain qualitative information common to all microelectrode designs may be obtained from these models, their usefulness is somewhat limited because the unique geometry of a particular microelectrode actually determines the character and extent of the PO_2 field disturbance induced by its operation and thus its performance (1). Furthermore, it is obvious that one cannot use spherical geometry to model the effects upon microelectrode performance of various geometric design criteria such as electrode taper, exposed tip length, recess length, or any of the other complex geometric characteristics of the several microelectrode configurations used experimentally. The present work was conducted so as to provide accurate simulations

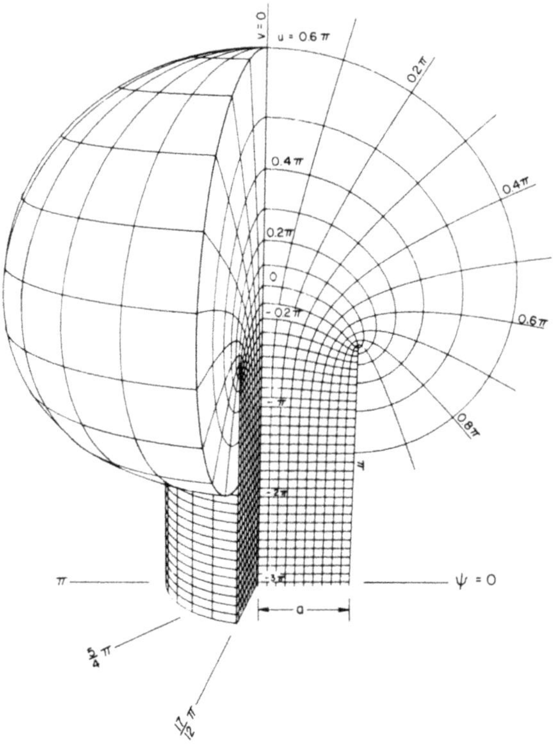

FIGURE 1: COORDINATE SYSTEM FOR RECESSED MICROELECTRODE
These Mushrooming Maxwellian Coordinates were obtained by rotation, about its axis, of the two-dimensional Maxwell conformal mapping system (7). Surfaces of approximately constant u and v simulate the geometry of recessed microelectrodes.

of electrode operation based upon the actual geometries of particular microelectrodes with and without membranes.

METHOD

The recessed microelectrode and the conically-shaped needle microelectrode were studied by simulating their operation in homogeneous media of initially uniform PO_2 (P_∞). The analyses of the induced PO_2 fields consisted of the numerical solution of Laplace's equation with appropriate boundary conditions.

A. Recessed Microelectrode

The geometry was based upon the microphotograph of an actual microelectrode (6) with the glass micropipette modeled near the tip as a right circular cylinder of negligible wall thickness. The gold, disc-shaped cathode, of diameter d = 2a, was recessed within at a distance ℓ from the "mouth" of the pipette. With this geometry, the analysis was greatly facilitated by the development and use of the new three-dimensional orthogonal coordinate system (1,7) shown in Figure 1. The recess was considered to contain a homogeneous membrane material with adjustable oxygen diffusion properties. Following the general methods of Moon and Spencer (7), Laplace's equation was derived in terms of u, v, and ψ and easily solved using standard finite difference methods (1).

B. Needle Microelectrode

Needle microelectrodes are made here by electrochemically etching a Pt/Ir wire to a fine taper and coating it, except for its tip, with a thin layer of glass (9). They are best described in prolate spheroidal coordinates as hyperboloids of revolution. This geometry makes it possible to model a wide variety of microelectrode tapers, tip sizes, and shapes. In addition, a membrane coating similar to the ones observed microscopically here could be modeled with its outer surface a hyperboloid of revolution confocal to the electrode surface.

RESULTS AND DISCUSSION

The performance characteristics studied depend upon the microelectrode geometry and the ratio, K, of the oxygen diffusivity-solubility product of the membrane material, $(Dk)_M$, to that of the external medium, $(Dk)_B$.

A. Recessed Microelectrode

The induced PO_2 fields are shown in Figure 2 as the cross-sections of the PO_2 equipotential surfaces (i.e. surfaces of constant PO_2). The cathode surface is the zero PO_2 equipotential and with increasing distances from the cathode the equipotential surfaces increase asymptotically to 100%, corresponding to the initially uniform PO_2 of the external medium, P_∞. The limiting case of zero recess corresponds to the flush-ended, cylindrically shaped gold wire in glass cathodes (prior to tip beveling or membrane applications) used experimentally (8). The accuracy of an electrode measurement depends upon the ability of the recess to contain all of the PO_2 disturbance such that it extends insignificantly into the external medium (1). The effect of a very shallow recess, $\ell/d = 0.5$, is dramatic. The 55% equipotential surface is contained entirely within the recess region. For $\ell/d = 10$, as used experi-

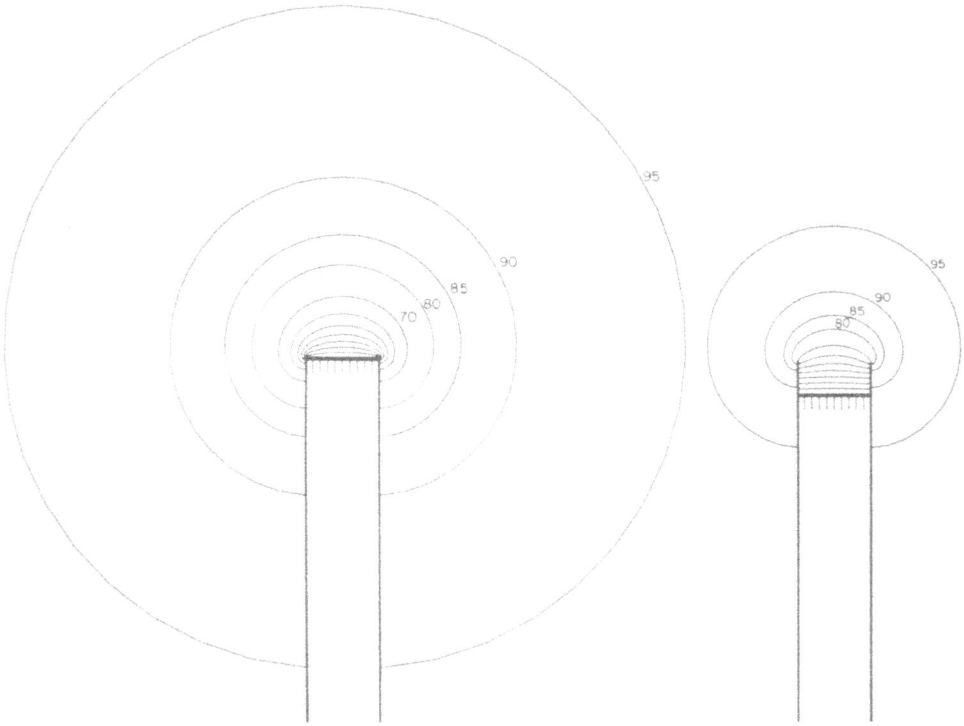

FIGURE 2: RECESSED ELECTRODE PO_2 EQUIPOTENTIALS
The equipotential PO_2 surfaces are for 0, 10, 20, 30, 40, 50, 60, 70, 80, 85, 90, 95 % of P_∞ for K = 1 and ℓ/d = 0 or 0.5.

mentally (6), the 96% PO_2 equipotential surface is contained entirely within the recess. With a lower K the accuracy is improved still further.

From the steady state simulations of the induced PO_2 field disturbance, the oxygen current sensitivities per micron of cathode radius, $\hat{S}_R$ (picoamps/mm Hg·μ), were numerically calculated and are shown as the curved lines in Figure 3. The dashed lines correspond to the idealized assumption that the induced PO_2 field is completely confined to the recess region. For this simple assumption, $\hat{S}_R$ is given (1) by:

$$(\hat{S}_R)_{IDEAL} = \frac{1}{a}\frac{dI}{dP_\infty} = 2.7048 \times 10^{-3} \frac{(Dk)_M}{(\ell/d)} \qquad [1]$$

For K = 1, the deviation of the actual curve from the ideal is large at small values of ℓ/d but, when $\ell/d > 10$, the deviation is less than 3% and so $\hat{S}_R$ can be calculated from equation 1. For K = 0.5, the deviation is less than 3% when $\ell/d > 6$. This deviation is actually

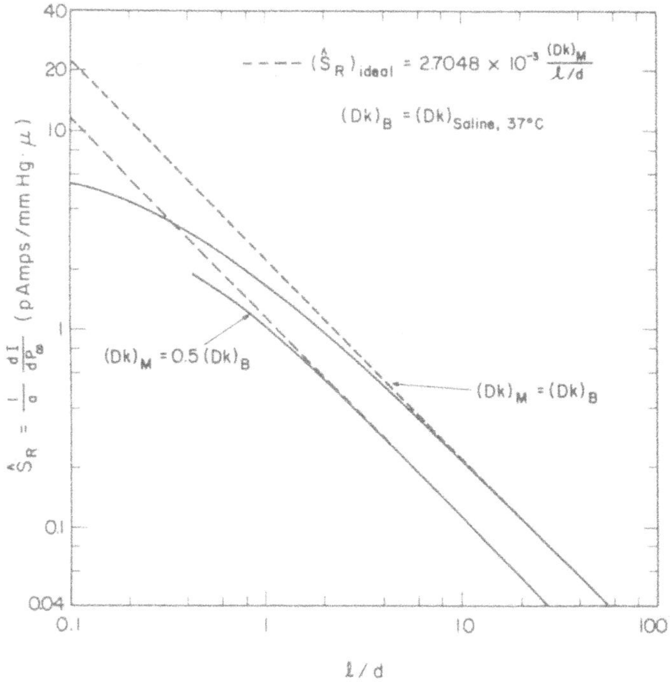

FIGURE 3: RECESSED ELECTRODE OXYGEN CURRENT SENSITIVITY
Medium is isotonic saline, at 37°C, and K is 0.5 or 1.

the stirring artifact. For K = 1, it drops from 70% at $\ell/d = 0.5$ to 3% at $\ell/d = 10$. For K = 0.5, the actual curve approaches more closely the ideal line and both are shifted making the stirring artifact correspondingly less. From the model it was also possible to calculate the measurement error resulting from the difference in physical properties between the calibration medium and the medium being probed. In general, for a given set of conditions, this error was found to decrease rapidly with increasing values of ℓ/d (1). The values for $\hat{S}_R$ shown are consistent with published experimental currents (6).

From the simulation for $\ell/d = 0$, $\hat{S}_R$ was computed to be 8.30 picoamps/mm Hg·μ in isotonic saline at 37°C [$(Dk)_B = 8.34 \times 10^{-10}$ cm^2/mm Hg·sec]. It is interesting to compare this value with the analytically obtained value of 5.74 picoamps/mm Hg·μ for a disc cathode on an infinite, insulated plane (1). The 45% higher value for the disc cathode on the end of an insulated cylindrical shaft would be expected because O_2 diffusion to this cathode is less restricted.

For a properly designed recess which contains essentially all

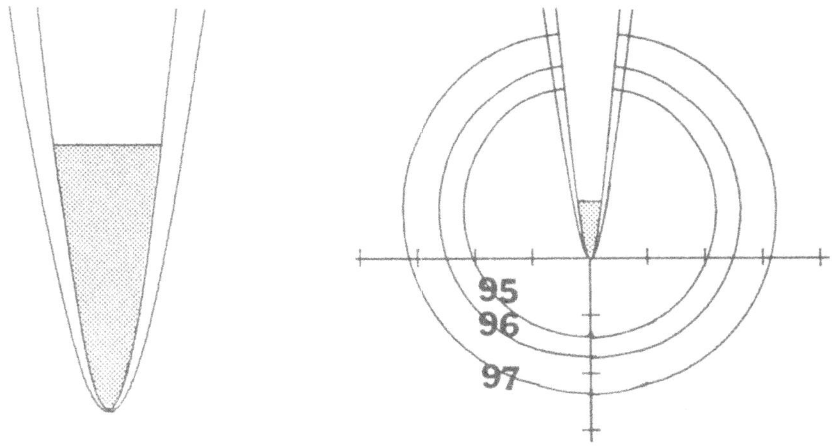

FIGURE 4: NEEDLE ELECTRODE TIP AND PO_2 EQUIPOTENTIALS FOR K = 0.1

of the induced PO_2 field, it is easy to calculate analytically (1) the 90% electrode response time (t_{90}) following a step change in PO_2 as:

$$t_{90} = \frac{2.996\ \ell^2 \times 10^{-8}}{\pi^2\ D_M} \qquad [2]$$

where D_M is the membrane O_2 diffusivity in cm^2/sec and ℓ is the recess length in microns. For $\ell = 10\mu$ and $D_M = 2.78 \times 10^{-5}$ cm^2/sec, the value for isotonic saline at 37°C, $t_{90} = 11$ msec. A response time to "full equilibration" of less than 25 msec has been reported (6) for a similar recess.

B. Needle Microelectrode

Figure 4 shows one particular tip shape and membrane as well as the PO_2 equipotentials for the case where K = 0.1. The tip shown looks almost exactly like those made here. Both the extent of penetration of the equipotentials and the current sensitivity decrease significantly with decreasing taper (1). Although the membrane coating shown is very thin, its effect is dramatic. The distance to the 95% PO_2 equipotential surface is reduced, by membrane application, from 3.9 exposed tip lengths to 1.3. With the very thin membrane shown, the 62% PO_2 equipotential surface is contained entirely within the membrane.

For this particular electrode and membrane geometry, the effect of changes in K on the induced PO_2 profiles are shown in Figure 5. Curve "d" with K = 1 corresponds to the bare cathode while curve "c"

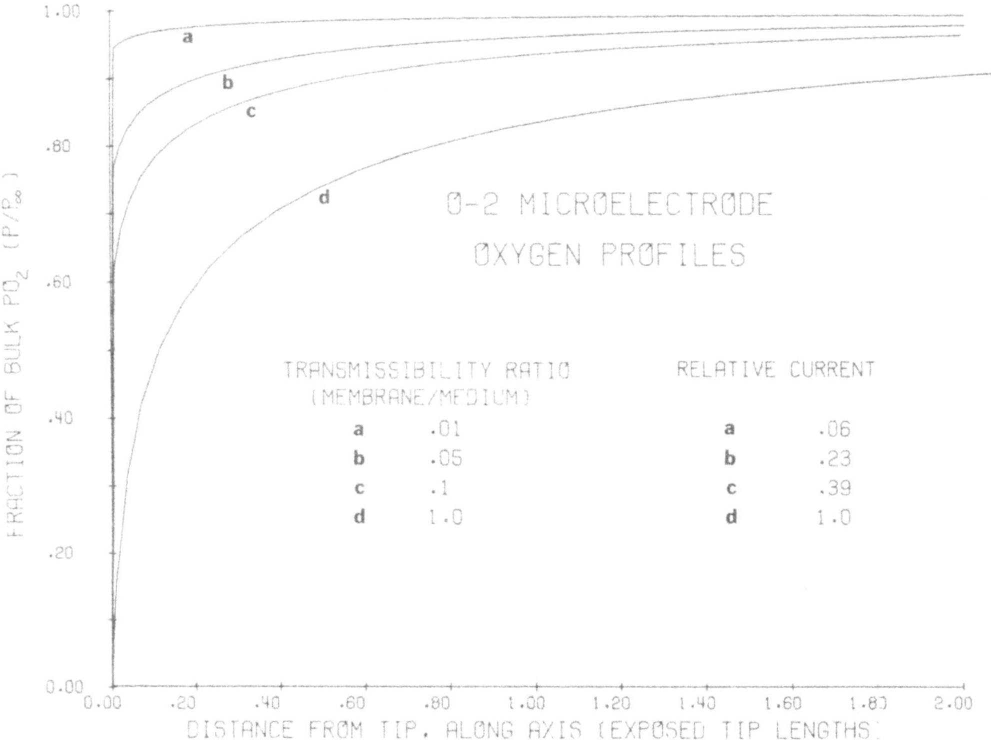

FIGURE 5: NEEDLE ELECTRODE PO_2 PROFILES
Distances are from electrode tip.

is for the membrane covered cathode illustrated in Figure 4. Accurate PO_2 measurement requires that the PO_2 disturbance induced by the cathode be confined to the membrane coating (1). Curve "a" with K = 0.01 would correspond to a polystyrene membrane (10) and a medium of isotonic saline. In this case, the effect of the membrane is even more dramatic. Even though the membrane is very thin, the 94% PO_2 equipotential surface is contained entirely within the membrane. Increasing the membrane thickness by only 1.5 times would increase this to 97%. The oxygen sensitivity per micron of exposed tip length, for the bare cathode (curve "d") in isotonic saline at 37°C, was computed as 5.05 picoamps/mm Hg·μ. This is consistent with experimental currents measured here. For the polystyrene membrane case (curve "a"), the O_2 sensitivity would be reduced, by the membrane application, to only 6% of the bare electrode value.

For the tip shown in Figure 4, the PO_2 drop from the bulk to the membrane surface and also the relative current changes caused by the membrane application are comparable within a factor of 2 to those calculated from Grunewald (5) for a spherical cathode with its radius equal to the exposed tip length and its membrane thickness equal to the average membrane thickness. The equipotentials, however, are very different. For example, with the spherical model the 95% equipotential for the electrode shown in Figure 4 would occur at 11.3 equivalent tip lengths while with the present model it occurs at 1.3. In the region closer to the membrane surface the agreement is even worse.

SUMMARY

Computer simulations of the operation of both the recessed and conically-shaped needle type microelectrodes were developed. The accurate portrayal of their geometries was greatly facilitated by the use of specialized three dimensional orthogonal coordinate systems with coordinate surfaces coincident with the geometry of the problem. From the simulations, calculations were made of the induced PO_2 fields, oxygen sensitivities, stirring artifacts, measurement errors, and time constants.

ACKNOWLEDGEMENTS

This research was supported by Evanston Hospital grants 3565 and 3595, NIH grants GM-00874, and HL-17517, Chicago Heart Association grant A74-37 and a Cabell Fellowship from Northwestern University to G.S. We gratefully acknowledge valuable discussions with C.G. Ellis and H.E. Guthermann and the technical assistance of L. Ebihara.

REFERENCES

1. Schneiderman, G., PhD thesis, Northwestern Univ., Evanston (1975).
2. Hudson, J.A., Med. & Biol. Engng., 5, 207-223 (1967).
3. Albanese, R.A., J. Theor. Biol., 33, 91-103 (1971).
4. Albanese, R.A., J. Theor. Biol., 38, 143-154 (1973).
5. Grunewald, W., Pflugers Arch., 320, 24-44 (1970).
6. Whalen, W.J., et al., J. Appl. Physiol., 23, 798-801 (1967).
7. Moon, P. and Spencer, D.E., "Field Theory Handbook", Springer Verlag, New York (1971).
8. Erdmann, W., et al., in "Oxygen Supply", ed. by M. Kessler et al., University Park Press, Baltimore, 169-174 (1973).
9. Silver, I.A., Med. Electron. Biol. Engng., 3, 377-387 (1965).
10. Baumgartl, H., et al., Microvas. Res., 4, 247-257 (1972).

THE APPLICATION OF HISTOLOGICAL ANALYSIS FOR THE LOCALIZATION OF TISSUE Po_2 AND LOCAL BLOOD FLOW WITH THE EXAMPLE OF THE GLOMUS CAROTICUM OF THE RABBIT (ORYCTOLAGUS CUNICULUS)

H. Weigelt, E. Seidl, H. Acker, D. W. Lübbers

Max-Planck-Institut für Systemphysiologie
46 Dortmund, German Federal Republic

The application of needle electrodes to oxygen pressure (Po_2) measurements in organs allows us to record Po_2 values in very small regions (1). Since these local measurements give information on the oxygen level in different depths of the tissue but do not permit the exact localization of the site of measurement, the question arose whether histological analysis may be helpful to correlate the measured values to the site of measurement. We studied this problem on the carotid body of the rabbit.

The length of the puncture channel measured from the first contact of the electrode with the organ surface is known from the physiological experiment. Both Po_2 and local flow measured with hydrogen slug injection are registered along the path of the penetrating electrode. After these measurements the carotid body is taken from the still alive and anaesthetized rabbit, fixated by immersion in Bouin's solution, embedded in paraplast after treatment with a clearing agent and cut in 7-μm slices. Trichrome staining is done according to Azan-Heidenhain or Masson-Goldner (2).

At first, the histological picture gives information on the state of the preparation and, if this is satisfactory, we assume that it was in the same or even a better state during the physiological experiment. Generally, the preparations are in a better state after Po_2 measurements than after hydrogen clearance experiments where, as a rule, highly acidophilic preparations were found.

Secondly, it is relevant to identify defective sites in the carotid body. Traces of defects caused by the puncture must be detectable through a series of subsequent slices. Fortunately, in a few cases we could follow the channel from its beginning in the connective tissue down to the specific tissue of the carotid body.

The next three figures demonstrate such a situation. In the first figure the puncture channel lies in the outer area, at a distance of 200 µm from the carotid body tissue.

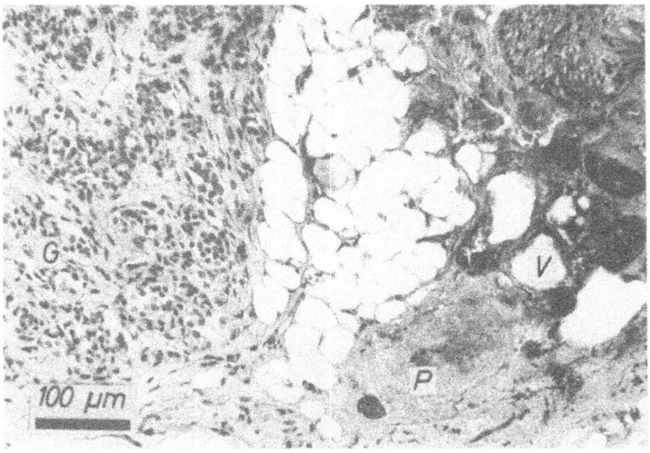

Figure 1
Puncture channel (P) in the outer area of the carotid body (G) close to some venules (V)

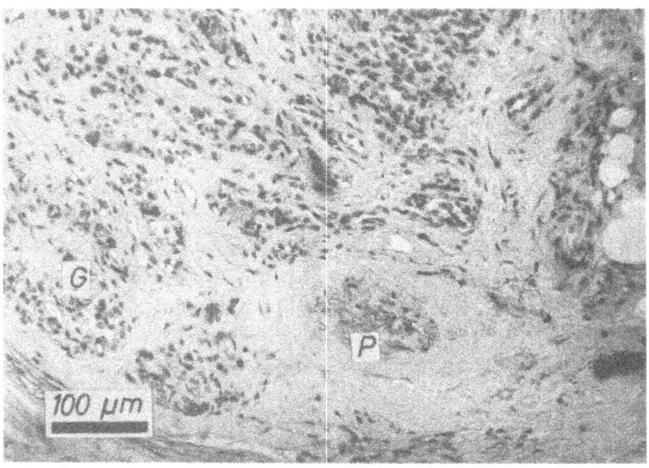

Figure 2
Puncture channel (P) near the glomoids (G)

In the second figure it passes through the interface near the functional subunits - we call them "glomoids". This picture shows the puncture channel clearly, and also reveals some of the problems due to the fact that the thicker upper part of the shaft of the advancing electrode widens the channel and destroys the sites of measurement which were only slightly affected by the previous measurement with the thin tip of the electrode. At the beginning of the electrode channel the diameter amounts to 40 µm. In the sequel - figure 3 - we approach the end of the puncture channel, which narrows down to about 15 µm and meets a glomoid which is only partly destroyed.

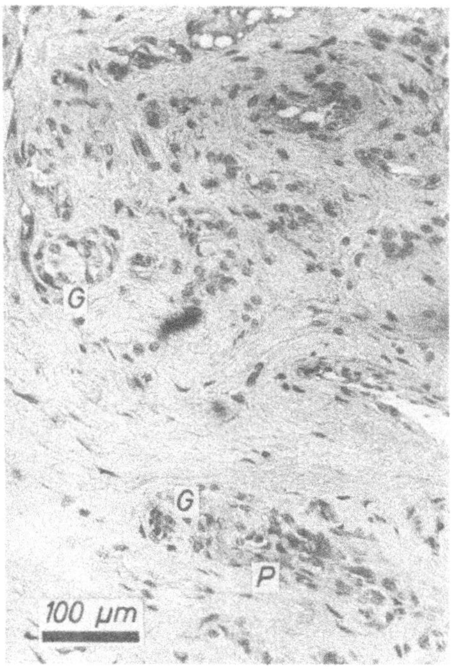

Figure 3
End of the puncture channel (P) in a glomoid (G)

According to the histological picture the reconstructed puncture channel does not proceed in a strictly straight line but describes a slight bend that is caused by various factors, such as the influence of fixation on the state of swelling and embedding, the cutting process and also the electrode itself which possibly follows more rigid structures of the carotid body tissue to a certain degree.

Figure 4 shows the measured Po_2 values and their correlation to the different tissue areas.

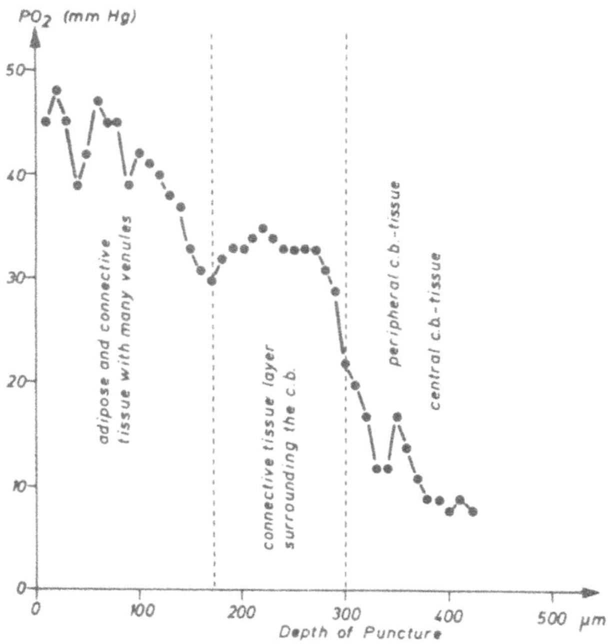

Figure 4
Tissue Po_2 of the carotid body shown in Figs. 1, 2, 3.

The first area includes measurements in the connective and adipose tissue which is rich in venules and extends as a large layer between vessels and nerves towards and finally into the carotid body (see Fig. 1).

The second area shows a lower Po_2 plateau and can be defined as a connective-tissue interface of the carotid body. We notice that here the tissue is more densely structured (see Fig. 2).

The third area belongs to the specific carotid body tissue where we only find low Po_2 values. Its beginning is characterized by a steep Po_2 slope occurring over a short distance of about 60 μm. The lowest values are to be found at the end of the puncture channel (see Fig. 3) (3).

Figure 5 shows an example for the correlation not of the Po_2 values but of the values of local flow to the tissue. Also here the electrode penetrates first the connective and adipose tissue. This tissue includes a great number of venules and, consequently, increased flow values are to be found here. Penetrating into deeper layers, a branch of the carotid body was met. Close to this branch the flow increases strongly at first and then decreases again as the electrode is inserted farther. The lowest flow values are regularly observed in the carotid body itself. However, we cannot discriminate whether these low flow values occur in the connective tissue between the glomoids or in the functional units themselves. The nearness of an arteriole is indicated by an increase in flow. In this experiment the mean flow is about 1200 ml/100 g . min and corresponds approximately to the mean value obtained from 199 individual measurements on 12 carotid bodies. As we saw in Fig. 5, an increase of flow indicates that a vessel is nearby; and from the histological picture we would expect an increased flow near a vessel.

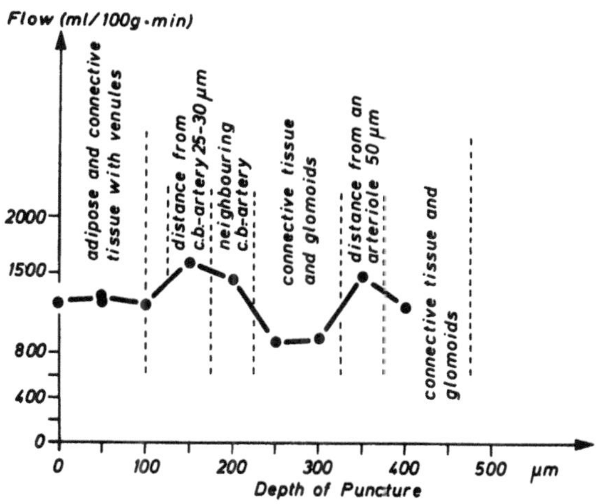

Figure 5
Flow distribution in the carotid body

Figure 6 shows Po_2 values measured in an artery and demonstrates a good correlation of the measured distance to the puncture channel. The onset of measurement is characterized by high Po_2 values. Because of the high speed of puncturing necessary to penetrate the arterial wall from outside, Po_2 measurements cannot be performed in this phase. As soon as the electrode enters the interior of the vessel, we notice high Po_2 values. After leaving the interior and penetrating into the vascular wall, the electrode indicates Po_2 values decreased by about 60 mm Hg.

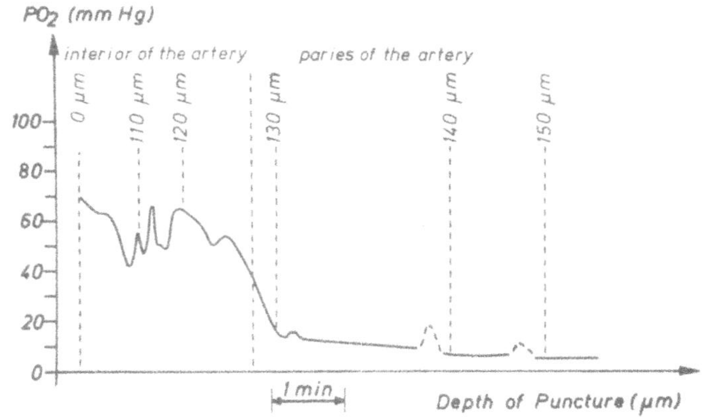

Figure 6
Po_2 measurement in an artery

Figure 7 shows the histological findings and clearly reveals the torn arterial wall.

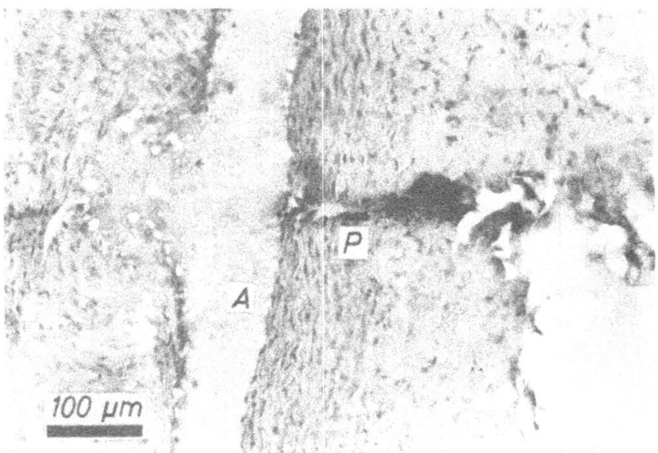

Figure 7
Histological picture of the artery (A) and the position of the puncture channel (P)

Summarizing we can say that we are able to ascertain whether the electrode entered into the specific tissue of the carotid body. With our Po_2 measurements in the carotid body of the rabbit we could clearly show that out of 24 puncture channels 16 were within and 8 outside the carotid body. In 16 puncture channels 461 individual measurements were performed, 311 of which were in the carotid body. The Po_2 values were not higher than 25 mm Hg; most values were between 5 and 10 mm Hg. The correlation between measured value and site of measurement cannot always be established, but in a few cases the position of the electrode could be measured with an accuracy of $\pm$ 30 μm.

References

1. Kessler, M., Bruley, D. F., Clark, L. C. Jr., Lübbers, D. W., Silver, I. A., Strauss, J. (Edts.): Oxygen Supply. Theoretical and Practical Aspects of Oxygen Supply and Microcirculation of Tissue. Urban & Schwarzenberg, München - Berlin - Wien 1973

2. Seidl, E.: Die Anwendung des Interferenz-Kontrast-Verfahrens am gefärbten Schnitt als Hilfsmittel bei der Rekonstruktion von Organellen. Leitz-Mitt. Wiss. Tech. VI, 57 - 58 (1973)

3. Weigelt, H., Acker, H., Seidl, E., Lübbers, D. W.: Oxygen pressure field in the carotid body of the rabbit (Oryctolagus cuniculus). Arzneimittel-Forsch. (Drug Res.) 23, 1607 - 1614 (1973)

4. Weigelt, H., Seidl, E., Acker, H., Lübbers, D. W.: Determination of local flow in the carotid body of the rabbit (Oryctolagus cuniculus). Pflügers Arch. 343, R 10 (1973)

A METHOD FOR MEASURING OXYGEN UPTAKE RATE DISTRIBUTIONS OVER THE SURFACE ZONE OF EXCISED TISSUES USING A 91-CATHODE ELECTRODE

N.T.S. Evans and T.B. Constable

Medical Research Council, Cyclotron Unit

Hammersmith Hospital, London

Existing methods for measuring the oxygen uptake rates of tissues require amounts of tissue in excess of 20mg or so, and provide no information on spatial variations in uptake rate. The method described here enables estimates of uptake rate to be made at known points on a tissue surface with a spatial resolution of better than 0.5mm.

THEORY OF THE METHOD

Consider a volume of uniformly respiring tissue having a plane surface S initially exposed to gas containing oxygen at a partial pressure p_0 mm Hg. Oxygen diffuses across S and is metabolised by the tissue at rate m mm Hg/sec. An equilibrium is reached within a few minutes, the oxygen tension falling from p_0 on S to zero at a distance x_0 in the tissue, where

$$x_0 = \sqrt{2sDp_0/m}$$

s and D being the solubility and diffusion constant respectively of oxygen in the tissue. The surface is then occluded by the end of a glass prism which has a platinum cathode sealed into it. The pO_2 at the tissue surface falls to zero as the dissolved oxygen is metabolised. The time course of the surface pO_2 is measured by the cathode current i(t). It can be shown theoretically (1,2) that the form of i(t), after the initial settling period immediately following the occlusion, is described quite accurately by:

$$i(t) = i_0(1 - \sqrt{8mt/\pi p_0})$$

where i_0 is the initial electrode current obtained by extrapolating back to zero time the linear part of the graph of i(t) against $\sqrt{t}$. If the slope of the linear part of this graph is k, m can be calculated from the expression:

$$m = \pi p_0 k^2 / 8 i_0^2$$

m is the mean uptake rate averaged over a distance of approximately x_0 from the cathode. By using a multi-cathode electrode, estimates of m at many points on the tissue surface can be obtained.

THE ELECTRODE ASSEMBLY AND MEASURING SYSTEM

The electrode consists of 91 platinum wires, 25μ in diameter, sealed into an hexagonal array of 0.5mm diameter glass capillaries. The capillaries are lightly sintered together and the lower ends are fused electrically and the surface polished to an optical finish. The electrode is mounted vertically over a cuvette which contains the piece of tissue to be measured (Fig.1). The tissue is covered with a 12μ polythene membrane, and a plunger in the lower part of the cuvette holds the tissue in firm contact with the membrane. The cuvette is mounted in a double gimbal suspension to facilitate automatic alignment of the tissue and electrode surfaces when they are brought into contact. Contact is brought about by raising the cuvette suspension vertically, using a linear bearing and a rubber diaphragm which can be deformed pneumatically. The end of the electrode and the cuvette are housed within a gas chamber which can be flushed with different gases. The entire assembly is in a thermostatically controlled box.

For the measurements, a drop of electrolyte is positioned on the end of the electrode, which is then lowered until the drop is 5mm above the cuvette surface. Gas containing oxygen is blown through the gas housing for a few minutes. Recording of the cathode currents is started and the cuvette brought into contact with the electrode. The currents are recorded until they have all reached low levels, and after a further few minutes, a short recording of the final currents is made.

The cathode currents are recorded using a 100-channel data logging system (Mycalex Instruments). The voltage across an 880KΩ resistor in series with each cathode is sampled once a second by one of four diaphragm relay scanner units operating in parallel and each scanning 25 channels sequentially. The voltages are amplified and converted to digital form by a voltage-to-frequency converter which integrates each voltage over a 20 msec period, thus achieving a very high 50Hz rejection. The digitized data are sequenced and recorded on an incremental magnetic tape unit. Automatic amplifier drift correction is applied by sampling the voltage developed across

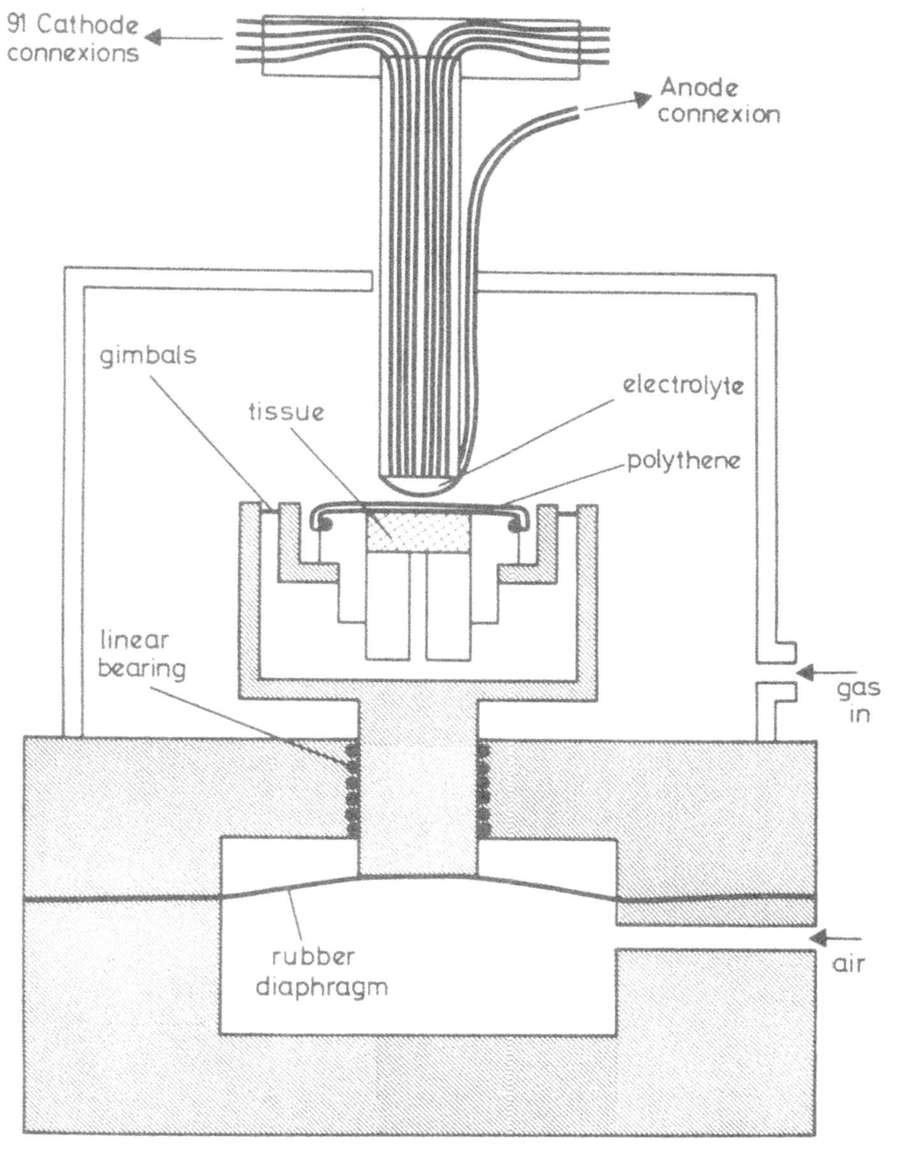

Fig. 1. The multi-cathode electrode assembly, with tissue in cuvette prior to measurement.

a dummy load of 880KΩ once a second and subtracting this value from the measured values. A visual monitoring system enables the digitized cathode currents to be reconverted to analogue form and displayed on a storage oscilloscope during the recording of the data.

DATA PROCESSING

Since a determination of oxygen uptake rate at 91 cathodes necessitates handling about 5000 current values, the data are transferred from magnetic tape to the magnetic disc store of an HP2116B

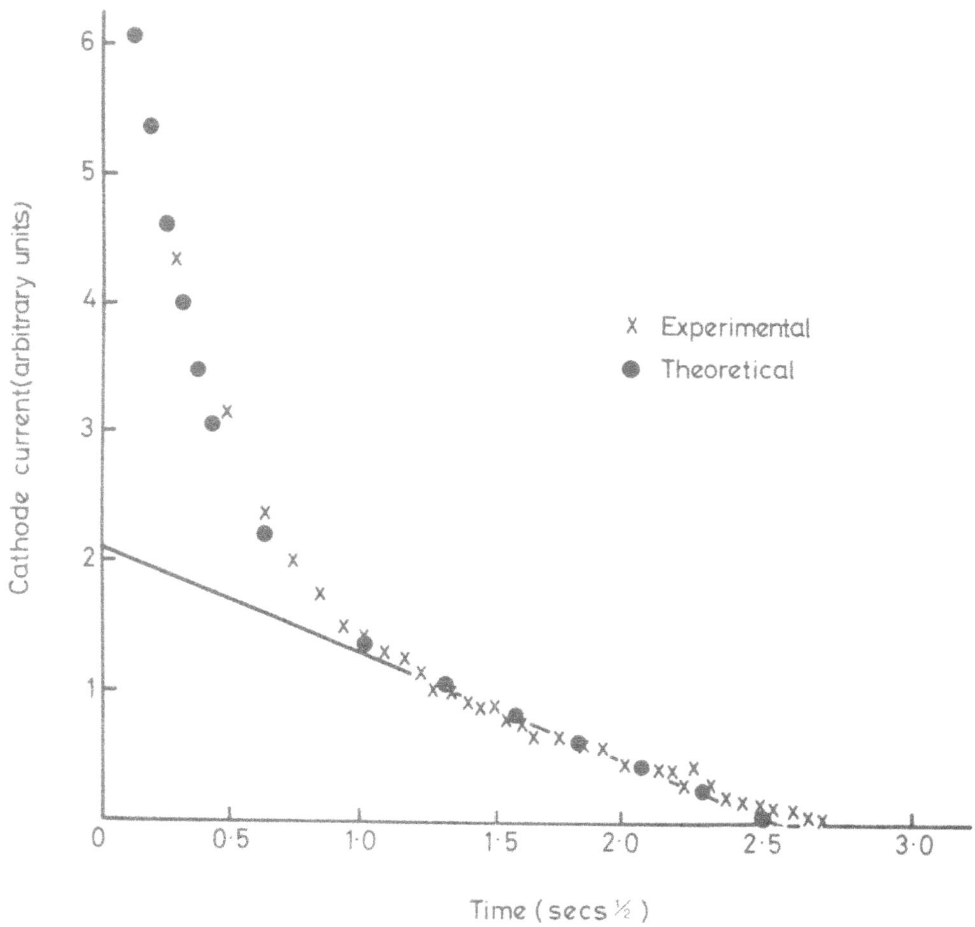

Fig. 2. Time course of cathode current after occlusion of tissue surface with electrode assembly.

computer for processing. After various checks for errors in recording, the data are sorted into separate channels for each cathode, and the time origin for the experiment found by detecting the time at which the current is 25% below the steady level obtained with the electrolyte drop. All current values are then related to $\sqrt{t}$ as measured from this time origin. Fig. 2 shows a set of current values plotted in this way. The solid circle points are theoretical ones calculated numerically (2). The slope k of the linear part of the current against $\sqrt{t}$ curve is computed by first setting a limit to exclude the data recorded during the settling time after occlusion. Progressively longer sections of the data centred on the point half-way between the initial and final currents are used to fit a series of regression lines. The slope estimates from these become more accurate as more data points are included until points beyond the limits of the linear part are used. Then the slope estimates begin to change rapidly. The estimates are averaged three at a time and the group showing minimal variance is taken as the best estimate of k. The procedure works well, although poor fitting occurs occasionally due to statistical anomalies. This is detected by testing for an unduly large standard error on the slope estimate or for a small number of data points used, and a modified calculation is performed. The final estimates of oxygen uptake rate can be printed out as a hexagonal pattern of values corresponding to the spatial position of each cathode on the electrode face.

MEASUREMENTS ON AN ARTIFICIAL TISSUE

In order to test the validity of the method, it was necessary to devise an artificial tissue with known oxygen uptake properties. Various concentrations of bacteria (E.Coli B/r) were mixed with agar (9.25g/l) and nutrient broth (25g/l) at 42°C, poured into the measuring cuvettes and allowed to set. Stabilisation of the oxygen uptake rate was achieved by inhibiting proliferation with 10µg/l of chloramphenicol. An independent measure of uptake rate of the bacteria/gel mixture was obtained in order to have a direct comparison with the values resulting from the multi-cathode system of measurement. For this the gel mixture was extruded as thin "worms" into a solution of nutrient broth containing chloramphenicol. The oxygen uptake rate of a known weight of this extruded gel was measured in a stirred closed vessel by estimating the rate of fall of pO_2 with a single cathode electrode (3).

Fig. 3 shows the oxygen uptake rates measured with the 91-cathode system using three different concentrations of bacteria. The standard deviation within the group of cathodes is 10% of the mean value.

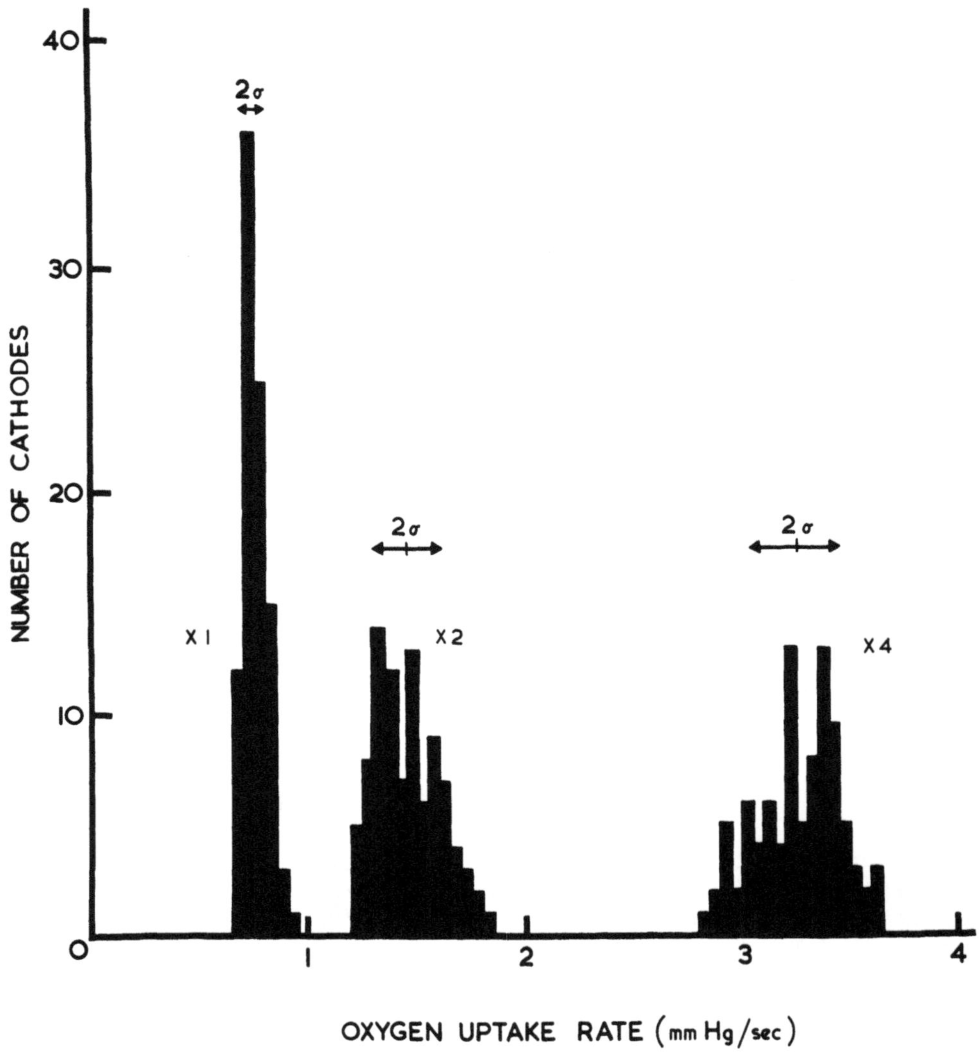

Fig. 3. Oxygen uptake rate distributions for different concentrations of bacteria in agar gel.

Fig. 4 shows the variation of uptake rate (solid points) with bacterial concentration, plotted on logarithmic scales to cover the range of concentrations used. The line has unit slope and indicates direct proportionality over a wide range of uptake rates. The open points show the uptake rates measured for gel "worms" in a stirred closed vessel. There is good agreement between the values obtained by the two methods.

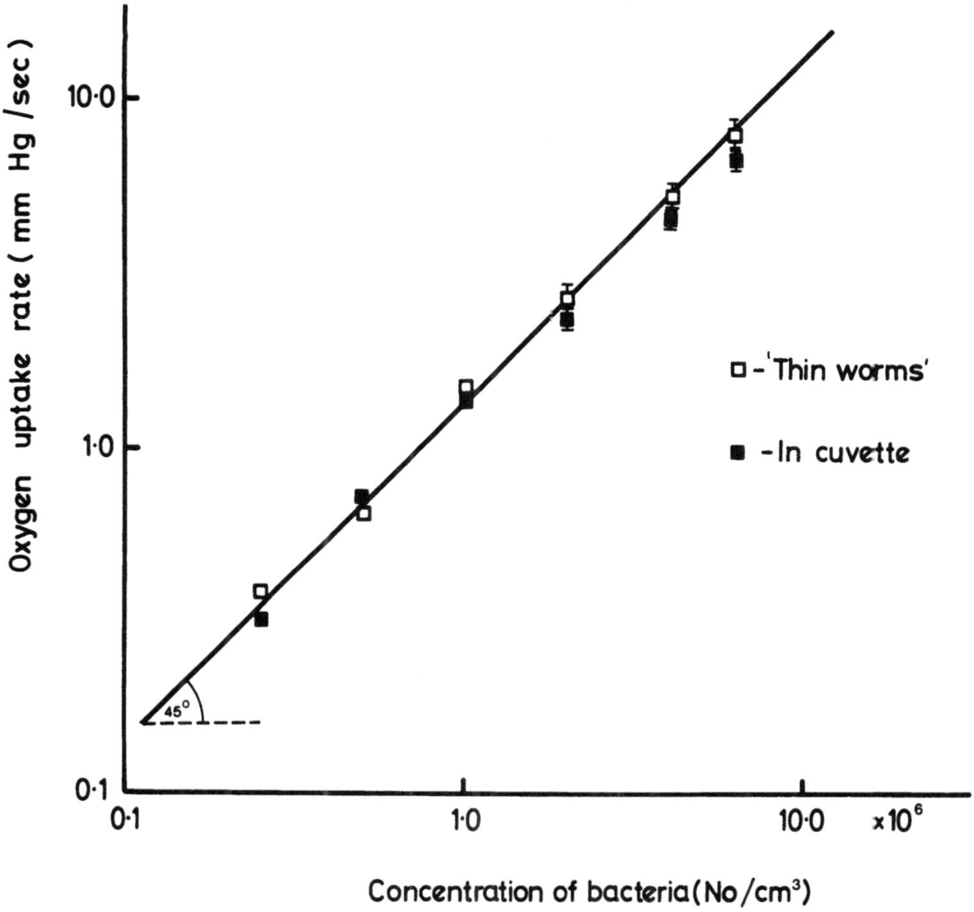

Fig. 4. Oxygen uptake rate as a function of bacterial concentration measured in a cuvette and directly in a closed vessel.

The spatial resolution of the system was assessed by measurements on a cuvette containing bacteria/gel mixture, a 1.5mm strip of which had been previously irradiated with 50Krad of 15MeV electrons. After incubation for 2 hours at 37°C there was a difference in oxygen uptake rate of about a factor 10 between the irradiated and unirradiated zones, and the change in measured values occurred almost completely within a single inter-cathode distance of 0.5mm.

APPLICATION TO TISSUES

The method described has been shown to give reliable estimates of oxygen uptake rate in a test system. Its use with mammalian tissues should be valid provided the measurements can be completed within a short enough time after removal from the organism for the uptake rate to be unchanged. It is possible to complete the estimations within 20 minutes of removal.

By varying the pO_2 of the gas used for equilibration, estimates of uptake rate averaged over different depths of penetration into the tissue are possible. The values are to a first approximation independent of the size of the oxygen diffusion constant in the tissue. The estimate of uptake rate is in the form of mm Hg/sec. If uptake rates in ml O_2/ml tissue/sec are required, it is necessary to know the oxygen solubility in the tissue.

A complication arises from the presence of significant amounts of haemoglobin or myoglobin in the tissue. This can be dealt with reasonably satisfactorily and will be discussed in a later paper (4).

REFERENCES

1. Crank, J. and Gupta, R.S. A moving boundary problem arising from the diffusion of oxygen in absorbing tissue. J.Inst. Maths.Applics. 10, 19-33, 1972.

2. Evans, N.T.S. and Gourlay, A.R. The solution of a two-dimensional time-dependent problem concerned with oxygen metabolism in tissue. In preparation.

3. Evans, N.T.S. Changes in the rate of oxygen consumption by mouse spleen following whole body X-irradiation. Rad.Res., 35, 465-471, 1968.

4. Constable, T.B. and Evans, N.T.S. The distribution of oxygen consumption rates in some tissues before and after X-irradiation. This symposium.

MONITORING OF PO_2 IN HUMAN BLOOD

H.P. Kimmich, F. Kreuzer, J.G. Spaan, K. Jank,
J. de Hemptinne, and M. Demeester
University of Nijmegen, Nijmegen, The Netherlands
University of Brussels, Brussels, Belgium

INTRODUCTION

The surveillance of arterial PO_2 in patients with pulmonary or cardiac failure by frequent sampling of blood has several obvious disadvantages. Alternatively the continuous monitoring of PaO_2 by use of catheter electrodes still poses numerous problems. However, from a continuous signal of a transducer able to follow variations in PaO_2 with respiration and heart activity, more useful information is gained. Under certain circumstances, as well as by studying the evolution of PaO_2 during controlled changes of inspired oxygen supply, continuous PO_2 monitoring can also be used as a diagnostic tool (e.g. for the detection of pathological shunts).

PROBLEMS OF APPLICATION OF PO_2 ELECTRODES TO CONTINUOUS MONITORING IN HUMANS

The requirements of continuous recording in vivo for the measuring system include technical as well as biological aspects. For evaluation and appreciation of such a system the following check list may be useful:

1) Sensitivity
2) Accuracy (linearity, reproducibility, short-term stability, long-term stability, transient response, zero current (value and drift), flow dependency, temperature dependency, sensitivity to CO_2, sensitivity to other gases, sensitivity to pressure, to acceleration, and to water (water deposition)).
3) Design - Constructive lay-out (miniaturization, safety, complexity of servicing and operation).

4) Sterilization
5) In vivo parameters (biocompatibility (toxicity, blood changes, tissue reactions, blood coagulation, etc), mechanical and electrical compatibility (flow distortion, tissue changes, electroshock, membrane potential changes), influences of the medium on sensor (protein deposition, blood coagulation at electrode, mechanical stress, galvanic reactions)).

The intensive research of the past years in the field of polarography has led to the solution of most problems connected with the technical parameters sensitivity, accuracy, constructive lay-out, and sterilization. For human applications, however, improvement of the constructive lay-out is still desirable, especially with respect to the size of the transducer. For prolonged monitoring of human PaO_2 the main issue, however, is the solution of the problems connected with the so-called in vivo parameters, especially the biocompatibility of the catheter electrode, and the influences of the medium on the sensor. But also the mechanical compatibility and the positioning of the transducer are important in some circumstances. Biocompatibility of a catheter electrode is never complete but it can be improved by incorporating a good lay-out and proper materials, e.g. by coating the tip of the catheter by silicone. Protein and blood cell deposition as well as blood coagulation at the tip of the electrode influence fast electrodes to a much greater extent than slow ones. Since these phenomena also involve a certain risk for the patient, it is advantageous that their effects on the fast electrodes become noticeable and thus provide a warning at an early stage.

Preliminary trials of monitoring PaO_2 in the radial artery with our "blood electrode" (Kimmich and Kreuzer, 1969) revealed the necessity of a transducer and catheter with smaller diameter. First this problem has been circumvented by measuring PaO_2 in an arteriovenous shunt, but simultaneously a new electrode with a diameter of 1.2 mm and essentially the same characteristics as previous designs has been developed.

PaO_2 MEASUREMENTS IN A SHUNT

The PaO_2 is measured inside a stainless steel holding block, connected to the radial artery and the antecubital vein by silastic tubes and Teflon needles. A slight disadvantage of this system is a possible reduction of the peripheral circulation due to the shunt.

On the other hand the blood flow in the shunt is markedly increased as compared to normal radial arterial flow. This has several advantages: 1) The risk of blood coagulation is decreased; 2) 2) The inevitable thermostating of the metal block is achieved by the blood itself (the temperature is checked continuously and is close to rectal temperature); 3) The well-defined flow situation (the blood flow was systematically measured at the beginning and end of the PaO_2 monitoring) excludes artefacts due to the remaining flow sensitivity of the polarographic cell.

Continuous recording of the PaO_2 was achieved for periods of 6 to 24 hours in more than 100 patients, mainly with respiratory failure. The PO_2 of blood samples taken from the shunt of each patient was compared with the continuous PaO_2 readings. The values tallied well up to 110 mm Hg. A systematically higher PO_2 measured in vivo in the shunt (from 110 mm Hg upwards) is likely due to leakage from the syringe and O_2 consumption by the erythrocytes during transport and analysis of the blood samples.

The system may be reliably used for monitoring of PaO_2 in patients up to 24 hours since no cutaneous or vascular reactions have been observed.

MINIATURE PO_2 ELECTRODE

It is well known that several parameters of polarographic electrodes are closely linked and oppose each other, such as flow dependency (size and shape of the cathode) and transient response (thickness and composition of the membrane and electrolyte layer, and shape of the cathode area), as well as stability of the electrode and transient response and size (especially diameter). To achieve a real progress, the design of a new smaller oxygen catheter should therefore not be to the detriment of other parameters of performance. The transient response of a new electrode with approximately 1 mm of diameter should be better than 2 sec (figure 1). Our new electrode has a diameter of 1.2 mm, a transient response of 0.4 sec and the lay-out is similar to previous designs (Kimmich and Kreuzer, 1969). The cathode is a platinum ring with a diameter of 0.3 mm and a thickness of approximately 3 μ. In order to guarantee a fast and sufficient electrolyte exchange in the space between the membrane and cathode area (which is important for the stability and small CO_2 dependency of the electrode) the ratio of the unsupported to total membrane area had to be increased from 4 to 6%. Since this might lead to an increased sensitivity to pressure, the static and dynamic sensitivity to pressure has been investigated with particular care. The characteristics of the miniature oxygen electrode are (all measurements at 37°C with a 6 u Teflon membrane) (figure 2):

Sensitivity = approximately 0.6 nA/mm Hg (figure 3),
Linearity = $\pm$ 0.2% (10 to 760 mm Hg),
Reproducibility = better than 0.1 mm Hg,
Short-term stability (2 h) = $\pm$ 0.25%,
Long-term stability (24 h) = $\mp$ 1%,
Transient response to a step function = 0.4 sec (figure 3),

Response (sec)	Diameter (mm)			
	⩽0.5	0.5 - 1.5	1.5 - 2.5	>2.5
0 - 0.05				
0.05-0.1			Kimmich and Kreuzer, 1968	
0.1 -0.5		Kimmich et al. 1975	Kreuzer and Schuler, 1965; Schuler and Kreuzer, 1967; Kreuzer and Kimmich, 1968; Kimmich, 1969; Huxtable and Fatt, 1974; Van Kempen & Kreuzer, 1975	
0.5 - 2		Parker et al. 1971	Kreuzer and Nessler, 1958; Kreuzer et al. 1960	
2 - 10		Charlton, Read and Read, 1963; Kunze, 1964; Huch et al., 1973/74	Rybak, 1964	
10 - 30		Johansen and Krog, 1959; Krog and Johansen, 1959	Grimnes, 1967	
30 - 120	Bicher et al. 1973			
>120				Sommerkamp and Oehmig, 1962

Figure 1: Catheter electrodes have been developed with small diameter (0.5 mm) as well as with short transient response (0.1 sec). The combination of both goals, however, presents increasing difficulties as we move in the direction of the upper left-hand corner of this scheme. The miniaturized catheter electrode presented here is a step towards this goal.

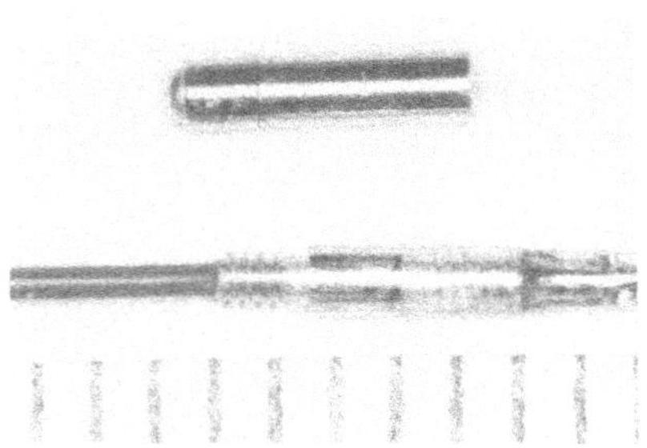

Figure 2: Miniaturized oxygen transducer. Diameter of the electrode and catheter: 1.2 mm. The anode chamber (upper part) is made of silver and carries the Teflon membrane tightened by a stainless steel ring. The cathode (lower part) is a platinum ring with a diameter of 0.3 mm and a thickness of 3 μ.

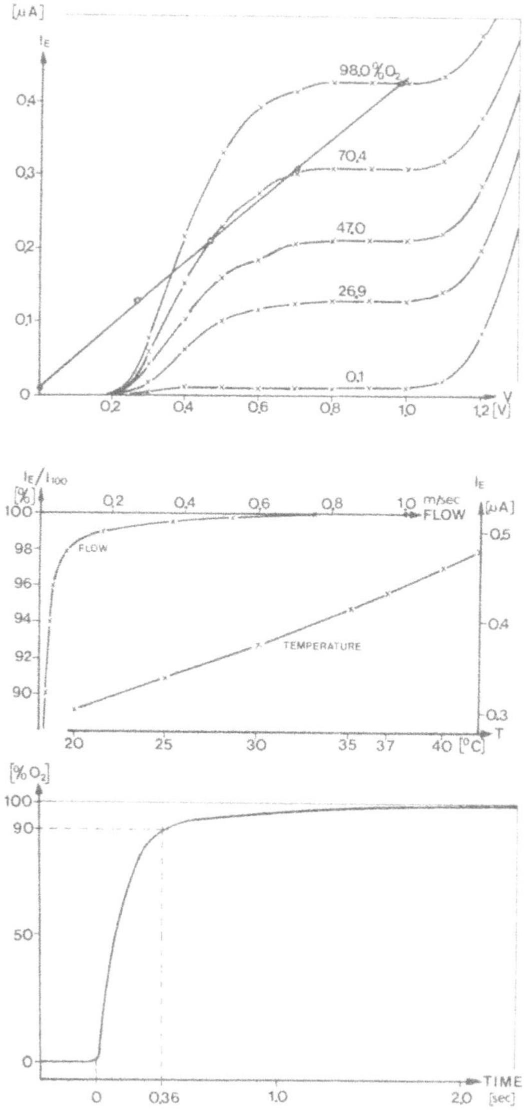

Figure 3:
(upper panel)
Calibration line and current-voltage curves (polarogram) of the miniature oxygen electrode. A slight double wave is noted but the horizontal part of the polarogram is still broad enough for a ring electrode of this size.

(middle panel)
Change of polarographic current as a function of the blood flow. The electrode current (I_E) has been related to the current measured with a flow of 1 m/sec. In the range of 20 to 45°C the temperature dependency varies from 2.5 to 2%/°C.

(lower panel)
Transient response of the miniature electrode to a step function in gas concentration. A slightly larger deviation from an exponential function is noted than in previous designs with larger diameter. It is assumed that this is incidental and not typical, as is the case with the double wave in the polarogram.

Zero current $\leqslant$ 15 mm Hg (drift 0.5 mm Hg/24 hours),
Flow dependency (7-100 cm/sec) = $\pm$ 1% (figure 3),
Temperature dependency: 2.05%/°C at 37°C, 2.45%/°C at 20°C, and 3.0%/°C at 10°C (figure 3),
Sensitivity to physiological CO_2 $\leqslant$ 2 mm Hg,
Sensitivity to pressure: static $\leqslant$ 0.2%, dynamic (DC to 5 Hz) 0 to 50 mm Hg $\leqslant$ 0.2%, 0 to 500 mm Hg $\leqslant$ 1% (figure 4),
Sensitivity to acceleration (0 to 10 g) $\leqslant$ 0.1%.

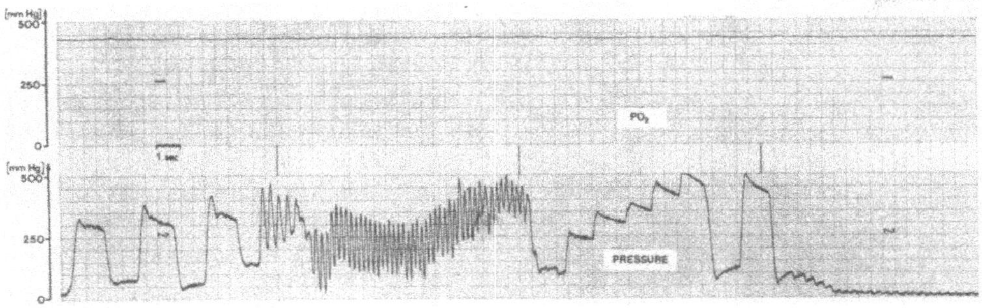

Figure 4: Recording of PO_2 in water (upper tracing) with changing pressure in the medium (lower tracing).

IN VIVO APPLICATIONS

The electrode has been applied to physiological studies in the dog and the cat (figure 5) as well as for continuous monitoring of human PaO_2 in the radial artery (figure 6). Introduction of the electrode into the radial artery was achieved through a Teflon needle. The electrode was used without any protection, which in some cases led to blood coagulation. If, however, no coagulation occurred in the first 15 minutes after insertion, the electrode was working perfectly for several hours. The animal experiments, where the catheter electrode tip was protected with silicone oil, were always successful.

CONCLUSIONS

The method of measuring in artificial arterio-venous shunts has proved to be applicable clinically for prolonged monitoring of human PaO_2, while the direct measurement with the miniaturized electrode still presents some problems. Animal experiments, however,

Figure 5: Tracings recorded in artificially ventilated cats during an investigation on the regulation of respiration. Two miniature electrodes were inserted into the aorta (close to the aortic arch) and into the carotid artery. The curves show the response to an increased respiratory PO_2 during a single breath on the PaO_2 in the aorta and carotid. The electrode has been inserted through the lingual artery into the carotid artery which may reduce the blood flow and induce additional mixing, resulting in apparent damping of the overall transient PO_2 response as well as of the respiratory and cardiac PO_2 fluctuations. If an electrode, however, is positioned through the subclavian artery up to but not into the carotid artery the magnitude of the oscillations of PaO_2 with respiration and heart activity is now practically identical to that in the aorta.

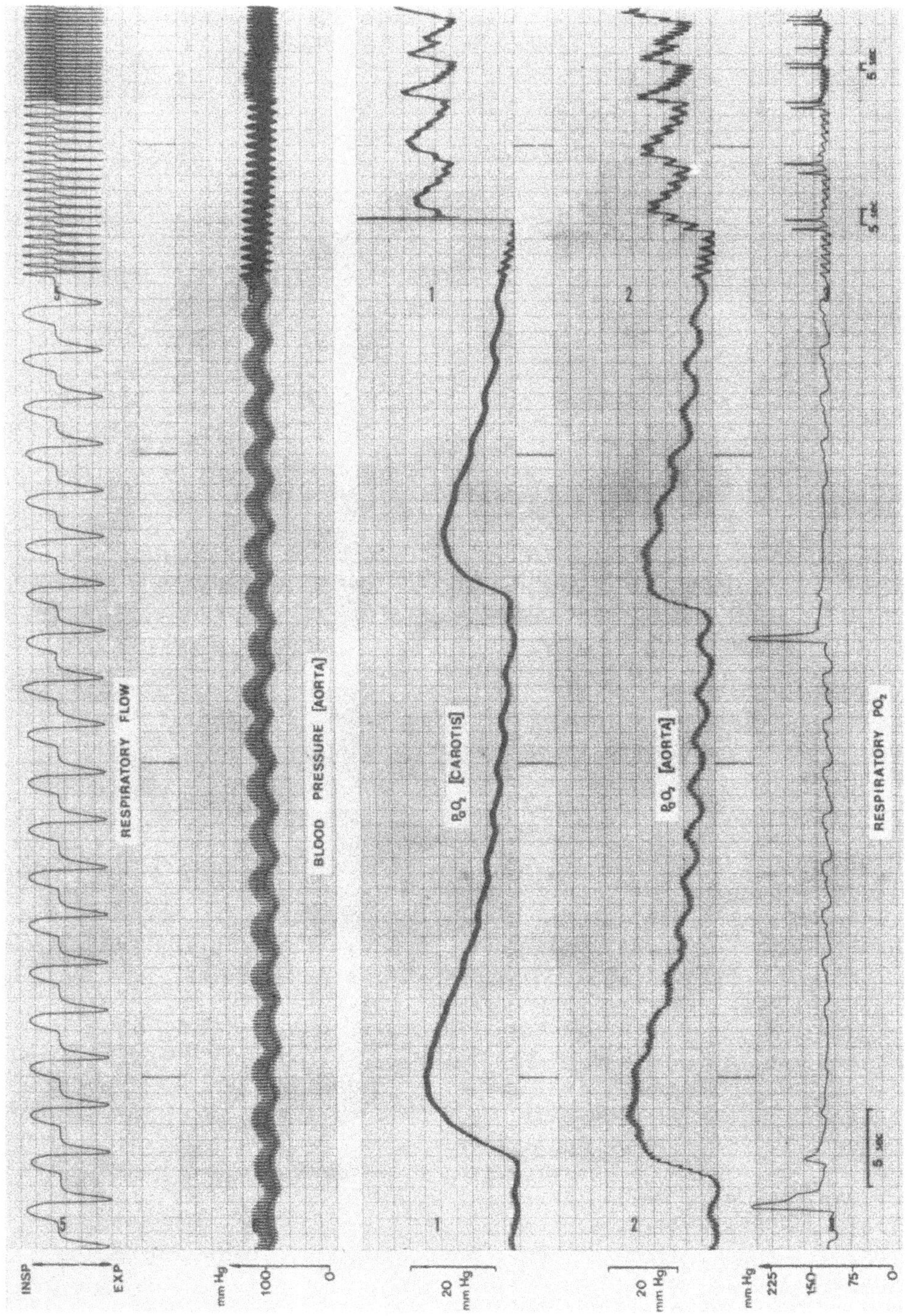

Figure 5: For explanation see opposite page.

show that clinical routine measurements with the miniature oxygen catheter should be possible as well, this has been proven in some patients.

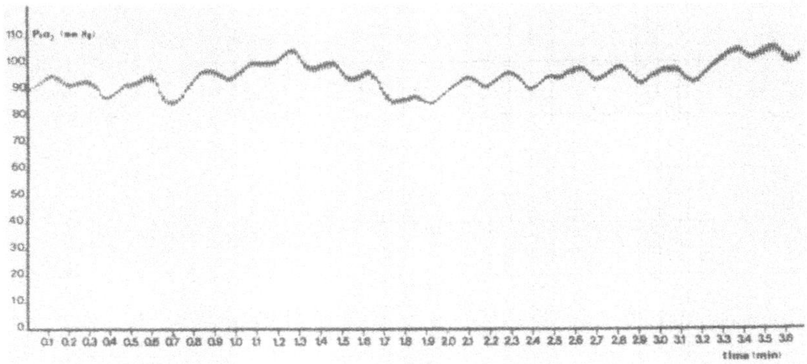

Figure 6: Recording of human PaO_2 in the radial artery.

Probably the direct method will be incorporated first in situations where the method with an artificial shunt is not applicable, e.g. for intracardiac monitoring.

Application of the miniaturized electrode by the "shunt method" may involve thinner connecting leads and needles and/or higher blood velocities in the shunt.

REFERENCES

Bicher, H.I., and D.F. Bruley, eds.: Oxygen Transport to Tissue. Adv. Exper. Med. and Biol., vol. 37A,B, Plenum Press, New York, 1973.
Charlton, G., D. Read and J. Read: J. Appl. Physiol. 18: 1247, 1963.
Grimnes, S.: Digest 7th ICOMBE, Stockholm, p. 278, 1967.
Huxtable, R.F., and I. Fatt: J. Appl. Physiol. 37: 435, 1974.
Johansen, K., and J. Krog: Acta Physiol. Scand. 46: 228, 1959.
Kempen, van, L.H.J., and F. Kreuzer: Respir.Physiol.,1975 (in press).
Kimmich, H.P.: Thesis University of Nijmegen, Holland, 79 pp., 1969.
Kreuzer, F., and C.G. Nessler, Jr.: Science 128: 1005, 1958.
Kreuzer, F., et al.: J. Appl. Physiol. 15: 77, 1960; 15: 1157, 1960.
Kreuzer, F., and R. Schuler: Digest 6th ICOMBE, Tokyo, p. 602, 1965.
Kreuzer, F., ed.: Oxygen Pressure Recording in Gases, Fluids, and Tissues. Progr. Resp. Res. 3, ed. H. Herzog, Karger, Basel, 1969.
Krog, J., and K. Johansen: Rev. Sci. Instrum. 30: 108, 1959.
Kunze, K.: Pflügers Archiv 279: 94, 1964.
Parker, D., A. Key and R. Davies: Biomed. Eng. 6: 313, 1971.
Rybak, B.: Life Sci. 3: 1123, 1964.
Sommerkamp, H., and H. Oehmig: Klin. Wschr. 40: 1112, 1962.

A NEW APPROACH TO THE EXPERIMENTAL MEASUREMENT OF MEAN TISSUE PO_2

R. E. Forster, C. W. Goodwin and N. Itada

Department of Physiology, University of Pennsylvania

Philadelphia, Pennsylvania 19174 USA

We have developed a method for the estimation of the total amount of reversibly bound + dissolved O_2 in a tissue based upon the differential exchanges of $^{16}O_2$ and $^{18}O_2$ between blood and the tissues through which it passes. While both isotopes enter the tissues and are metabolized to the same extent (the isotope effect is negligible), any O_2 outside the capillaries will appear as a distribution or dilution pool to the labelled but not the unlabelled O_2. This will cause a delay in the passage of a pulse of $^{18}O_2$ through the tissue relative to an indicator. Steady state conditions are maintained so that there is no significant alteration in the total concentrations of O_2 in blood or tissue.

METHODS

The experimental measurement was carried out in the skinned hind limb of an anesthetized dog by injecting into the femoral artery 1 cc of the animal's own blood which contained the same O_2 concentration but enriched with about 20% $^{18}O_2$, and 1 mgm/cc of indocyanine green (ICG). Venous samples were collected anaerobically and serially and analyzed for [HbO_2] and ICG by spectrometry, and P_{O_2}, P_{CO_2} and pH by electrode. [$^{18}O_2$]/[$^{16}O_2$] was determined on a mass spectrometer by means of a specially designed 1.5 ml glass chamber the bottom of which, consisting of a Teflon membrane supported on a sintered glass disc, separates the blood from the vacuum inlet system of the instrument. Any gas in the blood diffuses into the mass spectrometer ion source where it is measured. About 0.001 to 0.003 mm Hg of O_2 partial pressure in the blood can be detected at ambient pressure and temperature. An electro-magnetic flow meter was placed in the femoral artery providing a measure of arterial blood flow. The total limb tissue volume, primarily muscle, was estimated at the end of the experiment by gross dissection.

[Dye] was used to calculate the $^{18}O_2$ originally in each venous sample according to the equation:

$$\text{Calculated Venous } [^{18}O_2] = \left[\frac{\text{Venous [Dye]}}{\text{Injected [Dye]}} \text{ Injected } [^{18}O_2] + \left(1 - \frac{\text{Venous [Dye]}}{\text{Injection [Dye]}}\right) \times \text{ arterial } [^{18}O_2]\right] \times \frac{\text{Venous } O_2 \text{ content}}{O_2 \text{ Arterial content}} \quad (1)$$

The natural abundance of the doubly labelled $^{18}O_2$ is approximately zero.

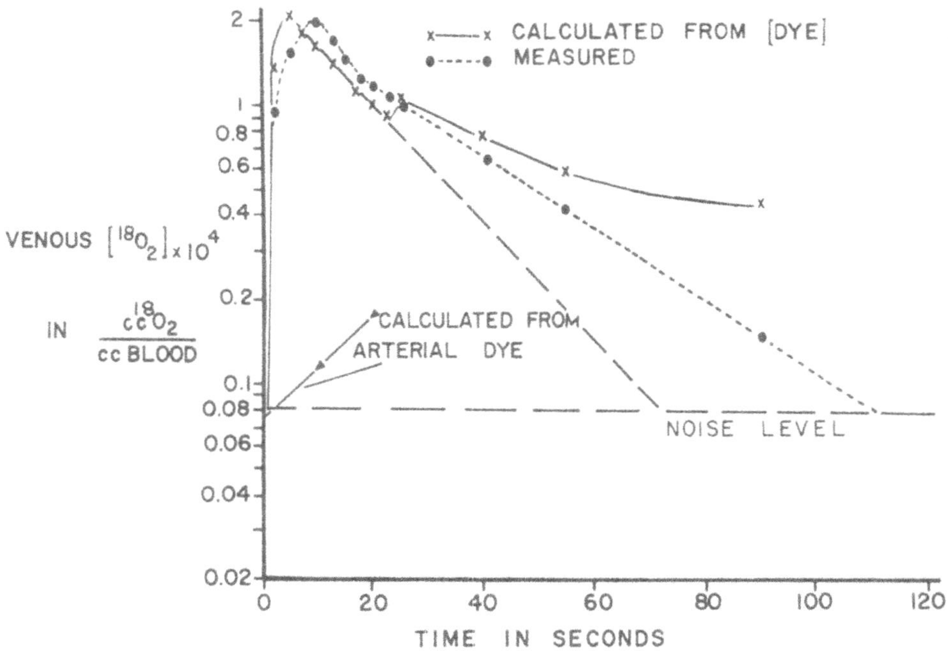

Figure 1. A graph of $^{18}O_2$ in venous blood, in cc gas/cc blood against time, following injection of 1 cc of autologous blood of the same CO_2 and O_2 content into the femoral artery of a skinned limb of a dog. The actual measured $^{18}O_2$ concentration is plotted as well as the value calculated from the venous dye according to Equation 1. $^{18}O_2$ in the inflowing arterial blood was also measured and a value calculated from the dye concentration. See text for further detail.

RESULTS AND DISCUSSION

The Log_{10} of the calculated venous concentration of $^{18}O_2$ as well as the actually measured concentrations in an experiment on a dog skinned hind limb are plotted against time in Figure 1. The labelled O_2 transient curve lagged behind the calculated curve in this, as well as in 7 other experiments on limbs and 6 in the kidney. Arterial blood was also sampled and analyzed for [Dye] and [$^{18}O_2$] and the calculated arterial [$^{18}O_2$] obtained using Equation 1 and the measured dye concentration. Recirculation of the dye occurred at least by 10 seconds. No measurable arterial concentration of $^{18}O_2$ was found in this or 6 other experiments.

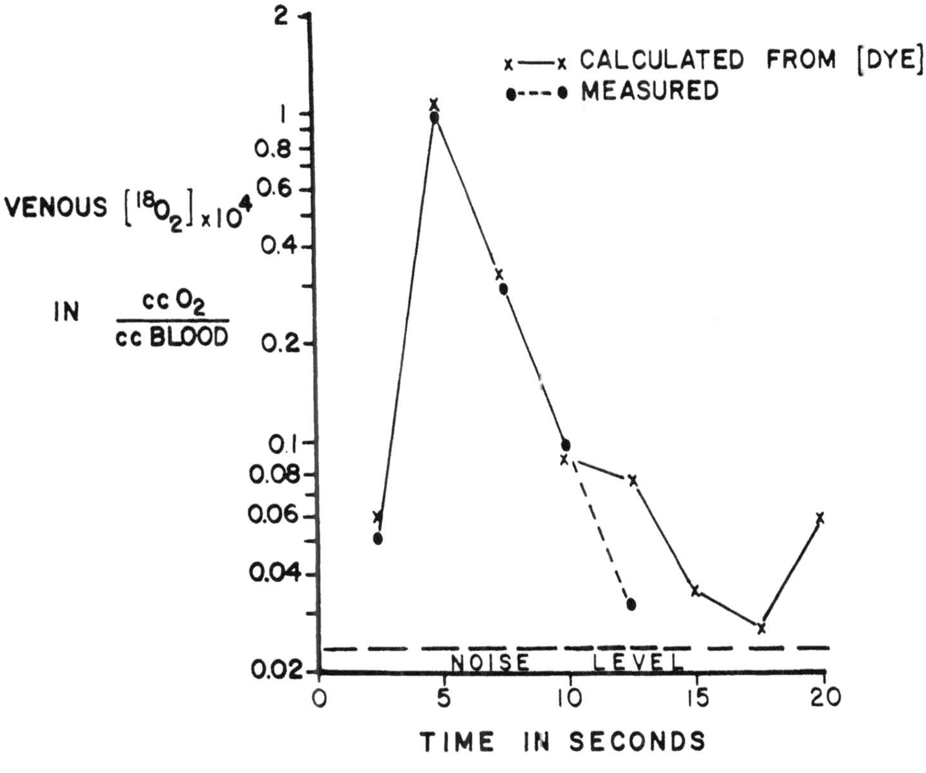

Figure 2. A graph of Log_{10} [$^{18}O_2$] in femoral arterial blood in cc gas/cc blood against time following injection of 1cc of autologous blood of equal O_2 and CO_2 content into the left ventricle. [$^{18}O_2$] actually measured as well as that calculated from femoral arterial [dye] is shown.

As controls, autologous blood containing ICG and $^{18}O_2$ was injected into the left ventricle or aorta in four experiments and serial samples obtained from the femoral artery. These experiments were more difficult in that the pulse passed so much more rapidly. The results of one typical experiment are shown in Fig. 2. There is no separation of the arterial $^{18}O_2$ curve from the calculated dilution curve. The measured $[^{18}O_2]$ curve would lag the expected or calculated curve if any process in the blood separated the two isotopes from each other or the labelled O_2 from the indicator dye. Taylor diffusion, radial diffusion within the flowing vessels, might cause the O_2 to mix better than the protein-bound dye. However, this effect does not seem to be very significant in the larger vessels. We conclude that there is no obvious technical cause for the lag seen in the limb venous $^{18}O_2$ curve.

Theoretically, once the injectate pulse in the arterial blood has passed, venous $^{18}O_2$ should follow an exponential curve as the labelled O_2 is washed out of the tissue. It can be shown that this relation is described by the equation:

$$\frac{\text{venous } [^{18}O_2]}{\text{venous } [^{18}O_2]_o} = e^{-\frac{\mathring{Q}\, C_A\, t}{C_V\, (V_B + V_T\lambda)\, 60}}$$

Where $\mathring{Q}$ = blood flow in cc per minute, C_A and C_V are the O_2 content of arterial and venous blood respectively, V_B is the blood volume in tissue, V_T is the tissue volume, λ is a partition coefficient equal to $\frac{\text{average } O_2 \text{ content of tissue}}{O_2 \text{ content of blood}}$, and t is in seconds. Q, C_A, C_V, V_B, V_T and λ are considered constant during the experiment, since the blood injected has approximately the same chemical composition as the arterial blood into which it is introduced.

The value of the exponential constant in Equation 2 can be obtained from the slope of the $^{18}O_2$ curve in Figure 1. C_A and C_V are known from the analysis of blood samples. Q can be obtained from the electromagnetic flow meter measurements of femoral arterial flow. In addition, Q/V_B can be obtained from the extrapolated exponential decrease in calculated venous $^{18}O_2$, because this curve has the same shape as the classical dye dilution curve (Hamilton-Stewart) and the exponential constant for this is Q/V_B. Thus we have the necessary data to calculate $V_T\lambda$ which is the size of the O_2 pool in the tissue, but in terms of cc of venous blood. Multiplying by the O_2 content of venous blood, usually about 0.15 cc/cc, we obtain the cc of O_2 in the whole tissue. Values for this datum are given in Table 1.

TABLE 1

Average P_{O_2} in Dog Hind Limb

Dog	Blood Flow	O_2 Pool	Average P_{O_2} as Dissolved O_2	Average P_{O_2} as Dissolved O_2 & Bound
	cc/cc X min	cc/cc	mm Hg	mm Hg
30A	0.097	0.00096	34.8	0.52
B	0.107	0.00100	36.2	0.54
C	0.112	0.00079	28.6	0.41
50A	0.125	0.00155	56.1	0.96
B	0.094	0.00134	48.5	0.79
C	0.056	0.00160	58.0	1.00
98A	0.096	0.0004	14.5	0.19
B	0.081	0.0019	68.8	1.09*

*Anesthetized animal also paralyzed with gallamine.

The average P_{O_2} of the tissue can be calculated provided the physical solubility of the gas in the tissue is known, as well as the extent of its binding by myoglobin. Average P_{O_2} calculated "as dissolved" O_2 was obtained by dividing the total O_2 pool by the solubility of O_2 in saline at 37 C. Average P_{O_2} as "dissolved + bound" gas was calculated from the physical solubility and the assumption that the Mgb P_{50} was 2.7 mm Hg (3) and that there was 0.004 gm myoglobin/cc tissue (2). The assumption is implicit that the kinetics of the reactions of O_2 with hemoglobin and myoglobin are not rate limiting.

We conclude that this indicator-dilution technique using $^{18}O_2$ can provide a measure of average P_{O_2} in a tissue. Although we hope to increase the accuracy, at present we believe we can detect as little as 0.0002 cc O_2/cc. The values of average P_{O_2} in Table 1 which take into effect the binding of O_2 by myoglobin, are lower than those estimated by Coburn using CO (3), the most comparable method. However it should be noted that the values we obtained included all the extravascular tissue and not just the myoglobin. There are many assumptions involved in our computations and further verification is needed.

We have not yet attempted to measure changes in average tissue P_{O_2} under various physiological conditions, particularly those in which it might be expected to alter.

ACKNOWLEDGMENT

We wish to recognize the help of Mr. James D. Graham, Jr. and Mr. Joseph Pili in the design and construction of the analytical chamber for the mass spectrometer, of Mrs. Ruth Manwaring for the preparation of the illustrations and of Mr. Henry John for technical assistance. This work was supported in part by a grant from the National Heart and Lung Institute (HL4108).

REFERENCES

1. Coburn, R.F. and L.B. Mayers. Myoglobin O_2 tension determined from measurements of carboxymyoglobin in skeletal muscle. Am. J. Physiol. 220:66-74, 1974.

2. Kagen, E.J. Myoglobin. New York: Columbia University, p. 42 (1973).

3. Rossi-Fanelli, A. and E. Antonini. Studies on the oxygen and carbon monoxide equilibria of human myoglobin. Arch. Biochem. Biophys. 77:478-492, 1958.

PYRENE BUTYRIC ACID: A NON-INVASIVE PROBE FOR IN SITU INTRA-CELLULAR OXYGEN CONCENTRATION

Frans F. Jöbsis, Michael H. Mitnick and Thomas R. Snow

Department of Physiology and Pharmacology

Duke University Medical Center, Durham, N.C., U.S.A.

Historically there have been two major problems facing researchers trying to measure the intracellular concentration of oxygen, $[O_2]_i$. The first is the cellular damage, however slight, concomitant with entry into cells by the (micro)electrodes used in polarographic techniques. The second drawback is the actual consumption, again however slight, of oxygen by the polarographic electrode. We could like to report at this time the successful application of pyrene butyric acid (PBA) as an alternative to the older methods as a quantitative tool for non-invasive, non-consumptive measurement of $[O_2]_i$.

Weber and Vaughn (1970) reported the in vitro data which indicated that PBA would be used in solutions as an indicator of $[O_2]_i$. They used the fact that PBA fluoresces in the region of 375-400 nm, when illuminated with light of wavelengths around 328 and 345 nm. This fluorescence is strongest when no oxygen is present, and is quantitatively quenched when oxygen concentration is increased. They showed that the Stern-Vollmer relationship described the difference in fluorescent intensities as a function of (O_2) as follows:

$$\frac{F_o}{F} = 1 + K\,[O_2]$$

F_o = unquenched intensity
F = quenched intensity
k = quenching constant
$[O_2]$ = in mm Hg

Longmuir and Knopp (1972) showed that PBA does not affect the respiratory quotient in liver cell suspensions, verified the Stern-Vollmer definition of PBA fluorescence in these suspensions, and also proved the PBA measured oxygen concentration and not partial pressure.

Until recently the PBA technique has only been applied to solutions and isolated cells but its use in excised tissues or organs *in situ* with normal circulation could provide data of such significance that we decided to launch a set of studies in this direction. The present article is a progress report on our efforts.

RESULTS

Isolated heart mitochondria have been used to study the possible effects of PBA on the respiratory chain and on oxidative phosphorylation. Steady state studies were performed with the wavelength-scanning differential ("split-beam") spectrophotometric technique (Yang and Legallais, 1954). Spectra were compared in metabolic states 1, 2, 4 and 5 of Chance and Williams (1955). None showed any difference after incubation in 5×10^{-6} M PBA. When exposed to suspension medium containing this PBA level, the mitochondria concentrate PBA to approximately 700 pico moles per mg dry weight. The suspension fluid typically shows, after incubation and centrifugation of the mitochondria, a 200-fold decrease in PBA concentration. This is in agreement with observations by Knopp and Longmuir (1972) of partition coefficients for PBA between cells and salt solutions.

Observations on state 3 were performed with the dual-wavelength or "double-beam" spectrophotometer of chance (1957) and the compensated double-beam fluorometer of Jöbsis and Stainsby (1968). For these observations, cycles of the redox responses of cytochromes *b* and *c* and of NADH to state 4-3-4 transitions were induced by additions of ADP in the presence of inorganic phosphate and substrates (usually pyruvate, occasionally β-OH butyrate) and with a continuous O_2 supply provided by dimpling the surface with a stream of 100% O_2. Two procedures were followed for the assessment of possible PBA effects. Either a series of ADP additions was made after which the PBA was added (to make 2 μM) and the identical series of ADP additions was repeated. Or, two equal aliquots of mitochondria were studied one with and one without PBA.

At the moment the study of fluorometrically observed cycles of NADH are most complete. No differences were noted in the transient redox cycles with 2 μM PBA (Fig. 1). When higher concentrations of PBA were used (100 μM, 1 mM), a general debilitation of the mitochondria occurred. At 10 μM the first signs of this effect might be present. But at concentrations below that (< 5 μM)

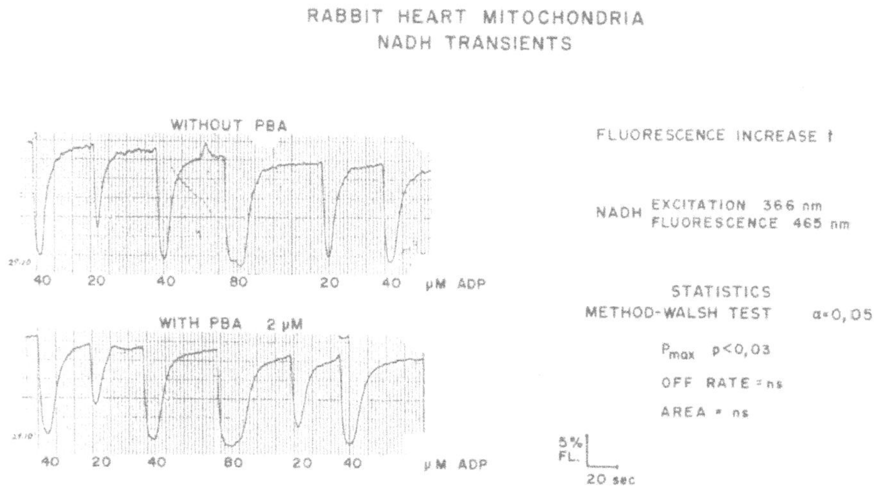

Fig. 1

there was no immediately observable difference between treated and untreated mitochondria.

In order to test whether more subtle, statistical differences might exist, a Walsh test was performed on the depth of the oxidation responses, on the rate of return to the baseline ("off-kinetics") and on the area under the curves (Fig. 1, right hand table). Consistently the outcome has been that there is no significant difference between the two populations of cycles analyzed for the last two parameters. For the depth of the fluorometric transient there was at times a P value of less than 0.03 for the hypothesis that the two populations were identical. This, however, holds true only if the PBA measurements are made later than the controls as was the case for the experiments shown in Fig. 1. When the data were pooled for a number of runs in which the sequences with and without PBA were randomly varied, there was no significant difference in this parameter also. Thus the presence of PBA does not affect the NADH oxidation responses occurring during state 4-3-4 cycles.

By means of double-beam spectrophotometry, we are studying similar cycles for cytochromes b and c. Again no observable differences were noted but the statistical analysis is still incomplete. Pending the outcome of the latter, it is nevertheless relatively safe to assert that PBA in the ranges stated above does not interfere with oxidative phosphorylation.

A quantitative study of the use of intramitochondrial PBA as an oxygen indicator is in the first stages. Our preliminary observations have not provided any qualitative discrepancies with expectations.

Papillary muscles from rabbit hearts have been studied to investigate the use of PBA as an in situ indicator of O_2 concentration. Double-beam fluorometry was used with 326 nm excitation and 397 nm recording of the emitted fluorescence. Observations on NADH fluorescence cycles (366 excitation, 465 emission) upon stimulation and contraction were used as one type of control experiment. Isometric tension development during PBA exposure and after washout provided other controls. All of these showed that PBA in concentrations up to 10 μM in the Ringer's solution does not produce a major effect. Occasionally a slight, slowly developing depression but sometimes an increase of tension production was noted which was reversible upon washout of the PBA.

Typically a 5 minute exposure to 10 μM PBA produces a large increment in 397 nm signal, in the range of 50% of the autofluorescence. After this exposure the excess PBA is washed out during which procedure the signal decreases to a stable 20 to 25% increase over the autofluorescence. This signal appears to originate from a more tightly bound fraction of PBA which washes out with a much more protracted time course (hours instead of minutes). After the rapid washout phase, observations on PBA fluorescence during and after series of contractions were performed. A typical record is shown in Fig. 2. The increase in fluorescence signal indicates a decrease of oxygen concentration (decreased quenching of PBA fluorescence).

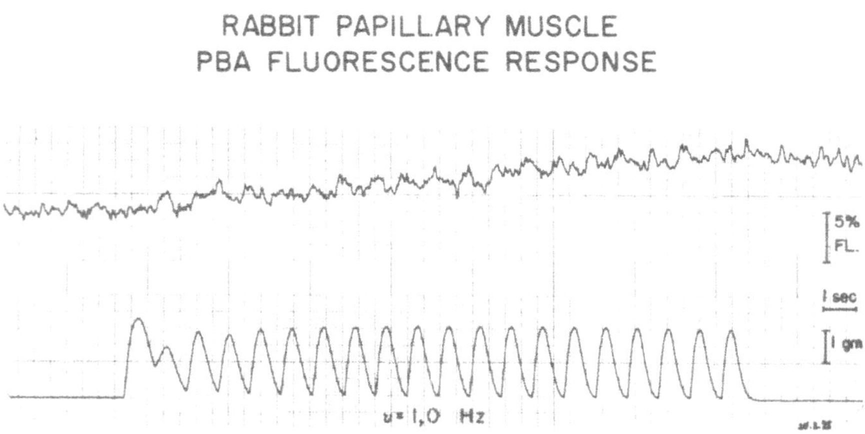

Fig. 2

It is important to note that in the absence of PBA sustained changes in the autofluorescence do not occur. A fair number of preparations do show rapid changes in signal during each contraction - usually increases - which are not always compensated by the subtraction of the reflectance trace in the double-beam instrument; but the return to the baseline is complete at the end of the tension relaxation. We ascribe these rapid fluctuations to motion of the preparation in the optical field.

Another important observation is the fact that the typical NADH fluorescence responses are not observed in the 397 nm channel: apparently the NADH emission is absent or minimal at this low wavelength. When NADH fluorescence is measured at 465 25 nm using 366±15 nm excitation, a clearcut decrease in fluorescence activity is observed in agreement with the expected NADH oxidation when going from state 4 to 3. In Fig. 3 such a response is shown for a series of ten contractions. The rapid increased intensity responses occur during the actual contraction and are again discounted as motion artifacts. The slower cumulative trend towards an oxidative shift of NADH has been identified with oxidative recovery metabolism (Chapman, 1972). The return to the resting baseline indicates the return to the state 4 metabolism. Similar but optically inverse cycles in O_2 concentration levels are obtained with PBA when the entire response is recorded (Fig. 4). Generally the return of the O_2 concentration changes does lag somewhat behind the NADH responses as could be expected. Since

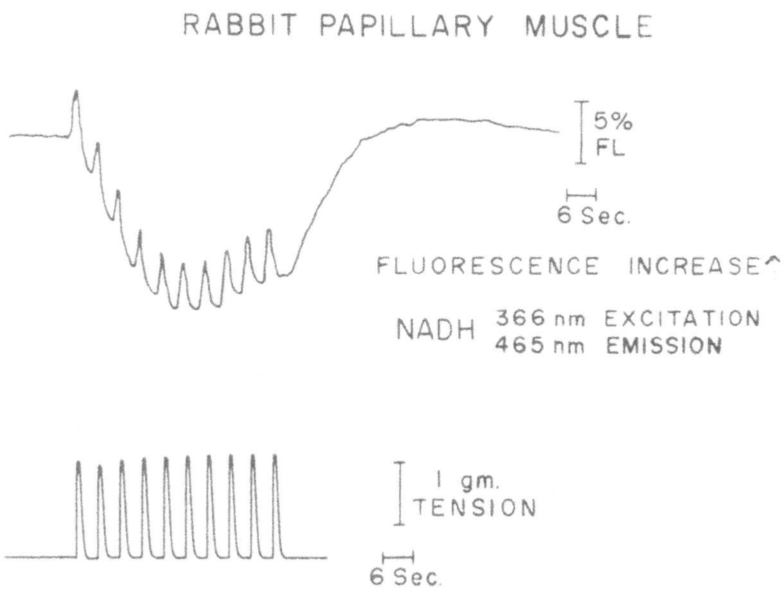

Fig. 3

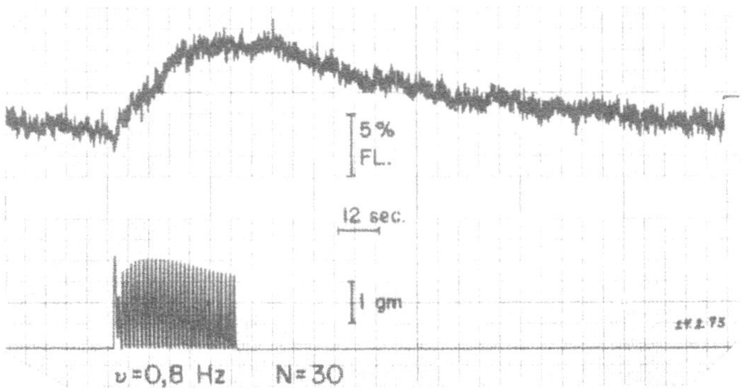

Fig. 4

front surface excitation and emission recording does tend to favor the more exterior layers, the signal is weighted against the core of the muscle which would return more slowly to resting O_2 concentrations. By varying illumination methods, we expect to be able to obtain signals emphasizing the deeper layers. By comparison data concerning the reactions in a hypoxic core and in the more accessible surface layers can be accumulated and the parameters of O_2 diffusion can then be studied.

The intact cerebral cortex of the cat *in situ* has been used in attempts to use PBA to normally circulated organs. Standardly we have used animals rendered comatose by electrolytic lesions in the brainstem at the intercollicular level. After several hours rest in order to allow the initial anesthetic (ether) to wear off, the supra sylvian gyrus is exposed and the pia covered with clear plastic film ("saran wrap"). The baseline level of autofluorescence is determined and several one to one and a half minute hypoxic to anoxic periods are recorded with the double-beam fluorometer. Through an intraperitoneal cannula Na-PBA dissolved in water is administered in doses ranging from 10 to 100 mg (4 to 50 μmoles per kg). Typically, the fluorescence at 397 nm starts to rise within a few minutes and comes to a new steady plateau 20 to 45 minutes after administration. This increased plateau is maintained unaltered for the duration of the experiment; the longest observations are now in the range of six to seven hours. PBA detoxification is apparently very slow in the cat, whereas it is much more rapid in the rat (Knopp and Longmuir, private communication).

The increase over the autofluorescence signal shows considerable variation between preparations. Administration of 100 mg to a 2.5 kg cat will increase the 397 nm signal 100 to 150%. The dose response relation is, however, not linear. Details of this relationship are being pursued by analysis of cortical samples. It might be important to emphasize that PBA appears to be transported adsorbed to serum proteins. In this condition its fluorescence is almost entirely quenched.

During the anoxic periods, considerable changes in both reflectance of the excitation and of the emitted light occur. The relationship appears to be different from the well studied situation for NADH recording (366 and 465 nm). The exact quantitative relationships are still under study. Qualitatively, it can be stated, however, that decreased O_2 levels, produced either by ventilation with N_2 or by dyspnea of the paralyzed animal, results in a net increase in PBA fluorescence as expected.

In conclusion, it appears that pyrene butyric acid can be utilized for studies on cellular oxygen concentration without interfering with oxidative metabolism or with normal physiological function of the tissue.

REFERENCES

Chance, B. 1957. Techniques for the Assay of the Respiratory Enzymes. Methods in Enzymology 4:273.

Chance, B. and Williams, G.R. 1955. Respiratory Enzymes in Oxidative Phosphorylation I-III. J. Biol. Chem. 217, 383-427.

Chapman, J.B. 1972. Fluorometric Studies of Oxidative Metabolism in Isolated Papillary Muscle of the Rabbit. J. Gen. Physiol. 59, 135-154.

Jobsis, F. and Stainsby, W.N. 1968. Oxidation of NADH during Contractions of Circulated Mammalian Skeletal Muscle. Respir. Physiol. 4, 292-300.

Knopp, J.A. and I.S. Longmuir. 1972. Intracellular Measurement of Oxygen by Quenching of Fluorescence of Pyrenebutyric acid. Biochim. Biophys Acta 279, 393-397.

Vaughn, W.M. and Weber, G. 1970. Oxygen Quenching of Pyrenebutyric Acid Fluorescence in Water. A Dynamic Probe of the Microenvironment. Biochemistry 9, 465-473.

Yang, C.C. and Legallais, V. 1954. A Rapid and Sensitive Recording Spectrophotometer for the Visible and Ultraviolet Region I. Description and Performance. Rev. Sci. Instr. 25, 801.

This work was supported by: 1 R01 H1 16828-01
MHM also received support from MH12333
TRS also received support from U.S. PHS NHLI - HF - 136 - 74.

KRYOMICROPHOTOMETRY AS A METHOD FOR ANALYZING THE INTRACAPILLARY HbO_2 SATURATION OF ORGANS UNDER DIFFERENT O_2 SUPPLY CONDITIONS+)

W. A. Grunewald and D. W. Lübbers

Abt. am Lehrstuhl für Physiologie der Universität
Regensburg, 84 Regensburg, GFR
Max-Planck-Institut für Systemphysiologie, 46 Dortmund,
GFR

During the last years we developed a method for the determination of the HbO_2 saturation in capillary blood. Until now, measurements of this important O_2 supply parameter were not possible. The developed method is a microkryophotometrical one. This method includes

1) the rapid-kryo-fixation of the HbO_2 saturation in the blood vessels of an organ sample,
2) the sectioning of the frozen samples,
3) the microphotometrical measurement of the hemoglobin absorption spectra in the transected vessels of the tissue sections.

Sectioning and photometrical measurement were done at low temperatures to maintain the kryofixated HbO_2 saturation.

Let us consider the individual steps of this method: an organ sample (e. g., myocardium tissue) with a diameter of 2 - 3 mm or a whole organ of this size (e. g. carotid body is extracted from the experimental animal by tongs which have been precooled in liquid nitrogen and then the sample is placed in Freon 13. By rapid-freezing the HbO_2 saturation is fixated as we have shown in preliminary experiments (GRUNEWALD, LÜBBERS 1969, 1975). The frozen sample is then sectioned in a kryotom into 10 - 15 μ thick sections at - 65 °C. Fig. 1 shows that the histological structure of the frozen and kryotomsectioned carotid body is well retained. I wish to thank Mrs. SEIDL of the Max-Planck-Institut in Dortmund for this picture. A frozen section is then brought into a microscope kryostat and there the frozen section is maintained at a temperature of -100 °C. The cooling of the microscope kryostat is

+supported by Volkswagen-Stiftung

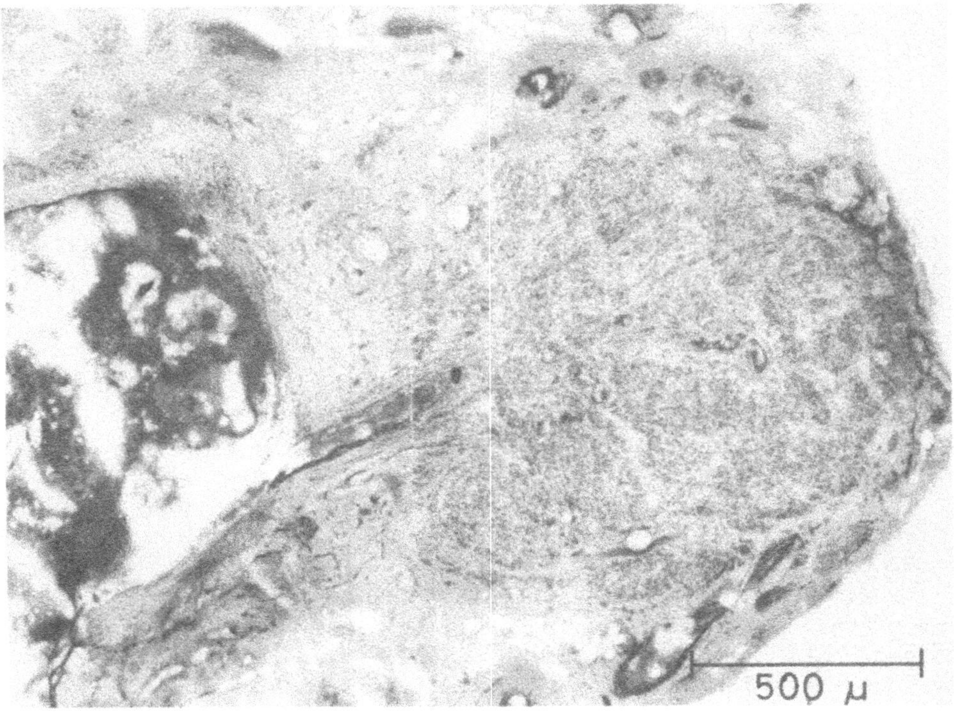

Figure 1

Histological slide of a kryofixated carotid body, sectioned at -65 °C, rewarmed and then fixated according to BOUIN and stained according to the MASSON-GOLDNER method. The figure shows that the histological structure of the tissue remains intact after kryofixation and kryosectioning. The erythrocytes hemolyse after rewarming the kryosections. (Fig. from E. SEIDL, Max-Planck-Institut für Systemphysiologie in Dortmund)

effected by a closed circulation system using isopentan at -130 °C. The microscope kryostat (Fig. 2) was built for us and is isolated between the objective and the condensor of the double-beam photometer UMSP1 by ZEISS. The object to be measured lies on a cooled copper disc which is enclosed in a vacuum for thermic isolation. The microscope kryostat can be opened at the top in order to change the samples. Above and below the sample are quartz windows. Near the object the temperature is measured. With a diaphragm diameter between 2 and 8 μ, the extinction of the hemoglobin in the transected capillaries and larger blood vessels in the frozen section is measured between 520 and 620 nm. The measured hemoglobin spectra are evaluated according to the weighted multicomponent

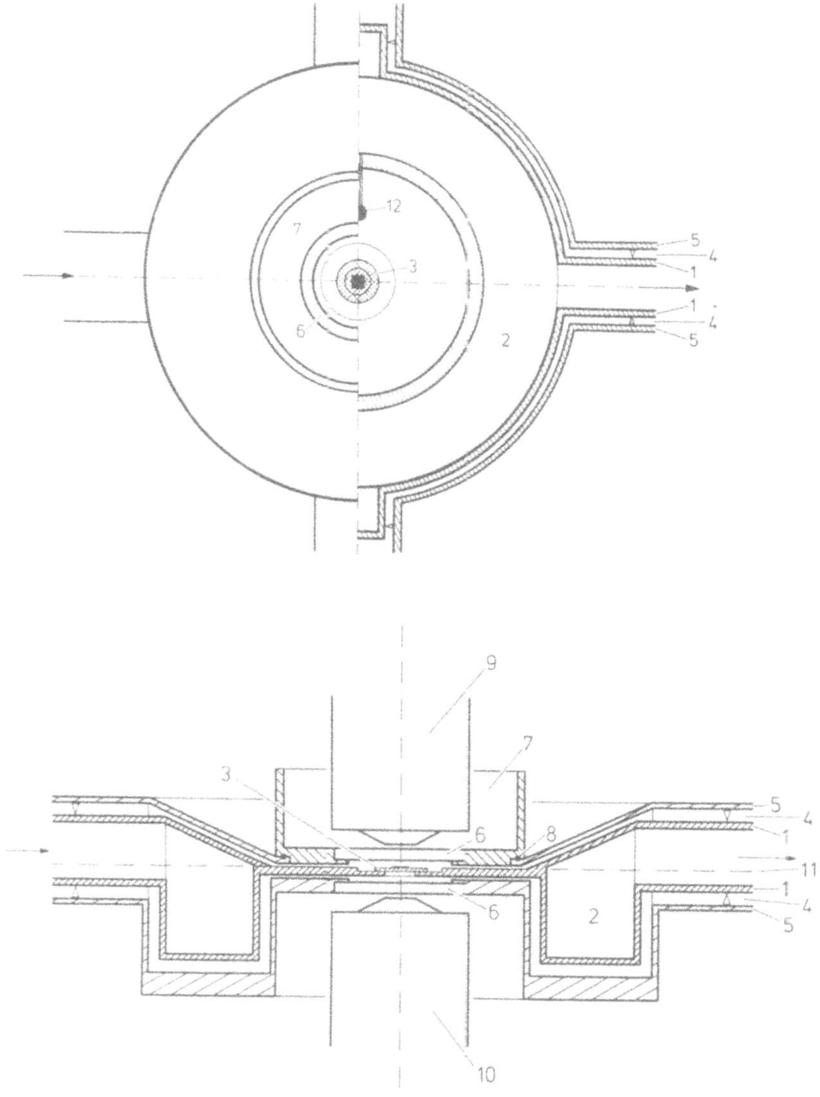

Figure 2

Vertical projection (above) and horizontal projection (below) of the microscope kryostat

1, cooled copper disc
2, isopentane container
3, slide with object
4, vacuum between 1 und 5 (for thermic isolation)
5, kryostat coat
6, quartz window
7, insertion for opening and closing the kryostat
8, O-ring-washer
9, and
10, objective or condensor, respectively
12, thermistor

analysis of WODICK and LÜBBERS (1969, 1971). The premise for this analysis is that a measured hemoglobin spectrum is a linear combination of the so-called basic spectra. The HbO_2 saturation is calculated from the coefficients of the basic spectra by a Least Square Fit. The basic spectra for such an analysis are shown in Fig. 3.

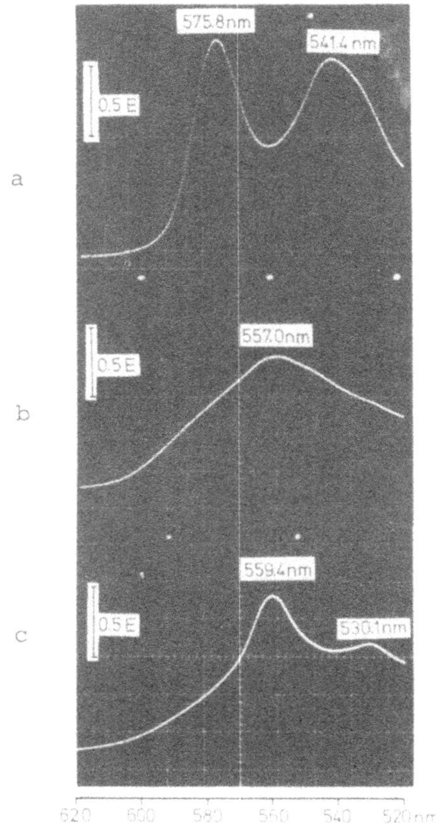

Figure 3
Hemoglobin basic spectra at -100 °C between 520 and 620 nm
(E: extinction unit) a: HbO_2 spectrum, b: Hb spectrum
c: dehydrated Hb spectrum

They are the absorption spectra of the oxygenated and deoxygenated hemoglobin at a temperature of -100 °C. Besides the normal oxygenated and deoxygenated hemoglobin spectra, a third basic spectrum has to be taken into account: that of the deoxygenated and dehydrated hemoglobin (GRUNEWALD 1972). It seems apparent that the dehydrated hemoglobin is formed by the removal of water during the ice crystal formation in the freeze period and under the influence of the vacuum in the microscope kryostat. That this third basic spectrum with its characteristic maxima is necessary, is shown in Fig. 4. By taking the three basic spectra into consideration, the approximation of the measured HbO_2 spectra is much better than by using just two basic spectra.

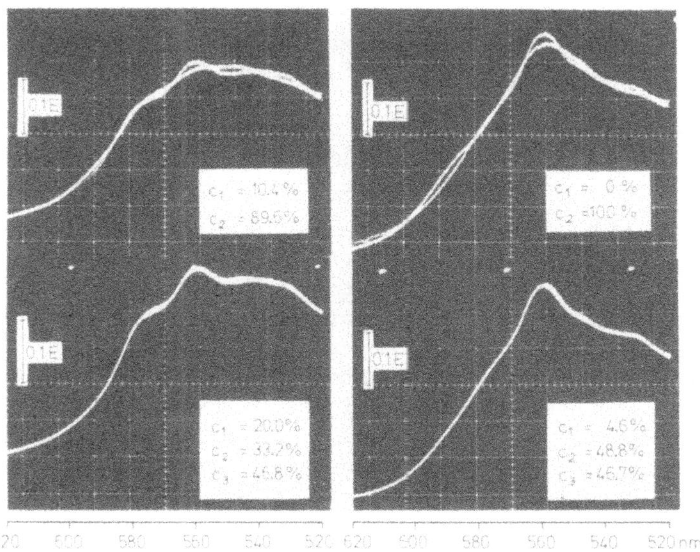

Figure 4

Approximation between the measured hemoglobin spectrum according to the weighted multicomponent analysis using the two basic spectra (above) and the three basic spectra (below). The three component analysis shows a better agreement between the measured and calculated spectra. c_i denotes the percentage portion of each basic spectrum from the measured spectrum

Before the microphotometric method could be used to determine the HbO_2 saturation of an organ, objects were used to test the method. The test objects were hemoglobin-filled glass capillaries, drops of hemoglobin and hemoglobin-loaded millipore membranes. Fig. 5 shows the HbO_2 saturation of a hemoglobin solution in glass capillaries at room temperature on the abscissa and on the ordinate

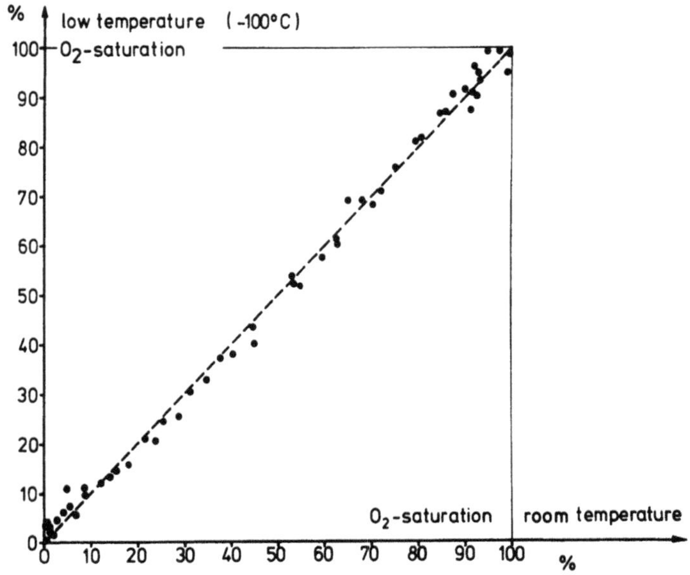

Figure 5

HbO_2 saturation of a hemoglobin solution in glass capillaries measured at room temperature (abscissa) and at kryostat temperature (ordinate). This figure shows that with n = 53 hemoglobin solutions in glass capillaries with differing O_2 saturations, a correlation r = 0.998 exists between the two measurements. A statistical difference is not significant.

is the HbO_2 saturation of the same test object at -100 $^{\circ}$C. From 53 measurements, a correlation coefficient of r = 0.998 resulted. A difference between HbO_2 saturation measured at room temperature and measured at kryostat temperature is statistically not significant.

If one compares the HbO_2 saturation from sectioned hemoglobin droplets with the HbO_2 saturation from hemoglobin solutions in glass capillaries, as systematic error is found. As we can see from Fig. 6, a saturation increase is found mainly at low HbO_2 saturations. It seems apparent that during the sectioning process the object is momentarily warmed at the knife edge and absorbs oxygen from the surrounding atmosphere. This systematic error is corrected in the following according to the curve of this figure.

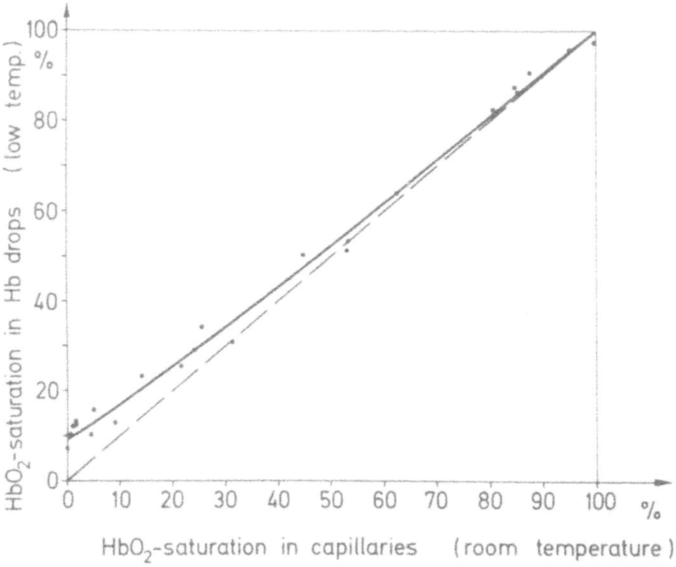

Figure 6

HbO_2 saturation of a hemoglobin solution in glass capillaries, measured at room temperature (abscissa) and of hemoglobin drops measured at the kryostat temperature (ordinate). The figure shows a systematic error of the O_2 saturation in the hemoglobin drops. This error is particularly large when the HbO_2 saturation is low.

As a third test object a hemoglobin-loaded millipore membrane is used which has different Po_2 values on either side of the membrane. When the steady-state has been reached, the membrane is kryofixated. As it can be seen in Fig. 7, with this method HbO_2 profiles can be fixated and measured (WEIGELT et al. 1973a, 1973b).

Fig. 8 finally shows the application of the kryophotometric method for measuring the intracapillary HbO_2 saturation in the rabbit myocardium at various O_2 supply conditions. The upper figure shows the frequency distribution of the intracapillary HbO_2 saturation while breathing room atmosphere (normoxie). The arterial saturation amounts to 98 %, the venous saturation to 24 %. The frequency maximum lies between 25 and 30 % HbO_2 saturation. HbO_2 saturation values lower than that were seldom found. The lower figure shows the frequency distribution by breathing a gas mixture with 5 % O_2 (hypoxia). The venous saturation value

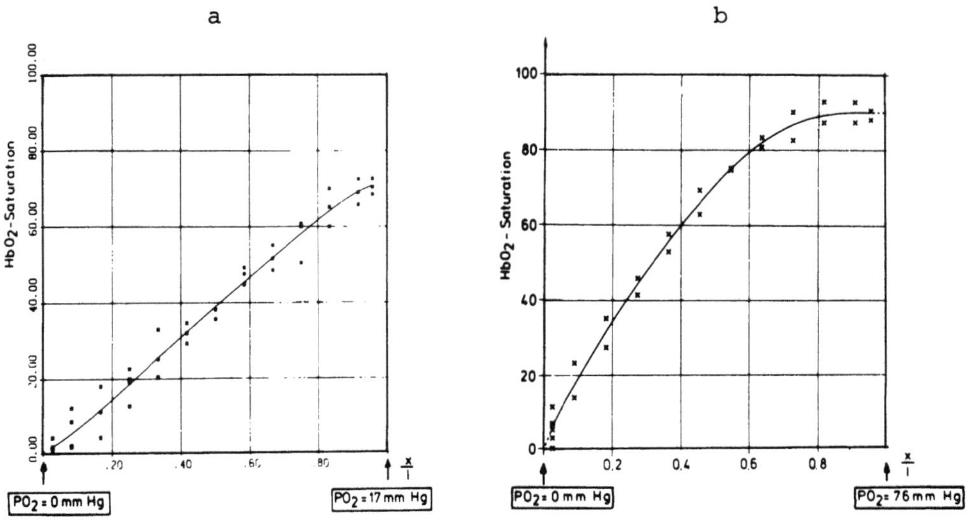

Figure 7

HbO_2-saturated profiles in a hemoglobin-loaded and kryofixated millipore membrane. Before kryofixation, the Po_2 was a) 0 mm Hg at the low pressure side and 17 mm Hg at the high pressure side; b) 0 mm Hg and 76 mm Hg, respectively

lies at 9 %. The frequency maximum is - compared to normoxie - shifted to the left. It lies between 0 and 5 % HbO_2 saturation.

From the results of the test measurements and the measurements from the rabbit myocardium we can see that the microkryophotometric method is a quantitative method that can be used to determine the intracapillary HbO_2 saturation. Thus, a parameter of the O_2 supply to the tissue has been revealed which up until now could not be measured.

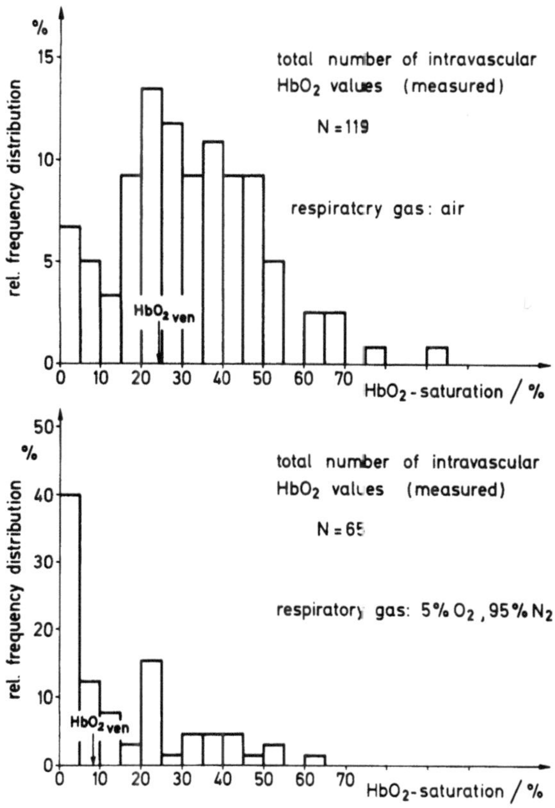

Figure 8

Frequency distribution of the intracapillary HbO_2 saturation of the rabbit myocardium under normoxic conditions (above) and hypoxic conditions with 5 % O_2 in the inspired air (below). The frequency maximum is shifted to the left from 20 - 25 to 0 - 5 % HbO_2 saturation during the change from normoxia to hypoxia

References

Grunewald, W. A.: Der Einfluß des deaquatisierten Hämoglobins auf die kryophotometrisch bestimmte HbO_2-Sättigung. Pflügers Arch. 335, R 4 (1972)

Grunewald, W. A., Lübbers, D. W.: Fixation of the O_2-saturation of the hemoglobin in the capillary blood by rapid freezing. Pflügers Arch. 307, R 12 (1969)

Grunewald, W. A., Lübbers, D. W.: Determination of intracapillary HbO_2-saturation with cryomicrophotometric method applied[+] to the rabbit myocardium. Pflügers Arch. 353, 255 - 273 (1975)

Lübbers, D. W., Wodick, R.: The examination of multicomponent systems in biological materials by means of a rapid scanning photometer. Appl. Optics 8, 1055 - 1062 (1969)

Lübbers, D. W., Wodick, R.: Schnelle Photometrie komplizierter biochemischer Mehrkomponentensysteme. Z. Anal. Chem. 261, 271 - 280 (1972)

Weigelt, Ch., Schneider, S., Grunewald, W. A., Lübbers, D. W.: Determination of HbO_2 gradients in thin layers - a method to quantify facilitated diffusion. Pflügers Arch. 339, R 4 (1973)

Weigelt, Ch., Grunewald, W. A., Lübbers, D. W.: Influence of back pressure on the course of the HbO_2 saturation gradient in HbO_2-loaded millipore membranes. Pflügers Arch. 343, R 5 (1973)

[+] for further literature

QUANTITATIVE FLUORESCENCE PHOTOMETRY WITH BIOLOGICAL FLUIDS AND GASES

D. W. Lübbers and N. Opitz

Max-Planck-Institut für Systemphysiologie
46 Dortmund, German Federal Republic

Longmuir and Knopp (1) have shown that the quenching of the fluorescence of pyrene butyric acid by oxygen (2) can be used to monitor oxygen concentration in tissue. However, since the fluorescence signal is also influenced by several other factors, such as

1) changes in the indicator concentration,
2) interaction of this indicator with other substances and
3) the filter effect of the tissue,

a quantitative evaluation meets with considerable difficulties. The error caused by concentration changes can be cancelled by using special indicators which change their spectra with the reaction. For example, Boldt and Lübbers (3) used ß-methyl umbelliferon as a pH indicator which has different excitation spectra for the dissociated and undissociated forms. The other errors cannot be taken into account without special measurements. The actual, possibly disturbed spectrum of the tissue can be related to the true indicator spectrum, if the indicator in the tissue is changed into its dissociated or undissociated form, e. g. on a deliberate change of the pH. Relating the relative intensity of the disturbed and the true spectrum wavelength by wavelength, we obtain a transformation by which the true indicator spectrum is obtained from the tissue spectrum (4, 5, 6). Unfortunately, this evaluation method is rather complicated and needs the registration of the total spectrum, or at least measurements at several wavelengths (7).

In a simple way the independence of all the disturbance factors can be achieved by separating the indicator from the measuring medium. For the blood gases the separation is brought about by a membrane which is impermeable to the medium, but permeable to the gases. Figure 1 shows a schematical drawing of such a measuring device, which we call in analogy to "electrode", "optode".

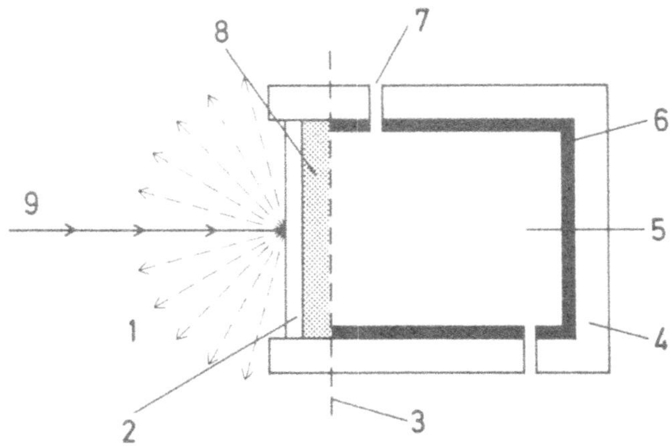

Figure 1

Schematic cross-section of the optode (not true to scale) for explanation, see text).

1 fluorescence
2 quartz window
3 membrane
4 plexiglass housing
5 gas or fluid chamber
6 light-trap
7 channel for gas or fluid conduction
8 solution chamber for the indicator
9 excitation radiation

The indicator pyrene butyric acid dissolved in dimethyl formamide forms an approximately 10-μm-thick layer between a quartz window and a 6-μm teflon membrane. The surface of the measuring space into which the medium is filled, is covered with black to reduce background fluorescence. The gas of the measuring medium diffuses into the indicator until an equilibrium is reached. The degree of fluorescence quenching is directly measured through the quartz window. The calibration curve obeys the Stern-Vollmer equation for fluorescence quenching. In the Po_2 range between 0 and 350 Torr a quotient, S_o'/S', of the fluorescence signal at 0 % oxygen, S_o', and the actual fluorescence, S', is linearly related to the Po_2 of the medium. If, instead of pyrene butyric acid, a solution of 10^{-3} M $NaHCO_3$ saturated with ß-methyl umbelliferon is used, the pH measured by the indicator can be related to the Pco_2 of the medium. Figure 2 shows the excitation spectra of both indicators.

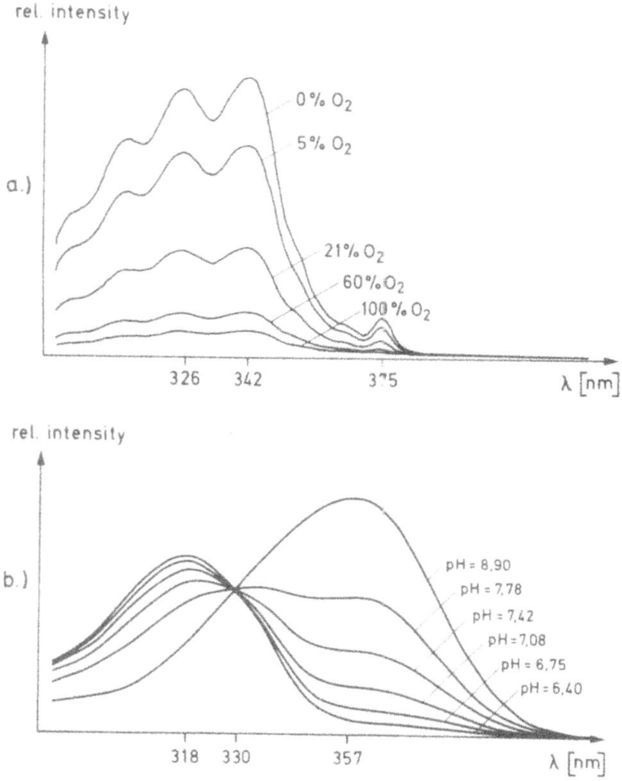

Figure 2
Corrected excitation spectra of a) pyrene butyric acid at an emmission wavelength of λ_{em} = 395 nm, and b) ß-methyl umbelliferon at λ_{em} = 445 nm

The isosbestic point of ß-methyl umbelliferon enables us to describe the pH dependence of the fluorescence by a quotient which, in a certain range, is independent of both concentration and amplification of the signal. However, with increasing concentrations the spectrum itself changes in dependence on the concentration. Figure 3 shows that the response time of the Pco_2 optode is quite short. It amounts to about 3 - 4 s. Addition of carboanhydrase reduces this time to about 1 s. For simultaneous measurements the two indicators can be mixed. With fixed concentrations the O_2 quenching can be measured at the isosbestic wavelength, whereas pH changes are given by the quotient.

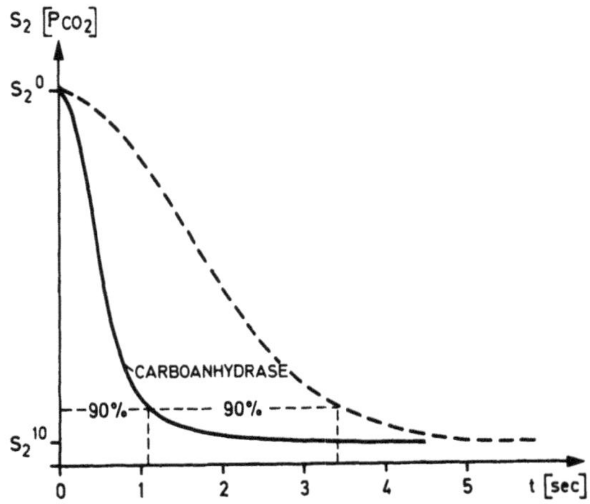

Figure 3
Equilibration curve of the P_{CO_2} optode monitored versus time during a CO_2 jump from 0 to 10 % atmospheric pressure (teflon 6-/um membrane, thickness 10/um, ß-methyl umbelliferon saturated in 10^{-3} M/ $NaHCO_3$)

The principle of this measurement is to separate the indicator from the measuring medium by a membrane which is permeable to the substance to be measured. In this way we guarantee that only this substance determines the fluorescence signal. For other applications it can be advantageous to deposit the fluorescence indicator on the membrane itself, or to use a small capsule filled with the indicator.

References

1. Knopp, J. A., Longmuir, J. S., Biochim. Biophys. Acta 279, 393 (1972)
2. Vaughan, W. M., Weber, G., Biochemistry 9, 464 (1970)
3. Boldt, M.: Ein korrigiert messendes Spektrofluorormeter zur Messung an trüben Medien. Dissertation Marburg 1971
4. Wodick, R., Lübbers, D. W., Hoppe-Seyler's Z. Physiol. Chem. 354, 903 (1973)
5. Wodick, R., Lübbers, D. W., Hoppe-Seyler's Z. Physiol. Chem. 354, 916 (1973)
6. Lübbers, D. W.: In: Oxygen Transport to Tissue. Instrumentation, Methods and Physiology, eds. H. I. Bicher and D. F. Bruley, Plenum Publ. Corp. New York 1973
7. Wodick, R., Lübbers, D. W., Pflügers Arch. 342, 41 (1973).

CONTROL OF ELECTRODE AGING BY A PERIODIC ANODIZATION TECHNIQUE

Vincent G. Murphy, Ronald E. Barr and Allen W. Hahn

The Dalton Research Center, University of Missouri

Columbia, Missouri 65201, U.S.A.

INTRODUCTION

The long-term use of noble metal electrodes for amperometrically monitoring oxygen tension in blood and tissue has been hampered by the unstable nature of the electrode calibration. Changes in sensitivity (current per unit oxygen tension) as rapid as 20% per hour have been reported [1]. If this drift were constant, it would, in principle, be simple to correct for; however, increasing and decreasing trends separated by plateau regions are most frequently encountered [2,3]. In some cases, changes in sensitivity have been attributed to protein deposition or to poisoning by sulfur-containing molecules [4], but such mechanisms cannot account for the drift observed with electrodes immersed in pure saline solutions [2,3]. The latter phenomenon, usually referred to as "electrode aging", can best (and perhaps only) be explained by supposing an interrelationship between the electrode's catalytic activity and its redox history. This, of course, is a concept well documented in the electrochemical literature [5]. Of particular importance here is that some electrochemical studies [6,7] suggest that, at least for Pt electrodes, strong oxidizing treatments, such as exposure to concentrated nitric acid or anodization at elevated potentials, may result in more stable electrode behavior. In this report, we present evidence, based on in vitro tests in physiological saline, indicating that the aging phenomenon can be controlled by periodically restoring the electrode surface to a pseudostable level of catalytic activity via in situ anodization.

MATERIALS AND METHODS

The design of the electrodes employed in this study was similar to that of the open or flush-ended electrode described by Davies and Brink [8]. Pt-Ir (80-20) wire, 50 μm in diameter, was silver soldered to a copper lead wire and then fused into one end of a soft glass capillary. After applying heat-shrinkable tubing at the opposite end to mechanically stabilize the wire within the capillary, the fused surface was ground flat and polished using a graded series of emery papers and polishing media. Residues from the polishing operation were then removed by ultrasonic cleaning in ethyl alcohol and distilled water. The use of deionized water was avoided since it is known [5] to cause erratic electrode behavior. Once an electrode had been cleaned, care was taken not to recontaminate its surface by direct handling.

All tests were conducted in a jacketed pyrex vessel equipped with a demountable plexiglass lid machined to accept a gas dispersion tube, a thermistor probe, a reference electrode holder and up to 10 test electrodes. The reference electrode was a saturated calomel half cell (SCE) electrically connected to the test solution by an agar bridge. As shown in the schematic in Figure 1, electrodes were monitored individually on Keithley Picoammeters (Models 416 and 610C) which were in turn connected to a Brush Multichannel Recorder to provide permanent documentation. Positive and negative D.C. voltage supplies connected to a manually operated DPDT switch

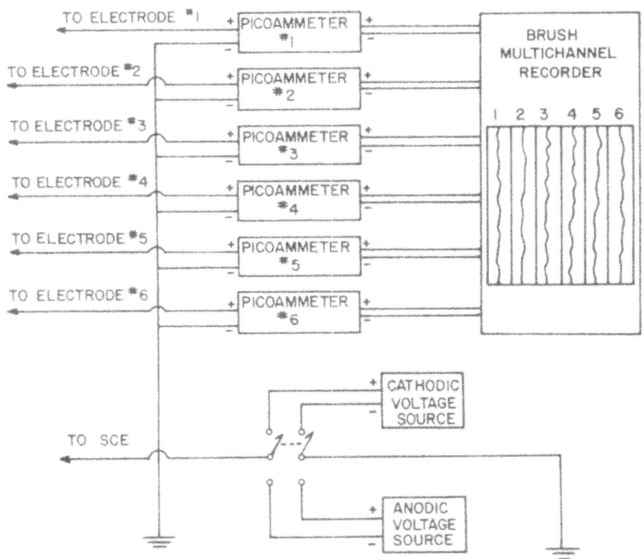

Figure 1. Block diagram of electronic system.

provided the anodic/cathodic polarization cycles. The test medium in all cases was sterile physiological saline (9 g/l NaCl) maintained at room temperature (22 ± 1°C).

RESULTS

In our early studies of factors affecting electrode stability, electrodes passivated with nitric acid for approximately 240 hours were noted to exhibit more stable behavior than untreated electrodes during the first 8-12 hours of operation in saline. In addition, we found that, after later periods of prolonged drift, the initial sensitivity could be restored for brief intervals (30-45 min) by an *in situ* anodization at +1450 mv (vs SCE). Subsequent experiments described below revealed that the somewhat inconvenient passivation procedure could be replaced, with equally good results, by a simple 30 minute anodization in saline if the electrodes were then reanodized *in situ* for 5 minutes at 90 minute intervals. Anodic and cathodic polarization levels in the latter tests were +1250 mv (vs SCE) and -700 mv (vs SCE) respectively.

An indication of the improvement in electrode stability resulting from periodic anodization is given in Figure 2. In this illustra-

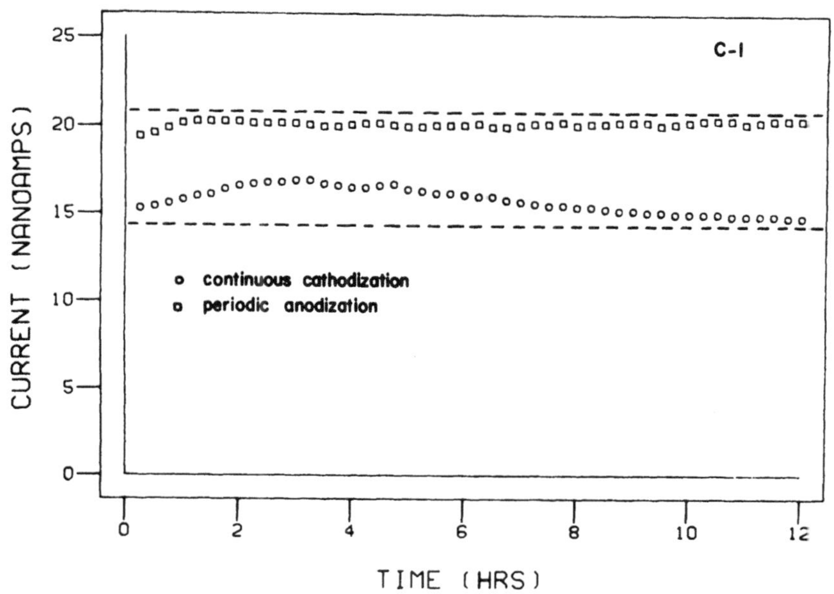

Figure 2. Electrode stability test comparing continuous cathodization and periodic anodization modes of operation. Dashed lines included for horizontal reference only.

tion, the open squares are data obtained using the polarization regimen described above (30 min preanodization followed by successive 90 min periods consisting of 5 min anodization/85 min cathodization), and the open circles are data for the same electrode under constant cathodic polarization. Although these data are for a single electrode, they are fully representative of the group of six tested in this manner. In all cases, electrode behavior was markedly more stable when the periodic anodization procedure was employed. Moreover, in tests prolonged to 30 hours, no degeneration in the effectiveness of the technique was detected.

Figure 3 presents data obtained from a still longer term experiment. On day 0, the electrode was calibrated (by equilibrating the saline with gases of known oxygen tension), and on days 1, 2, 4 and 6 thereafter, it was operated for 9.5 hours under ambient conditions using the periodic anodization procedure. In the figure, the dashed line represents the calibration value for air saturation, and the vertical bar at the upper right, the magnitude of a 5% deviation from this value. On any given day, at most a 1-2% variation in sensitivity occurred, and day to day reproducibility was within 2-3%. Over the first four days, there appeared to be an upward trend in sensitivity, but the data for days 4 and 6 were nearly identical, and, in any case, the overall drift from the calibration value over the en-

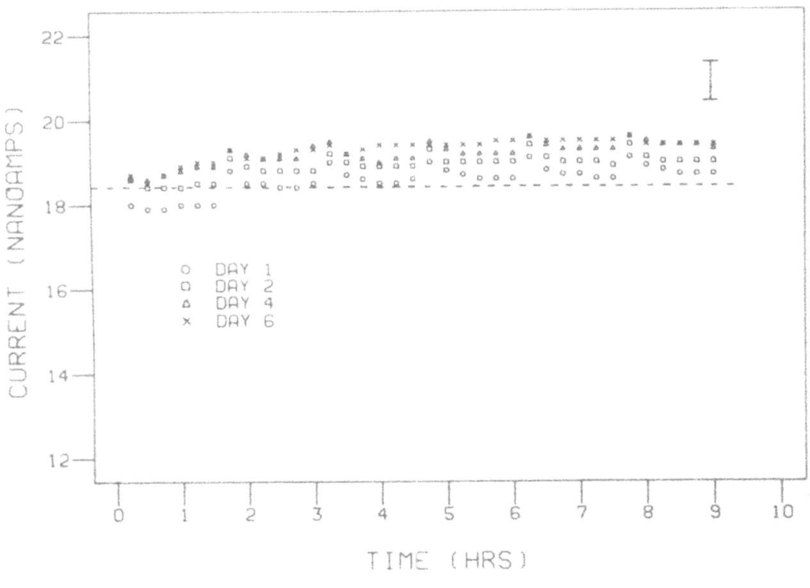

Figure 3. Long term test of effectiveness of periodic anodization technique. Dashed line represents calibration value obtained on day 0. Vertical bar (upper right) represents magnitude of 5% deviation from calibration level.

tire course of the experiment was within about 5-6%. Three other electrodes tested in this manner yielded similar results.

In another experiment, four electrodes were calibrated on day 0 and then left on open circuit in air-saturated saline for over a month. On day 35, two of the electrodes were anodized at +1250 mv (vs SCE) for 30 min and then all four were polarized cathodically at -700 mv (vs SCE). As shown in Figure 4, the preanodized electrodes, N-2 and N-3, exhibited almost no drift from their calibration values; whereas, the untreated electrodes, C-2 and C-3, ran well below their previous levels.

DISCUSSION

The results presented above strongly indicate that, although periodic anodization does not eliminate electrode aging, it does bring the process under control by permitting periodic _in situ_ restoration of a standard, pseudo-stable level of oxygen reduction activity. A complete discussion of the mechanism responsible for the improved stability following anodization is beyond the scope of this report, but we believe it to be the same as that proposed by Hoare

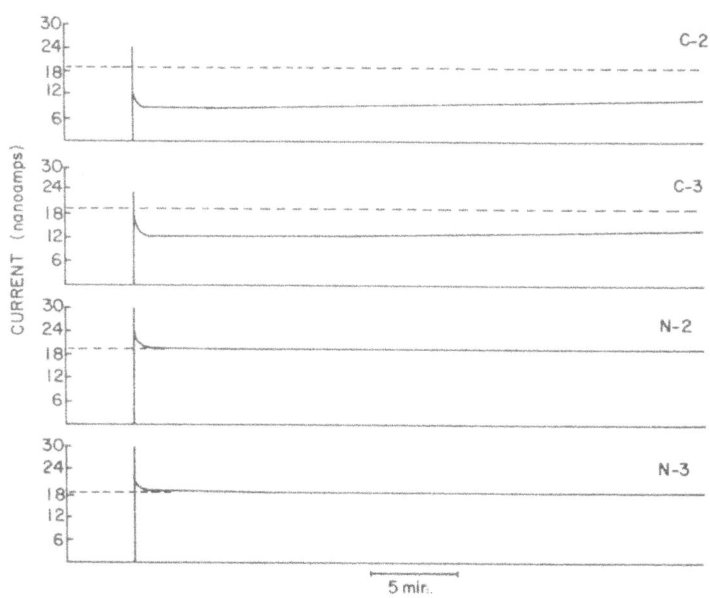

Figure 4. Electrode responses to recathodization (-700 mv vs SCE) after 35 days on open circuit in saline. N-2 and N-3 were anodized (1250 mv vs SCE) for 30 min just prior to cathodization; C-2 and C-3 were not. Dashed lines represent calibration values obtained on day 0.

[7] in explaining the superior performance of preanodized Pt indicator electrodes in various redox systems. Briefly, during anodization, oxygen atoms (resulting from the decomposition of water molecules), in addition to forming a surface film on the electrode, dissolve into the subsurface layers of the metal creating a Pt-O-alloy having catalytic properties superior to those of the pure metal.

Many years ago, Olson and co-workers [9] reported good results using an alternating polarization scheme in which the electrode was anodized for 1/4 of the cycle time; however, later workers [10] investigating pulsatile electrode operation found that no benefit was derived from including an anodic pulse between successive cathodic pulses. This seeming contradiction cannot be explained with certitude, but it may be that in the more recent work [10] the pulse width was too narrow or the voltage level too low to facilitate the dissolution of oxygen atoms into the metal during the anodic pulse. The latter seems especially likely since the quantity of oxygen dissolved by Pt has been shown [11] to depend strongly upon the applied potential.

Despite the very promising nature of the results presented in the preceding section, it might be worthwhile to note some limitations that must be placed on their interpretation. For one thing, all tests were conducted in sterile saline using bare electrodes; therefore, the applicability of the periodic anodization technique in the case of membrane covered electrodes operated in biological media remains to be demonstrated. Happily, initial attempts in that direction have been encouraging. Another potential limitation is that, following resumption of cathodic polarization after each 5 minutes anodization, about 5-10 min elapses before the current reaches its steady operating level. Thus, out of each 90 min operational interval, a period of 10-15 min is unavailable for monitoring oxygen tension. However, since the present polarization regimen was arrived at fortuitously, it may be possible to significantly decrease the percentage of "down time" by shortening the anodization phase and/or lengthening the cathodization phase.

ACKNOWLEDGMENT

The authors are indebted to Bonnie MacAlmon for technical assistance and to Chuck Jorgenson for preparing the illustrations. This work was supported in part by a contract from the U.S. Army Medical R & D Command (DADA-17-71-C-1104).

REFERENCES

1. H. Baumgärtl and D. W. Lübbers (1973), "Platinum needle electrodes for polarographic measurement of oxygen and hydrogen", in Oxygen Supply (M. Kessler et al., eds.), University Park Press, Baltimore, pp. 130-136.

2. M. Kessler (1973), "Problems with the use of platinum cathodes for the polarographic measurement of oxygen", in Oxygen Supply (M. Kessler et al., eds.), Unviersity Park Press, Baltimore, pp. 81-85.

3. I. A. Silver (1973), "The oxygen micro-electrode", in Oxygen Transport to Tissue (H. I. Bicher and D. F. Bruley, eds.), Plenum Press, New York, pp. 7-15.

4. D. B. Cater, I. A. Silver and G. M. Wilson (1956), "Apparatus and technique for the quantitative measurement of oxygen tension in living tissues", Proc. Royal Soc. London Sec. B., 151: 256-276.

5. E. Bishop and P. H. Hitchcock (1973), "The pre-treatment of solid electrodes and a review of the effects of oxidation of platinum", Analyst, 98:475-484.

6. J. P. Hoare, S. G. Meibuhr and R. Thacker (1966), "Some effects of nitric acid on Pt/O_2 cathodes", J. Electrochem. Soc., 113: 1078-1082.

7. J. P. Hoare (1966), "On the reversible Pt indicator electrode", J. Electroanal. Chem., 12:260-264.

8. P. W. Davies and F. Brink (1942), "Microelectrodes for measuring local oxygen tension in animal tissues", Rev. Sci. Instrum., 13:524-533.

9. R. A. Olson, F. S. Brackett and R. G. Crickard (1949), "Oxygen tension measurement by a method of time selection using the static platinum electrode with alternating potential", J. Gen. Physiol., 32:681-703.

10. K. Kunze and D. W. Lübbers (1973), "Absolute PO_2 measurements with Pt electrodes applying polarizing voltage pulsing", in Oxygen Transport to Tissue (H. I. Bicher and D. F. Bruley, eds.), Plenum Press, New York, pp. 35-43.

11. R. Thacker and J. P. Hoare (1971), "Sorption of oxygen from solution by noble metals. I. Bright platinum", J. Electroanal. Chem., 30:1-14.

SUMMARY OF DISCUSSION - SESSION I: OXYGEN MEASUREMENTS IN BLOOD AND TISSUE

Chairmen: W. J. Whalen and H. Hutten

Paper of Drs. Lehmkühler, et al.
The comments mainly concerned the size and impedance of the reference electrode. Of course, the larger it is the lower the resistance. By sputtering AgCl on the shaft of the electrode near the tip the errors are minimized.

Paper of Drs. Schneiderman and Goldstick
The questions concerned the geometry of the O_2 field around a nonrecessed electrode. The speaker replied that the spherical model does not apply to a recessed electrode. Stirring artifacts were brought up in discussion but according to the speaker would be expected to be negligible for the recessed tip. Also, that a slight change in the geometry of the reccess would not seriously alter the conclusions.

Paper of Drs. Seidl, et al.
The question as to whether H_2 clearance was a good indicator of blood flow was answered in a tentative way, i. e. that there was reasonable agreement with measurements of venous outflow.

Question of Dr. Goldstick:
The PO_2 profile you have measured in the arterial wall is quite different from published profiles (HUNT et al.) and from profiles we have measured in the rabbit thoracic aorta, with and without perfusion of the vasa vasorum. These other studies all show a gradual decrease in PO_2 (moving inward from the adventitia),

a minimum, a rapid rise in PO_2 as the lumen is approached, and finally a constant PO_2 in the lumen. Could you explain why your profile is so different?

Answer:
The artery with the high PO_2 shown in the figure, is a rather small one and is inside the tissue of the carotid body. It is surrounded by the specific tissue of the carotid body, which has a low oxygen tension kept in this range by the tissue respiration. The measured O_2-decrease is caused by these two factors.

Paper of Drs. Evans and Constable

The major question on this paper concerned the possible interaction between the cathodes. The speaker said that because of the 500 μm distance between them, there was none.

Paper of Drs. Forster, et al.

The question of a possible error being introduced depending on the value of PO_2 (50) of myoglobin. The speaker felt that this error would not exceed 100 %.

Papers of Drs. Jöbsis and Mitnick, and Drs. Longmuir and Knopp

The possibility that absolute PO_2 might be measured by this technique was discussed. The speaker said that O_2 concentration was being measured and partial pressure. The conversion could not be made since there were too many unknowns. Some doubt was expressed as to whether there might be extinction by the membrane and too much light scattering. The speaker admitted that were serious problems and they might have to resort to the laser method. A question was asked about the relevance to the measurement of the diffusion constant for O_2. This was answered affirmatively.

Paper of Drs. Grunewald and Lübbers

The question arose that it should be possible to make a good estimate of intercapillary distance from this preparation. The answer was that it could only be crude estimate since some capillaries, presumably open, contained only plasma.

Blood Oxygenation

EFFECTS OF 2,3-DIPHOSPHOGLYCERATE ON FUNCTIONAL PROPERTIES OF HEMOGLOBIN AND ON GLYCOLYSIS OF HUMAN ERYTHROCYTES

Jochen Duhm

Physiologisches Institut

Universität München, München, Germany

This report is divided into two parts. The first is concerned with the binding of 2,3-diphosphoglycerate (DPG) to deoxy- and oxyhemoglobin in the absence and presence of CO_2 under conditions comparable to those prevailing in intact erythrocytes. In the second part an attempt is made to analyze the mechanism by which glycolysis is inhibited in erythrocytes containing elevated concentrations of DPG.

BINDING OF DPG TO DEOXY- AND OXYHEMOGLOBIN: EFFECT OF CO_2

It is generally accepted that the affinity for DPG of deoxyhemoglobin exceeds that of oxyhemoglobin (1-4). Agreement has not yet been obtained, however, whether DPG is bound at all to oxyhemoglobin (5-10). Such a binding to oxyhemoglobin should decrease the efficiency of DPG in reducing the oxygen affinity of hemoglobin and should increase the concentration of free DPG in intact human erythrocytes. From studies on the effects of CO_2 on the functional properties of hemoglobin it is known that CO_2 inhibits the binding of DPG to hemoglobin (11) and, vice versa, that DPG inhibits the binding of CO_2 (1,12). Not enough binding data are available, however, to evaluate quantitatively the magnitude of the CO_2 effect on the affinity of hemoglobin for DPG.

A resolution of these open questions would be desirable for a better understanding of the allosteric properties of hemoglobin as well as of the regulation of

DPG metabolism and glycolysis in intact erythrocytes. Therefore, an attempt was made to estimate association constants of the hemoglobin-DPG complex from P_{50} values like those shown in Figure 1 and from similar results obtained at other DPG concentrations. The results strongly indicated that DPG is bound also to oxyhemoglobin (13).

Figure 1 demonstrates the pH dependency of the effects of physiological concentrations of DPG and CO_2 on the P_{50} of solutions containing about 70% of the hemoglobin concentration of intact erythrocytes. Obviously, both DPG and CO_2 decreased the oxygen affinity of hemoglobin. However, with rising pH the DPG effect decreased whereas the CO_2 effect increased, indicating that DPG and CO_2 change the Bohr effect of hemoglobin in the opposite direction (1,13). Figure 2 shows oxyhemoglobin dissociation curves determined at pH 7.2, i.e. at the red cell pH of human erythrocytes suspended at the normal plasma pH of 7.4. The curves demonstrate that normal concentrations of the two effectors are needed to shift the oxygen dissociation curve of "stripped" hemoglobin back to the normal

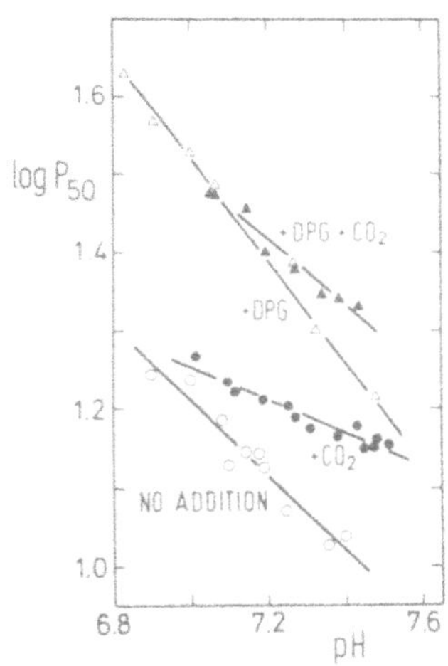

Figure 1

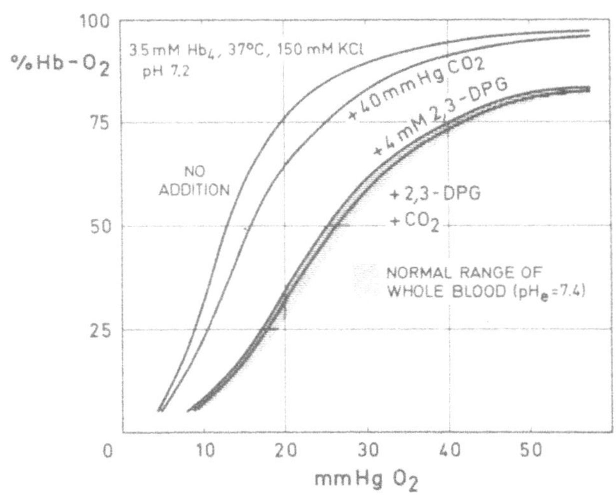

Figure 2

Figure 1: pH dependencies of the effects of 4 mM DPG and of 40 mmHg CO_2 on the P_{50} (partial pressure of O_2 at 50% O_2 saturation of hemoglobin) of human hemoglobin (37°C, 3.5 mmoles Hb_4/ml solution, 150-170 mM Cl^-). For experimental details see ref. 13 and 23.

Figure 2: Effects of physiological concentrations of DPG (4mM) and CO_2 (40mmHg) on the oxyhemoglobin dissociation curve. The curves were calculated from the data given in Figure 1.

Table 1: Comparison of DPG binding constants (liters/mole) of deoxy- and oxyhemoglobin (K_{deox} and K_{ox}) determined in concentrated hemoglobin solutions at 37°C and pH 7.2.

K_{deox}	K_{ox}	mmHg CO_2	Cl^- (mM)	Hb (mM)	Technique
5 000	250	0	150	1.5	Ultrafiltration (Berger et al., 1973, ref. 14)
9 710	210	0	120	0.6-4	Dialysis (Hamasaki and Rose, 1974, ref. 15)
9 800	164	0	170	3.5	Calculation from P_{50} values (Duhm,
2 850	66	40	150	3.5	1974, ref. 13)

range of whole blood. Furthermore it appears from Figures 1 and 2 that the efficiency of one effector becomes considerably reduced in the presence of the second one.

In Table 1 binding constants for DPG of deoxy- and oxyhemoglobin obtained by different techniques are compared. The data of Garby and DeVerdier (10) were not included since they have been determined in the presence of 3 mM $MgCl_2$. It is to be noted that all the binding constants given in Table 1 were determined in concentrated hemoglobin solutions at 37°C, pH 7.2, and at an ionic strength close to that of intact erythrocytes. The results obtained in the absence of CO_2 by the three different techniques agree surprisingly well. The data indicate concordantly that oxyhemoglobin exhibits a definite affinity for DPG. The ratios of the DPG binding constants of deoxy- and oxyhemoglobin were equal to or greater than 20. The results thus agree with the postulate that the affinity of deoxyhemoglobin for DPG should exceed that of oxyhemoglobin at least by one order of magnitude (8).

In the presence of CO_2 the binding constants of deoxy- and oxyhemoglobin for DPG were lowered markedly (Table 1). Because of the magnitude of the CO_2 effect it appears that the presence of CO_2 in human blood cannot be neglected when estimating the concentrations of free and hemoglobin-bound metabolites in oxygenated and deoxygenated erythrocytes (cf. 9,16,17).

The effects of CO_2 and of the oxygenation state of hemoglobin on the concentrations of bound and free DPG in solutions containing the hemoglobin concentration found in normal erythrocytes become evident from Table 2. The values given in this Table were calculated from the binding constants determined in our laboratory assuming a DPG, hemoglobin and water content of 4.5 and 5.2 µmoles/ml solution, and of 65%, respectively. The concentrations of free DPG in circulating human erythrocytes should exceed the values to be expected from the data given in Table 2 since the concentrations of free DPG have been calculated without taking into account the chelation of Mg^{++} by the DPG anion and the competition of DPG and ATP for the same binding sites of hemoglobin.

As a result of the marked effect of CO_2 on DPG binding by hemoglobin the concentrations of free DPG are considerably higher in the presence of CO_2 than in its absence (see Table 2). Furthermore it appears that CO_2 enhances the change of free DPG occurring upon oxygenation from 3.40 to 3.95 µmoles/ml water. This unexpected phenomenon results from the more pronounced alteration by CO_2 of DPG binding to oxyhemoglobin than to deoxyhemoglobin (Figure 3).

According to the linkage equations describing the reciprocal effects of oxygen and other ligands on hemoglobin (18) one would expect that a CO_2-induced increase of oxygen-linked DPG binding should be associated with an increased effect of the organic phosphate on the oxygen affinity of hemoglobin. In contrast, the magnitude of the DPG effect is found to be reduced in the presence of CO_2 (see Figures 1 and 2, and ref. 1). In interpreting this discrepancy it has to be taken into account that the concentration of free DPG is not independent of the

Table 2: Concentrations of bound and free DPG in solutions containing 5.2 µmoles Hb_4 and 4.5 µmoles DPG per ml. (37°C, pH 7.2). For details see text.

	0 mmHg CO_2		40 mmHg CO_2	
	deoxy	oxy	deoxy	oxy
DPG_{bound} [1)]	6.49	3.09	5.92	1.97
DPG_{free} [1)]	0.43	3.83	1.00	4.95
% free	6 %	45 %	15 %	71 %

[1)] The values are given as µmoles/ml water. To obtain values in terms of amount per ml of solution, the concentrations given in the Table have to be multiplied by 0.65.

oxygenation state of hemoglobin in concentrated hemoglobin solutions. Such an independence would be a prerequisite for an application of the linkage equations to the data. On the other hand, the lesser effectiveness of DPG in the presence of CO_2 might result from the DPG-induced reduction of oxygen-linked CO_2 binding (1,12). Then, the decrease of oxygen-linked carbamate formation in the presence of DPG should be of greater significance for O_2 binding than the CO_2-induced increase of oxygen-linked DPG binding. Finally it has to be considered that not only the oxygen-linked binding of DPG but also the DPG binding to oxyhemoglobin per se could influence the functional properties of hemoglobin.

From the results it is concluded that oxyhemoglobin exhibits a definite affinity for DPG in concentrated hemoglobin solutions at 37° and pH 7.2. CO_2 reduces the binding of DPG to both deoxy- and oxyhemoglobin. The CO_2-induced change in bound or free DPG is more pronounced in oxygenated than in deoxygenated solutions of high hemoglobin content. Consequently, the oxygen-linked DPG binding to hemoglobin is increased in the presence of CO_2 (see Table 2 and Figure 3). At the moment it is not understood why this increased differential DPG binding in the presence of CO_2 is not associated with an increased effect of DPG on the oxygen affinity of hemoglobin.

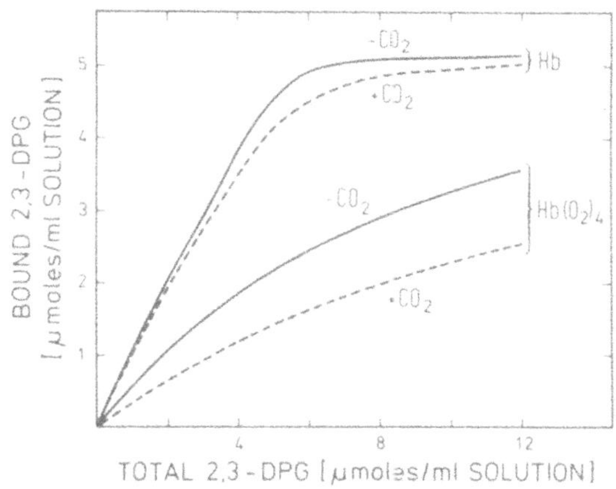

<u>Figure 3:</u> Effect of CO_2 (40 mmHg) on the concentration of bound DPG (37°C, pH 7.2). The curves were calculated from the binding constants given in Table 1 (13) assuming a hemoglobin and water content of 5.2 µmoles/ml solution and of 65%, respectively.

Table 3: Dependence of the inhibition of glycolysis[1] in "high-DPG" cells[2] on the extracellular pH (37°C).

	pH_e=7.0		pH_e=7.4		pH_e=8.0	
	Gluc	Lac	Gluc	Lac	Gluc	Lac
Normal cells	0.12 ±0.01	0.26 ±0.01	0.22 ±0.01	0.40 ±0.04	0.42 ±0.02	0.72 ±0.02
"High-DPG" cells	0.06 ±0.01	0.19 ±0.01	0.07 ±0.01	0.25 ±0.03	0.10 ±0.01	0.30 ±0.02
Inhibition	54 %	28 %	68 %	38 %	77 %	59 %

[1] Values given as μmoles glucose consumed (Gluc) or as μmoles lactate formed (Lac) per μmole hemoglobin tetramer per hour (mean values ± SEM from four to six experiments). This manner of presentation was chosen in order to eliminate apparent changes in the glycolytic rate per unit volume of erythrocytes which would result from changes of the cellular water content (26,27)

[2] DPG levels were elevated above the normal value of 4 to 5 μmoles/ml cells (normal cells) to 20 to 25 μmoles/ml cells ("high-DPG" cells) by a 100 min preincubation period in the presence of inosine, pyruvate, and inorganic phosphate (for methodical details see ref. 26 and 27). The cells were then washed several times to remove the substrates and to reduce the concentrations of accumulated metabolites other than DPG.

Table 4: Inhibition of glycolysis in "high-DPG" cells at different intracellular pH values[1] (37°C).

	pH_i=6.84		pH_i=7.20		pH_i=7.53	
	Gluc	Lac	Gluc	Lac	Gluc	Lac
Normal cells	0.12	0.26	0.22	0.40	0.42	0.72
"High-DPG" cells	0.07	0.25	0.13	0.35	0.31	0.60
Inhibition	40 %	4 %	42 %	12 %	26 %	17 %

[1] The values of the intracellular pH (pH_i) given in the Table are the red cell pH values determined in normal cells at the extracellular pH values of 7.0, 7.4, and 8.0, respectively. The glycolytic rates in "high-DPG" cells at the pH_i values indicated were taken from Figure 1 of ref. 27.

EFFECT OF DPG ON RED CELL GLYCOLYSIS

Several investigations showed that DPG can inhibit a number of glycolytic enzymes (19-21). This observation led to the conclusion that the inhibition of glycolysis in erythrocytes containing high concentrations of DPG is due enzyme inhibition by DPG (21,22). On the other hand, it is known that elevation of the red cell DPG content decreases the red cell pH (23-25). A decrease of the red cell pH, however, reduces the glycolytic rate due to the properties of the enzyme phosphofructo kinase. Thus, the the inhibition of glycolysis in "high-DPG" cells has been attributed to the pH effect (26). To differentiate between the two possible inhibitory mechanisms glycolysis was studied in normal cells and in erythrocytes containing elevated concentrations of DPG at different values of the intracellular and extracellular pH, respectively.

The results obtained are summarized in Tables 3 and 4. The rates of glucose consumption and of lactate production in "high-DPG" cells were almost independent of the extracellular pH (Table 3). Consequently, the inhibition of glycolysis increased with rising extracellular pH values. When the glycolytic rates were compared at identical intracellular pH values (Table 4), the inhibition of glycolysis in the "high-DPG" was far less pronounced. Thus it becomes apparent that the inhibition of glycolysis in "high-DPG" cells can be attributed in part to the DPG-induced decrease of the red cell pH.

The remaining part of the inhibitory effect must be caused by a DPG-induced inhibition of glycolytic enzymes. To identify the enzyme(s) which become(s) inhibited by DPG in "high-DPG" cells, concentrations of various glycolytic intermediates and glycolytic rates in the presence of methylene blue were determined (27). The results indicated that elevation of red cell DPG concentration leads to an inhibition of the enzymes hexokinase and pyruvate kinase. It appears unlikely, however, that the inhibition of the latter enzyme contributes in the DPG-induced reduction of the glycolytic rate.

From all these findings it is concluded that the inhibition of glycolysis in erythrocytes containing very high concentrations of DPG is the result of two independent DPG effects, namely 1) of the DPG-induced decrease of the red cell pH and the consecutive inhibition of the enzyme phosphofructo kinase, and 2) of a DPG-induced inhibition of the enzyme hexokinase.

REFERENCES

1) Kilmartin,J.V., L.Rossi-Bernardi: Physiol.Rev. 53: 836-890 (1973)
2) Arnone,A.: Ann.Rev.Med. 25:123-130 (1974)
3) Bauer,C.: Rev.Physiol.Biochem.Pharmacol. 70:1-31 (1974)
4) Duhm,J., E.Gerlach: In: The Human Red Cell in Vitro (T.Greenwalt, G.A.Jamieson,eds.), Grune and Stratton, New York-London, pp. 111-148 (1974)
5) Chanutin,A., E.Herman: Arch.Biochem.Biophys. 131:110-115 (1969)
6) Luque,J., D.Diederich, S.Grisolia: Biochem.Biophys. Res.Commun. 36:1019-1023 (1969)
7) Benesch,R.E., R.Benesch, C.I.Yu: Biochemistry 8: 2567-2571 (1969)
8) Benesch,R.E., R.Benesch, R.Renthal, W.B.Gratzer: Nature New Biology 234:174-176 (1971)
9) Bunn,F.H., B.J.Ransil, A.Chao: J.Biol.Chem. 246: 5273-5279 (1971)
10) Garby,L., C.-H.DeVerdier: Scand.J.Clin.Lab.Invest. 27:345-350 (1971)
11) Caldwell,P.R.B., R.L.Nagel, E.R.Jaffe: Biochem.Biophys. Res.Commun. 44:1504-1509 (1971)
12) Bauer,Ch.: Resp.Physiol. 10:10-19 (1970)
13) Duhm,J.: In: Erythrocyte Structure and Function (G.Brewer,ed.), IIIrd International Conference, Ann Arbor, Oct. 16-19, 1974. A.R.Riss, New York (in press)
14) Berger,H., G.-R.Jänig, G.Gerber, K.Ruckpaul, S.M. Rapoport: Eur.J.Biochem. 38:553-562 (1973)
15) Hamasaki,N., Z.B.Rose: J.Biol.Chem: 249:7896-7901 (1974)
16) Rose,I.A.: Exp.Eye Res. 11:264-272 (1971)
17) Gerber,G., H.Berger, G.-R.Jänig, S.M.Rapoport: Eur.J.Biochem. 38:563-571 (1973)
18) Wyman,J.: Advanc. Protein Chem. 4:407-531 (1948) and 19:223-286 (1964)
19) Brewer,G.J.: Biochim.Biophys.Acta 192:157-161 (1969)
20) Ponce,J., S.Roth, D.R.Harkness: Biochim.Biophys.Acta 250:63-74 (1971)
21) Beutler,E., F.Matsumoto, E.Guinto: Experientia 30: 190-192 (1974)
22) Keitt,A.S.: Clin.Res. 19:40(Abstract) (1971)
23) Duhm,J.: Pflügers Arch. 326:341-356 (1971)
24) Salhany,J.M., A.S.Keitt, R.S.Eliot: Febs Letters 16: 257-261 (1971)
25) Duhm, J.: In: Oxygen Transport to Tissue, Adv.Exp.Med. Biol. Vol 37A, Plenum Press, New York-London. pp. 179-186 (1973)
26) Deuticke,B., J.Duhm, R.Dierkesmann: Pflügers Arch. 326:15-34 (1971)
27) Duhm,J.: Biochim.Biophys.Acta (in press)

THE EFFECT OF RED CELL 2,3-DPG CHANGES INDUCED BY DIABETIC KETOACIDOSIS ON PARAMETERS OF THE OXYGEN DISSOCIATION CURVE IN MAN

Eberhard Standl and Jørn Ditzel

Department of Medicine, Aalborg Regional Hospital, Denmark and Diabetes Research Unit, City Hospital Schwabing, Munich, Germany (FRG)

INTRODUCTION

As early as in 1939 Guest and Rapoport reported a striking decrease of the red cell 2,3-diphosphoglycerate (2,3-DPG) concentration in patients suffering from severe diabetic ketoacidosis (1). This observation has been amply confirmed in more recent years (2,3,4,5), when interest was resurrected to investigate the regulation of red cell 2,3-DPG after Benesch and Benesch (6) and Chanutin and Curnish (7) had shown the effect of 2,3-DPG on the oxygen affinity of hemoglobin. 2,3-DPG is formed as an intermediary product of red cell glycolysis; increase in hydrogen-ion concentration decreases red cell glycolysis mainly through inhibition of the phosphofructokinase step (8) and it has been widely accepted that the remarkable low erythrocyte 2,3-DPG levels in diabetic ketoacidosis - as little as 2o per cent of the normal concentration is observed - are due to this mechanism and an additional inhibition of diphosphoglycerate mutase at lower pH (9). In diabetic ketoacidosis there is also a significant depletion of the body phosphorus stores and Ditzel (4,5) has demonstrated that 2,3-DPG resynthesis during recovery from diabetic ketoacidosis is closely correlated to the plasma concentration of inorganic phosphate (Pi). This has been attributed to the known effect of Pi on the activity of phosphofructokinase (1o) and glyceraldehyde-3-phosphate-dehydrogenase (11).

It has been assumed that the oxygen delivery capacity of red blood cells is probably unchanged in diabetic ketoacidosis, because a reduction of the hemoglobin oxygen affinity by acidosis, i.e. the Bohr effect, should oppose the adverse shift of the oxygen dissociation curve to the left induced by the effect of acidosis on red cell 2,3-DPG. In the past years, however, it has been shown by several groups using in vitro techniques that 2,3-DPG influences also the Bohr effect of hemoglobin (12,13,14,15,16). Although in most of these studies diluted hemoglobin solutions were investigated, it seemed worthwile to assess whether these results could be applied to human disease, e.g. diabetic ketoacidosis, where striking changes in red cell 2,3-DPG occur, and if so , how this would affect the shape and position of the oxygen dissociation curve (ODC) during ketoacidosis and recovery.

PATIENTS AND METHODS

Eight patients with newly diagnosed juvenile diabetes admitted to the hospital in ketoacidosis constituted our material. The ages of the patients varied from 15 to 51 years; 6 were males and 2 females. None of them had anemia or suffered from renal insufficiency.

The blood sampling was carried out immediately on admission and thereafter each morning prior to breakfast and insulin administration. Arterial blood samples were drawn for pH and blood gas measurements. Venous blood was collected in heparinized syringes and was analyzed for plasma inorganic phosphate (17) and for 2,3-DPG (18). Measurements of the ODC were performed at 37° and constant pCO_2 of 4o mmHg by the dissociation curve analyzer (type DCA-1, Radiometer, Copenhagen) providing a continous print out of the ODC of whole blood (19). The linear regression equations between the log O_2 half saturation pressures as recorded by the analyzer and the corresponding pH values were computed for blood samples at different concentration ranges of 2,3-DPG, whereby the linear regression coefficient gives the Bohr factor $\Delta \log P_{50}/\Delta$ pH in analogy to the method of Bauer (12). P_{50} act pH was calculated from the recorded curves according to the formula: $\log P_{50} = \log T + K$ (pH recorded - pH act), where T is the pO_2 corresponding to 5o % saturation and K represents various Bohr factors as found for different concentrations ranges of 2,3-DPG. The Hill-coefficient n was obtained according to the Hill equation at constant pH and pCO_2.

RESULTS

Table 1 shows the changes occurring in arterial pH and pCO_2, in the hemoglobin concentration, plasma inorganic phosphate and red cell 2,3-DPG on admission in ketoacidosis (Group I), the day after acidosis has been corrected (Group II), and the day before discharge (Group III). Due to dehydration on admission the hemoglobin concentration fell following the replacement with fluids. Pi was initially elevated above normal, but immediately after insulin administration there occurred a pronounced drop in Pi, not infrequently remaining at such low levels for several days. Slightly elevated Pi-values were observed before discharge. The red cell 2,3-DPG content was decreased in all ketoacidotic patients, averaging at 6.66 µmoles/g Hb on admission. At discharge values slightly above the normal range had been reached.

	Group I		Group II		Group III
art pH	7.19±0.13	+	7.41±0.06		7.42±0.02
pCO_2 (mmHg)	28.0 ±4.9		30.3 ±4.5	+	39.6 ±3.2
Hb (g/100 ml)	16.0 ±1.7	+	13.6 ±2.1		12.8 ±1.1
Pi (mmol/l)	1.50±0.37	‡	0.67±0.3	‡	1.31±0.14
2,3-DPG (µmoles/g Hb)	6.66±3.62	≢	8.73±2.11	+	17.10±1.70

Statistical differences between the respective groups
+ : p - value below 0.001
‡ : p - value below 0.005
≢ : p - value below 0.01

table 1: Mean values and SD of arterial pH and pCO_2, Hb, Pi and red cell 2,3-DPG concentrations in 8 diabetics during ketoacidosis (Group I), after correction of acidosis (Group II) and before discharge (Group III).

Fig. 1 shows the regression lines between log P_{50} and pH - both values as actually measured by the ODC analyzer - for two ranges of red cell 2,3-DPG concentrations, whereby the linear regression coefficients give the Bohr factors. At 2,3-DPG concentrations below 10 µmoles/g Hb - i.e. on admission in ketoacidosis - the Bohr factor was diminished to - 0.24. In contrast, an approximately normal Bohr factor of - 0.52 was obtained for blood samples with a 2,3-DPG concentration between 1o and 14 µmoles/g Hb. The analogous linear regression for blood samples with a 2,3-DPG content above 14 µmoles/g Hb was $y = -0.48x + 4.99$ ($r = -0.61$; $p < 0.01$), the Bohr factor being - o.48.

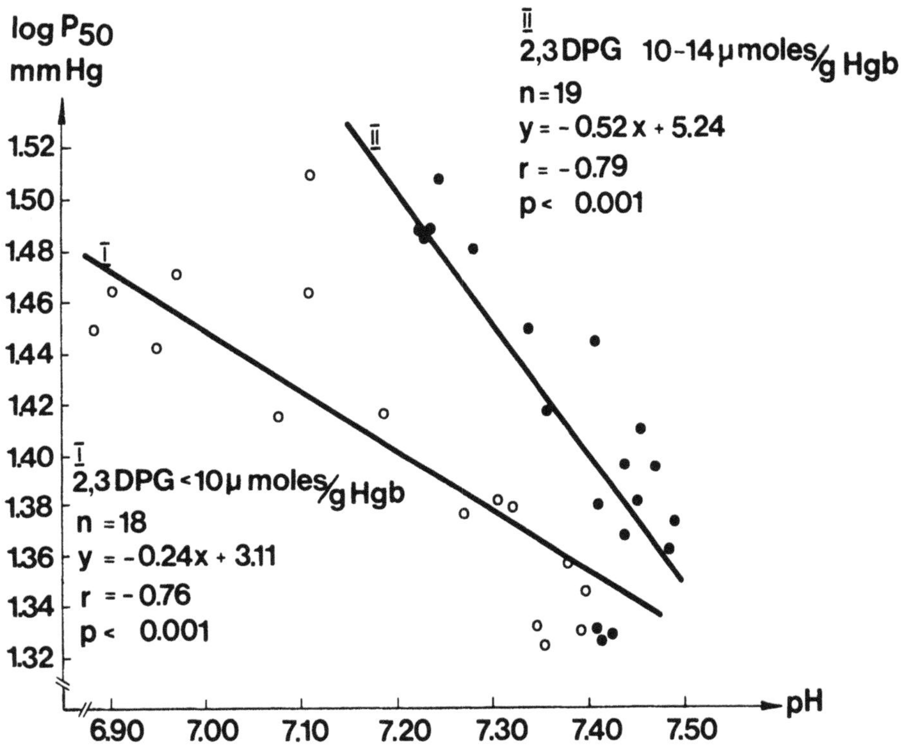

Fig. 1: Half saturation pressures (P_{50}) and pH-values at 37°C and a pCO_2 of 4o mmHg as recorded by the dissociation curve analyzer. The regression coefficient gives the Bohr factor.

Using these different Bohr factors P_{50} act pH and the Hill-coefficient were calculated for Group I (admission in ketoacidosis), Group II (the day after correction of acidosis), and Group III (before discharge). Table 2 reveals that the mean P_{50} act pH on admission and at discharge did not differ from each other, whereas after correction of acidosis P_{50} act pH decreased considerably. In addition to that, the shape of the ODC was altered as well. The Hill-coefficient

	Group I		Group II		Group III
P_{50} act pH (mmHg)	27.3±1.9	+	23.5±2.0	+	27.2±1.8
Hill-coeff. n	2.24±0.12	≠	2.04±0.14	+	2.51±0.11

Statistical differences between the respective groups

+ : p - value below 0.001
≠ : p - value below 0.005

table 2: Mean values and SD of P_{50} act pH and the Hill-coefficients n in 8 diabetics during ketoacidosis (Group I), after correction of acidosis (Group II) and before discharge (Group III).

was diminished already on admission and even more after correction of acidosis (Group II). There was a close correlation of n with 2,3-DPG for all values determined ($n = 0.04$ DPG $+ 1.83$; $r = 0.71$; $p < 0.001$) and with Pi for blood samples with a 2,3-DPG content of less than 10 µmoles/g Hb ($n = 0.31$ Pi $+ 1.85$; $r = 0.71$; $p < 0.001$).

DISCUSSION

This study clearly indicates that alterations in the shape and position of the oxygen dissociation curve take place during diabetic ketoacidosis and recovery. Variation of the Bohr factor of hemoglobin does occur in relation to different red cell 2,3-DPG concentrations; this finding suggests that results previously obtained from in vitro experiments mainly using diluted hemoglobin solutions (12,13,14,15,16) have significant physiological bearing for in vivo conditions as diabetic ketoacidosis. Interpreting this observation - without going into details - it should be mentioned that 2,3-DPG might effect the Bohr factor by a decrease of the oxygen linked carbamate formation (12,20). At 2,3-DPG concentrations below 10 µmoles/g Hb, i.e. on admission in ketoacidosis and for some time thereafter, the Bohr factor was diminished to approximately 50 per cent of the normal value. But even when this was taken into account in calculating the oxygen affinity of whole blood at actual pH, P_{50} values were not decreased during ketoacidosis. Comparing the results of P_{50} act pH in our patients obtained on admission and at discharge (table 2) the effect of decreased red cell 2,3-DPG concentrations was virtually balanced by the lowered pH during acidosis. This is somewhat in contrast to the study of Bellingham who found even elevated P_{50} - values in his 4 patients during ketoacidosis, but used a constant Bohr factor of - o.48 for calculations (2). In any case, after correction of acidosis the disproportion between pH and 2,3-DPG resulted in a considerable fall of P_{50} act pH, which might be of potential hazard to the patients in terms of tissue oxygenation.

The Hill-coefficient n has been shown to be related to the 2,3-DPG/Hb ratio in hemoglobin solutions in vitro (15,21). A decrease of n at low 2,3-DPG concentrations, similar to the lowered 2,3-DPG levels in our patients during ketoacidosis and after correction of acidosis, could be prevented by higher Pi concentrations (15). Again, our results agree favourably with these in vitro experiments as indicated by the close association of n with 2,3-DPG and additionally with Pi at 2,3-DPG levels below lo µmoles/g Hb. This gives an explanation, why n was slightly diminished in ketoacidosis, when high Pi levels counteracted low 2,3-DPG concentrations, and decreased further after Pi had fallen to very low values. As Benesch et al. (21) have shown, this decrease in n does probably not reflect a decrement in heme-heme interaction, but is rather the result of the successive oxygenation of two hemoglobin species, namely, 2,3-DPG devoid hemoglobin with a high oxygen affinity and 2,3-DPG complexed hemoglobin with a much lower oxygen affinity.

In summary then, the pronounced fluctuations of red cell 2,3-DPG during diabetic ketoacidosis and recovery from very low in acidosis to elevated levels at the time of discharge cause changes in the oxygen affinity of whole blood, in the Bohr factor of hemoglobin and in the Hill-coefficient of the ODC. Apparently this marked variation of erythrocyte 2,3-DPG makes diabetic ketoacidosis a unique tool to demonstrate the implications of 2,3-DPG on the oxygen transport system of blood in the living human organism as compared to results obtained in vitro.

ACKNOWLEDGEMENTS

Supported by a grant of the Municipal of Aalborg, the Nordic Insulin Foundation and the Deutsche Forschungsgemeinschaft.

REFERENCES

1. Guest, G.M., Rapoport, S.: Am.J.Dis.Child. 58, 1o72, 1939.
2. Bellingham, A.J., Detter, J.C., Lenfant,C.: Trans. Ass.Am.Phys. 83, 113, 197o.
3. Alberti, K.G.M.M., Darley, J.H., Emerson, P.M., Hockaday, T.D.R.: Lancet 1972 II, 391.
4. Ditzel, J.: Advanc.Exp.Med.Biol. 37 A, 163, 1973.
5. Ditzel, J.: Horm.Metabol.Res. 5, 471, 1973.
6. Benesch, R., Benesch, R.E.: Biochem.Biophys.Res. Commun. 26, 162, 1967.
7. Chanutin, A., Curnish, R.R.: Arch.Biochem.Biophys. 121, 96, 1967.
8. Rapoport, S.: in Campbell, P.N., Greville,G.D. (eds): Essays of Biochemistry 4, 69, New York, Academic Press, 1968.
9. Rose, Z.B.: Arch.Biochem.Biophys. 138, 9o3, 1973.
1o. Kühn, B., Jacobasch, G., Gerth, C., Rapoport, S.M.: Eur.J.Biochem. 43, 437, 1974.
11. Rapoport, S., Maretzki, D., Schewe, C.: in Rørth, M., Astrup, P. (ed.) Oxygen affinity of hemoglobin and red cell acid base status, p. 527-538. Copenhagen: Munksgaard, New York: Academic Press 1972
12. Bauer, Ch.: Life Sci. 8, 1o41, 1969.
13. Benesch, R.E., Benesch, R., Yu, C.I.: Biochemistry 8, 2567, 1969.
14. Siggaard-Andersen, O., Salling, N.: Scand.J.Clin. Lab.Invest. 27, 361, 1971.
15. Tomita, S., Riggs, A.: J.Biol.Chem. 246, 547,1971.
16. Duhm, J.: in Bicher, H.I., Bruley, D.F. (ed.) Oxygen transport to tissue. p. 179-186. New York: Plenum Publishing Corporation 1972
17. Parekh, A.C., Jung, D.H.: Clin.Chim.Acta 27, 373, 197o.
18. Ericsson, A., de Verdier, C.H.: Scand.J.Clin.Lab. Invest. 29, 85, 1972.
19. Duvelleroy, M.A., Buckles, R.C., Rosenkaimer, S., Tung, C., Laver, M.A.: J. Appl.Physiol. 28, 227, 197o.
2o. Riggs, A.: Proc.Nat.Acad.Sci. 68, 2o62, 1971.
21. Benesch,R., Benesch,R.E., Yu, C.J.: Proc.Nat. Acad.Sci. 59, 526, 1968.

THE INFLUENCE OF $MgCl_2$ ON THE O_2- Hb- BINDING CURVE OF HUMAN HEMOGLOBIN UNDER INTRACELLULAR CONDITIONS

Wolfgang Barnikol

Physiologisches Institut der Universität

6500 Mainz, Saarstr. 21, BRD

In 1969 a model was proposed (BARNIKOL et al.) to explain the effect of the Hb- concentration on the O_2- Hb- binding curve (GROTE, 1967). The existence of at least one low molecular substance (called Z) besides H^+ and CO_2 was postulated, which is equimolar with Hb ($\approx$ 5 mM) and which is bound preferentially to deoxy- Hb. From a simple stoichiometric consideration it follows, that a substance can only have a measurable influence on the O_2- Hb- binding curve, if its molar concentration is not to low compared with the molar Hb- concentration. For example, 2,3- diphosphoglycerate (= DPG), glutathione and Mg^{++} have intracellular concentrations of the necessary magnitude. Only a small part of Magnesium is bound to the membrane of the erythrocytes (HARRISON et al.). Principally all these substances are candidates for Z. In 1967 it was shown by BENESCH et al. and by CHANUTIN et al., that ATP and DPG influence the O_2- Hb- binding curve as was postulated for Z, and it was shown (BENESCH et al., 1968), that the organic phosphates are bound preferentially to deoxy- Hb. In our speculation on the chemical nature of Z first we prefered Mg^{++} because of its complex forming properties. It is known for a long time, that Mg^{++} forms a complex with ATP (MARTELL et al., 1956) and in 1970 it was found, that DPG forms also a complex with Mg^{++} (COLLIER et al.). In addition GARBY et al. (1969) showed, that Mg- ions reduce binding of organic phosphates to deoxy- Hb. Hence at least an indirect influence of Mg^{++} on the O_2- Hb- binding curve is expected. This was found by BUNN et al. (1971) : in diluted Hb- solutions (0.05 mM tetramer) Mg^{++} diminishes the P_{O_2} of half saturation ($P_{0.5}$), neither a direct effect was found nor an effect of Mg- complexed organic phosphates. Lateron these results were confirmed by BERGER et al. (1973). The aim of this investigation is to study the influence of $MgCl_2$ on the O_2- Hb- binding curve under intracellular conditions.

Many investigations on the O_2- Hb- equilibrium are carried out with modified systems, especially with concern to the Hb- concentration, perhaps due to methodical reasons. But the results achieved under modified conditions cannot be applied to the in vivo system in all cases. An example is the unexpected reduced binding of organic phosphates to Hb in concentrated Hb-solutions (GARBY et al., 1971), unexpected, when assuming a simple mass interaction between Hb and organic phosphates. Within recent times investigations, simulating intracellular conditions increase. In order to study the functional properties of the in vivo system it is best to take the system itself and to change exclusively one parameter. This usually involves the development of new techniques. As experimental approximation to the stated ideal erythrolysates are used, which were made of packed erythrocytes (centrifugation 5 min. at 450 g) by freezing with liquid air. Substances were added to the system in two portions (80 µL + 5 µL + 5 µL). So the system is disturbed by a dilution of only 11%.

The O_2- Hb- binding curve of the erythrolysates was measured by equilibration and photometry (λ = 578 nm) of thin layers (≈ 10 µ). It is possible to registrate the O_2- Hb- binding curve several times within 4 hrs. with the same layer. As an example in fig. 1 the $P_{0.5}$- values of a fresh erythrolysate (□ □ □) in dependence of time are shown (BARNIKOL et al., 1973).

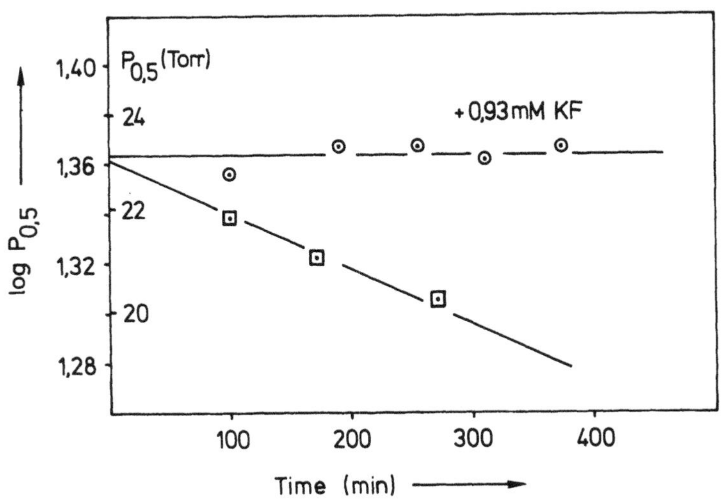

Fig. 1: The change of $P_{0.5}$ with time ; □ □ □ = fresh erythrolysate ; ooo = 0.93 mM KF added ; P_{CO_2} = 40 ± 1 Torr ; pH = 7.16 ; 37°C.

It is shown, that in a logarithmic scale as concerns $P_{0.5}$ this changes linear with time, so it is possible to extrapolate to time zero, i.e._time of venipuncture. Addition of 0.93 mM KF stabilises $P_{0.5}$ (ooo). F^- inhibits the enzyme enolase (WARBURG et al., 1942) and for this reason inhibits the the glycolysis. The cause for the change of $P_{0.5}$ is, that glycolysis goes on. The concentration of F^- is 5 times the value necessary for half inhibition. The molar ratio F^- / Hb (tetramer) remains 0.2. Thus a possible weak specific effect of F^- is not to be measured. The extrapolation of the two series of points results in the same $P_{0.5}$ - value. This legitimates the extrapolation procedure and excludes a specific effect of F^-. From fig.1 the standard deviation of $P_{0.5}$ may be estimated to 0.1 Torr. The ATP- measurements were done with an enzymatic method (test combination, Böhringer, Mannheim, BRD). pH- values were measured with an IL 113 (Instrumentation Laboratory Inc., Boston, Massachusetts, USA) at full oxygenation. The standard deviation was 0.01. For oxygenation 50 µL erythrolysate was brought in an equipment similar to the BMS 2 MK 2 (Radiometer, Copenhagen) and equilibrated with gas (5.6% CO_2 / 94.4% O_2). The shaking frequency was 2700 /min. and the amplitude was 2.5 mm. Within 15 min. equilibrium was achieved tested by pH measurements.

To study the effect of $MgCl_2$ on the O_2- Hb- binding curve 38.8 mM $MgCl_2$ were added to fresh erythrolysates. The normal intracellular concentrations of Mg^{++} is 4.6 mM (HARRISON et al., 1968). In an analog manner the experiments were performed with incubated blood (20 hrs at 37°C). Under these conditions the concentration of DPG decreases from the normal value 6.14 mM to zero (SIGGAARD- ANDERSEN, 1971). The concentration of ATP (normal value 1.84 mM) was still 0.18 mM after incubation. All stated concentrations values refer to free water assuming a partial volume of 71.4% (MURPHY, 1968).

In fig.2 the influence of $MgCl_2$ on the O_2- Hb- binding curve is illustrated. In case of fresh erythrolysate the curve is shifted to the left (upper part), in case of incubated blood the curve is shifted to the right (lower part). In fig.3 it is shown, that by addition of $MgCl_2$ the effect of incubation on the O_2- Hb- binding curve is eliminated.

To compare the effects quantitatively the values for $\Delta \log P_{0.5} / \Delta \log X$ were calculated, where X stands for the concentration of substances in question. Table 1 shows the results. It is seen, that under the experimental conditions the effects of $MgCl_2$ are of the same magnitude as those of the organic phosphates.

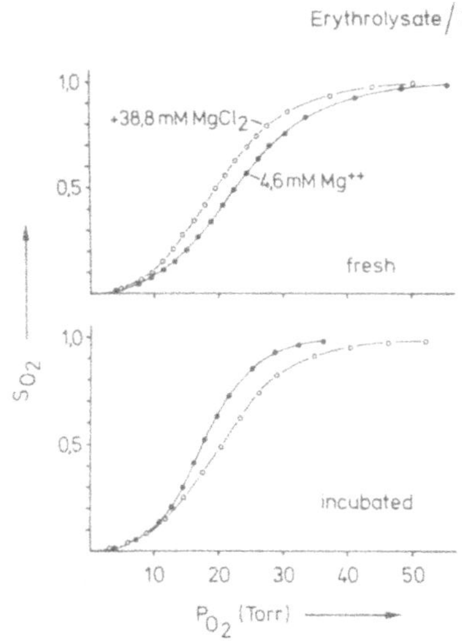

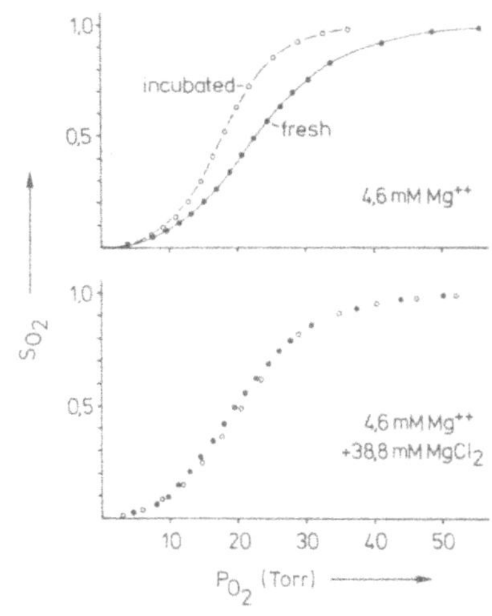

Fig.2: The influence of $MgCl_2$ on the O_2- Hb- binding curve of erythrolysates in case of fresh and incubated blood.

Fig.3: The influence of incubation on the O_2- Hb- binding curve. Upper part without and lower part with additional $MgCl_2$.

Table 1: Quantitative comparison of the influence of $MgCl_2$ and organic phosphates on the O_2- Hb- binding curve. X = concentration.

X	$\Delta \log P_{0.5} / \Delta \log X$	remarks
Mg^{++}	- 0.073	fresh blood
Mg^{++}	+ 0.070	incub. blood
DPG + ATP	+ 0.070	no $MgCl_2$ added
DPG + ATP	0	38.8 mM $MgCl_2$ added

The shift to the left of the O_2- Hb- binding curve of fresh erythrolysates on addition of $MgCl_2$ (fig.2 upper part) was also found in diluted Hb- solutions and may be interpreted as increased complex formation between Mg^{++} and organic phosphates, thus reducing the interaction between Hb and the organic phosphates.

If the O_2- Hb- binding curve is exclusively influenced by H^+, CO_2 and free organic phosphates, then the left curves of fig.2 should be identical. This is not the case. The lower part of fig.2 shows clearly, that $MgCl_2$ generates a shift to the right in erythrolysate depleted from organic phosphate.

By addition of $MgCl_2$ the ionic strength is increased and the question arises if this is the reason for the measured effect. To answer this question the effect may be compared with the influence of Na_2SO_4 on $P_{0.5}$. This was measured by AMICONI et al. (1969) in diluted Hb- solutions ($\approx$ 0.3 mM tetramer) at 20°C and pH = 7.0. From AMICONI's measurements one would expect an increase in $P_{0.5}$ of 0.3 Torr by adding the same molar amount of salt. This is only 1/10 of the increase found with $MgCl_2$.

In fig.3 the influence of $MgCl_2$ on the effect of the organic phosphates is shown. $MgCl_2$ eliminates the effect. This again may be understood as a binding of the organic phosphates by Mg- ions.

To conclude one can say, that $MgCl_2$ governs the effect of the organic phosphates on the O_2- Hb- binding curve and vice versa the organic phosphates govern direction and magnitude of the $MgCl_2$- effect.

I thank Miss Anne Deutschmann for skillfull technical assistance.

The support of the Deutsche Forschungsgemeinschaft is gratefully acknowledged.

Literature

G. Amiconi, E. Antonini, M. Brunori, J. Wyman
in "Hemoglobin and Myoglobin in thin Reactions with ligands", authors : E. Antonini and M. Brunori, North- Holland Publishing Company, Amsterdam - London, 1971, p.246

W.K.R. Barnikol, G. Thews
Zur Interpretation der O_2- Bindungskurve des Human- Hämoglobins. Pflügers Arch. 309, 232- 249 (1969)

W.K.R. Barnikol, W. Wahler
On the Accuracy of an Improved Method for the Measurement of O_2- Dissociation Curves According to NIESEL and THEWS, 1961.
Adv. in Exp. Medicine and Biology 37 A, 325- 331 (1973) (Editors : D.F. Bruley, H.I. Bicher), Plenum Press, New York- London

R. Benesch, R.E. Benesch
The Effect of Organic Phosphates from the Human Erythrocyte on the Allosteric Properties of Hemoglobin.
Biochem. Biophys. Res. Comm. 26, 162-167 (1967)

R. Benesch, R.E. Benesch, C.I. Yu
Reciprocal Binding of Oxygen and Diphosphoglycerate by Human Hemoglobin.
Proc. Nat. Acad. Sci. (Wash.) 59, 526-532 (1968)

H. Berger, G.R. Jänig, G. Gerber, K. Ruckpaul, S.M. Rapoport
Interaction of Hemoglobin with Ions. Interactions among Magnesium, Adenosine 5-Triphosphate, 2,3-Biphosphoglycerate, and Oxygenated and Deoxygenated Human Hemoglobin under Simulated Intracellular Conditions.
Eur. J. Biochem. 38, 553-562 (1973)

H.F. Bunn, B.J. Ransil, A. Chao
The Interaction between Erythrocyte Organic Phosphates, Magnesium Ion, and Hemoglobin.
J. Biol Chem. 246, 5273-5279 (1971)

A. Chanutin, R. Curnish
Effect of Organic and Inorganic Phosphates on the Oxygen Equilibrium of Human Erythrocytes.
Arch. Biochem. 121, 96-102 (1967)

H.B. Collier, A. Lam
Binding of Ca^{2+} and Mg^{2+} by 2,3 Diphosphoglycerate.
Biochim. Biophys. Acta 222, 299-306 (1970)

L. Garby, G. Gerber, C.H. de Verdier
Binding of 2,3-Diphosphoglycerate and Adenosine Triphosphate to Human Hemoglobin A.
Eur. J. Biochem. 10, 110-115 (1969)

L. Garby, C.H. de Verdier
Affinity of Human Hemoglobin to 2,3-Diphosphoglycerate. Effect of Hemoglobin Concentration and pH.
Scand. J. Clin. Lab. Invest. 27, 345-350 (1971)

J. Grote
Die Bestimmung der Sauerstoff-Bindungskurve von hochverdünnten Hämoglobinlösungen.
Pflügers Arch. 296, 202-211 (1967)

D.G. Harrison, C. Long
The Calcium Content of Human Erythrocytes.
J. Physiol. 199, 367-381 (1968)

A.E. Martell, G. Schwarzenbach
Adenosinphosphate und Triphosphat als Komplexbildner für Calcium und Magnesium.
Helv. Chim. Acta 39, 653-661 (1956)

J.R. Murphy
The Influence of pH on Physical Properties of the Erythrocyte.
in " Stoffwechsel- und Membranpermeabilitäten von Erythrocyten und Thrombocyten", Thieme, Stuttgart 1968, p. 452

O. Siggaard-Andersen
Oxygen-Linked Hydrogen Ion Binding of Human Hemoglobin. Effects of Carbon-Dioxide and 2,3-Diphosphoglycerate. I. Studies on Erythrolysate.
Scand. J. Clin. Lab. Invest. 27, 351-360 (1971)

O. Warburg, W. Christian
Isolierung und Kristallisation des Gärungsfermentes Enolase.
Biochem. Zeitschr. 310, 384-425 (1942)

OXYGEN TRANSPORT AND HEMODYNAMICS OF STROMA-FREE HEMOGLOBIN SOLUTIONS+

F. Jesch, B. Endrich and K. Messmer

Institute for Surgical Research, University of Munich, FRG

In contrast to conventional plasma substitutes properties as carrying and unloading of oxygen are expected from stroma-free hemoglobin solutions. Previous experiments with a 6 % stroma-free hemoglobin solution prepared according to BONHARD (2), however, have revealed that this solution exhibits major disadvantages: 1) inadequate intravascular persistence and thus volume retaining capacity and 2) a high affinity of hemoglobin for oxygen impairing the unloading of chemically bound oxygen at the tissue level (9). This series of experiments was designed to find out if the oxygen affinity of stroma-free hemoglobin can be influenced by either modifying the preparation procedure described by BONHARD (2) or on the other hand by introducing pyridoxalphosphate into the hb-molecule as originally described for in vitro conditions by BENESCH et al. (1).

METHODS

12 mongrel dogs of either sex (8 - 14 kg body weight) were splenectomized 4 - 6 weeks before the experiment. After premedication with Droperidol[R], Fentanyl[R] and Atropine[R] the animals were anesthetized intravenously with 20 ml/kg pentobarbital sodium and relaxed by succinylcholine. The animals were ventilated with air containing 30 % oxygen maintaining an endexpiratory PCO_2 of 40 mmHg (Uras). For pressure monitoring, blood-sampling and bleeding the femoral artery and for infusion the femoral

+Supported by Sonderforschungsbereich 37, Munich, FRG

vein were cannulated under aseptic conditions. A catheter was placed into the right atrium via the jugular vein and a thermistor probe into the ascending aorta via the carotid artery. 3.0 mg/kg heparin sodium were given intravenously.

After a control period of 30 minutes 20 ml/kg of whole blood were withdrawn and immediately replaced via femoral vein by an equal amount of normothermic hb-PLP (n=6) prepared by BONHARD (3) using a modified method of BENESCH et al. (1) or hb-W (n=6) according to KAPLAN et al. (6).

Characteristics of the hemoglobin solutions used

		hb-PLP	hb-W
Hemoglobin	g %	4,9	5,3
Methemoglobin	rel %	2,0	15,0
Sodium	meq/l	99	146
Potassium	meq/l	1,3	3,7
pH		7,3	7,3
Source		Biotest, Frankfurt, FRG	Warner-Lambert, Morris Plains, N.J.
Batch		740 220	WXb 8326

At control pressure recordings (Statham elements) and cardiac output measurements (thermodilution method) were performed; blood samples were taken for determinations of 2,3-DPG (enzymatically with phosphoglycerate mutase), P_{50} at standard conditions (3 different PO_2 and O_2-saturation determinations, plot according to Hill's equation), total and plasma hemoglobin (cyanhemiglobin method), arterial and central venous PO_2 (polarographically, Combitest, Eschweiler), O_2-saturation (AO-oxymeter) and O_2-content (Lex-O_2-Con) and central venous pH (Astrup equipment). Blood volume (^{51}Cr-tagged autologous red cells) and t/2 of hemoglobin (tagged with 125-iodine according to FRANKS et al. (5), removal of free 125-iodine activity by gel-filtration on sephadex) were determined after repeated injections and equilibration of the RBC's for 20 minutes. The animals were observed for survival until 7 days after the experiment. Mean values ± SEM have been calculated and analyzed for significance by student-t-test with $p<0.05$ as the level of significance.

RESULTS

Mean arterial blood pressure (MAP) remained fairly constant throughout the postdilutional observation period of 4 hours (Tab.1). Although 30 or 33 % of the measured circulating volume (BV) have been exchanged isovolemically in both groups BV was decreased to about 90, 86 and 77% at 10, 60 and 240 minutes after the exchange without any significant difference between both groups (Fig.1).

Initially there was a decrease in heart rate (HR) ($p<0,005$ after hb-W), but an increase again during the following observation period (Tab.1). Cardiac output (CO) declined progressively in the hb-PLP treated animals whereas a temporary normalization was observed in the hb-W treated dogs at 60 minutes after dilution. 240 min after exchange, however, identical low CO values were observed (Fig.2).

As seen from Fig.1 total hemoglobin concentration de-

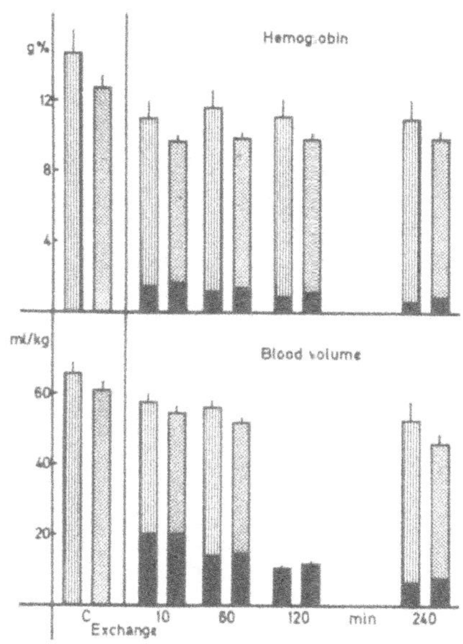

Fig.1: Changes in total hemoglobin-concentration (whole columns) plasma hemoglobin (black part), circulating blood volume (whole columns) and volume of plasma hemoglobin (black part) before and after isovolemic exchange of 20 ml/kg whole blood for hb-PLP (▥ ,●) and hb-W (▨,o).

Table 1: Changes in mean arterial blood pressure (MAP), heart rate (HR), arterial and central venous PO_2, arterial-venous oxygen saturation difference ($AVDO_2$) and central venous pH before and after isovolemic exchange of 20 ml/kg whole blood for hb-PLP (n=6) and hb-W (n=6).

		Time after exchange (min)				
		C	10	60	120	240
MAP mmHg	hb-PLP	143,3±8,1	142,5± 7,5	135,0±16,3	137,0±14,2	137,0± 9,8
	hb-W	137,5±5,7	145,0± 4,7	152,5± 5,0	144,1± 5,9	139,1± 7,3
HR min^{-1}	hb-PLP	161±14	136±14	153±14	145±17	147±20
	hb-W	166±13	112± 7	168±16	166±16	137±15
PO_2 a mmHg	hb-PLP	128,8±10,7	147,4±16,9	121,0± 6,8	113,3± 9,3	112,7± 9,8
	hb-W	116,5± 8,3	134,4± 8,9	118,6±10,5	112,8±11,7	111,1± 6,2
PO_2 v mmHg	hb-PLP	50,6± 2,0	42,3± 2,9	38,6± 3,7	34,7± 2,4	32,8± 2,6
	hb-W	50,8± 4,0	40,9± 4,6	43,5± 5,1	44,4± 5,0	34,8± 5,5
$AVDO_2$ sat%	hb-PLP	18,7± 1,9	26,8± 2,8	32,8± 2,9	34,7± 3,6	40,1± 2,7
	hb-W	20,0± 3,3	29,5± 2,6	28,0± 5,5	34,0± 3,2	40,0± 5,8
pH_{cv}	hb-PLP	7,318±0,023	7,255±0,028	7,237±0,042	7,234±0,026	7,172±0,043
	hb-W	7,309±0,028	7,269±0,030	7,272±0,025	7,242±0,029	7,167±0,048

creased immediately after exchange due to the low hb-content of the infused solution and remained at this level throughout the experiment. The plasma hemoglobin concentration reached about 15 % at 10 minutes, but only 7 % of total hemoglobin at 240 minutes. Circulatory half time t/2 for hb-PLP was 100.3 ± 6.3 minutes and 140.2 ± 6.7 minutes for hb-W.

P_{50} and 2,3-DPG concentration as well as the in vitro dissociation curves under standard conditions for both solutions are given in Fig. 3.

After exchange transfusion (lower part of Fig.3) the 2,3-DPG concentration decreased without significant differences between both groups. At the end of the experiments 2,3-DPG had increased above the initial values. 1 and 4 hours after exchange P_{50} was not different from control. Despite the decrease in oxygen availability (CO x arterial O_2-content) in both groups ($p<0,005$) the total oxygen consumption did not decrease significantly. For that the oxygen saturation difference had to increase

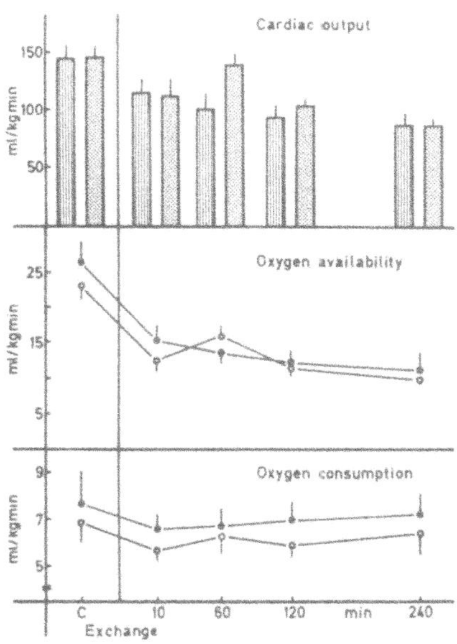

Fig.2: Changes in cardiac output, O_2-availability and O_2-consumption before and after isovolemic exchange of 20 ml/kg whole blood for hb-PLP and hb-W (see legend Fig. 1).

by about 100 %. Whereas arterial PO_2 remained essentially unchanged venous PO_2 had to decrease from control by 35 and 31 % respectively. Nevertheless, venous pH decreased (p<0,05) during the postdilutional period.

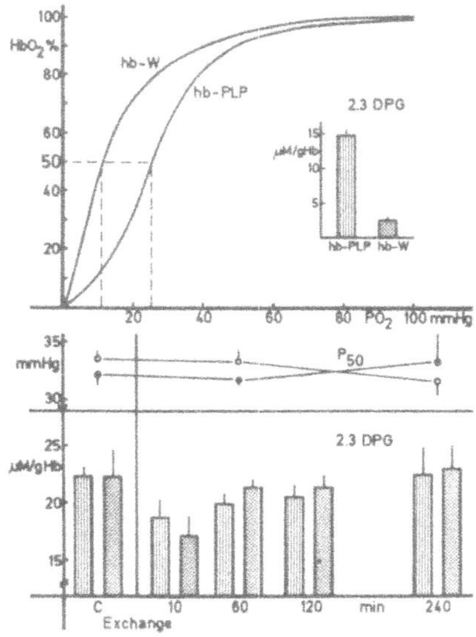

Fig.3: Oxygen dissociation curves (measured with the DCA_1 (Radiometer, Copenhagen) according to DUVELLEROY et al.(4)) and 2,3-DPG concentration of the hb-solutions infused (upper part).
Changes in P_{50} and 2,3-DPG concentration before and after isovolemic exchange of 20 ml/kg whole blood for hb-PLP and hb-W (see legend Fig.1).

DISCUSSION

In previous experiments the circulatory half time of conventionally prepared stroma-free hb-solution was found to be 110 min (7). Whereas hb-W, prepared without acidification step, yielded t/2 of 140 min, the pyridoxylation of hb did not prolong the intravascular persistence. However, no significant differences were observed with regard to the circulating BV measured by ^{51}Cr-RBC's. This emphasizes a different transcapillary refill rate in both groups and/or differences in the water binding capacity of both hemoglobins. This question has to be subject of further investigations. As a consequence of the volume loss amounting to 1/3 of the normal circulating volume at 240 min after exchange transfusion, cardiac output was reduced, whereas TPR rised inspite of the dilutional reduction in whole blood viscosity; this is indicative for hypovolemia and in agreement with data obtained with conventional stroma-free hb-solution (8). HR dropped significantly (10 min), but CO increased more (60 min) in the hb-W group, which might reflect a pharmacological effect on the heart exerted by hb-W, because identical exchanges of whole blood for conventional hb-solution and hb-PLP did not provoke similar changes (7,8). The maintenance of the O_2-consumption was only possible by a 100 % rise in $AVDO_2$ (Tab.1), while the O_2-availability was consistently reduced as result of blood replacement by the low concentrated hb-solutions and by the lack in cardiac response.

Since both solutions yield a reduced but at the same time different concentration of 2,3-DPG the concentration of this metabolite/g hb in whole blood was temporarily reduced by dilution but fully restored in both experimental groups 240 min after exchange transfusion.

As to notice from Fig. 3 the actual dissociation curves for both hb-solutions are different with regard to position and shape, which is also reflected in different P_{50}-values. The high oxygen affinity of hb-W, however, was fully compensated after 60 minutes by a still unknown mechanism in vivo; this is clearly emphasized by the unsignificant P_{50}-changes in whole blood after exchange transfusion with hb-W, which were not different from those observed after hb-PLP. It has, however, to be admitted that significant changes might have been prevented by either the already low oxygen hemoglobin affinity of the anemic (splenectomized) dogs or by the small exchange volume, or more likely by both factors. Inspite of unchanged P_{50} and 2,3-DPG levels and inspite of normal arterial and venous PO_2 values metabolic acidosis developed as reflected by the fall of both central venous pH and plasma bicarbonate concentration. The findings mentioned above lend further support to the already suggested hypothesis (7) that the occurance of hypovolemia after isovolemic exchange transfusions with hb-solution is more detrimental than the disadvantage of a high oxygen hemoglobin affinity.

SUMMARY

The intravascular persistence of hb-W is significantly longer than of pyridoxylated hb (hb-PLP), however, no significant differences in BV were observed after isovolemic exchange of 20 ml/kg b.w. Even though the oxygen affinity of hb-PLP in vitro was reduced when compared to the affinity of hb-W significant differences in vivo were lacking. The development of hypovolemia and thus the lack of an adequate increase in cardiac output have been recognized as the most relevant causes to explain the changes observed. Neither of the solutions is yet to be recommended for clinical blood replacement therapy.

REFERENCES

1. BENESCH,R.E., BENESCH,R., BANK,A., PENTHAL,R., BRAX, A.B.: Genetical, functional and physiological studies on haemoglobins. Proc. 1st Inter.-American Symp. on Hemoglobin, Caracas 1969, Karger, Basel, New York, 1971, p.134
2. BONHARD,K.: Preparation and examination of an infusable hemoglobin solution. In: Martin,H., Nowicki,L.: Synthesis, structure and function of hemoglobin,p.285 (Lehmann, München 1972)
3. BONHARD, K.: Personal communication
4. DUVELLEROY,M.A., BUCKLES,R.G., ROSENKAIMER,S., TUNG, C., LAVER,M.B.: An oxyhemoglobin dissociation analyzer. J. appl. Physiol. 28, 227 (1970)
5. FRANKS, J.J., TAKEDA,V., REEVE,E.B.: Preparation of autologous J^{131} albumin for metabolic studies in man. J. Lab. clin. Med. 60, 619 (1962)
6. KAPLAN,H.R. and MURTHY,V.S.: Hemoglobin solution: An attractive oxygen transporting candidate for plasma volume expansion. Fed. Proc., in press
7. SUNDER-PLASSMANN,L., DIETERLE,R., SEIFERT,J., JESCH, F., MESSMER,K.: Stromafree haemoglobin solution as a blood replacement fluid. Actual state and problems. Europ. J. Intensive Care Med. 1, 37 (1975)
8. SUNDER-PLASSMANN,L., JESCH,F., SEIFERT,J., GROHMANN, W.,MESSMER,K.: The hemodynamic and hemorrheological effects of a stroma-free hemoglobin solution. 7th Europ. Conf.Microcirculation,Aberdeen 1972,Part I, Bibl.Anat.11, 104 (Karger,Basel 1973)
9. SUNDER-PLASSMANN,L.,SINAGOWITZ,E.,RINK,R.,DIETERLE,R., MESSMER,K. and KESSLER,M.: The local oxygen supply in tissue of abdominal viscera and of skeletal muscle in extreme hemodilution with stromafree hemoglobin solution. Advanc. Exp.Med.Biol., 37A, 395 (1973)

Acknowledgement: The production and supply of hb-PLP by Dr.K.BONHARD,Biotest,Frankfurt, FRG,and of hb-W by Drs. J.DOCZI and M.WINBURY,Warner-Lambert Research Institute, Morris Plains, N.J.,USA, are gratefully acknowledged.

OXYGEN TRANSPORT ON MOUNT EVEREST: THE EFFECTS OF INCREASED HEMATOCRIT ON MAXIMAL O_2 TRANSPORT

Paolo Cerretelli

Centro Studi di Fisiologia del Lavoro Muscolare del C.N.R.

University of Milano, Milano, Italy

INTRODUCTION

Maximal oxygen consumption ($\dot{V}_{O_2}max$) undergoes a progressive reduction in hypoxia, both acute and chronic. Such decrease, for a pressure drop of half an athmosphere corresponding to a climb to about 5500 meters a.s.l., ranges, according to various Authors (1), between 30% and 45% and is apparently independent of the degree of acclimation (Fig. 1). Possible thoracic causes for the observed $\dot{V}_{O_2}max$ limitation in subjects exposed to low oxygen are:

1) the decreased arterial O_2 pressure (Pa_{O_2}) and blood O_2 percent saturation ($O_{2a}Hb\%$) of which, however, the latter may be more than compensated for in the acclimated, by the increased RBC and blood hemoglobin (Hb) concentration;
2) hypoxia of the myocardium, that may reduce maximal cardiac output ($\dot{Q}max$) both in acute and chronic hypoxia;
3) limited to the acclimated, the effects on $\dot{Q}max$ of the increased blood relative viscosity (from 5 to 11, according to personal measurements by the Ostwald viscometer) brought about by the high increase in the hematocrit (Hct).

The few direct measurements of $\dot{Q}max$ available in subjects exposed for several weeks to high altitude, performed by the acetylene method (5) or by N_2-CO_2 rebreathing (Cerretelli, Veicsteinas and Sassi, in preparation) seem to indicate, however, that $\dot{Q}max$ decreases only moderately, by the same relative amount as maximal

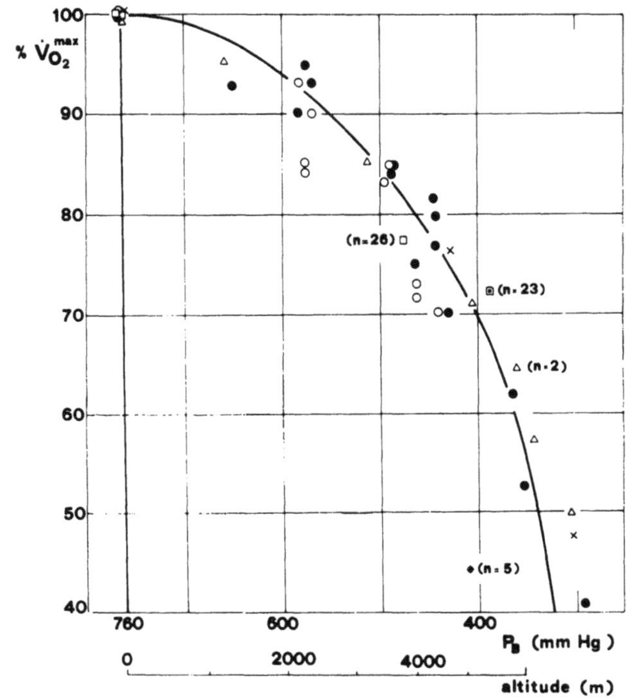

Fig. 1: Maximal O_2 uptake (% of sea level control, % $\dot{V}O_2^{max}$) as a function of altitude and barometric pressure (from 1)
● ▣ * acclimated newcomers ○ △ □ acute hypoxia
× " natives

heart rate (h.r.^{max}). At P_B = 390 mmHg the drop does not exceed about 12-15%.

After a prolonged sojourn at altitude, the decrease of muscular power exceeding that accounted for by the reduction of cardiac output may originate at the peripheral level from:

1) the limited O_2 diffusion rate, due to the lower mean O_2 gradient and/or to a change of the diffusion properties of the blood-tissue barrier;
2) a limitation of the O_2 transport to the exchanging vessels caused by altered hemodynamics;
3) an impaired O_2 utilization by the tissues.

In order to analyze the role played by the above factors in limiting maximal aerobic performance, the effects on $\dot{V}O_2^{max}$ of inhaling pure O_2 at P_B = 390 mmHg was investigated in 10 members of the 1973 Italian Expedition to Mount Everest after 8-10 weeks exposure to altitudes above 5500 meters.

RESULTS

The results of average blood measurements at rest together with the most significant exercise parameters recorded in three environmental situations, i.e. at sea level and at 5350 meters when breathing ambient air or O_2, appear in the Table. $\dot{V}O_2^{max}$ was determined by a direct method (closed circuit metabograph (3)).

subjects n°. 10	age years	weight kg	Hct %	Hb g%	$\%O_2$aHb rest	$\dot{W}^{max}$ kpm/min	$\dot{V}_E^{max}$ l/min	f^{max} a/min	h.r.^{max} b/min	$\%O_2$aHb max. exerc.	$\dot{V}_{O_2}^{max}$ l/min	$\dot{V}_{O_2}^{max}$ ml/kg·min
sea level 122 m a.s.l.	26.1 ±4.7	72.72 ±10.65	44.7 ±1.3	15.0 ±0.9	98.2 ±2.1	1500	97.5 ±13.6	36.42 ±5.68	184.9 ±9.4	97.8 ±2.8	3.213 ±0.27	45.26 ±8.58
altitude B.C. 5350 m a.s.l.		67.4 ±10.3	63.82 ±4.59	20.6 ±1.41	84.31 ±4.65	1200	145.1 ±21.5	47.0 ±10.1	160.6 ±15.4	79.8 ±5.4	2.260 ±0.24	34.42 ±6.67
altitude 5350 m a.s.l. in O_2					98.3 ±2.0	1440	141.7 ±43.1	50.2 ±10.15	169.3 ±14.5	98 ±1.5	2.946 ±0.413	43.1 ±9.16

Vital statistics, hematocrit, hemoglobin concentration, arterial O_2 saturation at rest and exercise, work load (bicycle), maximum heart rate and ventilation (BTPS) and maximum O_2 uptake when breathing air at sea level and at 5350 meters a.s.l. as well as O_2 at 5350 meters.

The effects of chronic hypoxia on blood composition are comparable to those reported in the literature for similar conditions. RBC increases by the same factor as Hb concentration. $\dot{V}O_2^{max}$, as a consequence of the prolonged sojourn at altitude, drops to 0.7 of sea level average value to resume 0.92 of the control, when breathing oxygen at P_B = 390 mmHg. This is shown in Fig. 2 where, in the left quadrant, mean $\dot{V}O_2^{max}$ (percent of sea level control) appears as a function of P_B together with the range of data from various Authors as from Fig. 1; the effects of O_2 breathing on both $\dot{V}O_2^{max}$ and h.r.^{max} are illustrated in the center and right quadrants: on shifting from air to O_2 breathing, $\dot{V}O_2^{max}$ increases from 0.7 to 0.92 of the sea level control, while h.r.^{max}, reduced in the course of acclimation from 185 to 161 beats/min, attains

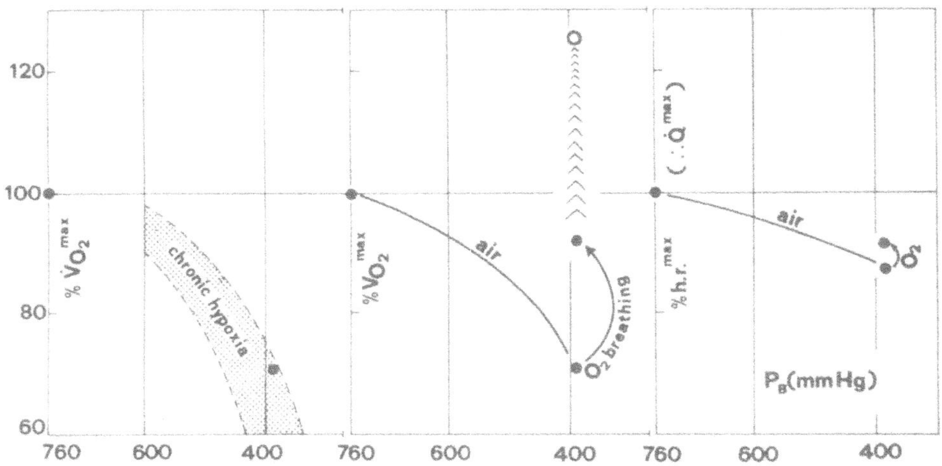

Fig. 2: $\dot{V}_{O_2}^{max}$ and h.r.^{max}(% of sea level) as a function of barometric pressure (P_B). • measured ○ estimated value.

169/min. The beneficial effect of O_2 breathing on $\dot{V}_{O_2}^{max}$ appears to be very modest. This finding is rather surprising in view of the high mean O_2 gradient, of the increase of RBC (40%), Hb concentration (20.6 g %) and Ca_{O_2} (38%). The increased Ca_{O_2}, even considering the reduction occurring in $\dot{Q}^{max}$, if $P_{\bar{v}O_2}$ were the same as in hypoxia or at sea level, could still account for an increase in $\dot{V}_{O_2}^{max}$ of 25-30% above sea level control (Fig. 2, center quadrant, open dot).

DISCUSSION

Before analyzing the various mechanisms possibly responsible for the failure of $\dot{V}_{O_2}^{max}$ to attain the expected high levels in O_2 breathing acclimatized individuals, it may be useful to examine the O_2 concentration and pressure values of both arterial and mixed venous blood, directly determined (with the exception of mixed venous blood O_2 pressure when breathing O_2 at altitude, which was estimated) for the various experimental situations. This is done in Fig. 3 where the "physiological" O_2 dissociation curves are drawn, respectively for 15 and 21 g % of Hb. The shape of the curve for the acclimated has been assumed to be unaffected by exposure to altitude on the basis of recent determinations made in newcomers to the Himalayas indicating that the known opposite effects

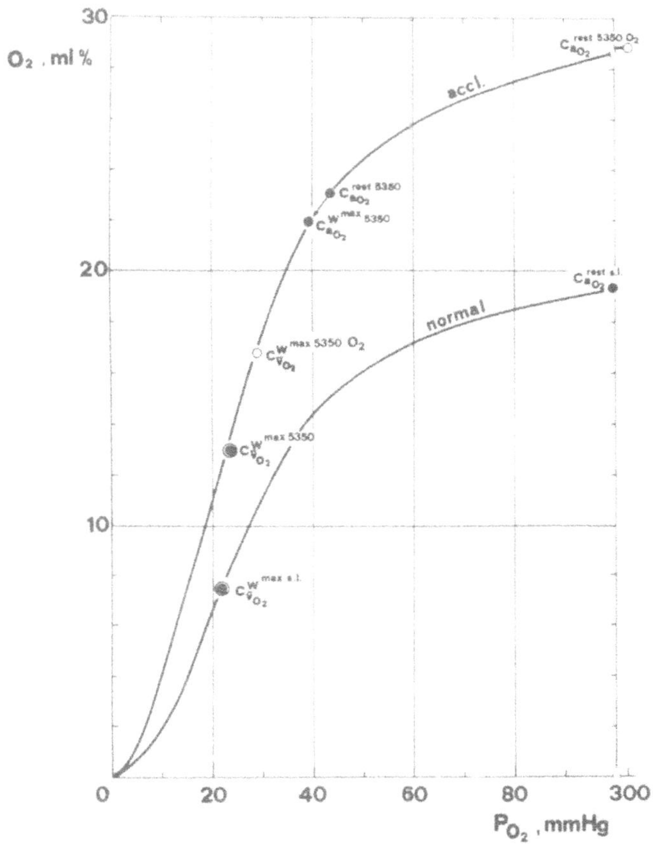

Fig. 3: "Physiological" O_2 dissociation curves for normal (Hb=15 g%) and acclimated subjects (Hb=21 g%). Arterial (a) and mixed venous ($\bar{v}$) points are indicated for resting (rest) and working (W) conditions when breathing air (•) and O_2 (o). The resting and working arterial points for air breathing conditions at sea level (s.l.) and O_2 breathing at altitude have been superimposed.

on the curve of increased blood 2-3-DPG concentration and reduced P_{CO_2} practically cancel out (4). Both $P_{\bar{v}O_2}$ values determined (in air breathing) or estimated (when breathing O_2) are relatively high in the acclimated. The maximal potential (a-$\bar{v}$) O_2 difference when breathing O_2 provided $P_{\bar{v}O_2}$ were the same, would be more than adequate for the observed cardiac output, to assure a $\dot{V}O_2^{max}$ much higher than at sea level.

Another necessary premise to any possible explanation of the present results is the observation that systemic pressure does not increase in working acclimated individuals more than it does in sea level controls. This finding, due to the relatively high cardiac output coupled with high Hct, necessarily implies a reduction of peripheral resistances to flow that could only be achieved by:

a) a dilatation of the arterioles, counterbalancing the increased resistance due to higher blood viscosity;
b) the opening of a number of arterio-venous anastomoses that could bypass a sizable fraction of blood from the high resistance districts to the veins, thus reducing the perfusion of the working muscles and the load on the heart.

In case (a) O_2 transport to the periphery when breathing oxygen would be high while the failure by the tissues to increase their oxidation rate could be the consequence of a change of the diffusion characteristics of the capillary-tissue barrier or of an hindrance of O_2 diffusion within the capillary, consequential to RBC plugging. In case (b), the transport of O_2 to the cells would be limited by the reduced blood flow and the improvement of maximal aerobic performance expected from the increased RBC would be minimized.

In both cases (a) and (b) the flow of O_2 to the tissues would be relatively more reduced when breathing air, due to the lower O_2 pressure head justifying the discrepancy between the observed percentage reduction of $\dot{V}_{O_2}{}^{max}$ and $\dot{Q}^{max}$. The high $P_{\bar{v}O_2}$ values found at maximal exercise both when breathing air and O_2 at altitude would also be explained.

The reduction of $\dot{V}_{O_2}{}^{max}$ found in the acclimated when breathing air as well as O_2 could also be attributed to a failure of the "power plant", i.e. to a limitation of the respiratory function of the mitochondria induced by chronic hypoxia or/and to a decrease of their number due to a reduction of the muscle mass. Experiments carried out in acclimated rats (2), however, indicate that the respiratory function of the mitochondria is not affected by chronic hypoxia. In addition, a decrease of the muscle mass of the order of magnitude as observed in the prolonged exposure to altitude does not seem to affect $\dot{V}_{O_2}{}^{max}$ to any measurable extent (personal observation).

The conclusion that may be drawn from the present experiments is that the limit to $\dot{V}_{O_2}{}^{max}$ at altitude is mostly peripheral. Whether the reduced O_2 flow to the muscles is attributable to a limitation of tissue perfusion, or to changes in the O_2 diffusion rate within the capillary or at the capillary-tissue barrier, is still matter of investigation. On the other hand, the respiratory characteristics of the muscle do not seem to be affected by chronic hypoxia and therefore to influence oxidative metabolism.

REFERENCES

1) Cerretelli, P. Effects of O_2 breathing on maximal aerobic power of man acclimatized to high altitude (Mt. Everest). XXVI Int.Congress of Physiol. Sciences, New Delhi, 1974 (in press).

2) Gold, A.J., T.F. Johnson and L.C. Costello. Effects of altitude stress on mitochondrial function. Am. J. Physiol. 224: 946-949, 1973.

3) Margaria, R., E. Galante and P. Cerretelli. An efficient CO_2 absorber for experiments on metabolism. J. Appl. Physiol. 14: 1066-1068, 1959.

4) Morpurgo, G., P. Battaglia, N.D. Carter, G. Modiano and S. Passi. The Bohr effect and the red cell 2-3 DPG and Hb content in Sherpas and Europeans at low and high altitude. Experientia 28: 1280-1283, 1972.

5) Pugh, L.G.C.E. Cardiac output in muscular exercise at 5800 m (19,000 ft). J. Appl. Physiol. 19: 441-447, 1964.

MEASUREMENT OF OXYGENATION AND DEOXYGENATION OF A SINGLE RED CELL OF CHICKEN EMBRYO BY MEANS OF A MICROPHOTOMETER

Masaji MOCHIZUKI and Hiroshi TAZAWA

Department of Physiology, Yamagata University

School of Medicine, Yamagata 990-23, Japan

In order to overcome difficulties inherent in the flow reaction apparatus so far used for kinetic studies of red cells, we have developed a technique of microphotometry. Since in a microphotometer a small light beam of about 10 μ is transmitted through a single red cell, the reactions with O_2 and CO can be measured by flushing a reacting gas onto the red cells. In the previous studies (1,2), the method of reaction measurement was elaborated and the CO reaction was determined in the red cells existing in the chorioallantoic capillary of chicken embryo. Since then, by using the same method and material, we have measured the oxygenation and deoxygenation rates and examined the velocity of combination and dissociation of O_2 due to the Bohr effect.

METHODS AND RESULTS

1. Calibration of O_2 Saturation

The influence of inhomogeneity of red cell thickness to the output signal was checked by comparing the O_2 saturation (So_2) determined by the present apparatus with that obtained by a Van Slyke analyzer. A freshly drawn human blood sample was tonometered at various Po_2 levels and the So_2 was measured by using a Van Slyke apparatus. At the same time, a small part of the sample was placed in a reaction cuvette of the microphotometer and covered with a silicon membrane of 25 μ thickness and, after flowing the same gases through the cuvette, the So_2 was measured by means of the photometer. The measurements were made at 0, 14, 26, 48 and 60 mm Hg Po_2, where Pco_2 was set at 40 mm Hg. In Fig. 1 is shown a pattern of So_2

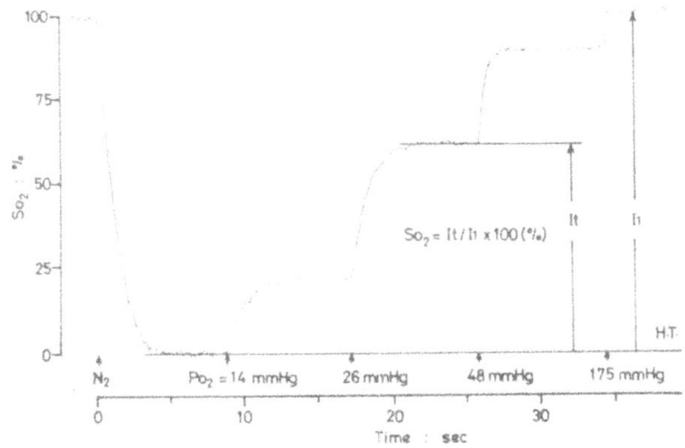

Fig. 1. Recorded pattern of So_2 change in human red cells covered with a silicon membrane.

recorded when the gas mixtures were made to flow successively. Since the red cell was equilibrated with the gas in a few seconds, the So_2 level was quantified by dividing an output current difference between 0 and any So_2 level (It) by that between 0 and 100 % So_2 (I_1). These So_2 values showed a fairly linear relation to those obtained from the Van Slyke analysis, but the former tended to be a little larger than the latter near 50 % So_2 as shown in Fig. 2. This fact suggests that the So_2 from the photometer shows an upward convexity, as expected from the theoretical consideration of Sirs and Roughton (3). Therefore, when the O_2 dissociation curve

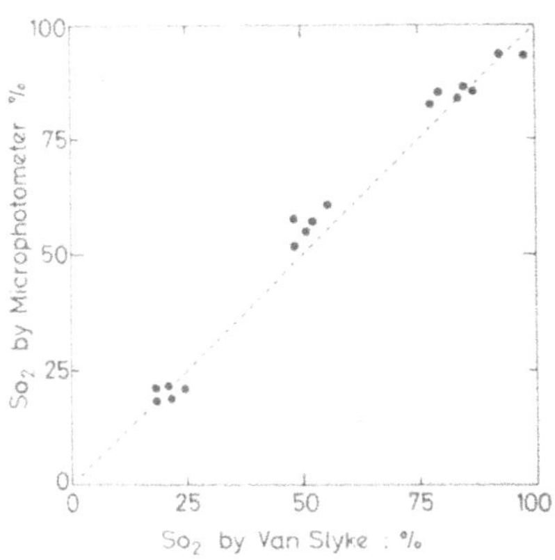

Fig. 2. Correlation between two So_2 values obtained from the photometer and Van Slyke analysis.

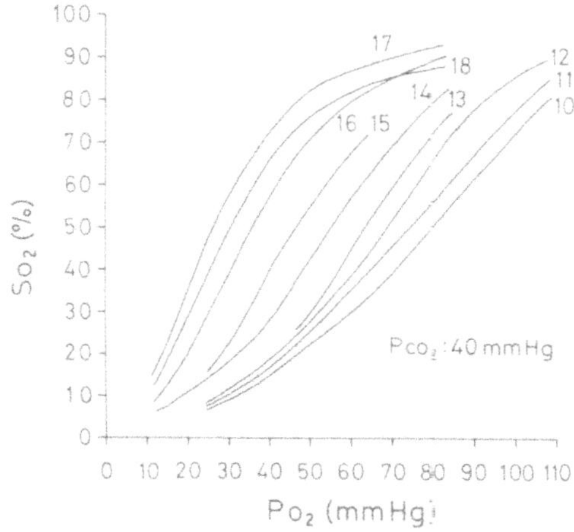

Fig. 3. O_2 dissociation curves at 40 mm Hg Pco_2 and at varying incubation days.

was measured, correction was made though slightly. When the oxygenation and deoxygenation rates were measured, however, the correction was abbreviated, because the slope of the dissociation curve corrected showed only a so small difference as to be neglected from that obtained with no correction.

2. O_2 Dissociation Curve of Chicken Embryo

The O_2 dissociation curve in chicken embryo blood was measured in the chorioallantoic capillary with progress of incubation days at 3 different Pco_2's of 10, 25 and 40 mm Hg. The measurements were performed according to the same manner as described in the previous paper (1). In Fig. 3 are shown the O_2 dissociation curves of 10 to 18 days of incubation obtained at 40 mm Hg Pco_2. The average values of about 10 measurements were taken to construct a curve. Though a scatter of each measurement was fairly large, the average values showed a drastic shift to the left side as the incubation proceeded. The P_{50} dropped from 79 mm Hg at 10 days to 26 mm Hg at 18 days. Furthermore, assuming that the relation of pH to Pco_2 in vitro is almost equal to that in vivo, we obtained the latter relation from the previous data on pH and Pco_2 in arterial and venous bloods of chicken embryo (4) as shown in Fig. 4. By referring to this relation we quantified the O_2 dissociation curve by using the modified Hill's equation (5) as follows;

$$(1) \quad \log Po_2 = K_1 - K_2 \cdot pH + K_3 \cdot \log (So_2/(100-So_2))$$

In Table 1 are shown the coefficients K_1, K_2 and K_3 during the course

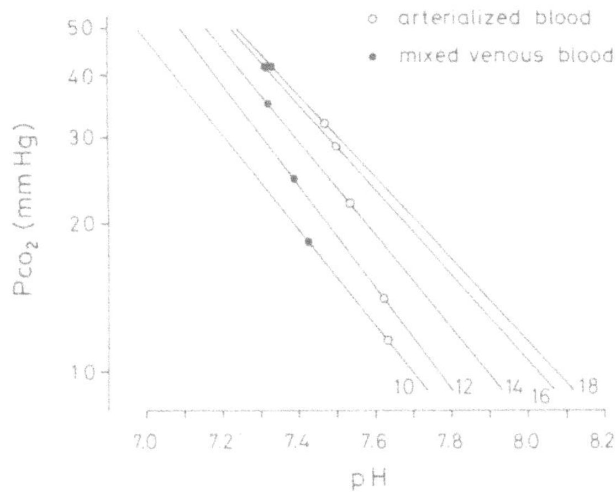

Fig. 4. In vivo relation between pH and log Pco_2 obtained from the data on gas analyses of arterial and venous blood of chicken embryo.

of incubation. A characteristic feature of the data in Table 1 is a change in K_3, which increased from 0.259 at 10 days to 0.464 at 18 days. Since the reciprocal of K_3 corresponds to the n value of the Hill's equation, the above data indicate that the heme-heme interaction is lowered as the embryo grows up. The coefficient K_2, on the other hand, represents the factor of the Bohr effect, which showed a maximum at 14 days. Although these values were not too low compared with those in mammalian blood, the effective Bohr effect (6) was enormously lowered because of low O_2 capacity.

3. Oxygenation and Deoxygenation Rates

From the So_2-time curves we further calculated the rate factor of oxygenation and deoxygenation according to the following formula:

Table 1. Coefficient values of the modified Hill's equation obtained at 5 incubation days.

age	Hill's equation			
10	$\log Po_2 =$ 4.250	− 0.334 pH	+ 0.259	log S/100−S
12	5.133	0.459	0.297	
14	5.232	0.482	0.310	
16	4.872	0.453	0.395	
18	4.216	0.373	0.464	

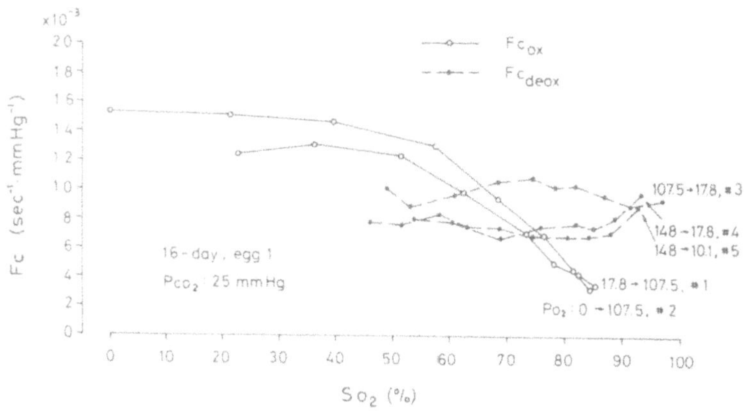

Fig. 5. Velocity factors of oxygenation (Fc_{ox}) and deoxygenation (Fc_{deox}) of the red cell in the chorioallantoic capillary of 16 days old chicken embryos.

$$(2) \quad Fc_{ox}\ (Fc_{deox}) = \frac{O_2\text{-capacity}}{\text{hematocrit}} \cdot \frac{dSo_2/dt}{100(Pa - Pc)}$$

where dSo_2/dt is the rate of change in So_2, Pa, the O_2 tension in a gas mixture and Pc, the back-pressure of the red cell which is estimated from the O_2 dissociation curve. Though both the factors largely scattered, the Fc_{ox} showed a plateau in a So_2 range below 60 % and decreased as the So_2 increased over 60 %. The Fc_{deox}, however, was almost independent of So_2 in the range of 90 to 45 %. Fig. 5 shows the Fc_{ox} and Fc_{deox} values obtained in 16 days old embryos. The Fc_{ox} in hypoxia was higher than the Fc_{deox}, suggesting that the inward diffusion was higher than the outward. In Table 2

Table 2. Velocity factors of oxygenation (in hypoxia) Fc_{ox} and deoxygenation Fc_{deox} at 4 incubation days.

	Days	Pco_2: mmHg			Av.
		10	25	40	
$Fc_{ox} \cdot 10^2$ $sec^{-1} \cdot mmHg^{-1}$	12	0.90	0.73	0.38	0.85
	14	1.06	1.13	0.33	1.01
	16	1.35	1.32	1.08	1.24
	18	1.34	0.99	1.04	1.11
	Av.	1.16	1.04	0.96	1.05
$Fc_{deox} \cdot 10^2$ $sec^{-1} \cdot mmHg^{-1}$	12	0.65	0.56	0.47	0.57
	14	0.70	0.94	0.70	0.81
	16	0.99	0.80	0.62	0.77
	18	0.65	0.93	0.48	0.70
	Av.	0.74	0.80	0.59	0.71

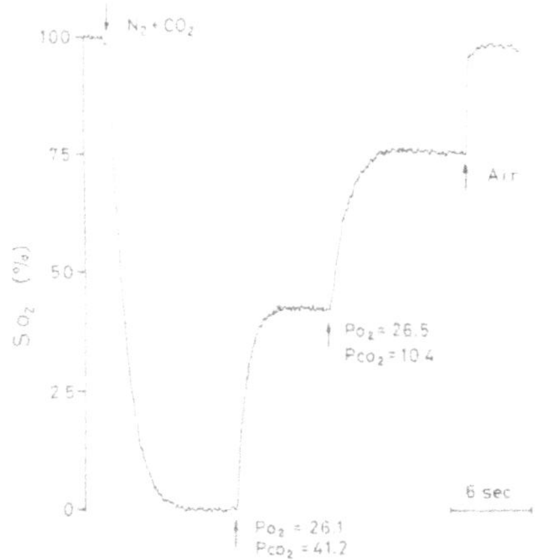

Fig. 6. Actual record of the Bohr shift of the red cell in the capillary of a 18 days old embryo.

are shown the Fc_{ox} in hypoxia and Fc_{deox} obtained in successive days of incubation at 3 different Pco_2's of 10, 25 and 40 mm Hg. The values of Fc_{ox} were certainly larger than the Fc_{deox}, but no significant dependency was observed on the age and Pco_2.

4. Bohr Shift

Such a change in So_2 as shown in Fig. 1 was also observed in the Bohr shift. In Fig. 6 is shown an actual record of the Bohr shift in 18 days old embryo. The fully oxygenated red cell was reduced to 0 % So_2 by flushing an O_2 free gas mixture with 40 mm Hg Pco_2, then, by flowing a gas mixture with 26.1 mm Hg Po_2 and 40 mm Hg Pco_2, the So_2 increased to 43.4 %. Next, by flushing a gas mixture with 10 mm Hg Pco_2 and the same Po_2 of 26.5 mm Hg, the So_2 elevated to 76.8 %. The change in So_2 was exponential in both on and off shifts as illustrated in Fig. 7, where the plots are average values of about 10 determinations in 16 days embryos. The experimental facts seem to suggest that the Pa, the O_2 back-pressure at the initial Pco_2, shifted very rapidly without changing any So_2 to that corresponding to another Pco_2, Pb. The subsequent reaction with O_2, however, was significantly retarded. Assuming that the physically dissolved O_2 content in the red cell is much less than the combined O_2, the So_2 increase is expressed approximately by the following equation;

$$(3) \quad \frac{dSo_2}{dt} = \alpha' \cdot \frac{dPc}{dt} = F_B \cdot (Pa \sim Pc)$$

where α' is the average slope of O_2 dissociation curve in a Po_2

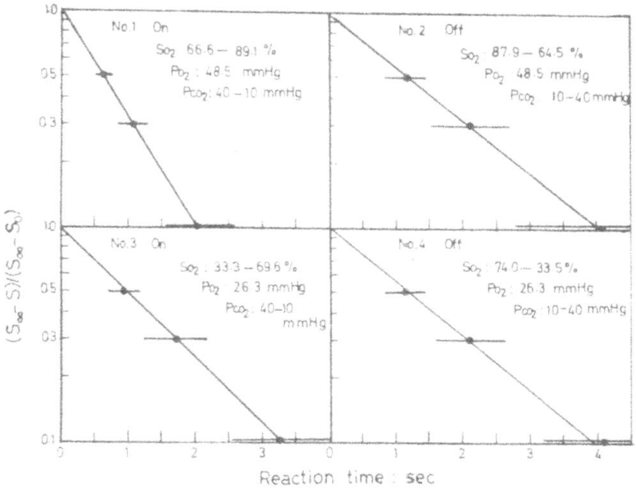

Fig. 7. Logarithmic expression of So_2 changes due to the Bohr shift in 16 days old embryos.

Table 3. Summarized data on the Bohr shift at 4 incubation days.

Days	Shift	Po_2	Pco_2	So_2	$t_{1/2}$	$\alpha' \cdot 10^2$	$Fc \cdot 10^2$	$F_B \cdot 10^2$	$K_B \cdot 10^2$
		mmHg	mmHg	%	sec	$mmHg^{-1}$	$sec^{-1} \cdot mmHg^{-1}$	$sec^{-1} \cdot mmHg^{-1}$	$sec^{-1} \cdot mmHg^{-1}$
12	On	48.5	40 → 10	27.2 → 63.7	1.72	0.90	0.85	0.36	0.52
	On	48.5	25 → 10	32.6 → 61.3	1.48	0.90	0.85	0.42	0.33
	Off	48.5	10 → 40	70.2 → 26.0	1.50	0.53	0.47	0.24	0.49
	Off	48.5	10 → 25	68.0 → 32.5	1.51	0.64	0.56	0.29	0.62
14	On	38.0	40 → 10	25.1 → 64.5	1.15	1.05	1.10	0.63	1.47
	On	38.0	25 → 10	39.9 → 64.3	1.04	1.05	1.10	0.70	1.93
	Off	38.0	10 → 40	65.3 → 24.6	1.06	0.55	0.70	0.36	0.74
	Off	38.0	10 → 25	67.4 → 37.3	1.17	0.74	0.94	0.44	0.82
16	On	48.5	40 → 10	66.6 → 87.1	0.60	0.43	0.90	0.50	0.86
	Off	48.5	10 → 40	87.9 → 64.5	1.14	0.24	0.62	0.15	0.20
	On	26.3	40 → 10	33.3 → 69.6	0.92	1.18	1.20	0.89	3.44
	Off	26.3	10 → 40	74.0 → 35.5	1.12	0.61	0.62	0.38	0.98
18	On	38.0	40 → 10	63.5 → 87.6	0.56	0.36	0.80	0.44	0.79
	Off	38.0	10 → 40	86.7 → 62.1	1.08	0.23	0.48	0.14	0.21
	On	26.3	40 → 10	42.7 → 73.4	0.92	1.00	1.00	0.75	3.00
	Off	26.3	10 → 40	74.3 → 41.7	1.12	0.56	0.48	0.35	1.29

range between Pa and Pb, and F_B is the oxygenation or deoxygenation rate due to the Bohr shift. The F_B was evaluated from Eq. (3) by dividing the gradient of lines of Fig. 7 by $1/\alpha'$. These values were generally smaller than the Fc_{ox} or Fc_{deox} in Table 2. Let the diffusion rate of O_2 into or out of the red cell be Kd, and the oxygenation or deoxygenation rate of hemoglobin by virtue of the Bohr shift be K_B. Then, the F_B may approximately be given by,

$$(4)\quad F_{\dot{B}} = Kd \cdot K_B/(Kd + K_B)$$

Since the simple oxygenation and deoxygenation reactions of hemoglobin proceeds very rapidly in hypoxia, the overall reaction rates are considered to represent the Kd values. Thus, putting Kd = Fc and by substituting the F_B values obtained from Eq. (3) into Eq. (4), we derived the K_B values. In Table 3 are tabulated the summarized data in 4 incubation days of 12 to 18 days. The K_B values in 12 days corresponded well with Fc values, but they increased significantly with age; especially in an on shift in hypoxia as shown in Fig. 8 and decreased as shown in Fig. 9.

DISCUSSION

According to Tazawa et al. (4), in chicken embryos of 16 days of incubation the mixed venous blood has about 20 mm Hg Po_2 and 40 mm Hg Pco_2, and the arterial blood has about 65 mm Hg Po_2 and 30 mm Hg Pco_2. From the O_2 dissociation curve shown in Table 1, the Po_2's of 20 and 65 mm Hg are read to be 23 and 93 % in So_2, respectively. On the other hand, according to Wangensteen and Rahn (7) the air space at the same incubation days has around 110 mm Hg Po_2. Thus, by referring to the Fc_{ox} value shown in Fig. 5, the

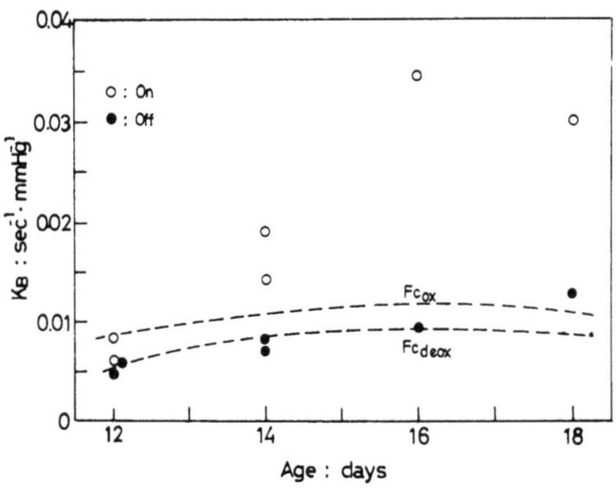

Fig. 8. Estimated rates of on and off Bohr shifts on hemoglobin inside the red cell at varying incubation days.

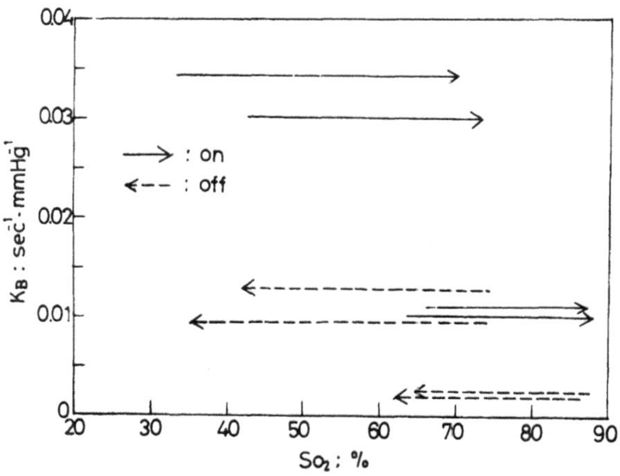

Fig. 9. Relationship between K_B and So_2. Arrows show the So_2 change observed in the Bohr shift.

transit time of red cells through the chorioallantoic capillary is estimated to be about 0.5 sec. This value agrees fairly well with the value obtained in the previous study (2), where it was calculated from the velocity factor of CO reaction (Fc_{CO}) by referring to the diffusing capacity measured by Temple and Metcalfe (8).

As shown in Table 3 the rate of the Bohr shift was lower than that of the usual O_2 reactions. This fact seemed to be explained by retardation of the transition of back-pressure. Provided that the transition of back-pressure had a similar time constant to the rates of oxygenation and deoxygenation of the red cell (Fc), the change in So_2 is considered to be given by a difference between two exponential curves and not to become a single exponential curve. Therefore, it may be safe to say that the combination and dissociation rates of O_2 with and/or from hemoglobin, more or less, become one of limiting factors in the Bohr shift unlike the usual O_2 reactions. Dependency of the K_B values on the So_2 shown in Fig. 9 seemed to support the above explanation. In any event, during the contact time of about 0.5 sec the contribution of the Bohr effect to the gas exchange through the capillary may not be so great as hitherto been expected.

REFERENCES

1) Mochizuki, M., H. Tazawa and T. Ono. Microphotometry fro determining the reaction rate of O_2 and CO with red cells in the chorioallantoic capillary. In: Oxygen Transport to Tissue. Ed. by D. F. Bruley and H. I. Bicher. New York, Plenum Pub. Co.,

1973, pp. 997-1006.

2) Tazawa, H., T. Ono and M. Mochizuki. Reaction velocity of carbon monoxide with blood cells in the chorioallantoic vascular plexus of chicken embryos. Respir. Physiol. 20: 161-170, 1974.
3) Sirs, J. A. and F. J. W. Roughton. Stopped-flow measurements of CO and O_2 uptake by hemoglobin in sheep erythrocytes. J. Appl. Physiol. 18: 158-165, 1963.
4) Tazawa, H., T. Mikami and C. Yoshimoto. Respiratory properties of chicken embryonic blood during development. Respir. Physiol. 13: 160-170, 1971.
5) Hellegers, A. E., G. Meschia, H. Prystowsky, A. S. Wolkoff and D. H. Barron. A comparison of the oxygen dissociation curves of the bloods of maternal and fetal goats at various pHs. Quart. J. Exptl. Physiol. 44: 215-221, 1959.
6) Bartels, H., P. Hilpert, K. Barbey, K. Betke, K. Riegel, E. M. Lang and J. Metcalfe. Respiratory function of blood of the yak, llama, camel, Dybowski deer and African elephant. Am. J. Physiol. 205: 331-336, 1963.
7) Wangensteen, O. D. and H. Rahn. Respiratory gas exchange by the avian embryo. Respir. Physiol. 11: 31-45, 1970/71.
8) Temple, G. F. and J. Metcalfe. The effects of increased incubator oxygen tension on capillary development in the chick chorioallantois. Respir. Physiol. 9: 216-233, 1970.

Supported by Ministry of Education, Japan. Grant No.948036.

SUMMARY OF DISCUSSION - SESSION II:

BLOOD OXYGENATION

Chairmen: R. F. Forster, J. P. Piiper

Paper by Duhm

Barnikol asks how the interpretation of the results would be modified if the intermeding steps of the oxygenation of Hb are taken into account and if the interactions with Mg^{++} have been considered.

Duhm estimates the errors due to neglect of the pressure of partially oxygenated Hb tetramers to be rather small. Binding constants in the presence of Mg^{++} or ATP have not been measured.

Versmold inquires about the possible role of O_2 saturation linked changes in the concentration of free 2,3-DPG in regulating the rate of glycolysis in red cells.

Duhm affirms stating that the higher concentration of free 2,3-DPG in deoxygenated red cells is expected to promote glycolysis.

Siesjö inquires about the experimental basis of the inhibition of hexokinase by high concentration of 2,3-DPG and about the factors involved in such an inhibition.

Duhm presents the experimental evidence and refers to literature data suggesting that chelation of Mg^{++} as well as direct interaction with enzyme protein are involved as mechanisms.

Paper by Standl and Ditzel

Forster inquired whether the main idea was that in acidosis red cell H^+ increased shifting $Hb\text{-}O_2$ equilibrium to the right, but the same decrease in pH reduced DPG in the cell, shifting the curve to the left so that both effects counteracted each other.

Standl replied that qualitatively this was so.

Forster then asked if hemoglobin carbamate was of importance in the changes occuring in acidosis. Standl believed it was not.

Siesjö asked whether small changes in P_{50} could be expected to produce alterations in tissue oxygenation of practical importance.

Forster commented that there is not ye t any clear-cut evidence that demonstrable changes in hemoglobin P_{50} alter P_{O_2} at the mitochondria, although there is a great deal of suggestive evidence.

Paper by Barnikol

Duhm asked whether Mg^{++} was really bound to the hemoglobin and whether also Cl^- was important.

Barnikol replied that he thought that the total ionic strength was a major factor.

Paper by Jesch, Enrich and Messmer

Forster inquired whether there was damage to the liver or kidneys in the experiments after infusion of hemoglobin solutions.

Jesch replied that urea and creatinine clearances were normal, but that no further specific tests were carried out.

Paper by Cerretelli

Siesjö asked if it was conceivable that the maximum working capacity might be limited by the glycogen concentration of muscles and that this content was decreased in hypoxia.

Cerretelli stated that glycogen concentration did not influence maximum O_2 uptake unless it was very low. He was unaware of any determinations of muscle glycogen in altitudeacclimated subjects. The ability to produce lactic acid in exhausting exercise, however, suggests that muscle glycogen content is not much reduced in individuals acclimated to high altitude.

Groom comments on the possible involvement of obstruction of small vessels by red cell aggregates of high hematocrit levels.

Coburn enquired whether some other factors than O_2 transport might limit O_2 uptake, for example H^+ transport.

Cerretelli remarked that muscle mass decreased under chronic hypoxic conditions in a manner similar to starvation.

Paper by Mochizuki, Tazawa and Ono

Thews pointed out that the size of the red cells could be an important factor producing differences in oxygenation of red cells when different animal species are compared.

Forster asked whether the chick embryo had more than one type of hemoglobin and whether the relative abundances of the types varied with age.

Mochizuki stated that this was unknown.

Tissue Respiration

CELLULAR CONTROL OF MITOCHONDRIAL RESPIRATION

David F. Wilson, Maria Erecińska, Marion Stubbs[1], J. Gordon Lindsay[2] and Charles S. Owen

Department of Biophysics and Physical Biochemistry, Medical School, University of Pennsylvania, Philadelphia, Pennsylvania 19174

[1]Metabolic Research Laboratory, Nuffield Department of Clinical Medicine, Radcliffe Infirmary, Oxford OX 2 6HE, U.K.

[2]Department of Biochemistry, Glasgow University, Glasgow, Scotland

THE PROBLEM

Oxygen delivery to tissues is essential for maintaining the oxygen tension at a level adequate to sustain the cellular energy supply via oxidative phosphorylation. The question is then how the cell regulates oxidative phosphorylation and, through this, the rate of oxygen consumption.

EXPERIMENTAL APPROACH

The control site(s) for any metabolic pathway must be a reaction(s) which is essentially irreversible (is accompanied by a large negative free energy change). Experimentally the search for the control site in mitochondrial oxidative phosphorylation requires three separate but sequential sets of measurements: 1) measurement of equilibrium constants for the reactions involved, including those for ATP hydrolysis and for the oxidation-reduction reactions (E_m values); 2) measurement of the metabolite concentrations under cellular conditions in order to determine which of the reactions are displaced from equilibrium; 3) a study of the properties of the reaction(s) displaced from equilibrium in order to discover and evaluate the control mechanism.

Measurement of the Equilibrium Constants

With respect to the measurement of the equilibrium constants, considerable progress has been made. As shown in Table 1, the half-reduction potentials are known for components in intact mitochondria at pH 7.2 ($E_{m7.2}$). The pH dependence of many of these components has also been measured, giving a comprehensive picture of the equilibrium constants for the oxidation-reduction reactions of the respiratory chain. As can be seen from Table 1, the $E_{m7.2}$ values fall into four groups. The values for the different groups are: near -0.300 V, 0.0 V, 0.24 V and 0.36 V. The $\Delta G^{\circ\prime}$ for ATP hydrolysis is -8.53 Kcal/mole at very low Mg^{++} concentrations and -7.60 Kcal/mole at cellular Mg^{++} concentrations (1 mM).

The Behavior Pattern for the Redox Reactions in Respiration

With respect to measurement of the metabolite concentrations, the steady-state reduction of several oxidation-reduction components of the respiratory chain have been measured in suspensions of isolated mitochondria. When the mitochondrial suspension was respiring in the presence of substrate, oxygen and the maximum [ATP]/[ADP][Pi] which could be formed from added ADP and Pi, the calculated E_h values show the presence of isopotential groups (23), that is, groups in which the reducing equivalents are transferred at near equilibrium ($\Delta E \rightarrow 0$). It is the transfer of reducing equivalents across the oxidation-reduction potential spans between these groups which is coupled to ATP synthesis (23,24).

Quantitative Evaluation of the Cellular Metabolite Levels and their Relationship with Respect to Equilibrium

In order to quantitatively evaluate the free energy relationship between the oxidation-reduction reactions and ATP synthesis, the mass action ratio has been measured for the reaction:

$$\text{NADH} + 2c^{+3} + 2\text{ADP} + 2\text{Pi} \longleftrightarrow \text{NAD}^{+} + 2c^{+2} + 2\text{ATP}$$

in which two reducing equivalents are transferred from NADH to oxidized cytochrome c (c^{3+}). The equilibrium constant for the reaction is expressed:

$$K = \frac{[\text{ATP}]^2}{[\text{ADP}]^2[\text{Pi}]^2} \times \frac{[\text{NAD}^+]}{[\text{NADH}]} \times \frac{[c^{2+}]^2}{[c^{3+}]^2}$$

This transfer is across two of the three phosphorylation sites and is coupled to the synthesis of two moles of ATP.

TABLE 1: MEASURED E_m VALUES FOR THE RESPIRATORY CHAIN COMPONENTS

Respiratory chain fragment	Component	$E_{m7.2}$	pH dependence < 7	pH dependence > 7	Reference
	Fe-S N1a	-0.380 ± .02			(1)
	" N1b	-0.240 ± .02			(1)
NADH	" N-3	-0.240 ± .02			(2,3)
dehydrogenase	" N-4	-0.240 ± .02			(2,3)
	" N-5,6	-0.260 ± .02			(1)
	" N-2	-0.020 ± .02			(2,3)
	Flavin	-0.045			(4)
Succinate	Fe-S S-1	0.030 ± .02			(5,6)
dehydrogenase	" S-2	-0.245 ± .02*			(6)
	" S-3	0.060 ± .02			(7)
Ubiquinone 10		0.045 ± .01		0.06 V/pH	(8)
	Cytochrome $\underline{b}_K$	0.030 ± .01	< 0.06 V/pH	0.06 V/pH	(9,10)
	Cytochrome $\underline{b}_T$	-0.030 ± .01	0.00 V/pH	0.06 V/pH	(9,10)
Cytochrome $\underline{b}$-$\underline{c}_1$ complex	Fe-S(Center 5)	0.040 ± .02			(3)
	Rieske Fe-S	0.280 ± .015		0.00 V/pH	(11,12)
	Cytochrome $\underline{c}_1$	0.225 ± .01		0.00 V/pH	(13,14)
Cytochrome $\underline{c}$		0.235 ± .005		0.00 V/pH	(14,15)
	Cytochrome $\underline{a}$	0.210 ± .01		0.02 V/pH	(16,17)
Cytochrome $\underline{c}$	Copper	0.245 ± .015		0.00 V/pH	(18)
oxidase	"invisible copper"	0.340 ± .015		0.00 V/pH	(19,20)
	Cytochrome $\underline{a}_3$	0.385 ± .010	0.00 V/pH	0.06 V/pH	(16,17)

* Probably not oxidized and reduced during respiration

In intact cells the mitochondrial $[NAD^+]/[NADH]$ must be measured indirectly using a metabolite couple which is in equilibrium with it. Depending on the cell type and experimental conditions, this criterion may be met by either the [3-hydroxybutyrate]/[acetoacetate] couple or the [glutamate]/[α-oxoglutarate][ammonia]couple. The intramitochondrial $[NAD^+]/[NADH]$ can then be calculated from the measured metabolite concentrations and the appropriate equilibrium constant (see for example 25). The cytochrome c reduction can be measured spectrophotometrically and the [ATP], [ADP] and [Pi] after quenching with perchloric acid.

The data obtained from two experiments on isolated rat liver cells are summarized in Table 2. The isolated cells were suspended in Krebs-Henseleit saline at 25° and incubated either in the absence or presence of added substrates. The measured [3-hydroxybutyrate]/[acetoacetate] ratios were 0.17 and 0.79 and the [reduced cytochrome c]/[oxidized cytochrome c] ratios were 0.23 and 0.31, while the [ATP]/[ADP][Pi] ratios were 1.7×10^3 M^{-1} and 2.6×10^3 M^{-1}. The E_m value for the NAD couple is -0.320 V (26), while that for the 3-hydroxybutyrate couple is 0.266 V (27), from which can be calculated $[NAD^+]/[NADH]$ ratios of 370 and 79 (see 25). The resulting mass action ratios were 5.5×10^7 M^{-2} and 5.2×10^7 M^{-2}, in agreement with the calculated equilibrium constant of 4.4×10^7 M^{-2}. Similar results have been obtained for perfused rat livers and suspensions of ascites tumor cells (24,28).

All three phosphorylation sites are coupled to a common pool of ATP, ADP and Pi and all three sites are fully reversible (for the reversal of Site 3; see 29). Near equilibrium between the oxidation-reduction reactions from NADH to cytochrome c and the cytoplasmic [ATP]/[ADP][Pi] under cellular conditions suggests that near equilibrium may exist for site 3 as well. The components on the oxygen "side" of site 3 consist of cytochrome a_3 and the "invisible copper" (19,20), the components responsible for reaction with molecular oxygen. The oxygen reaction itself is strongly displaced from equilibrium with the potential span from approximately 0.64 V to 0.8 V not coupled to ATP synthesis (23).

The information on respiratory control obtained from the measurement of the equilibrium constants and the metabolite concentrations may be summarized in two parts. 1) The rate of respiration is dependent on the mitochondrial $[NADH]/[NAD^+]$ and the cytoplasmic [ATP]/[ADP][Pi]. The dependence in each case is on the ratios of the reactants, not the concentration of individual reactants (30). 2) The reaction of cytochrome oxidase with molecular oxygen is the only reaction strongly displaced from equilibrium and is therefore the control site for mitochondrial respiration.

TABLE 2

THE REDOX STATE OF CYTOCHROME c AND THE MITOCHONDRIAL $[NAD^+]/[NADH]$ COUPLE, AND THE [ATP]/[ADP][Pi] RATIO IN SUSPENSIONS OF ISOLATED LIVER CELLS

Add Reactant or Reactant Ratio	Expt A No Added Substrate	Expt B 10 mM Lactate, 10 mM Ethanol
[3-Hydroxybutyrate]/ [acetoacetate]	0.17	0.78
[Cyt. c oxidized]/ [Cyt. c reduced]	4.43	3.21
ATP	2.36	2.08
ADP	0.64	0.46
P_i	2.16	1.74
[ATP]/[ADP][Pi]	$1.71 \times 10^3\ M^{-1}$	$2.6 \times 10^3\ M^{-1}$
$\frac{[ATP]^2}{[ADP]^2[Pi]^2} \times \frac{[NAD^+]}{[NADH]} \times \frac{[c^{2+}]^2}{[c^{3+}]^2}$	$5.5 \times 10^7\ M^{-2}$	$5.2 \times 10^7\ M^{-2}$
Calculated K_{eq}	$4.4 \times 10^7\ M^{-2}$	

Liver cells [17.2 mg wet wt/ml (A) and 20.5 mg wet wt/ml (B)] were incubated for 30 minutes at 25°. ADP, ADP and Pi are expressed as µmoles/g wet wt of cells. 3-Hydroxybutyrate and acetoacetate are expressed as µmoles/ml of incubation mixture. The values are the average of two experiments where duplicate incubations were made.

On the Mechanism and Kinetics of the Oxygen Reaction

Although considerable effort has been made to measure the kinetics and mechanism of the reaction of oxygen with molecular oxygen, the molecular mechanism remains a matter for speculation. Recently it has been observed (19,20) that potentiometric titration of the formation of the cytochrome oxidase-CO compound has an n value of 2.0 instead of 1.0 as would be expected for the simple formation of a reduced cytochrome a_3 CO compound. Detailed analysis of the CO concentration and pH dependence of the E_m value for the CO compound show that the CO binds with high affinity only when <u>both</u> cytochrome $\underline{a}_3$ and a component with an $E_{m7.2}$ of 0.340 V are reduced (see Figure 1 for a schematic representation). Since CO is competitive with respect to oxygen in its inhibition of respiration, oxygen also binds only when both components are reduced. If both metal atoms bind to the oxygen molecule to form a bridged compound, the bound O_2 would be reduced in a two-electron transfer ($E_{m7.0}$ approx. 0.7 V) to a bound peroxide, circumventing the thermodynamically unfavorable one-electron reduction to O_2^- ($E_{m7.0}$ approx. -0.45 V; see ref. 31). The bound peroxide could then be reduced to water in either a two-electron process or two one-electron processes. Kinetic analysis must take into account the unique requirement for both cytochromes $\underline{a}_3$ and the "invisible copper" before O_2 can react as well as the existence of a relatively stable bound peroxide intermediate.

The mechanism for the control of mitochondrial respiration will lie in the combination of the redox potential required for ATP synthesis at the existing [NADH]/[NAD$^+$] and [ATP]/[ADP][Pi] with the kinetic terms imposed by the mechanism and oxygen tension.

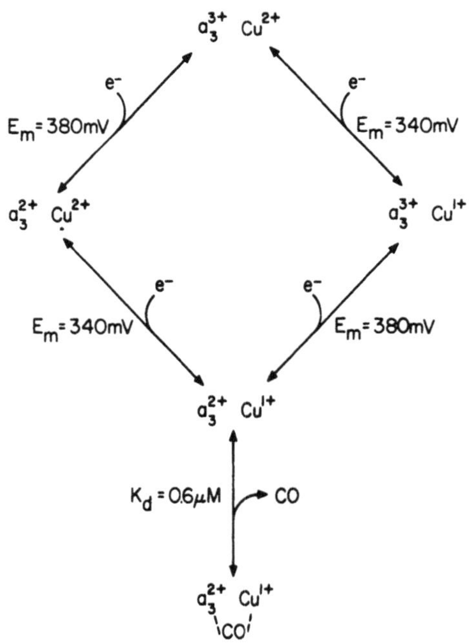

FIGURE 1: A schematic representation of the oxidation-reduction reactions associated with the reaction site of CO and oxygen with cytochrome $\underline{c}$ oxidase. The given E_m values are for pH 7.2.

REFERENCES

1. Ohnishi, T. and Pring, M. (1974) in "Dynamics of Energy Transducing Membranes (L. Ernster, R.W. Estabrook, and E.C. Slater, eds.) Elsevier Scientific Pub. Co., Amsterdam, pp. 169-180.
2. Ohnishi, T. (1975) Biochim. Biophys. Acta, in press.
3. Ohnishi, T., Wilson, D.F., Asakura, T. and Chance, B. (1972) Biochem. Biophys. Res. Commun. 46, 1631-1638.
4. Erecińska, M., Wilson, D.F., Mukai, Y. and Chance, B. (1970) Biochem. Biophys. Res. Commun. 41, 386-392.
5. Wilson, D.F., Erecińska, M., Dutton, P.L. and Tsudzuki, T. (1970) Biochem. Biophys. Res. Commun. 41, 1273-1278.
6. Ohnishi, T., Leigh, J.S., Jr., Winter, D.B., Lim, J. and King, T.E. (1973) Biochem. Biophys. Res. Commun. 53, 231-237.
7. Ohnishi, T., Winter, D.B., Lim, J. and King, T.E. (1974) Biochem. Biophys. Res. Commun. 61, 1017-1025.
8. Urban, P.F. and Klingenberg, M. (1969) Eur. J. Biochem. 9, 519-525.
9. Wilson, D.F. and Dutton, P.L. (1970) Biochem. Biophys. Res. Commun. 39, 59-64.
10. Wilson, D.F., Erecińska, M., Leigh, J.S. Jr. and Koppelman, M. (1972) Arch. Biochem. Biophys. 151, 112-121.
11. Wilson, D.F. and Leigh, J.S. Jr. (1972) Arch. Biochem. Biophys. 150, 154-163.
12. Prince, R.C., Lindsay, J.G. and Dutton, P.L. (1975) FEBS Letts., in press.
13. Green, D.E., Järnefelt, J. and Tisdale, H.D. (1960) Biochim. Biophys. Acta 31, 34-46.
14. Dutton, P.L., Wilson, D.F. and Lee, C.P. (1970) Biochemistry 9, 5077-5082.
15. Rodkey, F.L. and Ball, E.G. (1950) J. Biol. Chem. 182, 17-28.
16. Wilson, D.F. and Dutton, P.L. (1970) Arch. Biochem. Biophys. 136, 583-584.
17. Wilson, D.F., Lindsay, J.G. and Brocklehurst, E.S. (1972) Biochim. Biophys. Acta 256, 277-286.
18. Erecińska, M., Chance, B. and Wilson, D.F. (1970) FEBS Letts. 16, 284-286.
19. Lindsay, J.G. and Wilson, D.F. (1974) FEBS Letts. 48, 45-49.
20. Lindsay, J.G., Owen, C.S. and Wilson, D.F. (1975) Arch. Biochem. Biophys., in press.
21. Guynn, R. and Veech, R.L. (1973) J. Biol. Chem. 248, 6966-6969.
22. Benzinger, T., Kitzinger, C., Hems, R. and Burton, K. (1959) Biochem. J. 71, 409-414.
23. Erecińska, M., Veech, R.L. and Wilson, D.F. (1974) Arch. Biochem. Biophys. 160, 412-421.
24. Wilson, D.F., Stubbs, M., Veech, R.L., Erecińska, M. and Krebs, H.A. (1974) Biochem. J. 140, 57-64.
25. Williamson, D.H., Lund, P. and Krebs, H.A. (1967) Biochem. J. 103, 514-527.

26. Rodkey, F.L. (1959) J. Biol. Chem. 234, 188-190.
27. Krebs, H.A., Mellanby, J. and Williamson, D.H. (1962) Biochem. J. 82, 96-98.
28. Wilson, D.F., Stubbs, M., Oshino, N. and Erecińska, M. (1974) Biochemistry 13, 5305-5311.
29. Lindsay, J.G. (1974) Arch. Biochem. Biophys. 163, 705-715.
30. Owen, C.S. and Wilson, D.F. (1974) Arch. Biochem. Biophys. 161, 581-591.
31. George, P. (1965) in "Oxidases and Related Redox Systems" (T.E. King, H.S. Mason and M. Morrison, eds.) Vol. 1, Wiley, New York, pp. 3-33.

INFLUENCE OF HEMOGLOBIN OXYGEN AFFINITY ON OXIDATION REDUCTION STATE OF CYTOCHROME aa_3 IN PERFUSED LIVER [+)]

H.Versmold, B.Brauser, K.P.Riegel

Kinderklinik der Universität and Institut für Physiol. Chemie und Physikal.Biochemie der Universität München

The assumption that a decrease of the oxygen affinity of blood improves the delivery of oxygen to the tissues is still under debate. In vivo a variety of parameters cooperates in oxygen transport.. Therefore the use of a restricted model seemed to be justified in order to evaluate whether or not mitochondrial oxygenation is influenced by alterations of hemoglobin oxygen affinity.

The isolated perfused rat liver represents a system to study influences of defined changes of perfusion conditions on cellular respiration (1, 2, 3). The oxidation reduction state of mitochondrial respiratory chain components can be directly monitored by adapting the ingenious spectrophotometric methods to the intact organ (4, 5, 3) which were developed mainly by Chance, 1951 (6), for the study of isolated mitochondria. The intracellular oxygenation is best measured by registrating the redox state of cytochrome aa_3.I n the normoxic perfused liver, like in isolated mitochondria (7) cytochrome aa_3 is oxidized to 98% (3), therefore the redox state of cytochrome aa_3 quantitatively indicates the fraction of oxygen acceptors of the mitochondrial respiratory chain in anoxic regions of the tissue (3, 8).

A response to defined alterations of the oxygen affinity of the perfusate can therefore quantitatively be assessed at the molecular site of oxygen consumption.

+) Supported by Deutsche Forschungsgemeinschaft (SFB 51, Klinische Molekularbiologie und Biochemie).

METHODS

Livers of female Wistar rats, 100 to 200 g of weight, were perfused by the method according to Scholz and Bücher, 1965 (1), by a solution of hemoglobin A_1 (2.5×10^{-4} M in Krebs-Henseleit solution, pH 7.4) containing lactate 2.0 mM and pyruvate 0.2 mM, at 20° C. Perfusion rate was 2.5 ml/g liver wet weight. Hemoglobin A_1 was isolated and freed from 2,3-diphosphoglycerate (2,3-DPG) by DEAE Sephadex A 50 chromatography (9). Methemoglobin content was below 5%. A decrease in hemoglobin oxygen affinity was provoked by adding 2,3-DPG to the perfusate entering the liver (Fig. 1) to give a final concentration of 3.0 mM. 2,3-DPG (cyclohexyl ammonium salt; Boehringer, Mannheim) had been converted to the free acid by a Dowex WA X 8 chromatography and titrated to pH 7.4 by NaOH.

The oxidation reduction state of cytochrome aa_3 as well as the oxygen saturation of hemoglobin within the perfused organ was recorded by transmittance spectroscopy according to Brauser et al., 1972 (3). Light of a modified "Rapidspektroskop" (10) was transmitted through a liver lobe like through a cuvette. The obtained absorption spectra are summed up and analyzed by a Fabritec Instrument Computer (11).

For quantitative evaluation of the spectra molar extinction coefficients of 13.4 $cm^{-1}mM^{-1}$ (555 nm) for deoxy hemoglobin, and 15.2 $cm^{-1}mM^{-1}$ (577 nm) for oxy hemoglobin (12) were used.

Transition from hypoxic to anoxic perfusion by equilibrating the perfusate with argon (+ 5% CO_2)leads to a total deoxygenation of hemoglobin and a 100% reduction of cytochrome aa_3. The difference spectrum of the anoxic minus hypoxic liver (Fig. 2) illustrates that the absorption maximum of reduced cytochrome aa_3 (607 nm) can be seperated from the spectral changes due to the deoxygenation of hemoglobin (578 nm and 558 nm).

Hypoxic perfusion was performed by equilibrating the perfusate with a gas mixture of oxygen and argon (+ 5% CO_2) to yield a 50% reduction of cytochrome aa_3, which empirically was achieved at a pO_2 in the range of 100 to 150 Torr. The perfusion condition chosen to demonstrate an effect of changing hemoglobin oxygen affinity on intracellular oxygenation thus corresponds to an anemic hypoxia, hemoglobin in the artery being fully oxygen saturated.

RESULTS

Oxygen Unloading from Hemoglobin

Upon addition of 3 mM 2,3-DPG to the perfusate a deoxygenation of hemoglobin is recorded within the transilluminated liver lobe

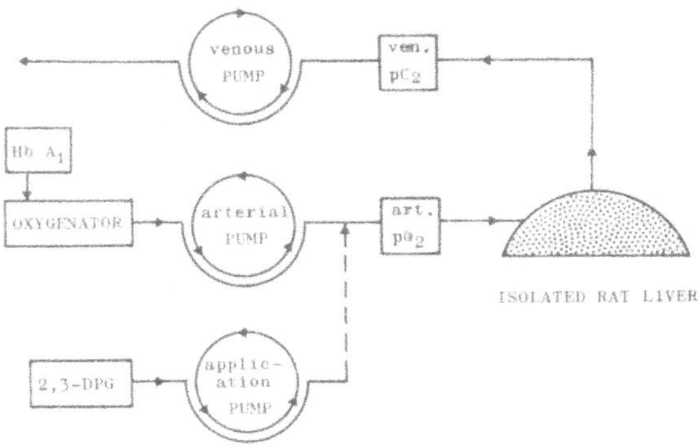

Figure 1: Diagram of the system for perfusion of isolated rat liver with a hemoglobin A_1 solution. Hemoglobin oxygen affinity changes are provoked by addition of 2,3-DPG to the perfusate. "Arterial" and "venous" pO_2 are recorded by Clark type electrodes.

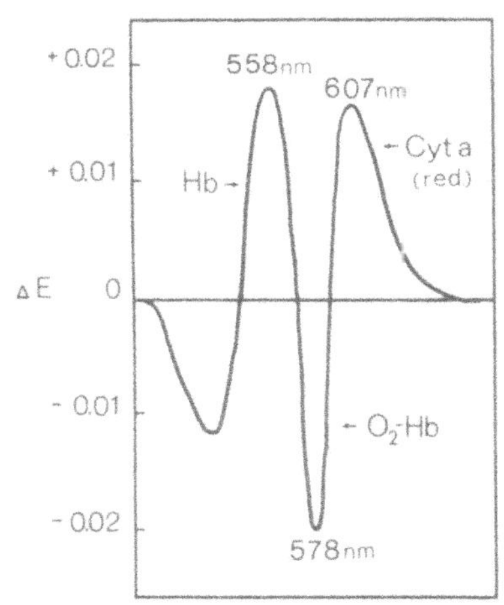

Figure 2: Difference spectrum of HbA_1 perfused liver. Transition from hypoxic to anoxic perfusion. For organ transmittance spectroscopy (Brauser, 1968) light is transmitted through a liver lobe like through a cuvette. Reduction of cytochrome aa_3 (absorption maximum at 607nm) and deoxygenation of hemoglobin (absorption minimum at 578nm, absorption maximum at 558nm) are simultaneously registrated.

(Fig. 3). The absorption minimum at 578 nm and the absorption maximum at 558 nm in the difference spectrum (hypoxia + 3 mM 2,3-DPG) minus (hypoxia without 2,3-DPG) represent a decrease of oxy hemoglobin concentration by 38.5 μM and a respective increase of deoxy hemoglobin concentration by 55,8 μM. Thus an additional oxygen unloading of o.31 μatoms O/ml perfusate (555 nm), or 0.44 μatoms O/ml (577 nm) occurs upon the addition of 2,3-DPG, with a mean of 0.27 μatoms O/ml perfusate in 3 experiments. The arterial hemoglobin bound oxygen content is 2.0 μatoms/ml perfusate.

The arterial and venous (7 - 10 Torr) pO_2 did not change upon 2,3-DPG addition, while the P_{50} value (pH 7.4; 20°C) rose from 7 to 13 Torr. From hemoglobin oxygen equilibrium curves an increase of oxygen unloading of 0.2 - 0.4 μatoms O/ml is calculated.

Oxidation Reduction State of Cytochrome aa_3

Simultaneously to the deoxygenation of hemoglobin an oxidation of cytochrome aa_3 occurs upon addition of 2,3-DPG to the perfusate (Fig. 3: negative peak at 607 nm). Quantitatively this cytochrome aa_3 oxidation represents about 15% of the cytochrome aa_3 present in the reduced state under the hypoxic perfusion conditions.

In control experiments 2,3-DPG was added to hemoglobin free perfused livers. No influence on O_2 uptake and redox state of cytochrome aa_3 was observed.

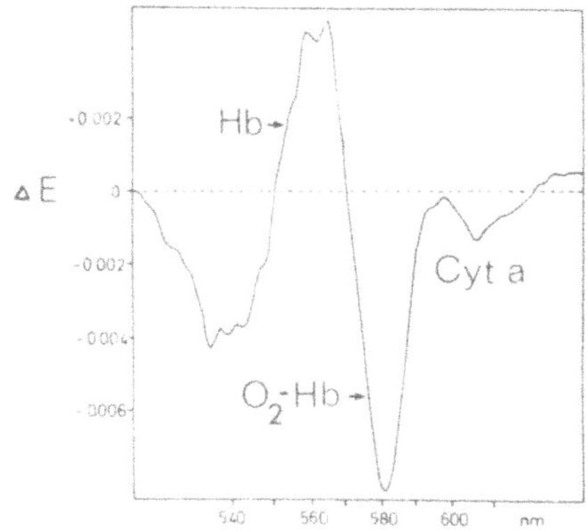

Figure 3: Spectral changes upon addition of 3mM 2,3-DPG to the perfusate of hypoxic liver (anemic hypoxia). Deoxygenation of hemoglobin (absorption minimum at 578nm, absorption maximum at 558nm) and oxidation of cytochrome aa_3 (absorption minimum at 607nm) are registrated, indicating improved mitochondrial oxygenation by a decrease in hemoglobin O_2 affinity of the perfusate. For quantitative data see text.

DISCUSSION

The present results demonstrate improved mitochondrial oxygenation in the intact organ, brought about by a decrease in hemoglobin oxygen affinity of the perfusate.

The dependence of the oxidation reduction state of cytochromes on the oxygen supply of the liver has been studied in livers perfused in the absence of hemoglobin (5, 3). Oxygen consumption of the perfused liver of (150-) 250 - 300 μatoms O/g liver x hour has been described (c.f.3). The additional oxygen unloading of 0.25 μatoms O/ml perfusate in presence of 2,3-DPG represents 45 μatoms O/g liver x hour and thus about 20% of the oxygen consumed by the liver under normoxic conditions. According to Brauser and coworkers (8) in the hemoglobin free perfused liver an oxygen supply of 75 μatoms O/g liver x hour results in 50% reduction of cytochrome aa_3. The present observation of 15% cytochrome aa_3 oxidation upon addition of 2,3-DPG to the perfusate are in agreement with these data.

Chance and Salkovitz (13), in a preliminary study, failed to demonstrate alterations of the intracellular NADH concentration in rat heart perfused by erythrocyte suspensions of different P_{50} values. It has to be stated, therefore, that conclusions from the present data are valid only for the conditions of this study. These conditions are characterized by low oxygen capacity, full oxygen saturation of hemoglobin in the artery and a venous O_2 tension in the range of the P_{50} value. Our results prove the validity of calculations of oxygen release to tissues from hemoglobin oxygen equilibrium curves. Such calculations have to be based on the O_2 parameters present under the specific experimental or clinical situation, which,of course, are different for different organs.

REFERENCES

1. Scholz,R., Bücher,Th., in: Chance,B., Estabrook,R.W., Williamson,J.R., Control of Energy Metabolism, Academic Press, New York, London 1965, p.393

2. Brauser,B., Versmold,H, Bücher,Th., Z.Physiol.Chem. 394, 1589 (1968)

3. Brauser,B., Bücher,Th., Sies,H., Versmold,H., in: Gaede,K., Horecker,B.C., Whelan,W.J.(eds.), Molecular Basis of Biological Activity, Academic Press, New York, London 1972, p.197

4. Brauser,B., Z.anal.Chem. 237, 8 (1968)

5. Brauser,B., Versmold,H., 5th FEBS Meeting, Prague 1968, Abstr. 248

6. Chance,B., Rev.Sci.Instr. 22, 634 (1951)

7. Chance,B., Williams,J.R., J.Biol.Chem. 217, 409 (1955)

8. Brauser,B., Sies,H., Bücher,Th., FEBS letters 2, 167 (1969)

9. Jonxis,I.H.P., Huisman,T.H.J.: A Laboratory Manual on Abnormal Hemoglobins (2nd ed.), Blackwell Sci.Publ., Oxford-Edingurg 1968

10. Niesl,W., Lübbers,D.W., Schneewolf,D., Botticher,W., Rev.Sci. Instr. 35, 578 (1964)

11. Brauser,B., Proc. SFB 51 der Deutschen Forschungsgemeinschaft, Vol.II, München 1973, p.815

12. Gratzer,W.B., in: UV-Atlas of Organic Compounds, Verlag Chemie, Weilheim 1969

13. Chance,B., Salkovitz,I.A., in: Chaplin,H., Jaffe,E.R., Lenfant, C., Valeri,C.R. (eds.), Preservation of Red Blood Cells, Nat. Acad.Sci., Washington 1973, p.73

PROBLEMS IN DETERMINATION OF OXYGEN DISSOCIATION OF AVIAN BLOOD

Peter Scheid, Takeo Kawashiro and Johannes Piiper

Max-Planck-Institut für experimentelle Medizin

Abteilung Physiologie, Göttingen, Germany

INTRODUCTION

Oxygen dissociation curves of avian blood have repetitively been reported to be shifted to the right with respect to mammalian curves, P_{50} values of the hen exceeding those of human blood by more than 20 torr. This shift has recently been propounded to be a methodological artifact produced by high O_2 consumption of nucleated avian red cells (Lutz *et al.*, 1973).

It is the purpose of this paper

(1) to report measurements on O_2 dissociation and

(2) on metabolic rates of duck blood;

(3) to assess quantitatively possible errors produced in blood gas analysis by the metabolic activity of avian blood.

METHODS

Details of the methods have been reported (Scheipers *et al.*, 1975; Scheid and Kawashiro, 1975). Blood was obtained by cardiac puncture from 22 adult ducks *(Cairina moschata)* and stored on ice until use. Addition of heparin prevented coagulation.

Oxygen Dissociation Curve

Blood samples were equilibrated at 41°C, the rectal temperature of the duck, with gas mixtures containing various fractions of O_2 with 5% CO_2 in N_2. O_2 and CO_2 content of whole blood, C_{O2} and C_{CO2}, were determined using Van Slyke manometric apparatus, pH was determined in electrodes. Determination was performed at different blood pH which was adjusted by addition of $NaHCO_3^-$. Equilibration at 35% O_2 was used to determine O_2 capacity in the Van Slyke apparatus. After correction for physically dissolved gas, saturation of O_2, SO_2, was calculated.

The Bohr effect factor, ϕ, was obtained using the half saturation partial pressure, P_{50},

$$\phi = \Delta log\ P_{50}\ /\ \Delta pH$$

and was used to group the results on S_{O2} into 3 different iso-pH groups. A Hill plot on the data of each group was performed to give an average Hill line which was converted into the corresponding O_2 dissociation curve, plotting S_{O2} against P_{O2}.

Metabolic Rates

Blood was equilibrated with 35% O_2, 5% CO_2 in N_2 and stored anaerobically in a syringe at 41°C. Samples were taken from the syringe in regular intervals for determination of C_{O2}, C_{CO2} and pH. O_2 consumption, $\dot{M}_{O2}$, and C_{O2} production rates, $\dot{M}_{CO2}$, were calculated as the slope of plots of C_{O2} and C_{CO2} against time of anaerobic storage.

RESULTS AND DISCUSSION

Oxygen Dissociation

The following P_{50} values were obtained in blood, whose O_2 capacity averaged 6.7 $mMol \cdot L^{-1}$, for various pH values (41 °C, P_{CO_2} = 35 torr):

pH =	*7.40*	*7.50*	*7.60*
P_{50} =	*41*	*37*	*32 torr*

The resulting Bohr effect factor is

$$\phi = -0.53 .$$

Figure 1 shows the O_2 dissociation curve for pH and P_{CO_2} values close to those measured in arterial blood of unrestrained, unanesthetized ducks (Kawashiro and Scheid, 1975). The slope of the dissociation curve, βb_{O_2}, in its steep portion, *viz.* around P_{50}, is

$$\beta b_{O_2} = 0.12\ mMol \cdot L^{-1} \cdot torr^{-1}.$$

The dissociation curve of fig. 1 is expected to virtually coincide with the *in-vivo* dissociation curve of ducks in the range of arterial P_{O_2}. An *in-vivo* dissociation curve extending to venous P_{O_2} values has been constructed on the basis of these results by Scheipers *et al.* (1975), account being given for P_{CO_2} and pH differences between venous and arterial blood. This curve is steeper than the iso-pH curve of fig. 1, βb_{O_2} around P_{50} being 0.14 $mMol \cdot L^{-1} \cdot torr^{-1}$.

It is evident from fig. 1 that our curve did not significantly differ from that obtained by Lutz *et al.* (1974) with a different method (Longmuir and Chow, 1970) in which both C_{O_2} and P_{O_2} were determined at the same time. We would take this as evidence for the applicability of the Van Slyke technique in determining O_2 dissociation curves even in the presence of high blood metabolic rates (see below).

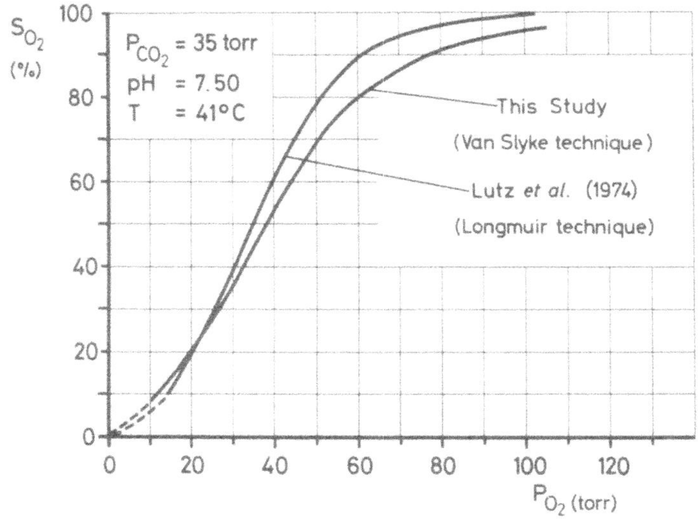

Fig. 1. Oxygen dissociation curves in duck blood obtained with different techniques.

The curve of Lutz *et al.* (1974) is steeper than ours in its upper portion. A Hill plot on their curve shows increasing slope as P_{O_2} increases, the Hill coefficient exceeding 4 in the upper part of the curve. For our curve, the Hill curve is steepest around P_{50}, Hill coefficient in this range being 2.9.

Metabolic Activity

Average values were $\dot{M}_{O_2}$ = 0.041 and $\dot{M}_{CO_2}$ = 0.036 mMol·(L blood)$^{-1}$·min^{-1} which is an order of magnitude higher than the corresponding values for man, 0.0036 and 0.0023 mMol·(L blood)$^{-1}$·min^{-1}, respectively (Greenbaum *et al.*, 1967). pH changes by 0.0014 unit·min^{-1} during anaerobic storage which is attributed to both lactic acid and CO_2 production (Scheid and Kawashiro, 1975), whereas for mammalian blood acidification, which is of similar magnitude (Greenbaum *et al.*, 1967), stems mainly from lactic acid production.

Blood Metabolism and Blood Gas Analysis

Systematic errors are possible in determination of any of the variables in blood that change with time elapsing between sampling of blood from the organism or from a tonometer and completion of analysis or chemical interruption of metabolism. These problems have been considered for human blood by Kelman and Nunn (1966) and have been made responsible for the shift to the right of dissociation curves, that were determined earlier by the Van Slyke method, in comparison with more recent techniques in which both P_{O_2} and C_{O_2} are measured simultaneously (Lutz *et al.*, 1973).

The errors are expected to be mainly dependent on the delay time between sampling and analysis and metabolic activity of the blood. For a quantitative assessment of the systematic error in determining O_2 dissociation curves in avian blood by the classical Van Slyke technique, the O_2 dissociation curve of this study will be used as the true one (fig. 2, continuous line), and the apparent dissociation curve will be constructed which would result if no correction was made for the O_2 consumption, $\dot{M}_{O_2}$, measured in this study, assuming a time delay of τ = 5 min between sampling and analysis.

The metabolic rate would result in a down-shift of all C_{O_2} values by $\tau \cdot \dot{M}_{O_2}$, which would be independent of P_{O_2} since $\dot{M}_{O_2}$ did not depend on P_{O_2} (see above). If one assumes that O_2 capacity is determined by an independent technique which is not subject to systematic errors, then the resulting dissociation curve, as the plot of S_{O_2} against P_{O_2}, would be down-shifted (s. fig. 2, dotted line) which would be particularly apparent in the upper portion of the curve.

If, however, as was done in our experiments, O_2 capacity is measured by the same technique and is thus subject to the same systematic errors, then the error would be much reduced and would

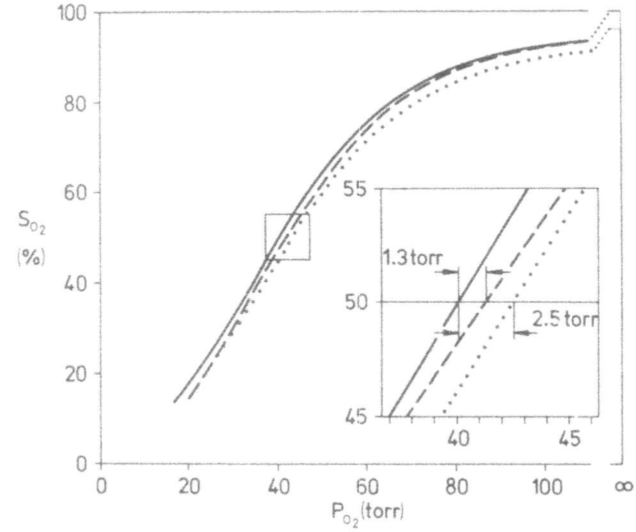

Fig. 2. Effect of metabolism on determination of O_2 dissociation curve. Continuous line, true curve; dotted line, apparent curve calculated using correct value of O_2 capacity; dashed line, aparent curve resulting if both O_2 content and O_2 capacity are subject to the same error. Inset gives enlargement around P_{50}.

virtually disappear in the upper part of the curve (fig. 2 , dashed line). The errors expected from metabolism in avian blood for determination of P_{50} would be 2.5 torr if calculated with the true O_2 capacity, but only 1.3 torr if O_2 capacity was obtained by the same technique (inset of fig. 2). In our experiments, the delay time was measured and never exceeded 1 min. Thus errors introduced by metabolism are expected to be insignificant in the entire range of the O_2 dissociation curve.

More significant errors are expected for determination of P_{O_2} or P_{CO_2} in blood samples. These errors depend largely on the slope of the respective dissociation curve. It can be assessed (Scheid and Kawashiro, 1975) that for a delay of 1 min, P_{O_2} will be underestimated by 0.5 torr around P_{50}, but by 2 torr at arterial P_{O_2} values and even by 30 torr for fully oxygenated blood, *i.e.* when all O_2 consumed is taken from physically dissolved gas. These errors will be much reduced if blood is stored on ice, or even at room temperature because metabolism declines with temperature (Q_{10} = 1.8 for chicken blood; Besch, 1966). Kawashiro and Scheid (1975) have found insignificant changes in P_{O_2} of arterial blood samples of ducks that were stored for 2 min at room temperature.

The absolute values of the errors in measuring C_{CO_2} and P_{CO_2} in avian blood using Van Slyke apparatus and electrodes are expected to be much less than those of the respective O_2 values due to the steeper course of the CO_2 dissociation curve. However, the relative error in P_{CO_2}, in relation, for instance, to the arterio-venous P_{CO_2} difference, may be of the same order of magnitude as the relative error for P_{O_2}.

CONCLUSION

No appreciable errors are expected in determination of blood gas values and pH using classical techniques provided time of anaerobic storage is kept small and is, if unavoidable performed on ice. In particular, dissociation curves may safely be analyzed with the Van Slyke technique which is in disagreement with the conclusions of Lutz *et al.* (1973). For measurement of P_{O_2} and P_{CO_2}, delay time is mainly dictated by response time of the electrodes; measurements may have to be corrected for metabolism, particularly in high P_{O_2} range.

REFERENCES

Besch, E.L. (1966). Respiratory activity of avian blood. *J. Cell. Physiol.* 67: 301-306.

Greenbaum, R., J.F. Nunn, C. Prys-Roberts, G.R. Kelman (1967). Metabolic changes in whole human blood (in vitro) at 37°C. *Respir. Physiol.* 2: 274-282.

Kawashiro, T., P. Scheid (1975). Arterial blood gases in undisturbed resting birds: measurements in chicken and duck. *Respir. Physiol.*, in Press.

Kelman, G.R., J.F. Nunn (1966). Nomograms for correction of blood P_{O_2}, P_{CO_2}, pH, and base excess for time and temperature. *J. appl. Physiol.* 21: 1484-1490.

Longmuir, I.S., J. Chow (1970). Rapid method for determining effect of agents on oxyhemoglobin dissociation curves. *J. appl. Physiol.* 28: 343-345.

Lutz, P.L., I.S. Longmuir, J.V. Tuttle, K. Schmidt-Nielsen (1973). Dissociation curve of bird blood and effect of red cell oxygen consumption. *Respir. Physiol.* 17: 269-275.

Lutz, P.L., I.S. Longmuir, K. Schmidt-Nielsen (1974). Oxygen affinity of bird blood. *Respir. Physiol.* 20: 325-330.

Scheid, P., T. Kawashiro (1975). Metabolic changes in avian blood and their effects on determination of blood gases and pH. *Respir. Physiol.*, in Press.

Scheipers, G., T. Kawashiro, P. Scheid (1975). Oxygen and carbon dioxide dissociation of duck blood. *Respir. Physiol.*, in Press.

METABOLIC AND ELECTRON MICROSCOPIC STUDIES POST MORTEM IN BRAIN MITOCHONDRIA

K. Ikrényi, E. Dóra, F. Hajós[+], A.G.B. Kovách

Experimental Research Department and [+]1st Anatomy Department, Semmelweis Medical University, Budapest, Hungary

Our earlier studies have demonstrated profound inhibition of cerebral mitochondrial oxidation processes in late hemorrhagic shock. (Ikrényi 1973). The most reasonable explanation for this would be the development of tissue hypoxia.

Short term (3 to 5 minutes) ischemic- anoxia leads to damage of the brain tissue: some of the mitochondria are swollen, some are losing their cristae and some are vacuolated (Hager et al. 1960, Brown et al. 1968, McGee-Russel et al. 1970). Data of Hossman (1970) and Kleihues (1974) demonstrated on the other hand that after as much as half to one hour of ischemia the electrical activity and metabolism of the cortex returned near to normal levels. Our present experiments were carried out to study the effect of ischemic-anoxia on the state 4; ADP activated, state 3; and DNP stimulated respiration of brain mitochondria isolated at different intervals after the start of ischemia. The metabolic changes of the mitochondria were correlated in time with the ultrastructural, electronmicroscopical changes.

Methods

The mitochondria were isolated from rat brains left in the skull at 20-22C^{o} for a period of 1, 4, and 12 hours after decapitation. The mitochondria were prepared according to Clark and Nicklas (1970). The oxygen uptake was measured polarographically. The incubation medium contained 0.01 M trisphosphate, 58 mM KCl, 26 mM NaCl, 6 mM $MgCl_2$, at pH:7.4. The respiration in St_4 and St_3 as well as DNP stimulated respiration was measured and the respiratory control ratio (RCR) was calculated.

For electron microscopy the mitochondrial fractions were fixed by adding a few drops of the fraction to Karnovsky's fixative (Karnovsky 1965). After fixation, fractions were pelleted and postfixed with 1% osmic acid and embedded in Durcupan (Fluka). Electronmicrographs were made with a JEOL 100B electron microscope.

Results and Discussion

The results of isolated mitochondrial respiration studies from the 1,4 and 12 hour groups in the presence of 1 mM malate + 5 mM glutamate and 2.5 mg/ml serum albumin are presented in figure 1.

The St_4 respiration did not change in the 1 hour group. In the other two groups there was a decrease of St_4 respiration. It decreased by 20% in the 4 hour group and by 48% in the 12 hour ischemic group. The St_3 respiration decreased progressively with time. It decreased by 33% in the 1 hour group, by 50% in the 4 hour group and by 80% in the 12 hour ischemic group.

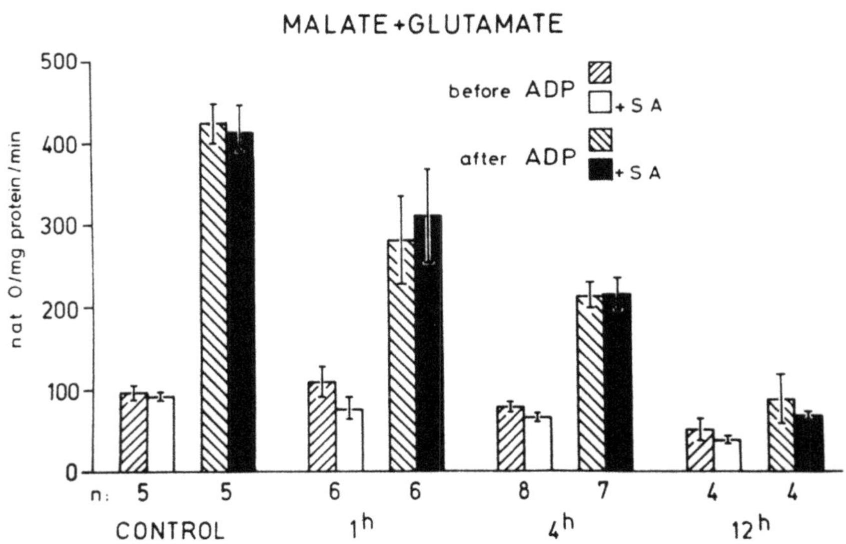

Figure 1.: The effect of 1, 4 and 12 hour ischemic anoxia on the oxidation of 1 mM malate + 5 mM glutamate with and without 2.5 mg/ml serum albumin. St_4 and St_3 respiration were measured. Incubation medium: 0.01 M trisphosphate, 58 mM KCl, 26 mM NaCl, 6 mM $MgCl_2$, pH:7.4; 37C°.

The uncoupling effect of free fatty acids was also studied. In the presence of serum albumin there was a slight decrease in the St_4 respiration in each group. The effect of serum albumin was more pronounced in the 1 hour group. The St_3 respiration was significantly elevated in the 1 hour group and unchanged or decreased in the other two groups after albumin treatment.

The effect of 2.5 mg/ml serum albumin on the RCR is demonstrated in figure 2. In the presence of serum albumin the RCR did not change in the control group. The addition of serum albumin had its maximal effect in the 1 hour ischemic group where the increase of RCR was 1.3. Thus the respiratory damage to mitochondria in the 1 hour group was mostly reversible. The increase of RCR was small in the 4 and 12 hour groups after serum albumin.

Our results support Hossman's observations (1970, 1974) and show that after 1 hour of ischemic-anoxia the function of the mitochondria is well preserved and the damage to them is reversible. However we can not exclude other possibilities, a: most of the non functioning mitochondria are lost during preparation and we measure only the activity of a selected population, b: during the preparation procedure the damaged mitochondrial function is regenerated.

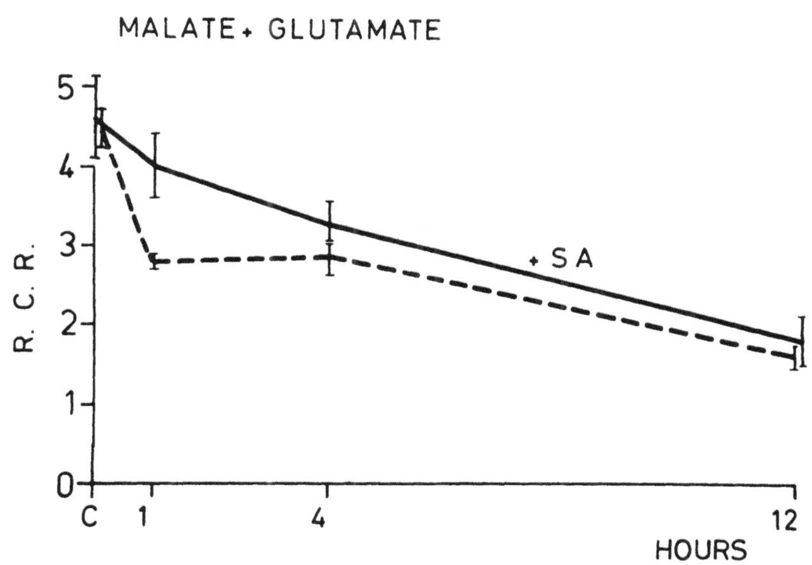

Figure 2.: The effect of 2.5 mg/ml serum albimin on the RCR in the 1, 4, 12 hour ischemic-anoxic groups. Conditions are those described in figure 1.

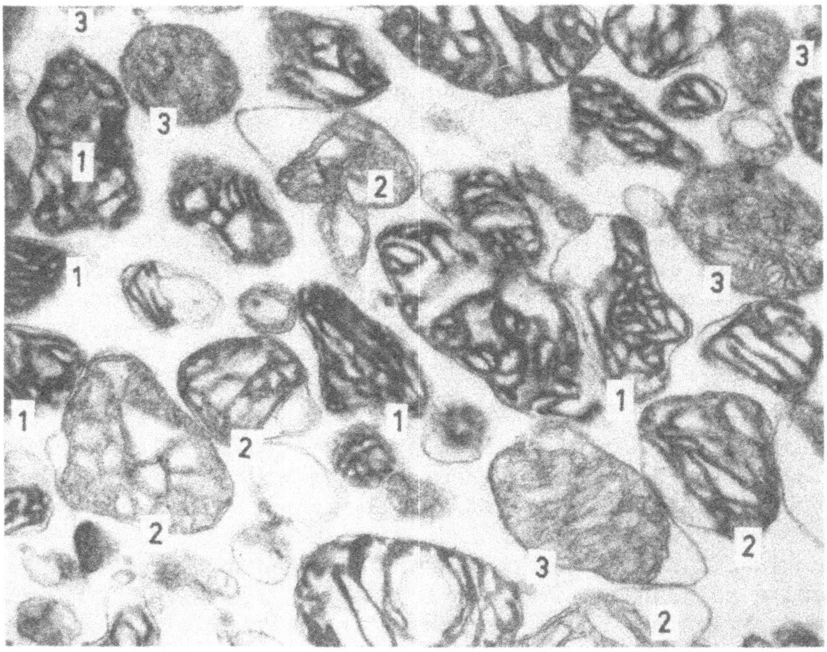

Figure 3.: EM picture from 4 hour ischemic - anoxic group.
1: dense, 2: light, 3: homogenous form.

Analysing the correlation between the mitochondrial function and morphological configuration Hackenbrock (1971) found that the liver mitochondria supplied with oxygen and substrate had a condensed structure. Hajós and coworkers (1975) found that electronmicrographs of brain mitochondria in the coupled state showed them to be in the condensed and not the orthodox form.

Mitochondria prepared from the three ischemic-anoxic groups of our present experiments were examined by EM. Two main mitochondrial structures were differentiated, namely the condensed or dense and the light or orthodox forms. The condensed form is characterized by dark, electron dense matrix and ovoid shape. The light mitochondria were subdivided further into two forms. One of them was characterized by a light matrix, but cristae were present, whereas the other form had more or less lost its inner organization and had a homogeneous light appearance. These forms are illustrated in Fig. 3.

The distribution of dense and light forms as well as RCR in the presence of serum albumin is demonstrated in Fig.4.

As can be seen, the number of light mitochondria increased proportionally with the decrease of the number of the dense type. After one hour of brain ischemia the EM picture of the isolated mitochondria remained unchanged in comparison with the control. The number of dark, electron dense mitochondria decreased by 82% in the 12 hour anoxic group, parallel with the RCR decrease. Our results are in good agreement with the data of Hajós (1975) and Hackenbrock (1971).

The post ischemic transformation of dense to light mitochondria was also observed in the case of EM fixation of brain in situ after 1 hour of anoxia. The isolation procedure could reverse the ratio of light to dense mitochondria in this group but in the case of 4-12 hour in situ anoxic damage the in situ picture showed predominantly the light type only.

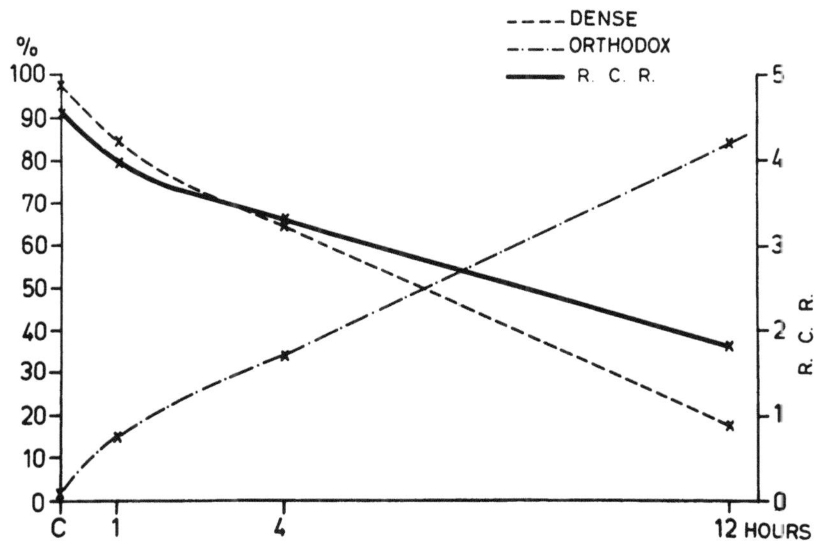

Figure 4.: The distribution of dense and orthodox forms of mitochondria in the different ischemic groups as well as the RCR in the presence of 2,5 mg/ml serum albumin.

Summary

The RCR of malate+glutamate oxidation of isolated rat brain mitochondria decreased with increasing duration of anoxia and it ceased completely in the 12 hour ischemic group. After one hour of ischemic anoxia neither the respiration of mitochondria nor their morphology altered irreversibly. There is a strong correlation between the ultrastructural changes and RCR value of mitochondria, namely the RCR decreased proportionally with increasing number of light type of mitochondria. From our results we can conclude that the dense form seems to be the functional form, while the light mitochondrial structure is a transition to the non functioning homogenous type of brain mitochondria.

References

1./ Brown, A.W., Brierley, B.J.: Brit. J.Exp.Path.49.87.1968.

2./ Clark, J.B., Nicklas, W.J.: J.Biol.Chem. 245. 4724, 1970.

3./ Hackenbrock, C.R., Rehn, T.G.: J.Cell.Biol.51. 123. 1971.

4./ Hager, H. In: Selective Vulnerability of the Brain in Hypoxemia. Schade, J.P., Mc Menemy, W.H.(Eds.) Oxford, Blackwell. p. 125, 1963.

5./ Hajós, F., Csillag, A.: J.Cell. Biol. 1975. In press.

6./ Hossman, K.A., Sato, K.: Z. Neurol. 198. 33. 1970.

7./ Ikrényi, K., Kovách, A.G.B., Somogyi, J.: 39th Meeting of the Hungarian Physiol.Soc. Pécs. 87. 1973.

8./ Karnovsky, M.J.: J. Cell. Biol. 27. 137 A. 1965.

9./ Kleihus, P., Kobayashi, K., Hossman K-A.: J.Neurochem.23. 417, 1974.

10./ Mc Gee-Russel, S.M., Brown, A.W., Brierley, J.B.: Brain Res. 20. 193. 1970.

This work was partially supported by NINDS 10939.

EARLY STRUCTURAL CHANGES IN MITOCHONDRIA IN RESPONSE TO ACUTE REDUCTIONS IN CAPILLARY FLOW

David R. Antonenko and William J. Gibson

Department of Surgery, Royal Alexandra Hospital and Surgical Medical Research Institute, University of Alberta, Edmonton, Alberta, Canada

Swelling of cells after prolonged shock whether septic or hemorrhagic is well accepted. Evidence for cell edema reflected by swelling of mitochondria and sarcoplasmic reticulum is not evident before the late stages of shock (6). However, reductions in cell membrane potential implying interference with the membrane pump and consequent cell edema occur very early after an acute hemorrhage (4).

Because of this discrepancy between physiological and ultrastructural evidence for cell edema in early shock we elected to evaluate the ultrastructural changes in skeletal muscle both quantitatively and qualitatively from the moment of hemorrhage until shock had been established.

Adult male Wistar rats were rapidly hemorrhaged for approximately 40% of their estimated blood volume. Serial biopsies of hind limb thigh muscle were taken as the mean arterial pressure (MAP) decreased and then fixed for electron microscopy. Electron micrographs were used to assess any ultrastructural changes. Application of principles of stereology (8) enabled accurate estimation of capillary and mitochondria volumes. Cell volume was estimated by measuring either the distance between the thick myofilaments of the muscle cell or by calculating the unit cell volume which accounts for any changes in sarcomere length (1). Since capillary diameter can be roughly equated to the conductance (7) some indication of capillary pressure and flow could be obtained with this method.

Capillary volume follows a predictable pattern as the MAP decreases following the hemorrhage (Figure 1). With an initial

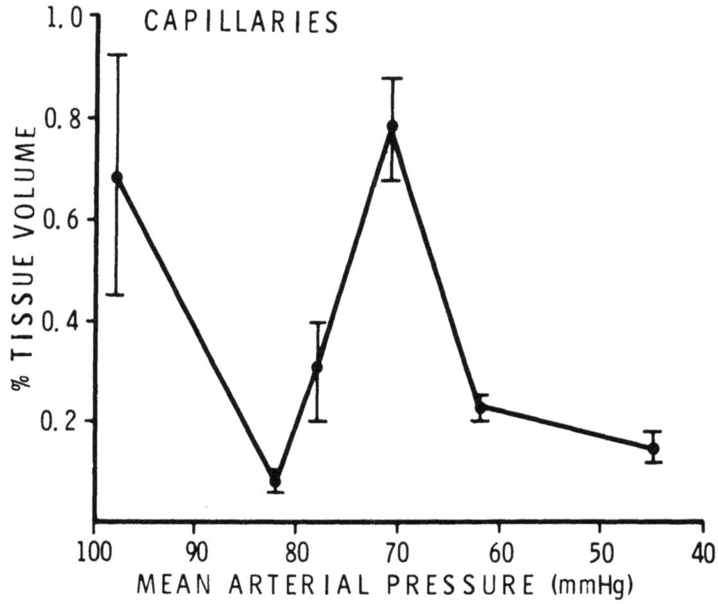

Figure 1. Effect of acute hemorrhage on the volume of capillaries in skeletal muscle.

drop in MAP to 80 mm Hg, there is an 80% reduction in capillary volume ($P < 0.05$). This is followed by a secondary rise to normal volume at 70 mm Hg and then a decrease to only 24% of normal when the MAP decreases to 45 mm Hg ($P < 0.05$). The small variation at the lowest levels of capillary volume implies a general reduction in capillary volume, pressure and flow in contrast to the irregular pattern of flow in normal muscle. This change in capillary volume after hemorrhage follows a course which is compatible with the vascular effects of the sympathetic nervous system's response to hemorrhage (5) or with the capillaron concept advanced by Rodbard (7).

As the MAP decreases cell volume does not change when estimated by either the spacing between thick myofilaments or by the unit cell volume (Figure 2). Even when the cell volume was measured one hour after the MAP had reached 40 mm Hg no change was evident. These results are inconsistent with the studies demonstrating decreases in membrane potential and the cell edema very early in shock but agree with previous ultrastructural studies.

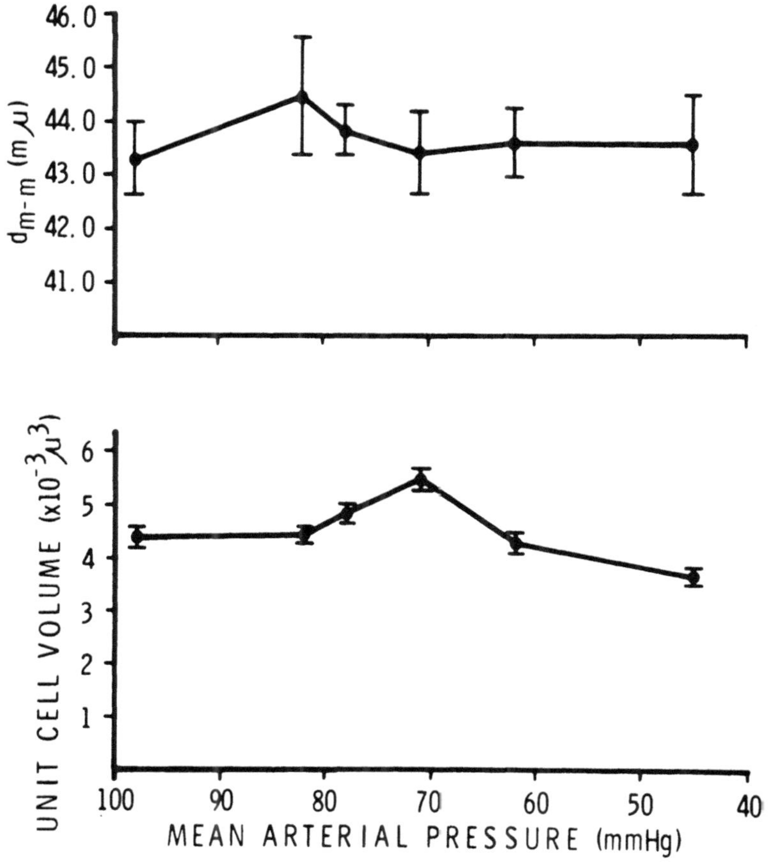

Figure 2. Response of cell volume to acute hemorrhage and reductions in capillary flow. Cell volume, estimated by the spacing between thick myofilaments (d_{m-m}) and by unit cell volume, does not change after hemorrhage.

In contrast to cell volume, mitochondria volume expressed as a percentage of cell volume changes significantly as the MAP decreases (Figure 3). The pattern of variation for mitochondria volume after hemorrhage correlates more with the variation in capillary volume suggesting a direct association between the two independent of any direct effect of hemorrhage on the cell. The secondary rise in mitochondrial volume to 2.5 times normal follows very closely the initial decrease in capillary volume and coincides with the secondary rise in capillary volume and pressure at 70 mm Hg MAP. At 45 mm Hg the volume of the mitochondria has returned to normal.

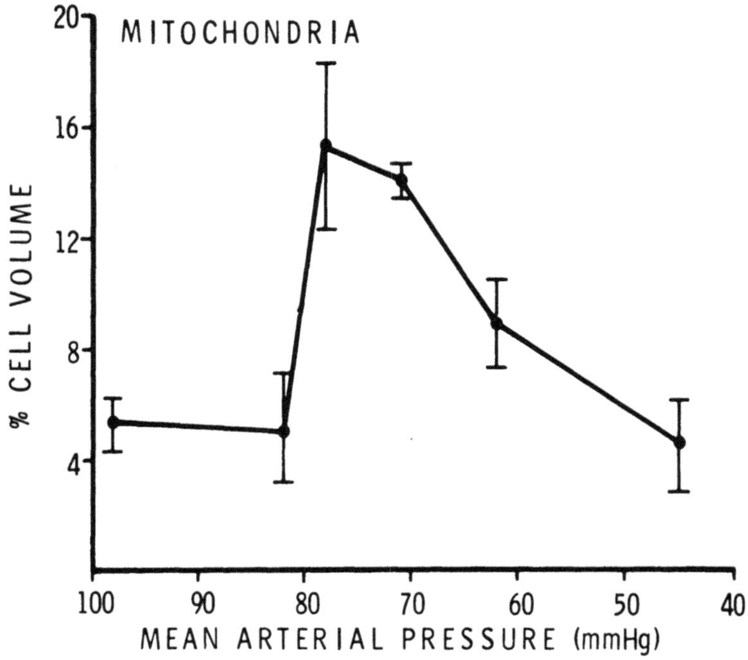

Figure 3. Volume of mitochondria in skeletal muscle cells following an acute hemorrhage. Note significant increase in volume at 75 mm Hg arterial pressure in contrast to no change in cell volume.

Ultrastructural changes during this early phase of shock are confined mainly to the mitochondria. There is either general enlargement of the mitochondria with loss of matrix density but intact cristae (Figure 4,a) or swelling confined to the cristae and intermembranous space with compression of the matrix and occasional disruption of the inner mitochondrial membrane (Figure 4,b). The outer mitochondrial membrane remains intact at all times. Mitochondrial volume and structure at 45 mm Hg MAP is normal.

Differences in the response of cell volume and mitochondrial volume are difficult to explain if mitochondria are intracellular even assuming some translocation of cell water. The explanation is simplified when the association of mitochondria with other cell organelles is examined. Birks and Davey (3) have suggested that sarcoplasmic reticulum communicates directly with the extracellular space. In normal and shock muscle direct luminal continuity between sarcoplasmic reticulum and the intermembranous space of the mitochondria can be frequently seen (Figure 5,a). On occasion we have observed direct membrane continuity of the sarcolemma with the

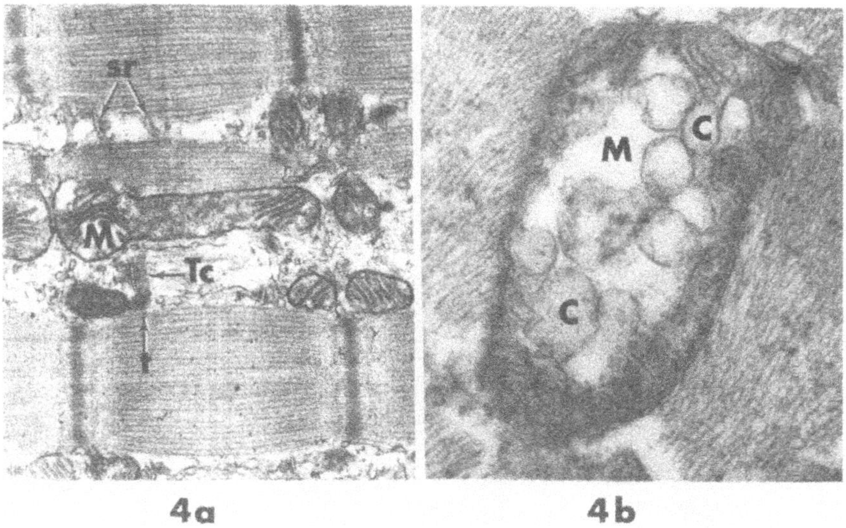

Figure 4. a: Skeletal muscle, longitudinal section, showing enlargement of mitochondria (M) at 70 mm Hg. Sarcoplasmic reticulum (sr), terminal cisternae (Tc) and transverse tubules (t) appear normal (X 6,300). b: Mitochondrion at 70 mm Hg MAP, swelling confined to cristae (c) with compression of matrix (X 50,000).

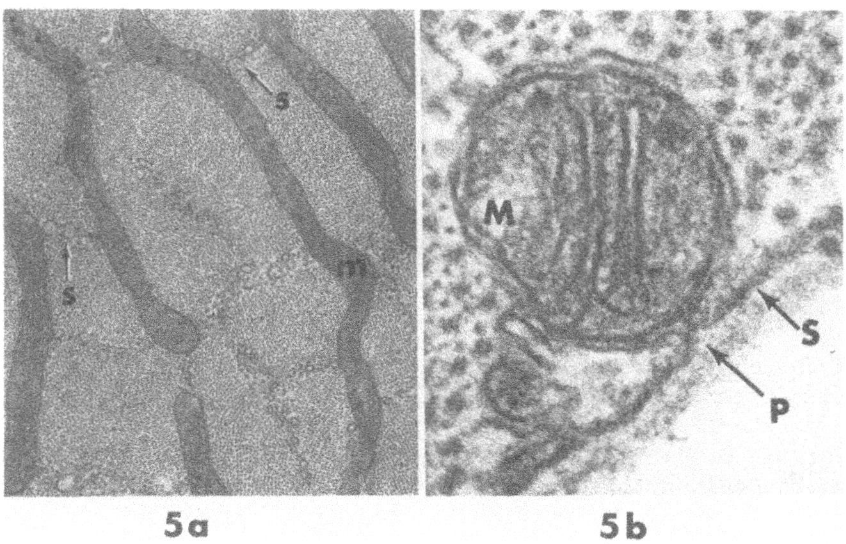

Figure 5. a: Skeletal muscle, I-band cross-section. Note tubular structures (s) connecting adjacent mitochondria (M). (X 23,000). b: Mitochondrion, A-band. Note pore-like communication between the intermembranous space and the sarcolemma (S). (X 141,000).

outer mitochondrial membrane and a pore-like communication of the mitochondrion with the extracellular space (Figure 5,b). Whether this access of the mitochondrion to the extracellular space is continuous or transitional varying with the metabolic activity of the cell remains speculative.

We propose that the endo-membrane system of the skeletal muscle cell, particularly the mitochondrion, has direct access to the extracellular space. Swelling of mitochondria following shock does not reflect cell edema. It reflects the direct effects on mitochondria of variations in the ionic, osmotic, diffusional and pressure characteristics in the extracellular space and capillaries.

REFERENCES

1. April, E. W., P. W. Brandt, G. F. Elliott. The myofilament lat tice studies on isolated fibers, J. Cell. Biol. 53: 53, 1972.

2. Baue, A., and M. S. Mohammed. Alterations in the functional capacity of mitochondria in hemorrhagic shock. Surg. 68: 40, 1970.

3. Birks, R.I., and D. F. Davey. Osmotic responses demonstrating the extracellular character of the sarcoplasmic reticulum. J. Physiol. Lond. 202: 171, 1969.

4. Campion, D.S., L.J. Lynch, F.C. Rector, Jr., N. Carter and G.T. Shires. Effect of hemorrhagic shock on transmembrane potential, Surgery 66: 1051, 1969.

5. Chien, S. Role of the sympathetic nervous system in hemorrhage, Physiol. Rev. 47: 214, 1967.

6. Holden, W.D., R.G. DePalma, W.R. Drucker, A. McKalen, Ultra-structural changes in hemorrhagic shock: Electron microscopic study of liver, kidney and striated muscle cells in rats. Ann. Surg. 162: 517, 1965.

7. Rodbard, S. Capillary control of blood flow and fluid exchange, Circ. Res. 29: 51 Suppl. 1, 1971.

8. Weibel, E. R. Stereological principles for morphometry in electron microscopic cytology. Int. Rev. Cytol. 26: 235, 1969.

THE INDUCTION OF CYTOCHROME P-450 BY HYPOXIA

I. S. Longmuir and Laura Pashko

Department of Biochemistry
North Carolina State University
Raleigh, North Carolina 27609 USA

A number of apparently unrelated observations have led us to look for daily fluctuations in the level of liver cytochrome P-450. We have observed that there seems to be a rather wide variation in P-450 concentrations in different animals of the same sex, age, and species. In addition the Chouteau phenomenon is pronounced in men after midnight, whereas the same stress has no effect in the afternoon. The third observation is that the response to certain drugs is greater in man after midnight than during the day, whereas in nocturnal species the same phenomenon is seen twelve hours out of phase. Since cytochrome P-450 appears to play an important role in both tissue oxygen transport and drug inactivation, these latter effects could be associated with a diurnal variation in the concentration of this pigment.

Our first approach was to examine the validity of the standard analytical method for determining P-450. Estabrook and his colleagues (1970) have shown by direct measurement in tissue slices that the level of P-450 is about four times higher than the figure found by isolation of microsomes. This is partly due to failure to remove all the endoplasmic reticulum as microsomes and partly due to degradation of the cytochrome during the isolation procedure. Unfortunately, the direct measurement in slices has two drawbacks; imperfections in the slice introduce optical errors, and the method cannot be easily adapted to correct for errors due to both haemoglobin and other CO-binding pigments. We, therefore, developed a method using crude homogenate which ensured that all the P-450 was present and which could be conducted quickly so that degradation was minimal. By the use of a third cuvette, a correction could be made for haemoglobin and cytochrome oxidase. It was found that addition of both haemoglobin and heart muscle preparation to the crude liver homogenate did not significantly affect our results.

We used this technique to measure P-450 levels in the livers of seven-week old male Dublin ICR strain white mice at various times during the day and night. The results are shown in Fig. 1. There is a large peak at midnight and a smaller one at midday. In this experiment the lights were on in the animal house from 6:00 a.m. to 6:00 p.m. When we reversed the light cycle for a week, the cyclical changes also reversed as shown in Fig. 2. Subsequent experiments showed that the reversal is complete in three days. In other words, this is an exogenous cycle apparently independent of endogenous factors.

The possibility that this could be due to some direct effect of light was investigated by using light of various wave-lengths. However, preliminary experiments were inconclusive; and it appeared that light was acting indirectly. It seemed reasonable to suggest that feeding might be stimulating P-450 synthesis. However, direct observation of the feeding habits did not show any clear pattern here; and starvation of the animals for 24 hours did not abolish the cycle, although it did diminish the amplitude. Continuous light or dark does, however, completely abolish the cycle whether the mice are fed or not. We found that in continuous darkness the level is uniformly at a value equal to the troughs found in the light cycle. Those kept in continuous light, on the other hand, showed a level equal to the peaks. There was no difference in the food intake or weight gain in the two groups. However, we did think that those in the continuous light were much more active than those in the dark. We, therefore, conducted experiments in which the animals were constrained continuously but fed ad lib. and kept in a twelve-hour illuminated and twelve-hour dark cycle. This group showed an invariant low level of P-450. It thus appeared that it is physical activity that stimulates P-450 synthesis. One of the effects of physical activity is to lower the oxygen tension of the liver (Bishop, Donald, and Wade, 1955). We thought, therefore, that liver hypoxia might be the stimulus to P-450 synthesis as it is for haemoglobin synthesis. We, therefore, exposed mice to hypoxia for periods of six hours and measured the liver P-450. The mice were placed in a vacuum desiccator in the dark with an adequate supply of food and water at a temperature of 27°. The chamber partially evacuated and had a continuous leak to flush out carbon dioxide. When the ambient pressure was atmospheric, the P-450 remained at the same low level found in other mice kept in the dark. However, when the pressure was lowered the level rose but fell at pressures approaching the lethal one. In no experiment did the carbon dioxide level rise above 1%, and separate experiments with 5% carbon dioxide in the chamber showed the synthesis of P-450 was inhibited. The results are shown in Fig. 3.

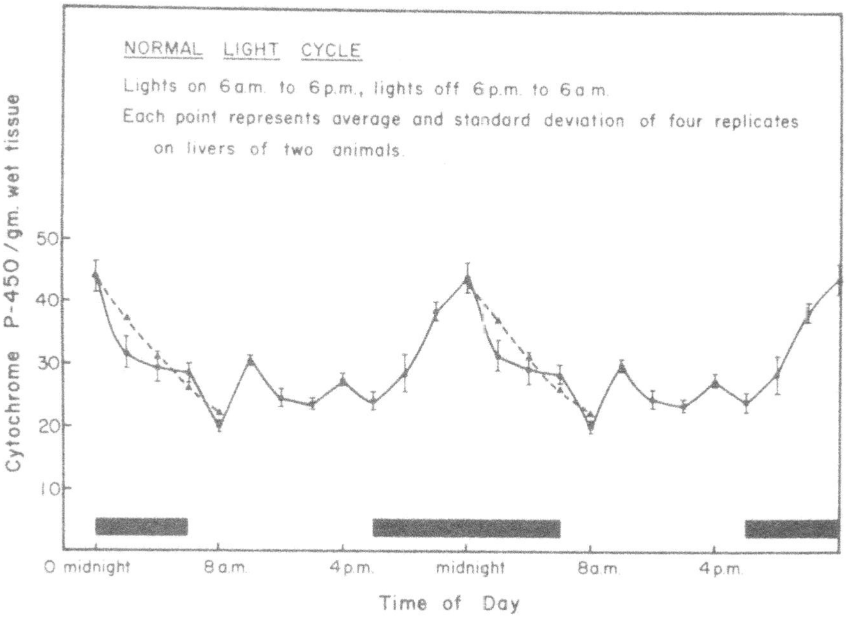

Fig. 1 Variation of cytochrome P-450 concentrations during normal daylight cycle.

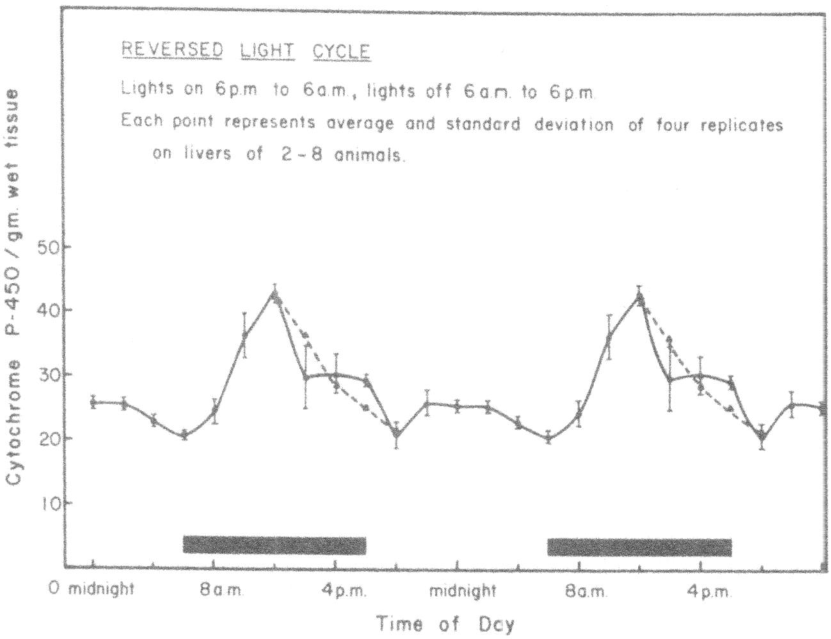

Fig. 2 Same as Fig. 1 but with reversed light cycle.

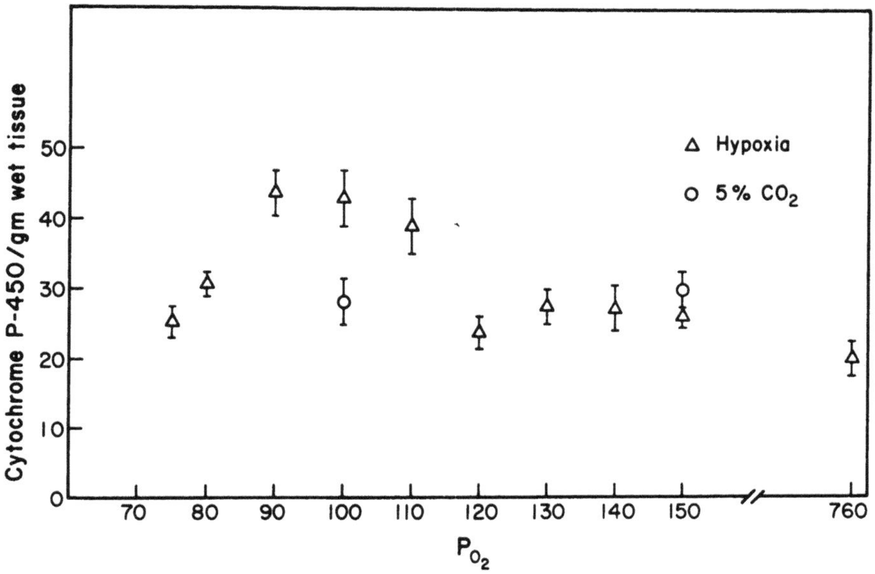

Fig. 3 Cytochrome P-450 levels in mouse livers following 6 hours exposure to varying ambient P_{O_2}. The effect of CO_2 is also shown.

DISCUSSION

It appears that the daily variation in sensitivity to oxygen lack and drug response is associated with daily fluctuations in the level of cytochrome P-450. It is known that this pigment is involved in drug inactivation, and it has been proposed as a tissue carrier of oxygen (Longmuir, 1970). In addition, administration of some drugs will induce its synthesis, thus increasing its ability to detoxify these substances. We have shown in this paper that hypoxia will also induce its synthesis, and it is tempting to hypothesize that this induction will also increase its ability to facilitate the transport of oxygen. It is interesting to note that, whereas the induction of P-450 by phenobarbiturate is a relatively slow process showing little effect until 24 hours, the induction by hypoxia after only 6 hours is quite considerable. We have not yet conducted experiments for longer periods but plan to do so.

Experiments on the acclimation of organisms to hypoxia have shown that there are a number of mechanisms involved. Hyperventilation raises the alveolar P_{O_2}; in residents at high altitudes, there is an increase in lung diffusing capacity, and in acclimated individuals there is an increase in blood oxygen capacity and a decrease in affinity for oxygen. All these acclimations go some way towards increasing the tension at which oxygen is delivered to the tissues over that in unacclimated individuals. However, mechanisms of acclimation at the tissue level are not so clear. The P_{O_2} at the mitochondria is very low, so to deliver the same amount of oxygen to them when the P_{O_2} of the tissue supply is lowered can only be done by facilitating the intracellular transport. Thus the same amount of oxygen can be delivered despite a lowered gradient. We propose that there is such a mechanism. Cytochrome P-450 in normoxic conditions is responsible for transporting an appreciable proportion of the oxygen used by the mitochondria, and it increases in amount in hypoxia and so can transport an increased proportion of oxygen.

Acknowledgements. This work was supported by N.I.H. Biomedical Sciences Support Grant No. RR 07071.

REFERENCES

Bishop, J. M., K. W. Donald, and O. L. Wade (1955) J. Clin. Invest. 34:1114.

Estabrook, R. W., A. Sligematsu, and J. B. Schenkman (1970) Advances in Enzyme Regulation 8:121.

Longmuir, I. S. (1970) 6th Europ. Conf. Microcirculation, Aalborg. (Karger, Basel) p. 3.

SUMMARY OF DISCUSSION - SESSION III:

TISSUE RESPIRATION

Chairmen: D. W. Lübbers and F. F. Jöbsis

Regarding the paper of D. F. Wilson, Philadelphia, the discussion was centered on the transition of this approach from the *in vitro* studies to the intracellular situation. In this respect Wilson pointed out that cellular pH and free Mg^{++} concentrations can be considered constant and that the $NADH/NAD^+$ ratios obtained from tissue analysis are not applicable since only the intramitochondrial fraction associated directly with oxidative phosphorylation is relevant but cannot be identified by tissue analysis. In addition, the speaker pointed out that the K_M values for cytochrome a_3 to O_2 are actually apparent K_M values only, since the existence of a peroxide intermediate must be postulated. Except for this complication, which should also affect the apparent V_M, the (ATP)/(ADP)·(P_i) should control the cytochrome $\underline{a}_3$ reaction. The result of increasing this ratio should qualitatively increase the apparent K_M and decrease the apparent V_M. Lack of sufficiently detailed data at defined (ATP)/(ADP)·(P_i) and of mitochondrial (NADH)/(NAD^+) prevents a quantitative expression at this time. Dr. Wilson also pointed that the use of uncouplers produces complex situations. With increasing dinitrophenol concentrations, for example, a region of mixed ATP-ase-like activity and oxidative phosphorylation must be passed until the latter function is completely abolished. At this point the respiratory rate is determined by a complex function of substrate availability, steady-state reduction of the respiratory chain and of "high energy" intermediates. It is highly questionable whether equilibrium conditions exist. At even higher uncoupler concentrations the mitochondrial integrity is lost and further effects develop by direct influence of the uncoupler dehydrogenases and other components.

Regarding the paper of H. Versmold, B. Brauser and K. Riegel, München, the discussion brought up the question of 2-3 DPG produced recruitment of capillaries. The possibility was rejected, since in control experiments without hemoglobin no direct influence on the O_2 uptake or the redox state of cytochrome a/a_3 could be seen. Neither penetration of 2-3 DPG into the hepatocytes nor a direct effect on mitochondrial reactions was considered likely as an explanation of the presented results. It was emphasized that proof for increased O_2 unloading derives boths from the unchanged venous Po_2 after DPG addition and from the spectra. In fact it is possible to calculate the amount of increased O_2 delivery from the hemoglobin spectra and from knowledge of the total vascular volume in the transilluminated tissue. The value is about 0.3 µm atoms of oxygen released per ml blood by the DPG treatment. It agrees with the value calculated from the P_{50} and the venous Po_2.

In addition it was pointed out that an indication of a cytochrome oxidation during perfusion with DPG blood and that the lack of clear indication in the difference spectrum of anoxic minus hypoxic conditions may only be due to the large hemoglobin peak that occurs under such conditions in the 555 nm region. It is encouraging to note that during normoxic perfusion cytochrome c is approximately 15 % reduced, in agreement with the scheme of Chance and Williams (1955) for isolated mitochondria.

Regarding the paper of P. Scheid, T. Kawashiro and J. Piiper, Göttingen, it was pointed out that the O_2 dissociation of human red cells is left-shifted when the measurements are made in isotonic phosphate since the intracellular pH increases in response to the new Gibbs-Doman conditions. Since Lutz et al. used isotonic phosphate as suspension medium for the duck red blood cells, it is highly likely that their left-shifted data exhibit the same effect. Thus the difference between the two sets of results might to a large part be due to differences in the suspension media.

The discussion of the paper of D. R. Antonenko and W. J. Gibbs, Edmonton, was both intensive and extensive. In summary, the problems of fixation technique, possibly persisting microcirculation at 80 mm Hg and occurrence of hypothermia were rejected as causes for the observed effects mainly on the basis of comparisons with parallel studies and with different methods. Questions concerning the mechanisms of mitochondrial swelling other than the possibility mentioned in the paper were not as easily answered. Thus the well-known swelling which takes place during Ca^{++} accumulation could play a rôle. So could changes in the pumping of other ions. These questions remain to be answered. Another persistent topic was the absence of previous reports on possible continuity of the sarcoplastic reticulum (SR) with the ECF or of mitochondrial membranes with the sarcolemma. Dr. Antonenko pointed out that indications of penetration of markers into the SR have been found by Davey and Bicks but denied by Franzini-Armstrong. Sperelakis and his group have demonstrated penetration of ruthenium red into the SR but not (yet ?) into the mitochondrial outer compartment. Thus a question of pore size may be involved since horse-radish peroxidase, the most commonly employed marker, has a much larger size. Walker et al. have previously demonstrated continuity between SR and mitochondria. Again, however, this is not a generally accepted notion at this moment. It was generally agreed that the possible "extracellular location" of mitochondria would require a considerable revision in our thinking.

Oxygen Diffusion in Blood and Tissue

DIFFUSION OF OXYGEN IN PLASMA AND BLOOD

Thomas K. Goldstick, Vincent T. Ciuryla, and
Leon Zuckerman
Chemical Engineering Department, Northwestern University
and Research Laboratories, Evanston Hospital
Evanston, Illinois 60201, USA

Quantitative analysis of oxygen transport in blood requires accurate values for the oxygen diffusion coefficient (D) in blood plasma and in whole blood. There has been a controversy over the effect of plasma composition on D. One group [1] has found a precipitous drop in plasma D with small changes in the concentrations of various common plasma proteins. This would have profound physiological and pathological consequences [2,3]. Other groups [4,5,6] have found D in solutions of plasma proteins to be well-behaved, decreasing regularly with increasing protein concentration. None of these measurements, however, have been made on natural human plasma. The present study, which used freshly drawn human plasma, found that D decreased almost linearly with total protein content, even in very abnormal plasmas. It also found that the D in plasma and its serum were identical and that serum could be stored frozen for several months without changing its D. From measurements of D in plasma, and literature values for D in packed red blood cells, D in whole blood was estimated.

METHOD

D was determined by an unsteady state technique employing a Clark-type oxygen electrode positioned beneath a thin layer of plasma, approximately 1 mm thick, in a closed diffusion cell (Figure 1). After the plasma layer had equilibrated with an initial gas, usually air, the PO_2 of the gas in the cell was abruptly changed, usually to 5% O_2 in N_2. The dissolved O_2 then diffused out of the layer until a new equilibrium was attained. During the unsteady state period, about 15 mins, the oxygen electrode continuously monitored the PO_2 at the bottom of the layer. Elaborate precautions were taken

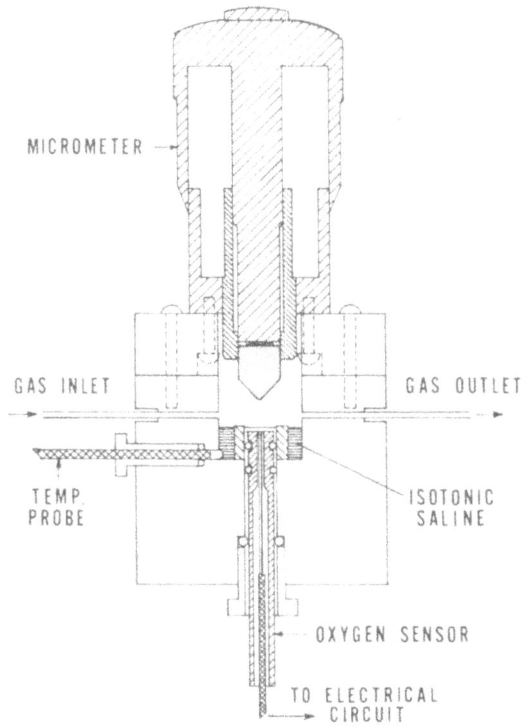

FIGURE 1: APPARATUS FOR DETERMINATION OF D

to avoid both mechanical and thermal convection. The thickness of the plasma layer was measured, to ±10μ, by slowly lowering the micrometer tip shown in Figure 1 until it just touched the liquid surface. All tests were made at ambient temperature, usually close to 25°C, and corrected to other temperatures using the experimentally verified coefficient of 2.5%/°C. The temperature variation during an acceptable test had to be < 0.3°C.

A mathematical analysis of the electrode transient was used to calculate D. It has been shown [5] that the solution of the diffusion equation for the conditions employed in this experimental procedure is:

$$\frac{P - P_\infty}{P_0 - P_\infty} = \frac{4}{\pi}\sum_{n=0}^{\infty} \frac{(-1)^n}{(2n+1)} \exp\left[-\frac{(2n+1)^2 \pi^2 D t}{4\ell^2}\right] \tag{1}$$

where P is the PO_2 at the closed bottom surface of the layer, torr

P_0 and P_∞ are the initial and final values of P

D is the oxygen diffusion coefficient, cm^2/sec

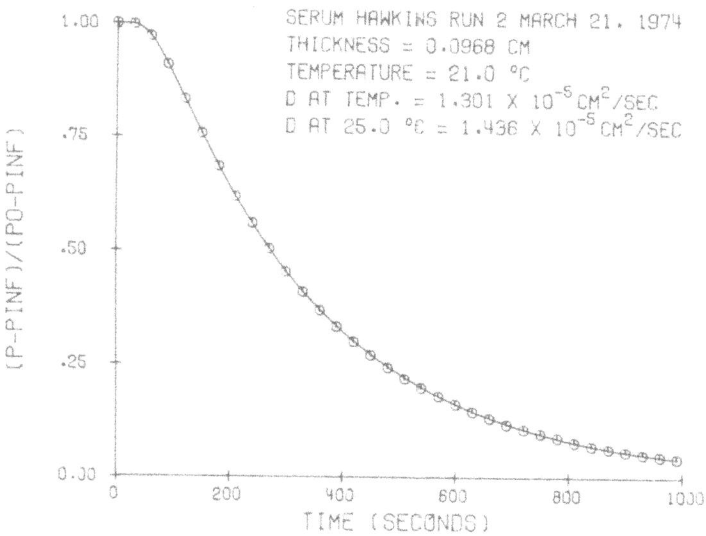

FIGURE 2: TYPICAL DIFFUSION TEST
The points are experimental and the line is the first five terms of equation 1 with D adjusted to give the best fitting curve.

t is time, sec
and ℓ is the thickness of the layer, cm.

The oxygen electrode current was always linear with P and so the left hand side of equation 1 is actually the relative current. A nonlinear least square fitting routine [7] was used to fit the experimentally measured transient current to the first five terms of equation 1 to find D. D was the only arbitrary parameter in this fitting procedure. It is significant to note that the transient solution given in equation 1 contains neither the oxygen solubility coefficient nor any arbitrary constants. The method used to evaluate D was therefore absolute.

For a diffusion test to be acceptable, the results had to agree almost exactly with equation 1. Figure 2 shows typical agreement. When a test was disturbed by convection the agreement was invariably very bad and the results rejected.

Total protein content (TP, g/100 ml) was determined using a modified Folin phenol method [7] with an estimated accuracy of ±5%. A polyacrylamide gel disc electrophoresis method [7] was used to determine the concentrations of 10 common plasma proteins (prealbumin, albumin, postalbumin, transferrin, haptoglobin, γ-globulin, α_2-macroglobulin, LDL, VLDL, HDL). Fibrinogen was also determined using a standard method [7].

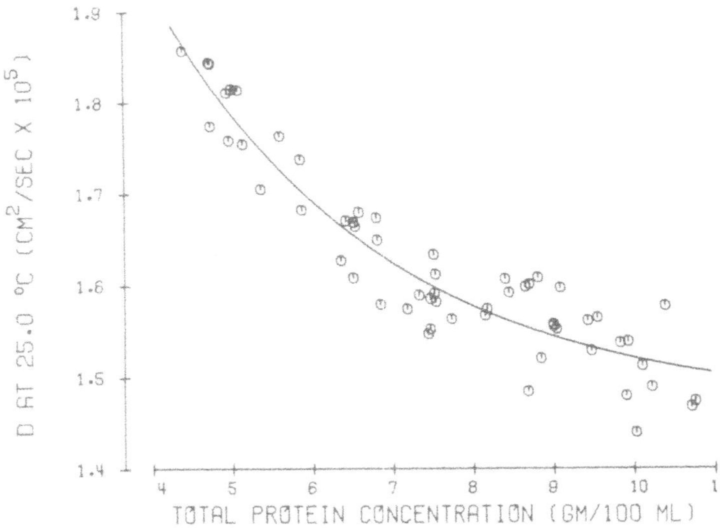

FIGURE 3: D IN HUMAN PLASMA AT 25°C

RESULTS AND DISCUSSION

To confirm the accuracy of the experimental method, D was determined in distilled water. From 43 separate determinations, D ± one standard deviation was found to be $2.11 \pm 0.02 \times 10^{-5}$ cm^2/sec, at 25°C, in good agreement with previously published values [5]. To verify the internal consistency of the method, D was measured in distilled water under different conditions. D did not vary significantly over a considerable range of ℓ or with different gas regimes. An important measure of internal consistency, of course, was also the excellent agreement between the experimental data and equation 1. D was also found to be the same in plasma and serum, in fresh and stored serum, and in samples of fresh plasma from the same individual drawn months apart. Citrate when used also had no affect on D.

Figure 3 shows the values for D in 57 different human plasmas (or sera), 13 normal and 44 abnormal. The scatter of the data, ±4%, is approximately what would be expected from errors in the experimental methods for both D and TP. The curve is the best nonlinear least squares regression fit of the data. It has the equation:

$$D = 1.8688\ (0.7841 + 0.7033^{TP}) \times 10^{-5} \qquad 4 < TP < 11 \quad (2)$$

In normal human plasma, D ranged from only 1.55 to 1.67×10^{-5} cm^2/sec with a mean of 1.62×10^{-5} cm^2/sec. From over 3000 samples drawn routinely from hospital patients, 21 had extremely abnormal protein content, TP < 5 or TP > 9. For these abnormal plasmas, D was found to range from 1.44 to $1.86 \times 10^{-5} \cdot cm^2/sec$. This is probably close to

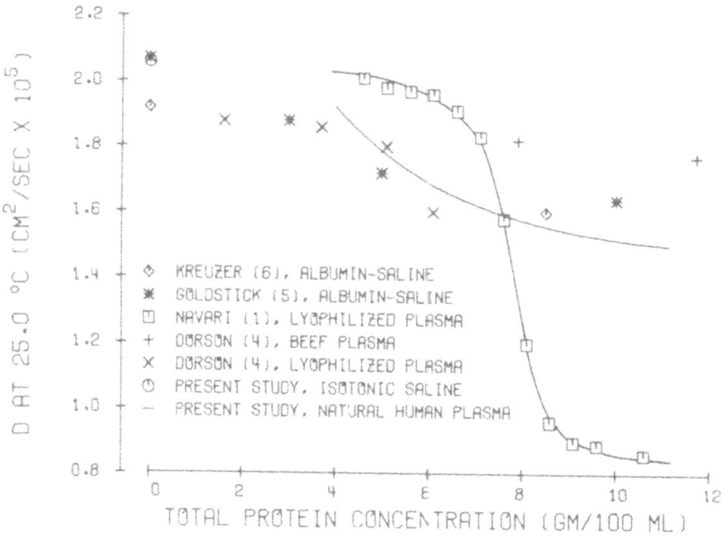

FIGURE 4: D IN HUMAN PLASMA AND COMPARABLE SOLUTIONS

the maximum range for D in plasma because, from demographic data, one might expect to encounter an individual outside this range only extremely rarely. Values of D at 25°C may be adjusted to 37°C using 2.5%/°C, i.e., by multiplying by 1.345.

A multiple linear step-wise regression analysis of D with the individual protein concentrations indicated a rather uniformly well-behaved system, with no one individual regression coefficient having an overwhelming effect. A predictive equation for D in terms of the various major protein fractions did not show any significant predictive advantage over equation 2. Both equations could predict D to ±3% (for 90% of the values) with no statistically significant difference in their predictive ability. This suggests that no single plasma component is conspicuously more important than another in determining D. Only the sum of all the protein concentrations appears to be important.

It has been suggested [1] that differences in D between serum and plasma might be expected because of the non-globular shape of the fibrinogen molecule. In the present study no substantial differences were noted in D whether measured in serum or plasma, indicating that the usual fibrinogen levels have little, if any, effect upon oxygen diffusion.

Figure 4 compares the curve of Figure 3 (equation 2) with other previously reported values of D measured in comparable protein solutions. Although the present results are in marked disagreement with those of Navari et al. [1], they are in reasonable agreement with

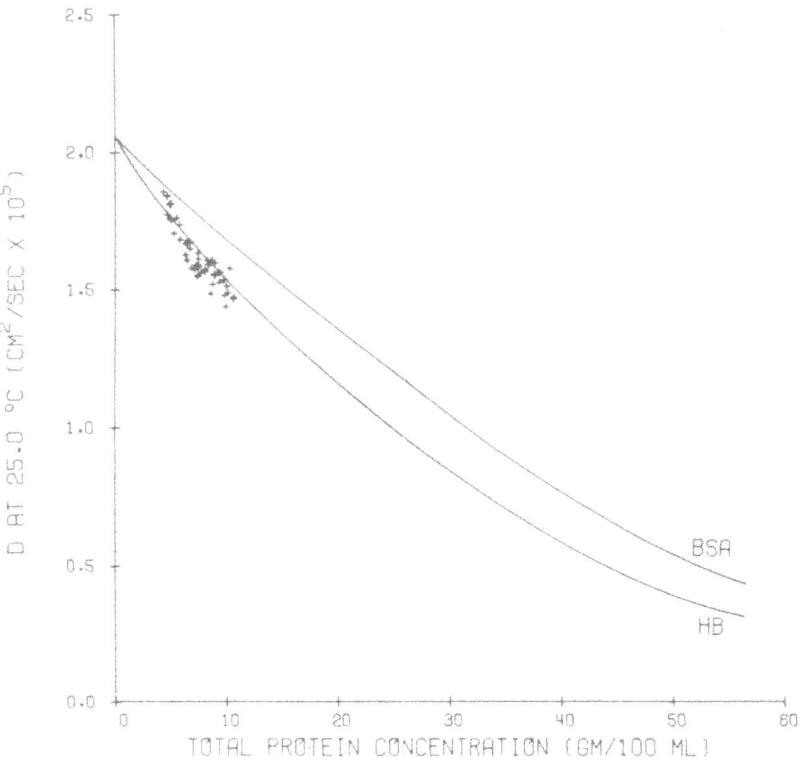

FIGURE 5: COMPARISON OF D IN HUMAN PLASMA WITH D IN BOVINE SERUM ALBUMIN AND HUMAN OXYHEMOGLOBIN SOLUTIONS [5]

other published data [4,5,6]. All of the data shown in Figure 4, except those of Navari et al. [1], were obtained by different unsteady state methods. However, only the present data were obtained on fresh human plasma. There are three major differences between the present method and that of Navari et al. [1]: 1. the use of natural plasma rather than simulated plasma solutions reconstituted from lyophilized protein constituents; 2. the use of an inert cell rather than a sintered glass diaphragm cell which could have caused protein denaturation; 3. the use of a rapid method (15 mins) rather than one which took many hours during which protein deterioration could have occurred. Perhaps these differences in method account for the different results obtained. The present results may also be compared with measurements of D in protein solutions over a much wider range [5] as shown in Figure 5. Again the agreement is quite good.

Based on the measured values for D in human plasma, literature values for D in hemoglobin solutions [5] and packed red cells [8], and oxygen solubility estimations [9], D in normal whole blood was calculated [7] using a Fricke-type [10] model (Figure 6). The red

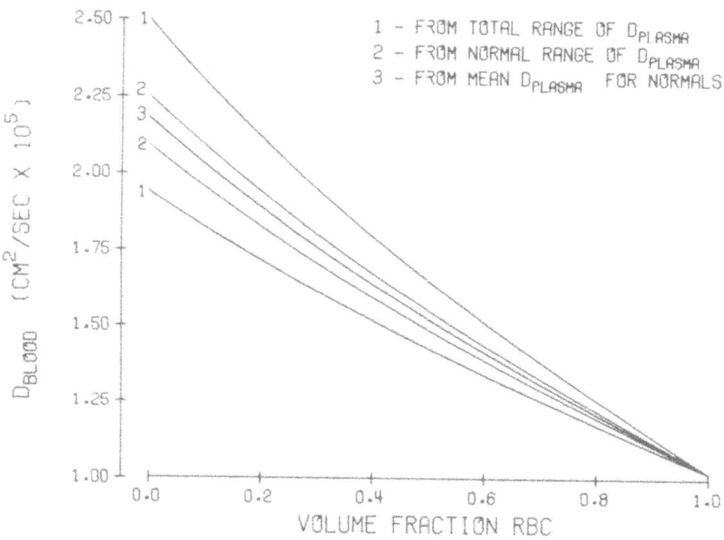

FIGURE 6: EFFECTIVE D IN WHOLE BLOOD AT 37°C
All parameters except D in human plasma were taken from the literature (see text).

blood cell membrane was considered to offer a negligible resistance [8]. The red blood cell was modelled by an oblate spheroid of axial ratio 4.25. Variations in the assumed red blood cell shape have been found [8] to have little effect on this calculation. In blood of average hematocrit (42%), at 37°C, D exhibits a mean value of 1.62 x 10^{-5} cm^2/sec. At this hematocrit, D within the normal range (curves 2) varies from only 1.57 to 1.65 x 10^{-5} and within the abnormal (curves 1), from 1.50 to 1.77 x 10^{-5} cm^2/sec.

SUMMARY

D in fresh human plasma has been found to decrease almost linearly with total protein content over a wide range of concentration and to vary only ±4% in normals and ±13% in abnormals. The average values for D in normal human plasma, at 25 and 37°C, are 1.62 and 2.18 x 10^{-5} cm^2/sec respectively. For normal human blood at 42% hematocrit, the values of D, at 25 and 37° C, are 1.20 and 1.62 x 10^{-5} cm^2/sec respectively.

ACKNOWLEDGEMENTS

This research was supported by Evanston Hospital grants 3565 and 3595, NIH grants GM-17115, GM-00874, and HL-17517, and Chicago Heart Association grant A74-37. We are also grateful to Dr. D.

Forman for providing some serum samples and to C.G. Ellis and G. Schneiderman for their advice and assistance.

REFERENCES

1. Navari, R.M., Gainer, J.L., and Hall, K.R., "Effect of Plasma Constituents on Oxygen Diffusivity", in "Blood Oxygenation" ed. by D. Hershey, pp. 243-261, Plenum Press, New York (1970).
2. Bryant, S.C. and Navari, R.M., "Effect of Plasma Proteins on Oxygen Diffusion in the Pulmonary Capillaries", Microvasc. Res., 7, 120-130 (1974).
3. Chisolm, G.M., Gainer, J.L., Stoner, G.E., and Gainer, J.V., Jr., "Plasma Proteins, Oxygen Transport and Atherosclerosis", Atherosclerosis, 15, 327-342 (1972).
4. Dorson, W.J., Yee, R., Larsen, K.G., Elgas, R.J., and Voorhees, M.E., "Oxygen Diffusion in Blood and Plasma", Proc. 24th ACEMB, 13, 280 (1971); Dorson, W.J., Personal Communication (October 29, 1974).
5. Goldstick, T.K. and Fatt, I., "Diffusion of Oxygen in Solutions of Blood Proteins", Chem. Eng. Prog. Symp. Ser. No. 99, 66, 101-113 (1970).
6. Kreuzer, F., "Über die Diffusion von Sauerstoff in Serumeiweisslösungen verschiedener Konzentration", Helv. Physiol. Acta, 8, 505-516 (1950).
7. Ciuryla, V.T., "Oxygen Diffusion in Human Blood Plasma", Ph.D. thesis, Northwestern University, Evanston, Ill. (1975).
8. Stein, T.R., Martin, J.C., and Keller, K.H., "Steady-State Oxygen Transport Through Red Blood Cell Suspensions", J. Appl. Physiol., 31, 397-402 (1971).
9. Goldstick, T.K., "Oxygen Transport", in "Engineering Principles in Physiology", Vol. II, ed. by J.H.U. Brown and D.S. Gann, pp. 257-282, Academic Press, New York (1973).
10. Fricke, H., "Electrical Conductivity and Capacity of Disperse Systems; Mathematical Treatment I. Conductivity of a Suspension of Homogeneous Spheroids", Phys. Rev., 24, 575-587 (1924).

FACILITATED DIFFUSION OF OXYGEN IN RED BLOOD CELL SUSPENSIONS

Pieter Stroeve, Kenneth A. Smith, and Clark K. Colton

Department of Physiology, University of Nijmegen, Holland and Department of Chemical Engineering, Massachusetts Institute of Technology, USA

A general model that treats the problem of diffusion with reversible chemical reaction in heterogeneous media has recently been developed (12, 11). This theory has been applied to the theoretical analysis of oxygen diffusion in red blood cell suspensions (13). Blood is modeled as a suspension of uniform spheres containing hemoglobin, which are suspended in a second continuous phase. In order to predict the steady state transport in such a medium, first the mass conservation equations are solved for a single reactive sphere located in an infinite nonreactive continuous medium in which a constant linear flux of the diffusing species A is imposed at a large distance from the center of the sphere. If the oxygen-hemoglobin reaction is modeled as a single step reaction of the form,

$$A + B \underset{k_2}{\overset{k_1}{\rightleftharpoons}} AB \qquad (1)$$

the equations inside the sphere and outside the sphere are nonlinear and must be linearized in order to be solved analytically. For a small sphere in a medium the partial pressure drop of A across an individual sphere is usually small so that a single point linearization technique is applicable (3). The equations are linearized about a single point by neglecting second order terms. By solving the linearized equations analytically, one can obtain the variation of the potential of A due to the presence of the sphere in the continuum. Second, for the analysis of a dilute suspension of spheres, the suspension is considered to be confined to a spherical region and located in an infinite continuous medium. By assuming the perturbation associated with each of the smaller spheres inside this spherical suspension to be independent of each other, an effective permeability for the reactive suspension can be obtained

$$\overline{P} = P_c \frac{2\,P_c + P_d\,(1 + F_d) - 2\,\Phi\,\left[P_c - P_d\,(1 + F_d)\right]}{2\,P_c + P_d\,(1 + F_d) + \Phi\,\left[P_c - P_d\,(1 + F_d)\right]} \qquad (2)$$

where P_c is the continuous phase permeability, P_d is the dispersed phase permeability, and Φ is the volume fraction of suspended spheres. The dispersed phase facilitation factor F_d is a measure of the contribution of the flux of A by the carrier molecules in the dispersed phase and for reaction 1 is given by

$$F_d = \frac{F_d^{eq}\left[\dfrac{(3\frac{\lambda^2}{a^2} + 1)\tanh\frac{a}{\lambda} - 3\frac{\lambda}{a}}{(2\frac{\lambda^2}{a^2} + 1)\tanh\frac{a}{\lambda} - 2\frac{\lambda}{a}}\right]}{1 + F_d^{eq}\left[1 - \dfrac{(3\frac{\lambda^2}{a^2} + 1)\tanh\frac{a}{\lambda} - 3\frac{\lambda}{a}}{(2\frac{\lambda^2}{a^2} + 1)\tanh\frac{a}{\lambda} - 2\frac{\lambda}{a}}\right]} \qquad (3)$$

The dispersed phase characteristic length, λ, gives a measure of the thickness of a shell at the inside of each sphere where deviations from chemical equilibrium are significant. For reaction 1

$$\lambda = \left[\frac{k_1\,\alpha_A p_A + k_2}{D_B} + \frac{k_1\,\alpha_A k_2 C_T}{P_d(k_1\,\alpha_A p_A + k_2)}\right]^{-\frac{1}{2}} \qquad (4)$$

where α_A is the solubility of A inside the sphere, C_T is the total carrier concentration, and D_B is the carrier diffusivity. When the ratio of sphere radius to characteristic length, a/λ, approaches infinity, the reaction is at equilibrium throughout the sphere and F_d approaches its equilibrium value

$$F_d^{eq} = \frac{D_B\,k_1 k_2 C_T\,\alpha_A}{P_d(k_2 + k_1\,\alpha_A p_A)^2} \qquad (5)$$

When a/λ approaches zero the reaction deviates from equilibrium throughout the sphere and F_d approaches zero. In this case eq.2 reduces to Maxwell's equation for inert heterogeneous media (8).

The effective permeability as given by eq.2 is defined only at a local point within the suspension, or for the total suspension when the driving force across the total physical system is very small. If one considers a slab composed of such a suspension which has imposed upon it a large partial pressure gradient of A, then the average effective permeability of the slab may be calculated by integrating the local expression over the thickness of the film

$$\overline{P}_{AVE} = \int_{p_A^L}^{p_A^o} \overline{P}\, dp_A / (p_A^o - p_A^L) \qquad (6)$$

The total flux of A across the film is given by

$$N_A = \overline{P}_{AVE}\, (p_A^o - p_A^L) \;/\; L \qquad (7)$$

where p_A^o and p_A^L are the partial pressures of A at the upstream and downstream side of the layer.

In this work the theory is utilized to analyse the steady state oxygen transport data obtained in thin films of red blood cell suspensions at 25°C (12, 14). Oxygen transport rates were measured with driving forces in the unsaturated regime of the oxygen-hemoglobin saturation curve for a variety of volume fractions. Using available physico-chemical constants, the comparison of theory with data suggests that the oxygen-hemoglobin reaction is not at equilibrium at 25°C. Previously published data are then analyzed. Based on this comparison predictions are made for the oxygen transport at physiological conditions. The effect of hemolysis on oxygen transport rate is discussed.

EXPERIMENTAL

Red blood cells were removed from fresh whole blood by centrifugation, washed thrice, and resuspended in isotonic phosphate buffer. Thin liquid films of the red blood cell suspensions were supported on each side by thin silicone support membranes in a sample holder. The mass transfer resistance of the membrane to O_2 was small and was taken into account in the data reduction. The experimental apparatus was designed as a modification of Barrer's classical time-lag apparatus (9). The experiments involved the introduction of O_2 gas at one side of the liquid layer and recording the downstream O_2 change with time as the gas emerged at the other side. Oxygen permeabilities were obtained from the steady-state mass transfer rate for known conditions of driving force, thickness of liquid film, and total mass transfer area (12).

RESULTS, DISCUSSION, and CONCLUSIONS

Experimental data points obtained from the measurement of steady state oxygen transport in red blood cell suspensions are shown in figures 1 and 2 for two different driving force conditions and various hematocrits(Hct = 100 Φ). The driving forces were chosen such that large saturation differences existed across the films. In such cases the one-step reaction scheme is expected to give reasonable predictions of the average effective permeability if compared to a more elaborate scheme such as that proposed by Adair (15). The theoretical lines in figures 1 and 2 were obtained by numerical integration of the analytical expression for the local effective permeability and are shown as a function of sphere radius. The inert line is equivalent to Maxwell's equation and corresponds to a suspension of very small spheres or a suspension with nonreactive hemoglobin. The line was obtained from oxygen diffusion experiments in red blood cell suspensions where the hemoglobin was completely saturated (14). The intercept at a hematocrit of 100 is equal to P_{RBC}/P_{saline}. Also on the figures is given the minimum and maximum red blood cell radii, which are 1 μ m and 4 μ m respectively. The equilibrium line is predicted for spheres of a larger size. The hemoglobin diffusivity employed in these calculations is 7.0 x 10^{-8} cm^2/sec and is consistent with data compiled by Kreuzer (5) at C_T = 33 gr/100 ml. The forward reaction rate is 3.0 x 10^6 1/mole/sec (4) and the backward rate was chosen such that the hyperbolic saturation curve predicted by equation 1 gave the same p_{50} as that measured experimentally (p_{50} = 13.5 mm Hg(12)). The data show, that for the reported conditions, oxygen transport is facilitated, and the results scatter in the region defined by the a = 1 μ m and 4 μ m curves. Other hemoglobin diffusivity values were also used but the value employed here gave the best results compared to these and additional data (12, 14).

There exist other published data with which to compare the theoretical model. Kutchai and Staub (7) reported steady state oxygen transport experiments through films of packed red blood cells at 21.5°C, in which the oxygen partial pressure at one side of the film was maintained near zero and the partial pressure at the other side was varied. The liquid films were supported by a thin wire screen with a thickness approximately one third of the total thickness of the films. The data points were compared with the theory by the following procedure. First, using the parameters employed previously as a basis, the physico-chemical parameters were calculated at 21.5°C and a hemoglobin concentration of 29.6 gr/100 ml. The temperature coefficient for the oxygen diffusivity is 2.5%/°C and 3.3%/°C for the hemoglobin diffusivity, and the oxygen solubility was obtained from literature (1). Second, the experiments obtained for oxygen diffusion through nonreactive packed red blood cells were compared with diffusion data reported in the literature in order to

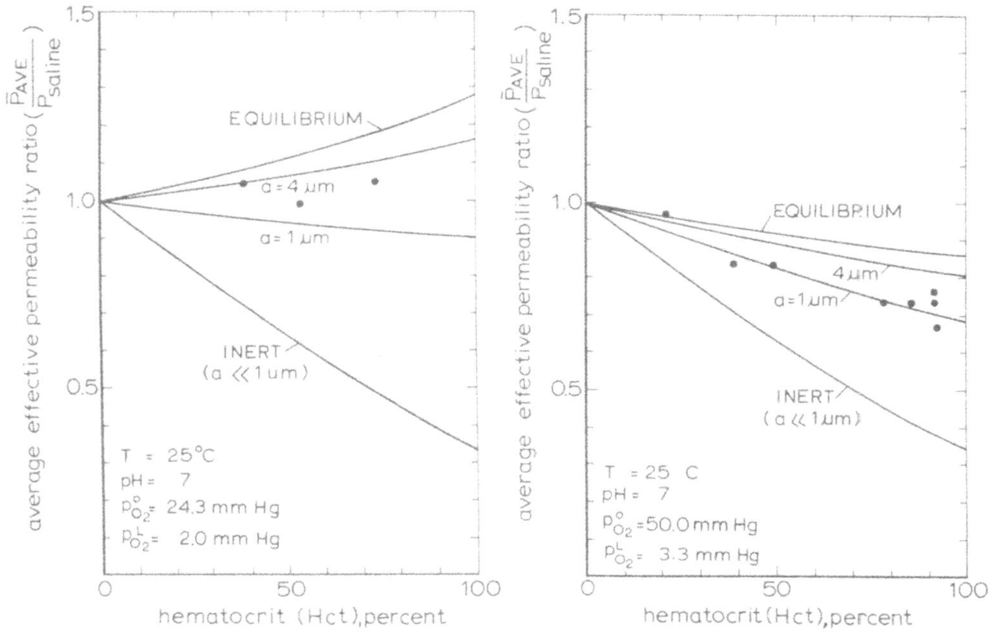

Figures 1 and 2. Average effective permeability ratio in red blood cell suspensions. Values for parameters are $P_{saline} = 3.52 \times 10^{-14}$ moles/cm/sec/mm Hg, $P_{RBC} = 1.20 \times 10^{-14}$ moles/cm/sec/mm Hg, $\alpha_{RBC} = 1.60 \times 10^{-6}$ moles/l/mm Hg. Other values given in text.

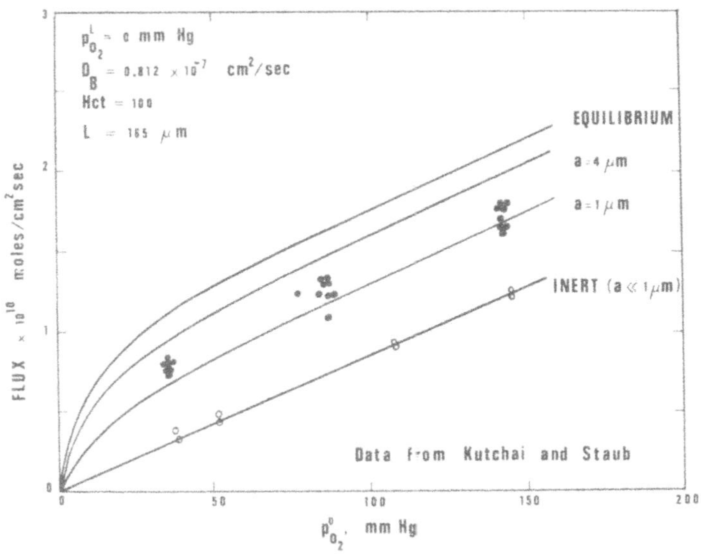

Figure 3. Comparison of Kutchai and Staub's data at 21.5°C with the theoretical model. Values of parameters are $P_{RBC} = 1.39 \times 10^{-14}$ moles/cm/sec/mm Hg, $\alpha_{RBC} = 1.71 \times 10^{-6}$ moles/l/mm Hg, $k_1 = 2.5 \times 10^6$ l/mole/sec, $k_2 = 35.7$ l/sec.

calculate an effective area. It was found to be 92% of total screen area. Experimental data and theoretical results are compared in figure 3. The open circles correspond to experiments where the hemoglobin reaction was inactivated. The filled circles scatter in the region between the 1 and 4 μm lines in agreement with the data presented earlier. It is tempting to cite this as supporting validation of the theoretical model. However when Kutchai and Staub hemolyzed the red cells, the oxygen flux through the resulting hemoglobin solution was the same at equivalent partial pressure. For the thickness of the films employed homogeneous media facilitation theory predicts the reaction to be at equilibrium. Kutchai and Staub concluded that the reaction inside the red blood cell is at equilibrium, and calculated a hemoglobin diffusivity of 0.54×10^{-7} cm^2/sec. If this value is employed in the theory, it can be shown that the data fall in the regime defined by the equilibrium and the $a = 1$ μm line. Because of the scatter of the data the conclusion of equilibrium is not justified.

The comparison of theory and the experimental results suggest that the oxygen-hemoglobin reaction is not at equilibrium at 25°C. However, for whole blood (Hct = 45) the equilibrium assumption is still a reasonable approximation. Before proceeding to predict the average effective permeability at physiological conditions and driving forces, it should be pointed out that hemolysis of blood samples during mass transfer experiments can significantly increase the oxygen mass transfer rate. When hemoglobin is released into plasma two important effects occur. First, hemoglobin will be a carrier in the continuous phase. The critical dimension for the continuous phase is the film thickness, which is usually of such an order that the reaction will be at equilibrium. Second, the hemoglobin concentration in the continuous phase will be diluted, although total concentration in the media is constant, and as a consequence the diffusivity will be higher. This is a problem of diffusion in heterogeneous media with two reactive phases which has been treated by Smith et al. (11). Figure 4 shows the increase of the average effective permeability ratio if 10% of the total red cells hemolyze, for the conditions of figure 2. In the experiments here hemolysis was less than 1%.

Theoretical predictions for the average effective permeability for blood at various hematocrits and physiological conditions are given in figure 5. The plasma diffusivity at 25°C was taken as 1.67×10^{-5} cm^2/sec (2) and was corrected for temperature. Other parameters were taken from the literature or predicted as previously. For whole blood the reaction is virtually at equilibrium. The maximum contribution of facilitated transport for this plasma diffusivity is approximately 15%. For higher diffusivities the relative contribution of facilitated transport decreases, reducing to 8% if the diffusivity is taken to be that of saline. The facilitated contri-

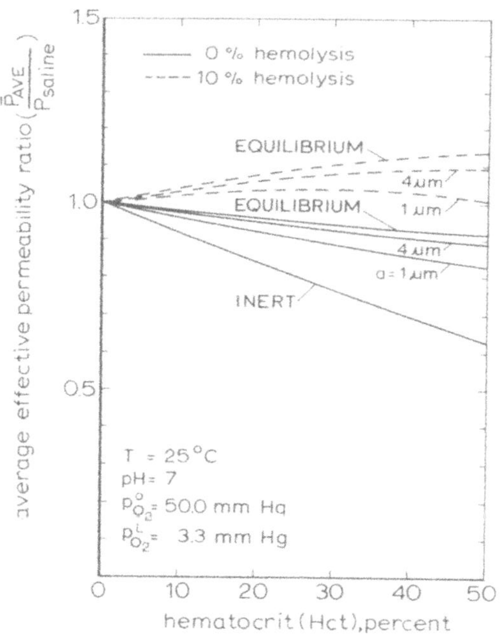

Figure 4. Effect of hemolysis on the average effective permeability ratio. Hematocrit is the initial hematocrit before hemolysis. Hemoglobin diffusivity in saline phase was taken from the correlation of Kreuzer (5), and oxygen permeability in the saline phase was adjusted for the presence of hemoglobin.

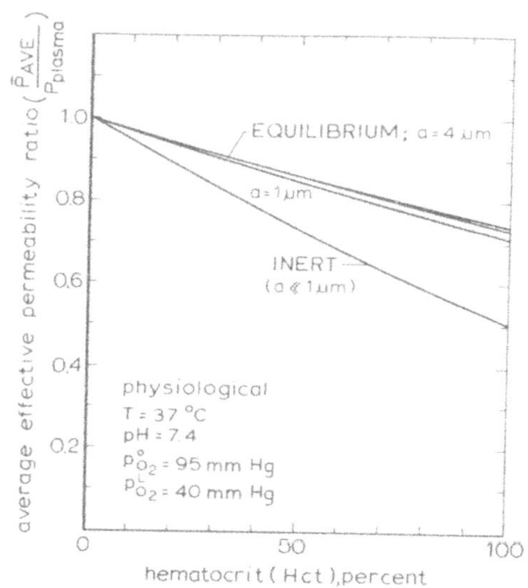

Figure 5. Average effective permeability ratio calculated for physiological conditions and driving forces. Values for the parameters are: $k_1 = 7.0 \times 10^6$ l/mole/sec, $k_2 = 240$ l/sec ($p_{50} = 26.5$ mm Hg), C_T = 33 gr/100 ml, $\alpha_{RBC} = 1.39 \times 10^{-6}$ moles/l/mm Hg, $P_{RBC} = 1.38 \times 10^{-14}$ moles/cm/sec/mm Hg, $P_{plasma} = 2.73 \times 10^{-14}$ moles/cm/sec/mm Hg ($D_{plasma} = 2.17 \times 10^{-5}$ cm^2/sec, $\alpha_{plasma} = 1.275 \times 10^{-6}$ moles/l/mm Hg).

bution is valid only for large dimensions of the system relative to the red blood cell radius such that small gradients exist. For large gradients across the red blood cell, such as in the capillaries, a second order analysis (6, 10) must be carried out to predict facilitation effects.

The theory presented here shows satisfactorily agreement with data when a one-step reaction scheme is used. Predictions can be made for a variety of conditions. It is likely that better results can be achieved if an improved kinetic model is used (12, 15). The accurate knowledge of the hemoglobin diffusion coefficient inside the red blood cell is further desirable.

REFERENCES

1. Altman, P.L., and D.S.Dittmer, Respiration and Circulation, Fed. Am.Soc.Exp.Biol., Bethesda, Md. (1971).
2. Ciuryla, V.T., Goldstick, T.K., and L.Zuckerman. This conference.
3. Friedlander, S.K., and K.H.Keller, Chem.Engr.Sci., 20, 121 (1965).
4. Gibson, Q.H., Prog.Biophys.Biophys.Chem., 9, 1 (1959).
5. Kreuzer, F., Respir.Physiol., 9, 1 (1970).
6. Kreuzer, F., and L.J.C.Hoofd, Respir.Physiol., 15, 208 (1972).
7. Kutchai, H., and N.C.Staub, J.Gen.Physiol., 53, 576 (1969).
8. Maxwell, J.C., A Treatise on Electricity and Magnetism, Vol.I, Clarendon Press, London (1881).
9. Skirrow, G., and R.M.Barrer, J.Polym.Sci., 3, 549 (1948).
10. Smith, K.A., Meldon, J.H., and C.K.Colton, AIChE J., 19, 102 (1973).
11. Smith, K.A., Stroeve, P., and C.K.Colton, in preparation.
12. Stroeve, P., Sc.D.Thesis, M.I.T., Cambridge, Mass. (1973).
13. Stroeve, P., Smith, K.A., and C.K.Colton, 72nd Annual AIChE, paper 25a, St.Louis, Missouri (1972).
14. Stroeve, P., Smith, K.A., and C.K.Colton, in preparation.
15. Stroeve, P., Smith, K.A., and C.K.Colton, in preparation.

ACKNOWLEDGMENTS

At the Massachusetts Institute of Technology, this study was supported in part by fellowships from the NSF and the NIH (number 4-F01-GM-49, 254-03) to Pieter Stroeve. At the University of Nijmegen Stiftung Volkswagenwerk provided funds.
We would like to thank Professor Dr.F.Kreuzer for the review of this paper. Graphic art by Ir.J.de Koning is appreciated.

MEASUREMENT OF DIFFUSIVITY AND METABOLIC RATE OF O_2 AND CO_2 IN RESPIRING TISSUE

Takeo Kawashiro, Peter Scheid and Johannes Piiper

Max-Planck-Institut für experimentelle Medizin

Abteilung Physiologie, Göttingen, Germany

INTRODUCTION

Diffusivity of respired gases in tissue is an important parameter in the study of tissue gas exchange. Most authors have measured O_2 and CO_2 diffusivity in dead tissue in which metabolism was blocked by pharmacological or physical interference.

This paper describes a method that allows determination of both Krogh's diffusion constant and metabolic rate for O_2 or CO_2 in freshly excised, intact muscle. Values obtained for rat abdominal muscle will be reported. The methods used and the results obtained will be presented in full detail elsewhere (Kawashiro *et al.*, 1975)

PRINCIPLE OF METHOD AND THEORY

A thin layer of tissue separates 2 chambers. One chamber is flushed and thus kept at constant partial pressure, P_o. The other chamber is closed after equilibration with given P_{O_2} and P_{CO_2}, and the rate of change of the partial pressure is measured by electrodes (fig. 1A).

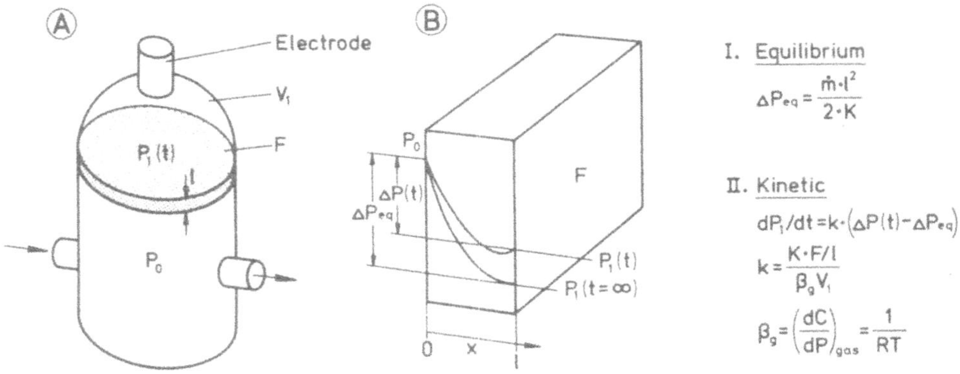

Fig. 1. Schema of set-up (A) and model for calculation (B).

Diffusion can quantitatively be analyzed in this system (fig. 1B) under the assumption of homogeneity of the tissue in respect of thickness, of metabolic rate, $\dot{m}$, and of Krogh's diffusion constant, K. Both K and $\dot{m}$ are furthermore assumed to be independent of P_{O_2} and P_{CO_2}.

Equilibrium

The partial pressure difference across the tissue at equilibrium is given by the metabolic rate, $\dot{m}$, Krogh's diffusion constant, K, and the thickness of the muscle, l,

$$\Delta P_{eq} = \frac{\dot{m} \cdot l^2}{2K} \qquad \ldots(1)$$

Equation (1) was first derived by Warburg (1923).

Kinetic

The partial pressure in the closed chamber, $P_1(t)$, will attain its steady value, $P_1(t{=}\infty)$, at a rate that is proportional to the deviation of the partial pressure difference across the tissue,

$\Delta P(t)$, from its equilibrium value, ΔP_{eq},

$$dP_1/dt = k\ \{\Delta P - \Delta P_{eq}\} \qquad \ldots(2)$$

The rate constant, k, is given by the ratio of the tissue conductance (Piiper *et al.*, 1971)

$$G = K \cdot F\ /\ l$$

to the capacity of the closed chamber, of volume V_1,

$$C = \beta g \cdot V_1 \quad .$$

Thus

$$k = \frac{G}{C} = \frac{K \cdot F/l}{\beta g \cdot V_1}$$

F is the area of tissue that is accessible for diffusion; β_g is the capacitance coefficient in gas phase, its value, 0.0517 mMol·L^{-1}·$torr^{-1}$ at 37°C, being constant for all gases.

From a plot of dP_1/dt against ΔP, according to eq.(2), ΔP_{eq} can be obtained as the abscissa intercept and k as slope; and $\dot{m}$ and K can be calculated therefrom using eqs. (1) and (3).

METHODS

A sheet consisting of abdominal transverse and internal oblique muscles was excised from rats and mounted in the diffusion apparatus, which was submerged under water at 37°C. Two different series were performed, one in which O_2 and another in which CO_2 partial pressure was measured in the closed chamber by respective electrodes. The open chamber was flushed with humidified gases, pure O_2 for the O_2 experiments and 3% CO_2, 40% O_2 in N_2 for the CO_2 experiments.

After a period of 30 min for attainment of steady temperature conditions, various diffusion periods were performed. In each of these periods the chamber in which P_1 was measured was equilibrated with gas mixtures and then closed, and the rate of change was observed during 3 min (CO_2 experiments) or 15 min (O_2 experiments). Several such measurements at various initial gas mixtures in the closed chamber were performed in one tissue. At the end of the experiment the area that was available for diffusion was cut out and weighed. Division by the specific gravity of 1.08 pond·cm^{-3} (T. Kawashiro, A. Campos Carles, S.F. Perry, J. Piiper, in preparation) yielded tissue volume and thus its thickness. The total time from excision of the tissue from the rat until completion of the experiment lasted between 120 and 150 min.

dP_1/dt was calculated over a period of 3 min (for CO_2) or 10 min (for O_2) and was plotted against the mean value of P_1 in the respective period.

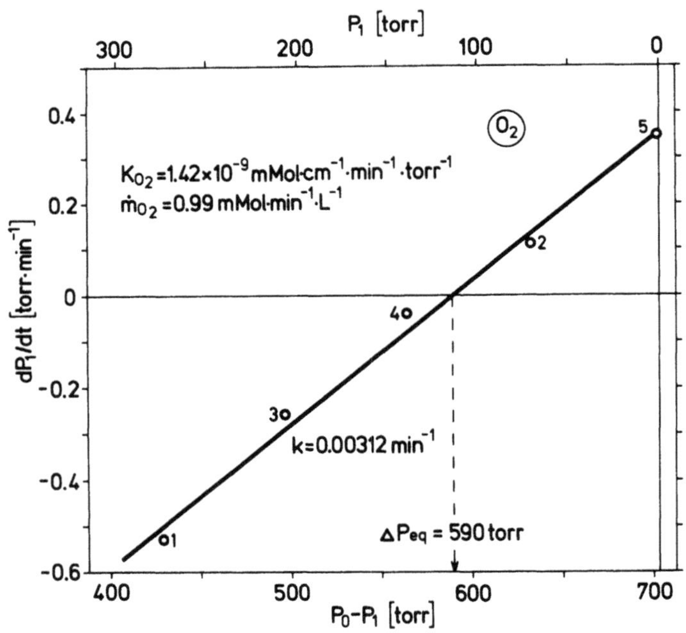

Fig. 2. Plot of dP_1/dt against $\Delta P = P_o - P_1$ (lower abscissa) and P_1 (upper abscissa) for O_2. The numbers at the individual measuring points indicate sequence of measurement.

RESULTS

Figures 2 and 3 show typical plots of dP_1/dt against $\Delta P = P_o - P_1$ for CO_2 and O_2. It is apparent that the measuring points can well be approximated by a straight line, as suggested from eq. (2). The sequence in which the data points were obtained, which is indicated by numbers in figs. 2 and 3, does not show any trend to deviate from the best fitting straight line.

Mean values ($\pm$ S.E.) for K and $\dot{m}$ in rat abdominal muscle of 410 µm average thickness were

$$K_{O_2} = (1.31 \pm 0.10) \times 10^{-9} mMol \cdot cm^{-1} \cdot min^{-1} \cdot torr^{-1}$$
$$K_{CO_2} = (28.9 \pm 0.7) \times 10^{-9} mMol \cdot cm^{-1} \cdot min^{-1} \cdot torr^{-1}$$
$$\dot{m}_{O_2} = 0.87 \pm 0.09 \; mMol \cdot min^{-1} \cdot L^{-1}$$
$$\dot{m}_{CO_2} = 0.74 \pm 0.04 \; mMol \cdot min^{-1} \cdot L^{-1}$$

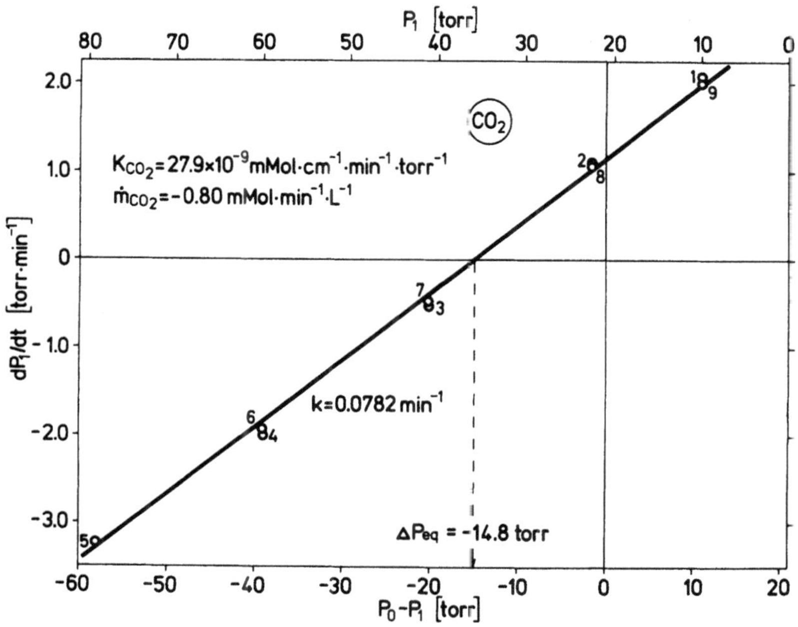

Fig. 3. Plot of dP_1/dt against $\Delta P = P_o - P_1$ (lower abscissa) and P_1 (upper abscissa) for CO_2. Numbers indicate sequence at which data were obtained.

Average respiratory quotient for the muscle,

$$R = \dot{m}_{CO_2} / \dot{m}_{O_2} = 0.85 \quad ,$$

did not differ significantly from unity.

DISCUSSION

Assumptions

The assumptions stated above shall now be critically reviewed.

Homogeneity of muscle thickness was checked histologically. Mean harmonic thickness differed from arithmetic mean by only 1.4%.

It is realized that the tissue, on a microscopic level, is inhomogeneous in respect of both K and $\dot{m}$. However, for solution of the diffusion equation volume elements have to be considered which may be large enough so that the average values of K and $\dot{m}$ therein are constant throughout the tissue. Thus K and $\dot{m}$ have to be considered average, effective values in the tissue.

It is generally held (Gore and Whalen, 1968) that tissue metabolism is independent of P_{O_2} down to very low P_{O_2} values. Since this critical P_{O_2} was never reached anywhere in the tissue in our experiments, $\dot{m}_{O_2}$ and $\dot{m}_{CO_2}$ may be considered independent of P_{O_2}. Any dependence on P_{CO_2} remains unknown at the moment.

Further assumptions, not listed above, where the constancy of closed chamber volume, V_1, during the diffusion period. It can be shown that V_1 in our experiments did not change much more than by 1%. Furthermore, it had to be assumed that the attainment of steady partial pressure profile in the tissue with changing P_1 was fast as compared with the rate of change of P_1 itself. This assumption is fulfilled, mainly because of the rather big capacity of the closed chamber as compared with the tissue capacity, V_1 being 0.43 ml.

Literature Values

K values have mostly been determined in tissue whose metabolism had been suppressed. Only Van Liew (1971) has determined K_{CO_2} in respiring cat urinary bladder. It appears, however, that the results on both K_{O_2} and K_{CO_2} of all authors fall into a quite narrow range comprising our values. Thus K does not appear to depend much on tissue metabolism.

The K values for O_2 and CO_2 in muscle tissue are only about 50% of the respective water values. This reduction is presumably due to the muscle proteins that hinder free diffusion (Gros and Moll, 1971).

Literature values on O_2 consumption in rat skeletal muscle fall into a narrow range comprising our value. Data on muscle slices appear, however, to be reduced when compared with intact tissue. We have checked our value of $\dot{m}_{O_2}$ on the same preparation using the Warburg manometric method. The result, ($\dot{m}_{O_2}$ = 0.74 $\pm$ 0.03 $mMol \cdot min^{-1} \cdot L^{-1}$) did not differ significantly from that obtained with the diffusion method.

CONCLUSION

The method described is apt to measure, at the same time, Krogh's diffusion constant and specific metabolic rates for O_2 and CO_2 in intact, respiring tissues. Due to metabolism tissue thickness for this method is limited to about 500 μm unless hyperbaric conditions are used. The results suggest that both K_{O_2} and K_{CO_2} are similar in alive and in dead tissue. Due to tissue inhomogeneity and to possible facilitation of O_2 or CO_2 transport our values of K have to be considered as effective mean values for the physiological range of P_{O_2} and P_{CO_2} in muscle at rest and at exercise.

REFERENCES

Gore, R.W., Whalen, W.J. (1968). Relations among tissue P_{O_2}, Q_{O_2}, and resting heat production of frog sartorius muscle. *Am. J. Physiol.* 214: 277-286.

Gros, G., Moll, W. (1971). The diffusion of carbon dioxide in erythrocytes and hemoglobin solutions. *Pflügers Arch. ges. Physiol.* 324: 249-266.

Kawashiro, T., Nüsse, W., Scheid, P. (1975). Determination of diffusivity of oxygen and carbon dioxide in respiring tissue. *Pflügers Arch. ges. Physiol.*, submitted.

Piiper, J., Dejours, P., Haab, P., Rahn, H. (1971). Concepts and basic quantities in gas exchange physiology. *Respir. Physiol.* 13: 292-304.

Van Liew, H.D. (1971). Diffusion constant for CO_2 through urinary bladders of cats. *Respir. Physiol.* 13: 372-377.

Warburg, O. (1923). Versuche an überlebendem Carcinomgewebe. *Biochem. Z.* 142: 317-333.

Acknowledgement Figures reproduced from Pflügers Archiv with permission by Springer Verlag, Heidelberg.

FACILITATED DIFFUSION OF CO AND OXYGEN IN THE PRESENCE OF HEMOGLOBIN OR MYOGLOBIN

F.Kreuzer and L.J.C.Hoofd

Department of Physiology, University of Nijmegen

Nijmegen, The Netherlands

Kreuzer and Hoofd (1970, 1972) presented an approximate analytical solution of the basic equations of facilitated diffusion including chemical reactions for the systems Hb + O_2 and Mb + O_2, and investigated the effects of various factors of possible importance including the values of the diffusion coefficients, the chemical reaction rates, the actual diffusion path length, a possible back pressure of oxygen on the low-pressure side, and nonequilibrium versus equilibrium approach. They assumed the presence of three regions in the layer: a middle core very near equilibrium and two marginal regions not at equilibrium (similar treatment by Smith et al., 1973). In their recent review Schultz et al. (1974) showed that this analysis leads to solutions which are valid over a wide range of Damköhler numbers (which, in diffusion-reaction problems, is the ratio of certain characteristic times for diffusion to certain characteristic or relaxation times for chemical reaction). This group successfully applied the same type of method to other, quite different situations, i.e., to the system CO + O_2 (Suchdeo et al., 1973), to analyze a single-reaction model for the bicarbonate-facilitated transport of CO_2 (Suchdeo and Schultz, 1974), and to carrier-mediated heat transport in chemically reacting media (Goddard et al., 1974). Furthermore these authors suggested a generalization of this analytical method for potential application to carrier-mediated systems with multiple reactions and several volatile species (Goddard et al., 1974). In the present paper we investigate the system CO + Hb or Mb in the absence and presence of oxygen by an improved mathematical approach, and present numerical calculations for certain specific situations.

THEORY

When trying to apply our method (Kreuzer and Hoofd, 1972) to the system CO + Hb or Mb it turned out that the interesting situations were near or even beyond the limitations of the method, i.e.: 1) there is lower limit for the membrane thickness L where the boundary layers begin to overlap and no middle core is left; 2) there is an upper limit for the gas partial pressure applied since the extrapolated equilibrium core solutions in the boundary layers become so steep, above a certain pressure, that they no longer may be assumed constant over the whole boundary layer. We therefore tried to modify the method of solution in such a way that it might be applied beyond these limitations. We start out from the same set of equations relating species transport to chemical reactions of CO, assuming one-step reactions and $D_{Hb} = D_{HbCO}$ (for notation see list of symbols at the end):

1) $$\mathrm{Hb + CO} \underset{\ell}{\overset{\ell'}{\rightleftharpoons}} \mathrm{HbCO}$$

so that at steady state:

2) $$D_{CO}\frac{d^2[CO]}{dx^2} = \ell' \,[Hb][CO] - \ell \,[HbCO]$$

3) $$D_{Hb}\frac{d^2[HbCO]}{dx^2} = \ell \,[HbCO] - \ell' \,[Hb][CO]$$

We define total Hb concentration as C_T:

4) $$C_T = [Hb] + [HbCO]$$

The boundary conditions are, applying Henry's law:

5) $$[CO]_{x=0} = \alpha_{CO}p_{CO,o} \; ; \; [CO]_{x=L} = \alpha_{CO}p_{CO,L}$$

and noting that the boundaries are impervious to each Hb species:

6) $$\left.\frac{d\,[HbCO]}{dx}\right|_{x=0} = \left.\frac{d\,[HbCO]}{dx}\right|_{x=L} = 0$$

These equations form a complete set from which the concentration profiles (and so the flux) are completely defined. Unfortunately, there is no obvious analytical solution for this system, so that approximations had to be made. Yet, by adding eqs. 2) and 3) the reaction terms cancel and we may integrate twice to achieve the exact result:

7) $$D_{CO}[CO] + D_{Hb}[HbCO] = J_{CO}x + K_{CO}$$

where J and K are integration constants and J is the total flux. By applying the boundary conditions and subtracting we get the exact solution:

8) $$J_{CO}L = D_{CO}\,\alpha_{CO}(p_{CO,L}-p_{CO,o}) + D_{Hb}([HbCO]_{x=L}-[HbCO]_{x=0})$$

As was pointed out in our first paper, in layers 'thick' enough there has to be a region ('middle bulk') where the concentration profiles must be at equilibrium. However at the boundaries, because of the impermeability for Hb there must be a non-equilibrium zone. Since $d[HbCO]/dx=0$ at $x=0,L$ there will be no more than minor deviations in [Hb] and [HbCO] in these regions. So we try to approximate [CO] by:

9) $$[CO] \approx [CO]^e - C_o e^{-\beta_o x/L} + C_L e^{-\beta_L(1-x/L)}$$

where the superscript e denotes an equilibrium profile, extended from the core to the boundaries. From eq. 7) we get:

10) $$D_{CO}[CO]^e + D_{Hb}[HbCO]^e = J_{CO}x + K_{CO}$$

where:

11) $$\ell'[Hb]^e[CO]^e = \ell[HbCO]^e$$

Substituting in eq.2) and ignoring the minor deviations leads to (β^2 = Damköhler number):

12) $$\beta_o = L\sqrt{\frac{\ell'[Hb]_{x=0}}{D_{CO}}}\;;\quad \beta_L = L\sqrt{\frac{\ell'[Hb]_{x=L}}{D_{CO}}}$$

Combining eqs. 9) and 10) with 7) shows that:

13) $$[HbCO] \approx [HbCO]^e + \frac{D_{CO}}{D_{Hb}}\{C_o e^{-\beta_o x/L} - C_L e^{-\beta_L(1-x/L)}\}$$

Applying eq. 6) now gives:

14) $$\frac{d}{dx}[HbCO]^e\Big|_{x=0} = \frac{D_{CO}}{L\,D_{Hb}}(C_o\beta_o + C_L\beta_L e^{-\beta_L})$$

We define a 'weighted derivative' ρ:

15) $$\rho = (D_{CO}/D_{Hb})(d[CO]^e/d[HbCO]^e)$$

so that:

16) $$\frac{d[CO]^e}{dx} = \frac{d[CO]^e}{d[HbCO]^e}\,\frac{d[HbCO]^e}{dx} = \frac{D_{Hb}}{D_{CO}}\,\rho\,\frac{d[HbCO]^e}{dx}$$

By differentiation of eq. 7) and applying 6) at x=0 we get:

$$17)\qquad J_{CO} = D_{CO}\frac{d[CO]}{dx} + D_{Hb}\frac{d[HbCO]}{dx} = D_{CO}\frac{d[CO]}{dx}\bigg|_{x=0}$$

Substituting the approximate eq. 9) now leads to an approximation for J_{CO} which is called J'_{CO}:

$$18)\qquad J'_{CO} = D_{CO}\left\{\frac{d[CO]^e}{dx}\bigg|_{x=0} + \frac{C_o\beta_o + C_L\beta_L e^{-\beta_L}}{L}\right\}$$

$$= \frac{D_{CO}}{L}(C_o\beta_o + C_L\beta_L e^{-\beta_L})(1 + \rho_{x=0})$$

The same procedure applied at x=L leads to:

$$19)\qquad J'_{CO} = \frac{D_{CO}}{L}(C_o\beta_o e^{-\beta_o} + C_L\beta_L)(1 + \rho_{x=L})$$

We may relate $p_{CO,L}$ and $p_{CO,o}$ in eq. 8) by applying eq. 5) to eq. 9) and approximate $[CO]^e$ at x=0,L:

$$20)\qquad [CO]^e = \frac{\ell}{\ell'}\frac{[HbCO]^e}{[Hb]^e} \simeq \frac{\ell}{\ell'}\frac{[HbCO]}{[Hb]} \quad \text{at } x=0,L$$

so that:

$$21)\qquad J'_{CO}\left\{1 - \frac{1}{1-e^{-\beta_o-\beta_L}}\left[\frac{1}{1+\rho_{x=0}}\left(\frac{1-e^{-\beta_o}}{\beta_o} - \frac{e^{-\beta_o}(1-e^{-\beta_L})}{\beta_L}\right) + \right.\right.$$

$$\left.\left.\text{same term with } 0 \rightleftharpoons L\right]\right\}$$

$$= \frac{D_{CO}}{L}([CO]^e_{x=L} - [CO]^e_{x=0}) + \frac{D_{Hb}}{L}([HbCO]_{x=L} - [HbCO]_{x=0})$$

Equations 9) at x=0,L, 12) and 19)-21) form a completely solvable set, but for small L the approximations turn out to be too crude to provide us with the correct solution, due to the fact that J'_{CO} comes out below the value for plain diffusion, resulting in negative facilitated fluxes of CO. Therefore we modified eq. 21) by trying to solve it in a situation where it really is exact. If the total Hb concentration C_T is made very large ($C_T \rightarrow \infty$), while keeping $\ell' C_T$ at the same value in order to maintain the same β and so the same boundary effect, an infinitely large change in [CO] is needed to alter the saturation. So in this situation an approximation of [CO] as established in eq. 9) will not affect the saturation profile anymore. Furthermore ℓ'[Hb] and so β now will indeed be constant across the boundary regions. With $C_T \to \infty$, $\rho \to 0$, so that eq. 21) becomes:

$$21') \quad J'_{CO}\left\{ 1 - \frac{(1-e^{-\beta_o})(1-e^{-\beta_L})}{1-e^{-\beta_o-\beta_L}}\left(\frac{1}{\beta_o}+\frac{1}{\beta_L}\right)\right\}$$

$$= \frac{D_{CO}}{L}([CO]^e_{x=L}-[CO]^e_{x=0}) + \frac{D_{Hb}}{L}([HbCO]_{x=L}-[HbCO]_{x=0})$$

The set of equations 9) at x=0,L, 12), 19), 20) and 21') leads to a correct behavior in all limiting regions: $L \to 0$, $p \to 0$, $L \to \infty$, and probably also (since the equilibrium profiles are no longer assumed constant over the boundary layers) $p \to \infty$. Note that J'_{CO} is used to solve e.g. [HbCO] at x=0,L from the above set of equations while after this procedure these values can be substituted in the exact equation 8) to solve for J_{CO} as the correct flux.

If now oxygen is added to the system the same procedure can be applied for solving $[O_2]$. Only eq. 16) for CO must be extended to:

$$22) \quad \frac{d[CO]^e}{dx} = \frac{\partial[CO]^e}{\partial[HbCO]^e}\frac{d[HbCO]^e}{dx} + \frac{\partial[CO]^e}{\partial[HbO_2]^e}\frac{d[HbO_2]^e}{dx}$$

This will not affect eq. 21') but it does affect eq. 18) and so eqs. 19) and 20) and the corresponding equations for $[O_2]$. However, in this paper we only calculate situations where $[O_2]$ will be approximately constant over the whole layer and we try to account for this by introducing virtual reaction rates ℓ'_v and ℓ_v for CO. We furthermore assume that the reaction with hemoglobin here takes place at the fourth step only, so that dissociation of CO from Hb will be at a rate:

$$23) \quad \ell_v = \tfrac{1}{4}\ell_4$$

We calculate ℓ'_v from the chemical equilibrium:

$$24) \quad \frac{\ell'_v}{\ell_v} = \frac{[HbCO]^e}{\{C_T-[HbCO]^e\}[CO]^e} = \frac{4[Hb_4(CO)_4]^e}{[Hb_4(CO)_3]^e[CO]^e} = \frac{4\ell'_4}{\ell_4} \text{ if } p_{O_2} = 0$$

$$= \frac{[HbCO]^e}{[HbO_2]^e[CO]^e} = \frac{M}{[O_2]^e} \quad \text{if } p_{O_2} \neq 0$$

so that, assuming $[O_2]^e \simeq \alpha_{O_2}p_{O_2}$:

$$25) \qquad \ell_v' = \ell_4' \text{ if } p_{O_2} = 0; \; \ell_v' = \frac{\ell_v M}{\alpha_{O_2} p_{O_2}} \text{ if } p_{O_2} \neq 0$$

Note that ℓ_v', ℓ_v here are derived for a situation not far from chemical equilibrium whereas the description by other authors using m' and m refers to the initial reaction rates of the displacement reaction of CO against O_2.

RESULTS AND DISCUSSION

Theoretically one should expect a facilitation of CO movement across a film of Hb or Mb even greater than that of O_2, provided the partial pressure of CO is low, due to the large concentration gradients for HbCO as compared with those for dissolved CO. We first studied the simpler system Mb + CO and plotted the calculated flux of CO in an 18 g% Mb solution being exposed to CO on one side (no back pressure) against the layer thickness for five CO pressures. The constants used at 20°C were: solubility of CO = 1.37 10^{-9} M/ml mm Hg, D_{CO} = 0.93 10^{-5} cm²/sec, D_{Mb} = 3.1 10^{-7} cm²/sec, ℓ' = 5 10^8 ml/M sec, ℓ = 0.017 sec^{-1}. The results are shown in fig. 1. The curves show a maximum or a plateau in the middle range of layer thicknesses, approach the chemical equilibrium asymptote with very thick layers (roughly at a layer thickness of about 10 cm), and the near-diffusion regime with very thin layers (below 1 μ). In the middle range the facilitated flux reaches a maximum at a CO pressure of about 2.5 mm Hg when increasing this pressure, and gradually declines when increasing CO pressure further. The maximum reached at the often used layer thickness of 150 μ is, however, only 8% of the value predicted from assuming chemical equilibrium across the entire layer, i.e., a system with CO is much farther removed from equilibrium than is the case with O_2.

Wittenberg (1966) experimentally found no augmented diffusion of CO in various pigment solutions including Hb and Mb. Murray and Wyman (1971) tried to explain this finding and concluded from their calculations that the presumed absence of any observed facilitation of CO diffusion by either Hb or Mb results from the very high affinity of both pigments for CO. However, their study, apart from neglecting previous evidence to the contrary (see below), considered only the special case of very high CO pressure (100 mm Hg), as did Wittenberg (1966; 70 to 760 mm Hg); their conclusion therefore cannot be generalized and does not present a solution to the problem. We calculated that with a CO pressure of 100 mm Hg the facilitation of CO diffusion is indeed only a few percent for both Hb and Mb but this is an abnormal situation since physiological CO pressures are much lower and there is appreciable facilitation in this low range.

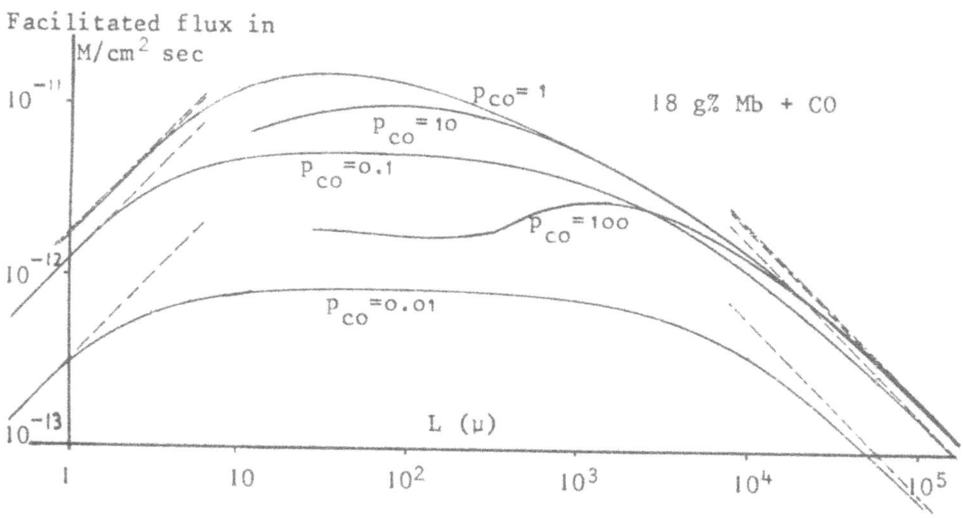

Fig.1. Facilitated CO flux against layer thickness for CO + Mb for five different CO pressures applied on one side of the layer (no back pressure). See text for constants used.

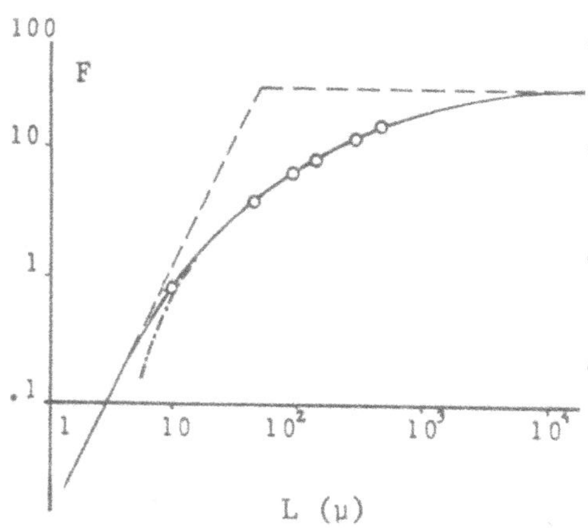

Fig.2. Facilitation against layer thickness calculated (————) for the data of Kutchai et al. (1970; open circles) and compared with calculations of Smith et al. (1973;second order theory —·—·—·) and asymptotes (– – – – – –).

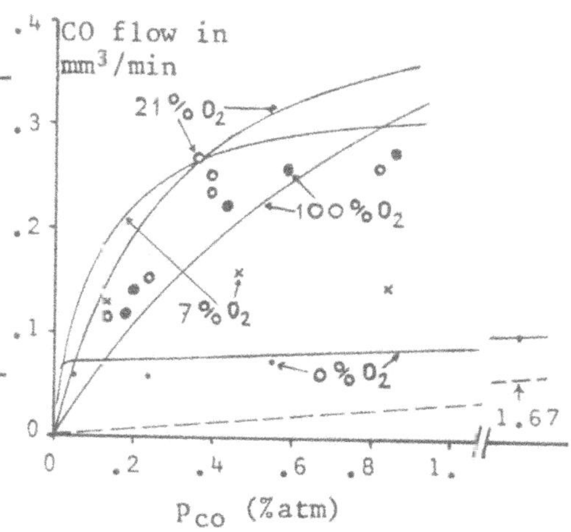

Fig.3. CO flow against pressure calculated for the experimental situation of Mochizuki and Forster (1962;points). See text for constants used. Conversion of CO flux into CO flow was so as to yield the same unfacilitated diffusion (– – – – –).

Figure 2 demonstrates the perfect agreement of our present new calculation of the facilitated flux of CO with the second-order theory of Smith et al. (1973) and with the points of Kutchai et al. (1970) down to a layer thickness of about 10 μ; with layer thicknesses below 10 μ the two curves diverge, and our curve reaches the near-equilibrium asymptote.

Mochizuki and Forster (1962) experimentally found that the facilitation of CO through a Hb solution was much greater than that for O_2, but was still only one-tenth that predicted from calculation, if one assumed chemical equilibrium. There was an increase in facilitated CO flux when the calculated equilibrated concentration gradient of HbCO across the film decreased in the presence of an increased O_2 concentration. It was concluded that the reaction velocities of CO and Hb, in particular the rate of dissociation of CO from HbCO which is favored by increased O_2, are limiting the overall process and that chemical equilibrium does not exist between Hb and the gases at the film surfaces. We compared our calculations with the experimental data of Mochizuki and Forster (1962). The constants used for a Hb solution of 10.8 g% at pH 7.4 and at 37°C were: solubility of CO = $1.11\ 10^{-9}$ M/ml mm Hg, solubility of O_2 = $1.44\ 10^{-9}$ M/ml mm Hg, $D_{CO} = 1.7\ 10^{-5}$ cm²/sec, $D_{O_2} = 2.1\ 10^{-5}$ cm²/sec, D_{Hb} = $5.33\ 10^{-7}$ cm²/sec, $\ell_4' = 3\ 10^{10}$ ml/M sec, $\ell_4 = 0.25$ sec^{-1}, M = 230. Figure 3 compares our calculated values with the data points of Mochizuki and Forster (1962). There is fair agreement with the exception of the case of a P_{O_2} of 50 mm Hg; we have no explanation for the divergence in this case.

We also calculated for the system Mb + CO + O_2 that increasing addition of O_2, to the same CO pressures, on both sides of the layer first increases CO facilitation in this range and then decreases it because most of the Mb becomes saturated with O_2; at the same time a counter-diffusion of O_2 is induced by the difference in MbO_2 in the absence of any difference in O_2 pressure (or, in other situations, even against an O_2 pressure gradient), as described previously by La Force (1966) and La Force and Fatt (1967).

In conclusion, the present new mathematical approach has extended the applicability of our previous approximate analytical solution of the equations for the facilitated diffusion of oxygen or CO in the presence of Hb or Mb over a wider range of layer thicknesses (in both directions) and of gas pressures (particularly for the case of high gas pressures). The situation of the simultaneous presence of CO and oxygen (the latter being approximately constant over the whole layer) was also considered. Comparison of these calculations with other previous computations or experimental data has shown good agreement in most cases.

LIST OF SYMBOLS

C_T	= total monomeric hemoglobin concentration
D_{CO}, D_{O_2}, D_{Hb}, D_{Mb}	= diffusion coefficients of CO, O_2, Hb and Mb
J_{CO}	= total CO flux
ℓ', ℓ	= overall forward and backward reaction constants of Hb (or Mb) with CO
ℓ_v', ℓ_v	= virtual forward and backward reaction rates for CO
ℓ_4', ℓ_4	= fourth-step forward and backward reaction constants of Hb_4 with CO
L	= layer thickness
M	= $[O_2]$ $[HbCO]/[CO]$ $[HbO_2]$= equilibrium constant of fully saturated Hb for concentration of CO relative to that of O_2
α_{CO},α_{O_2}	= solubilities of CO and O_2, respectively
ρ	= $(D_{CO}/D_{Hb})(d[CO]^e/d[HbCO]^e)$

REFERENCES

Goddard, J.D., J.S. Schultz and S.R. Suchdeo: AIChE J. 20: 625, 1974.
Goddard, J.D., J.S. Schultz and S.R. Suchdeo: Chem. Eng. Sci. 29: 2041, 1974.
Kreuzer, F., and L.J.C. Hoofd: Respir. Physiol. 8: 280, 1970.
Kreuzer, F., and L.J.C. Hoofd: Respir. Physiol. 15: 104, 1972.
Kutchai, H., J.A. Jacquez and F.J. Mather: Biophys. J. 10: 38, 1970.
La Force, R.C.: Trans. Faraday Soc. 62: 1458, 1966.
La Force, R.C., and I. Fatt: In: Chemical Engineering in Medicine and Biology, ed. D. Hershey, p. 107, Plenum Press, New York, 1967.
Mochizuki, M., and R.E. Forster: Science 138: 897, 1962.
Murray, J.D., and J. Wyman: J. Biol. Chem. 246: 5903, 1971.
Schultz, J.S., J.D. Goddard and S.R. Suchdeo: AIChE J. 20: 417, 1974.
Smith, K.A., J.H. Meldon and C.K. Colton: AIChE J. 19: 102, 1973.
Suchdeo, S.R., J.D. Goddard and J.S. Schultz: In: Oxygen Transport to Tissue, eds. D.F. Bruley and H.I. Bicher. Adv. Exper. Med. and Biol., vol. 37B, p. 951, Plenum Press, New York, 1973.
Suchdeo, S.R., and J.S. Schultz: Biochim. Biophys. Acta 352: 412, 1974.
Wittenberg, J.B.: J. Biol. Chem. 241: 104, 1966.
Yung, D., and R.F. Probstein: J. Phys. Chem. 77: 2201, 1973.

ACKNOWLEDGMENTS

This work was supported in part by a grant from the Stiftung Volkswagenwerk. Discussions with Prof. Dr. J.S. Schultz are appreciated.

THE MEASUREMENT OF THE FRACTION OF OXYGEN CARRIED BY FACILITATED DIFFUSION[1]

I. S. Longmuir

Department of Biochemistry

North Carolina State University, Raleigh, N.C. 27607 USA

Evidence has been presented that the cytochrome P-450 in the endoplasmic reticulum can facilitate the diffusion by oxygen through tissue (Longmuir, 1970). This hypothesis is based on the observation that the respiration rate of liver slices as a function of ambient oxygen tension more closely fits a model equation based on purely passive diffusion. However, the fit is not perfect at higher oxygen tensions, and it seems highly improbable that there can be no passive diffusion proceeding concomitantly. The respiration rate of a slice in which there is only passive diffusion would rise as the square root of the ambient oxygen tension, whereas if transport is purely by carrier, the respiration rate would show "saturation" kinetics. That is, the rate of rise would fall off rapidly, becoming asymptotic to a maximum rate. Thus it seems certain that both passive and facilitated diffusion are proceeding simultaneously. That this is the case can be shown by the application of specific inhibitors to tissue slices. Their effect is to reduce the respiration rate of slices somewhat and, depending on how much of the cytochrome P-450 is bound, alter the data obtained by measuring the respiration rate as a function of ambient oxygen tension from a set which fits the facilitated diffusion equation to one which fits the passive diffusion equation.

If the two processes do not interfere with one another to an appreciable extent, then it should be possible to measure the fraction carried by facilitated diffusion by deleting facilitated diffusion and measuring the rise in tension necessary to keep the respiration rate of the slices constant. This can be done experimentally with a cell devised to measure the role of catalase in oxygen transport (Longmuir, Soucie, and Sun, 1970). The rationale is as follows: Let X equal the amount of oxygen carried by passive diffusion and Y that by facilitated diffusion, then:

$$X = 2A\alpha \sqrt{\frac{2DP_{O_2}}{\alpha}} \qquad (1)$$

Where A is the area of the slice, α is the respiration rate of unit volume, D is the diffusion coefficient in Krogh's units, and P_{O_2} is the ambient partial pressure of oxygen. And:

$$Y = \frac{\bar{V}P_{O_2}}{K + P_{O_2}} \qquad (2)$$

Where $\bar{V}$ is the maximum respiration rate of the slice and K is a constant. Then if passive diffusion is deleted and the oxygen tension allowed to rise by an amount ΔP_{O_2} until the respiration rate becomes the same as before, it will be given by the following equation:

$$X + Y = 2A\alpha \sqrt{\frac{2D\ (P_{O_2} + \Delta P_{O_2})}{\alpha}} \qquad (3)$$

Thus, the fraction of oxygen carried by passive diffusion will be given by:

$$\frac{Y}{X + Y} = 1 - \sqrt{\frac{P_{O_2}}{P_{O_2} + \Delta P_{O_2}}}$$

MATERIALS AND METHOD

Seven-week old male Wistar strain rats were killed by cervical dislocation and their livers removed and cut into slices 0.4 mm thick. The slices were then suspended in saline (Longmuir and Bourke, 1960) and placed in the polarographic cell (Fig. 1). As the slices respired, the tension fell as shown in Fig. 2. When all the oxygen had been removed, a potential was applied between the platinum anode and the collodion-coated palladium cathode. The potential was adjusted so that the current remained constant. Then, provided the rate of generation of oxygen did not exceed the maximum respiration rate of the slices, the tension will rise to a constant value when the rate of generation exactly balances the respiration rate. When some P-450 inhibitor is added to the cell,

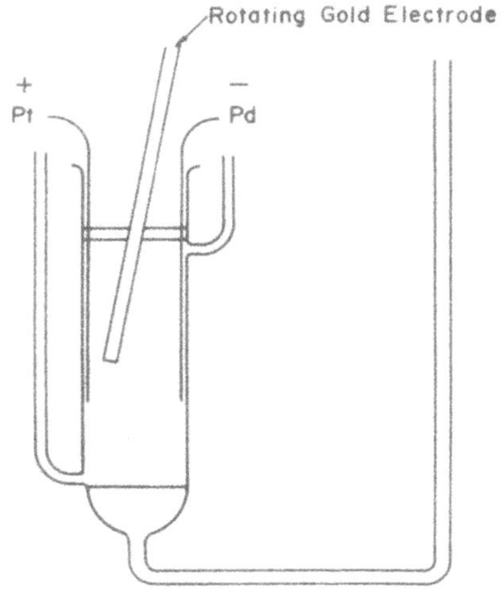

Fig. 1 Polarographic cell (Longmuir, 1957) with addition of generating electrode system; a platinum anode and palladium cathode.

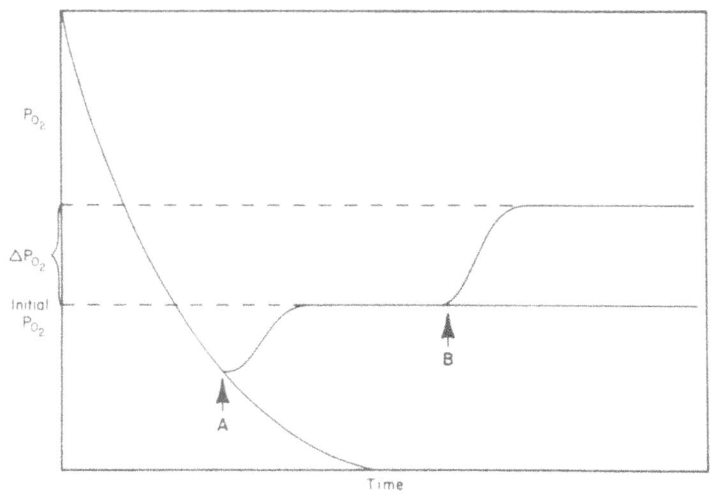

Fig. 2 Plot of oxygen tension against time. In the initial part of the trace, the generating system is off. When it is switched on, the tension rises and plateaus at a constant value. On addition of the inhibitor, the tension rises to a new plateau.

the P_{O_2} rises by ΔP_{O_2} to become constant at a new level. Further additions can then be made to determine the Ks of the inhibitor with respect to the carrier. A number of inhibitors specific to P-450 were studied. Unfortunately most of the classical ones are rather insoluble. Nicotinamide was found to be the most suitable.

In separate experiments, this substance was found to have no significant effect on cytochrome oxidase nor is it polarographically active at the potentials employed. That is to say, it neither interfered with the signal from the measuring electrode nor affected the coulombmetric efficiency of the generating system.

RESULTS

When the reciprocal of ΔP_{O_2} was plotted against the reciprocal of nicotinamide concentration, the points lay on a straight line; and from the intercept and the slope, the Ks was measured to be 2.6 mM (Fig. 3). This agrees with the literature value for the binding constant of nicotinamide to P-450 obtained spectroscopically (Schenkman, Remmer, and Estabrook, 1967).

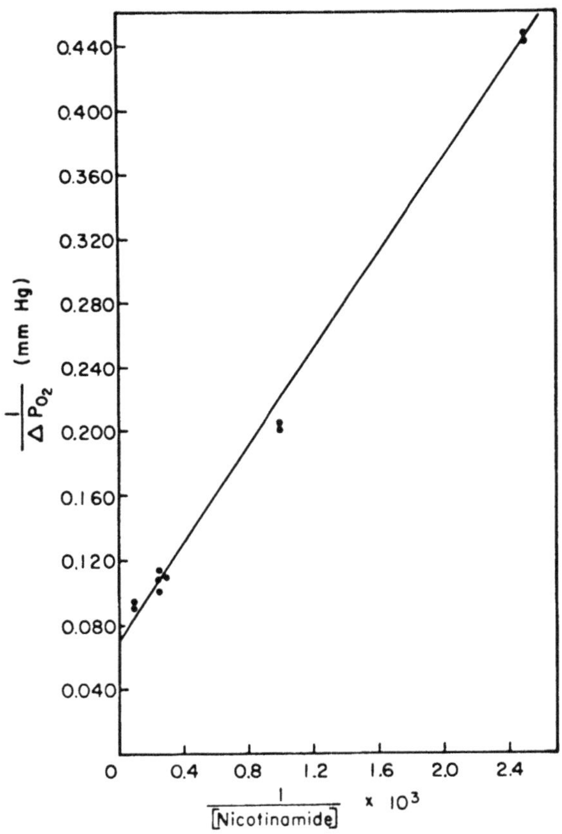

Fig. 3 Plot of $1/\Delta P_{O_2}$ against reciprocal nicotinamide concentration (millimolar)$^{-1}$.

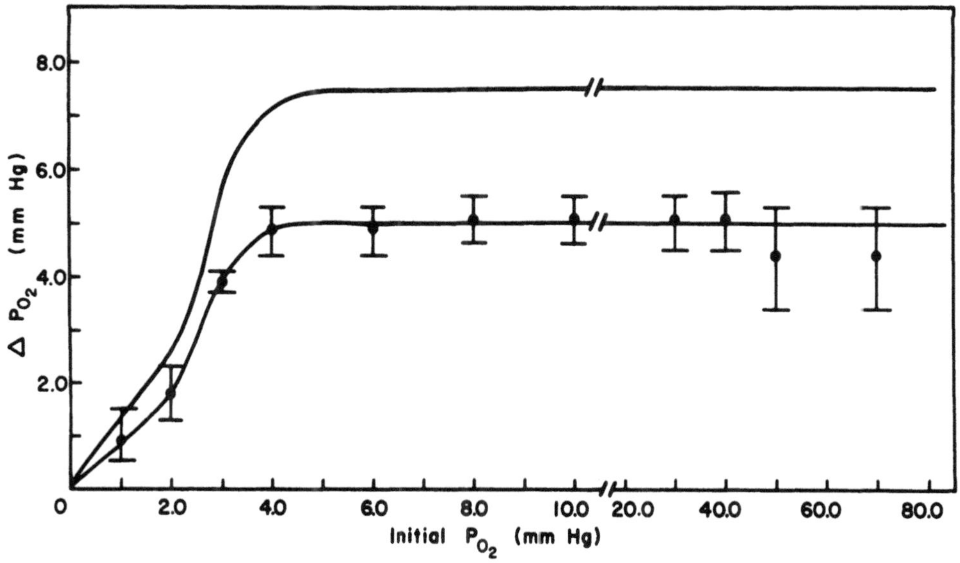

Fig. 4 Lower curve plot of experimentally determined P_{O_2} against ambient P_{O_2}. Upper curve values calculated if all the carrier was inhibited.

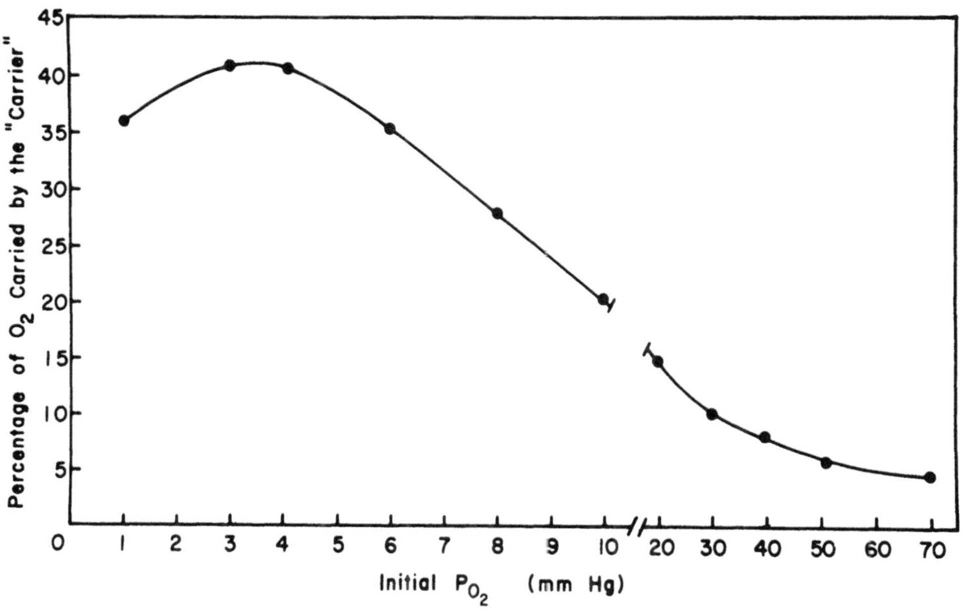

Fig. 5 Plot of fraction of oxygen carried by facilitated diffusion as a function of ambient tension.

Fig. 4 shows a plot of P_{O_2} against initial P_{O_2}. The concentration of nicotinamide used was 3 mM, an amount able to bind little more than half the P-450. The upper line is calculated assuming there is complete inhibition. Fig. 5 is a plot of the fraction of oxygen carried by facilitated diffusion as a function of the initial ambient tension of oxygen.

DISCUSSION

Cytochrome P-450 in tissue exists in both the oxidized and reduced state. In the reduced state, it can react reversibly with oxygen (Longmuir, Sun, and Soucie, 1971). Even if only a quarter of the cytochrome is reduced, the molecules will still be close enough to permit oxygen molecules to jump from one to the next over a smaller energy barrier than they would in diffusing from one quasi-equilibrium position to the next as described by current theory on the mechanism of passive diffusion. If a substance binding only to the oxidized form of P-450 is added, it will decrease the amount of reduced P-450 available for facilitated diffusion. Since the concentration of nicotinamide necessary to raise ΔP_{O_2} to half its maximum value is of the same order as that necessary to bind half the P-450, this seems to support the hypothesis that this substance is involved in the facilitated diffusion of oxygen.

It will be seen from Fig. 4 that the carrier shows saturation kinetics, that above about 10 Torr, ΔP_{O_2} does not rise any more and that at about 2 Torr, ΔP_{O_2} is half maximum. The latter figure compares with most published figures for the Ks of P-450 of 1 Torr.

From Fig. 5, it appears that facilitated diffusion would be most effective at low tensions of oxygen such as are found in liver which receives 80% of its oxygen supply from portal venous blood which in many species has a tension less than 20 Torr. Facilitated diffusion can thus be seen as an adaptive mechanism to enable the liver mitochondria to receive enough oxygen from a rather luxurious blood flow containing oxygen at low tension. As we show in another paper in this symposium, this is an adaptation which can also acclimate to decreasing oxygen supply by a substantial increase of P-450 in a remarkably short time.

REFERENCES

Longmuir, I. S. (1957) BIOCHEM. J. 65:378.

Longmuir, I. S. (1970) 6TH EUROP. CONF. MICROCIRCULATION, Aalborg. (Karger, Basel) p. 3.

Longmuir, I. S., and Ann Bourke (1960) BIOCHEM. J. 76:225.

Longmuir, I. S., W. G. Soucie, and S. Sun (1970) FED. PROC. (Abs) 2123.

Longmuir, I. S., Stella Sun, and W. Soucie (1971) OXIDASES AND RELATED SYSTEMS. (King, Mason and Morrison, Eds.) Vol. II, p. 451.

Schenkman, J. S., H. Remmer, and R. W. Estabrook (1967) MOL. PHARMACOL. 3:113.

FOOTNOTE

[1]Contribution from the Schools of Agriculture and Life Sciences and Physical and Mathematical Sciences. Paper No. 4739 in the Journal Series of the North Carolina Agricultural Experiment Station, Raleigh, North Carolina 27607.

MEASUREMENT OF DIFFUSION PARAMETERS WITH NOBLE METAL ELECTRODES

Wilhelm Erdmann and Wolfgang Krell

Department of Anesthesiology

University of Alabama in Birmingham

After closing of the electric circuit in the beginning of a PO_2-measurement with a bare noble metal electrode, the primary current is high but decreases rapidly in form of a first steep, then gradually flattening curve and approaches a decisively lower value finally (fig. 1).

This characteristic time course of the diffusion limited current is due to the development of an oxygen diffusion (gradient) field around the electrode surface. Finally at any time there are diffusing as many O_2 molecules to the electrode as are reduced. This is the secondary stable state part of the curve.

As the electrode is counting and eliminating the arriving molecules, the primary decrease of the current is defined by D_{O_2} (as it is dependent on D_{O_2} and K_{O_2}) and the stable final value is defined by K_{O_2} (O_2-conductivity coefficient) and the PO_2 of the medium (Krell, 1972).

The diffusion coefficient D is, according to Thews (1960),

$$D = \frac{K}{60 \cdot \alpha}$$

directly proportional to the conductivity coefficient K and reciprocally proportional to the solubility coefficient α.

Changes of D_{O_2} in a medium can only be recognized out of the time course of the first part of the diffusion limited current curve. Changes of K_{O_2} must be assumed when during a constant P_{O_2} and elimination of all influences as there are temperature, convection, etc., a change of the stationary part is perceived.

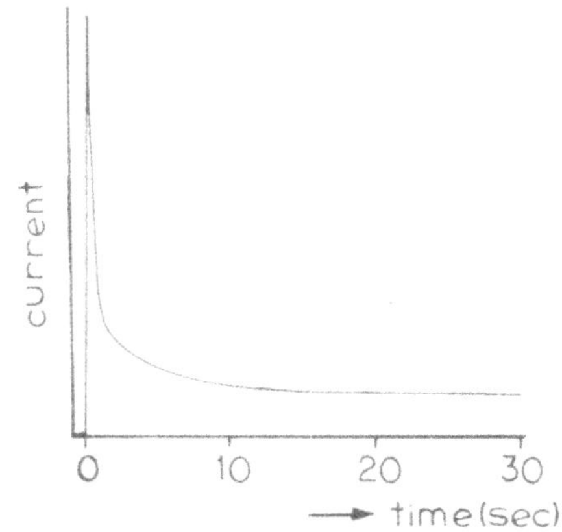

Figure 1: Time course of the diffusion limited current after closing of the electric circuit for PO_2-measurement

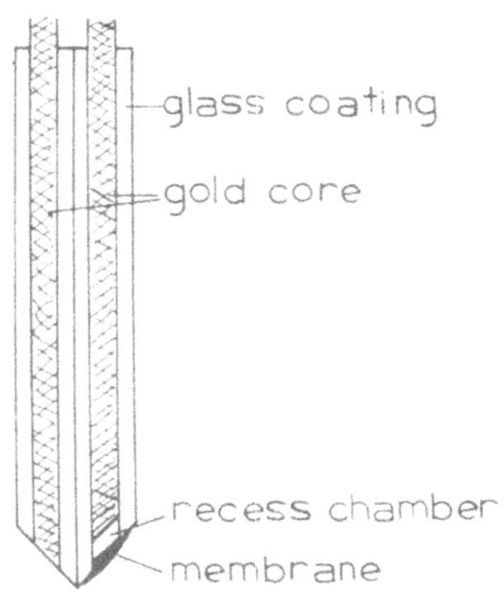

Figure 2: Electrode system consisting of bare O_2-concentration measuring noble metal electrode and a membrane covered O_2-partial pressure measuring electrode for determination of diffusion parameters

Predicted, a continuous measurement of the actual P_{O_2} is exactly performed by membrane covered electrodes, it would be possible to measure the D_{O_2}, K_{O_2} and $\measuredangle O_2$ with a second bare electrode (fig. 2).

Determination of D_{O_2}:

As according to the second Fick's law, the relation of diffusion coefficient and diffusion time is reciprocal. The hyperbel function was taken for mathematical analysis of the time course of the adjustment curve:

$$1) \quad Y = \frac{a}{X} + b$$

where X = time passed from the beginning of the curve
Y = current values registered

b can be calculated according to: $b = \frac{X_1 Y_1 - X_2 Y_2}{X_1 - X_2}$

a can be calculated with known b according to: $a = (Y - \bar{b}) \cdot X$

For the calculation of the unknown diffusion coefficient of a medium $\bar{a}$ is measured in physiological NaCl with known $D_{O_2} = 2.0 \cdot 10^{-5}$ $(\frac{cm}{sec})$ (Goldstick, 1966). Then $\bar{a}$ of the medium with unknown D_{O_2} is measured and D_{O_2} is calculated according to:

$$2) \quad D_{O_2} = \frac{2.0 \cdot 10^{-5}}{\bar{a}_1} \cdot \bar{a}_2$$

$\bar{a}_1$ = mean value of n constants of a in physiological NaCl
$\bar{a}_2$ = mean value of n constants of a in analyzed medium

Determination K_{O_2}:

Bare and membrane covered electrode tips are calibrated in a glycerin concentration with known K_{O_2} (Gmelin, 1958) ($K_{O_2(1)}$) and the output voltage of the two amplifiers is adjusted to the same value. The measurement is repeated in a second glycerin concentration with $K_{O_2(2)}$ and the difference between the output voltages ($V_{d(1)}$) of the two electrodes is registered, which is proportional to the difference of K_{O_2} in the two solutions. The K_{O_2} ($K_{O_2(3)}$) of the medium to be analyzed is calculated according to:

$$3) \quad K_{O_2(3)} = K_{O_2(1)} + \frac{K_{O_2(1)} - K_{O_2(2)}}{V_{d(1)}} \cdot V_{d(2)}$$

$V_{d(1)}$ = difference of output voltages in second glycerin solution
$V_{d(2)}$ = difference of output voltages in analyzed medium

REFERENCES

Gmelin Handbuch der anorganischen Chemie. Hrsg. Deutsche Chemische Gesellschaft, Weinheim/Bergstr.: Chemie, Nr. 3, 446-495, 1958.

Goldstick, T. K.: Diffusion of oxygen in protein solutions. Ph.D. Thesis, University of California. Berkeley, 1966.

Krell, W.: Die polarographische Messung des Sauerstoffpartialdruckes mit Mikroelektroden. Untersuchung der methodischen Voraussetzungen für die Anwendung in vivo. Med. Diss., Mainz, 1972.

Thews, G.: Ein Verfahren zur Bestimmung des O_2-Diffusionskoeffizienten, der O_2-Leitfähigkeit und des O_2-Löslichkeitskoeffizienten im Gehirngewebe. Pflugers Arch. ges. Physiol. 271, 227-244 (1960).

SUMMARY OF DISCUSSION - SESSION IV:

OXYGEN DIFFUSION IN BLOOD AND TISSUE

Chairmen: F. Kreuzer and I. S. Longmuir

In reply to a question by Dr. Ditzel on the effect of lipoproteins on the diffusion of oxygen Dr. Goldstick stated that they had separated 57 samples of plasma on polyacrylamide gel and could find no one protein had a disproportionate effect despite the fact that many of the samples were of grossly abnormal plasma containing a wide range of concentrations of lipoprotein. It seemed that all the proteins studied had about the same effect on the diffusion coefficient of oxygen. Thus this effect seems to be directly proportional to protein concentration although there might be some proteins not encountered in this study which could behave differently, but it seemed unlikely.

Dr. Goldstick went on to say that he felt the dramatic results reported by Grainer could be due to protein interaction with the glass frit or the lyophylisation and prolonged period of measurement in that study.

In reply to a question by Dr. Meldon on the applicability of his theoretical model to pulmonary capillaries Dr. Stroeve stated that it was really only valid for small driving forces whereas in the pulmonary system the driving forces were much larger.

Consideration of the role of mixing within the red cell is difficult to evaluate but models which assumed no convective stirring yield numbers which agree with experimental determinations. If mixing did occur, large discrepancies would be expected.

Dr. Stoeve replied to the suggestion that he should have considered various other factors by saying that it was possible to incorporate such factors as failure to reach equilibrium into his model, but it seemed experimentally these would introduce only a very small perturbation.

Dr. Moll asked Dr. Kawashiro how his ratios of diffusion coefficients of oxygen and carbon dioxide in muscle and water compared with those of Krogh, Wright, and Grote. In his reply he gave for oxygen 0.47 which compares with Krogh's figure of 0.96 and Grote's of 1.47. However, in the case of carbon dioxide there was very close agreement with all four authors. There seemed to be some anomaly in the case of oxygen transport in tissue.

Dr. Evans expressed some concern about the variation in tissue thickness in Dr. Kawashiro's experimental arrangement. It seemed to him that the harmonic mean of the thickness should be used not the arithmetic. However, it appeared that these two means differed by only 1.4%.

Dr. Kreuzer in reply to a question from Dr. Meldon said that he felt the strange behavior of his figure for facilitated diffusion in thin films could be accounted for by the boundary layer thickness approaching that of the film in these experiments.

Dr. Lubbers wondered whether some of the effects seen by Dr. Longmuir might not be due to the presence of damaged cells and if this might not be overcome by using isolated cells. Dr. Longmuir assured him that all damaged cells were removed and that the experiment had been repeated with isolated cells. These gave qualitatively the same results but the measurements had to be made at much lower partial pressures which greatly increases the error. Dr. Lubbers also asked a further question on the possibility that other oxidative processes might be going on in the slices and it was on these that nicotinamide was exerting its effect. Dr. Longmuir explained that before measurements were begun the slices were aged for about thirty minutes so that all endogenous substrates could be exhausted. The slices were then supplied with succinate as the only substrate. As aging does not affect the rate of electron transport until a much longer period has elapsed, it appeared that only succinate was being oxidized. A further advantage of this substrate is that being independent of adenine dinucleotides their loss from the slices during the experiment has no deleterious effect. Separate experiments showed that nicotinamide in the concentrations used has no effect on electron transport; thus, the effect it has on tissue oxygen uptake must be on oxygen transport. As it is unlikely this effect could be on passive diffusion it must be on facilitated diffusion.

Mathematical Models to Describe Oxygen Transport in Blood and Tissue

A GENERALIZED ADVANCING FRONT MODEL DESCRIBING THE OXYGEN TRANSFER IN FLOWING BLOOD

J.M.M. Oomens and J.A.E. Spaan

Department of Mechanical Engeneering, University of Technology, Eindhoven, the Netherlands

INTRODUCTION

It is well known from literature that under certain conditions the steady state transport of oxygen in flowing blood can be described relatively simple when a sharp boundary (advancing front) is assumed between oxygenated and unoxygenated blood (4). Advancing Front (A F) theories have been used to predict oxygen transfer rates in membrane oxygenators (e.g. 2,5). Advancing Front models presented in literature (2,3,4,5,6) have been derived for specific geometries of the flow channel and well defined velocity profiles. A general A F theory would be useful to predict oxygen transport performance for the variety of flow geometries and flow conditions encountered in experimental studies with membrane oxygenators and to analyse the data of existing oxygenators. In this work a general A F theory is presented.

The derivation of the more general A F theory will be done for an oxygenation situation as given in Fig. 1 and under the following conditions: the flow in the oxygenation channel is fully developed laminair flow, the hemoglobin distribution in the blood is considered to be uniform, the diffusion of oxygen in the flow direction is neglected with respect to the diffusion perpendicular to the flow, the oxygen tension outside the flow channel is constant, and the diffusion of hemoglobin and oxyhemoglobin is neglected. The basic assumptions for the A F theory are the following: the oxygenation reaction is instantaneous, a large difference exists between the initial oxygen partial pressure in the blood and the partial pressure in the gas side, and the oxygen flux through the membrane and the saturated blood layer is considered to be constant by given z*.

MASS TRANSFER EQUATIONS

The dimensionless transfer equations which determine the O_2 transfer in flowing blood can be given by (1,2,3 and 6)

$$\frac{\partial^2 C}{\partial x^{*2}} = f(x^*)\cdot\frac{\partial}{\partial z^*}(C + h.S) \qquad \text{flat duct (1)}$$

$$\frac{1}{r^*}\cdot\frac{\partial}{\partial r^*}\left(r^*\cdot\frac{\partial C}{\partial r^*}\right) = f(r^*)\cdot\frac{\partial}{\partial z^*}(C+h.S) \qquad \text{tube (2)}$$

Equations 1 and 2 represent a differential mass balance where at steady state the diffusion of oxygen into a blood volume is balanced against the convective removal. In the above equations z^*; $f(x^*)$, $f(r^*)$; and x^*, r^* are the dimensionless flow channel length, the dimensionless velocity profile, and the depth in the blood layer, respectively, and are given by

flat duct		tube	
$z^* = \frac{z.Dv}{d^2.\bar{V}}$	(3)	$z^* = \frac{z.Dv}{R^2.\bar{V}}$	(4)
$f(x^*) = V_z(x)/\bar{V}$	(5)	$f(r^*) = V_z(r)/\bar{V}$	(6)
$x^* = x/d$	(7)	$r^* = r/R$	(8)

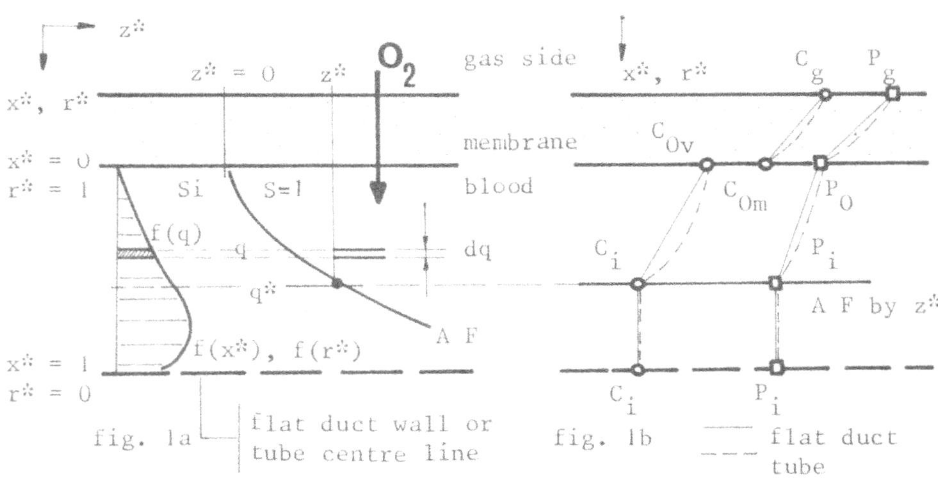

Figure 1. Schematic diagram of an oxygenation channel. The blood is separated from the gas side by a permeable membrane.
a) Path of the A F front with a general velocity profile.
b) Corresponding O_2 concentration-partial pressure profiles in the blood and the membrane by given channel length z^*.

The corresponding boundary conditions for equations 1 and 2 are (see also figure 1)

flat duct		tube	
All x^*; $z^*<0$; $C = C_i$	(9)	All r^*; $z^*<0$; $C = C_i$	(10)
blood membrane interface			
$C_{ov}/\alpha_v = C_{om}/\alpha_m$	(11)	$C_{ov}/\alpha_v = C_{om}/\alpha_m$	(12)
$x^*=0; z^*\geq 0; D_v(\frac{\partial C}{\partial x^*}) = D_m(\frac{\partial C}{\partial x^*})$	(13)	$r^*=1; z^*\geq 0; D_v(\frac{\partial C}{\partial r^*}) = D_m(\frac{\partial C}{\partial r^*})$	(14)
conditions of no flux in the solid wall or center line			
$x^*=1$; All z^*; $D_v \frac{\partial C}{\partial x^*} = 0$	(15)	$r^*=0$; All z^*; $D_v \frac{\partial C}{\partial r^*} = 0$	(16)

Because of the A F assumptions the following equations obtain within the saturated part of the blood layer

$$\frac{d}{dx^*}\left[D_{v,m}\left(\frac{dC}{dx^*}\right)\right] = 0 \quad (17) \qquad \frac{d}{dr^*}\left[r^* \cdot D_{v,m}\left(\frac{dC}{dr^*}\right)\right] = 0 \quad (18)$$

Integration of equations 17 and 18 result in the following formulas for the O_2 concentration profiles

$$C = C_i + (C_{ov} - C_i)(1 - \frac{x^*}{q^*}) \quad (19) \qquad C = C_i \cdot \frac{\ln r^*}{\ln q^*} + C_{ov}(1 - \frac{\ln r^*}{\ln q^*}) \quad (20)$$

The A F equations may be obtained by integration of the differential equations 1 and 2, from the blood membrane interface to the A F and from the front to the unpermeable wall respectively the tube centre line (6). In performing the integration procedure, the O_2 concentration and saturation profiles as well as the boundary conditions have to be used. This results for the tube in

$$dz^* = \left[H \cdot q \cdot f(q)(\ln q - 2M) + \frac{1}{q(\ln q - 2M)}\left(\int_0^{q^*} q \ln q \, f(q)dq - 2M \cdot \int_0^{q^*} q \cdot f(q)dq\right)\right] dq \quad (21)$$

The flow averaged saturation at a dimensionless distance z^* is

$$\overline{S} = 2\int_{q^*}^{1} q \cdot f(q)dq + S_i \cdot 2\int_0^{q^*} q \cdot f(q) \cdot dq \quad (22)$$

Integration of equation 21 together with 22 results in the general A F model for the tube. It is given in terms of four dimensionless numbers L^*, H, M, and f and three integral formulas I_1, I_2 and I_3. For the flat duct and the tube the general A F equations become

$$\boxed{L^* = H(I_2 + M\, I_1) + I_3} \quad (23) \qquad \boxed{f = I_1} \quad (24)$$

Where L^* is the dimensionless length of the flow channel, H is the ratio of the remaining O_2 uptake capacity of the entering blood and the concentration difference between the entering blood and the gas side, M is the relative membrane resistance, and f the fractional saturation change. I_1, I_2 and I_3 depend only on the velocity profile and the chosen flow channel geometry. Equations 23 and 24 are presented for a general velocity profile and geometry of the flow channel. Tabel I gives an overview and comparison of the terms of the equations for the tube and the flat duct geometry. Equation 23 can be subdivided in three characteristic parts wich represent the three influences that determine the depth of penetration of the oxygenation front in the bloodlayer at a given dimensionless length of the flow channel L^*.

$H \cdot I_2$	represents chemical reaction	(23a)
$H \cdot M \cdot I_1$	represents the membrane resistance	(23b)
I_3	represents physically dissolved oxygen	(23c)

The effect of the membrane resistance or the physically dissolved oxygen can be neglected simply by setting M or I_3 equal to zero. Under normal conditions the chemical reaction term determines for 85% the required flow channel length, the membrane resistance for 10% and the physically dissolved oxygen for 5%. Therefore a closer examination of the integral term I_2 in the equation 23 is necessary.

The physical significance of the integral term I_2 and the effect of the velocity profile will be investigated for the flat duct geometry. I_2 can be defined from figure 1a as the dimensionless saturated flow moment. It is the sum of the flow in parallel differential saturated layers (f(q) dq) times the diffusion pathways q travelled by the O_2 to reach these layers,

$$I_2 = \Sigma\ (f(q)dq) \cdot q = \int_0^{q^*} q \cdot f(q)dq \qquad (41)$$

The saturated flow moment allows to quantify the (intuitive) supposition that a large part of the flow close along the blood gas interface achieves more effective oxygenation than flow far from this interface. In terms of a flow moment, one can say that by a fixed saturated flow (a fixed amount of O_2 uptake in the blood), the smaller I_2 the shorter the needed dimensionless flow channel length. Since I_2 is only determined (for a given f) by the function f(q) it is clear that the influence of f(q) on I_2 can be studied by a velocity distribution that depends on one parameter only in which the flow can be brought either close or far from the blood gas interface by change of that parameter. Such a velocity profile for example is represented by the formula

TUBE

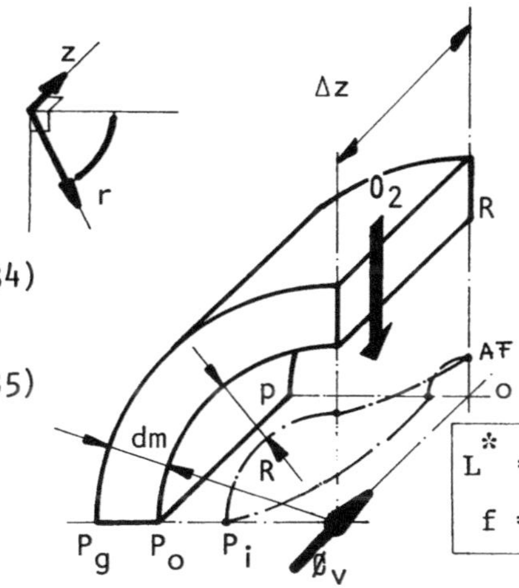

$$f(q) = \frac{V_{z(r)}}{\overline{V}} \quad (34)$$

$$q^* = \left(\frac{R-P}{R}\right) \quad (35)$$

$$f = \frac{\bar{S}-Si}{1-Si} \quad (27) \qquad I_1 = -2\int_1^{q^*} q.f(q)dq \quad (31)$$

$$L^* = \frac{L \cdot D_v}{d^2 \cdot \overline{V}} \quad (28) \qquad I_2 = \int_1^{q^*} q.\ln q.f(q)dq \quad (32)$$

$$H = \frac{h \cdot (1-Si)}{(P_g-P_i)\alpha_v} \quad (29) \qquad I_3 = \int_0^{q^*} \frac{I_2+MI_1}{q(\ln q-2M)} dq \quad (33)$$

$$M = \frac{1}{2}\, \frac{\alpha_v.D_v}{\alpha_m.D_m} \ln\left(1 + \frac{dm}{R}\right) \quad (30)$$

$L^* = H(I_2+MI_1) + I_3$
$f = I_1$

FLAT DUCT

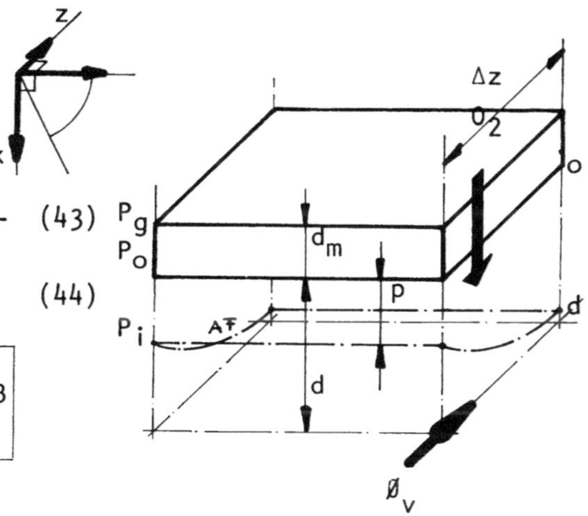

$$f(q) = \frac{V_z(x)}{\overline{V}} \quad (43)$$

$$q^* = \frac{p}{d} \quad (44)$$

$$f = \frac{\bar{S}-Si}{1-Si} \quad (36)$$

$$L^* = \frac{L.D_v}{R^2.\overline{V}} \quad (37) \qquad I_1 = \int_o^{q^*} f(q)\, dq \quad (40)$$

$$H = \frac{h \cdot (1-Si)}{(P_g-P_i)\alpha_v} \quad (38) \qquad I_2 = \int_o^{q^*} q.f(q)dq \quad (41)$$

$$M = \frac{\alpha_v.D_v}{\alpha_m.D_m} \cdot \frac{dm}{d} \quad (39) \qquad I_3 = \int_0^{q^*} \frac{I_2+MI_1}{q+M} dq \quad (42)$$

TABLE I. Overview and Comparison of the Dimensionless Numbers and Integral Terms in the General A F Equations 23 and 24.

$$V_z(x)=A\cdot\left(\frac{x}{d}\right)^n \tag{45}$$

and the reversed function

$$V_z(x)=A\cdot\left(1-\frac{x}{d}\right)^n \tag{46}$$

with 0 = n = ∞ and coupled by n=0. The mean velocity for both profiles is given by

$$\bar{V} = A\cdot\left(\frac{1}{n+1}\right) \tag{47}$$

$V_z(x)$ divided by $\bar{V}$ yields the dimensionless velocity function $f(x^*)$. For equation 45 and 46 $f(x^*)$ becomes respectively

$$f(x^*) = (n+1)\cdot(x^*)^n \tag{48}$$

$$f(x^*) = (n+1)\cdot(1-x^*)^n \tag{49}$$

The corresponding integrals I_2 can be calculated for eq. 45 as

$$I_2=(n+1)\cdot\int_0^{q^*} q\cdot(q)^n\,dq = \left[(n+1)/(n+2)\right] q^{*\,n+2} \tag{49}$$

and for 46 as

$$I_2=(n+1)\int_0^{q^*} q(1-q)^n dq=(n+1)/(n+2)\left[(1-q^*)^{n+2}-1\right]-\left[(1-q^*)^{n+1}-1\right] \tag{50}$$

In figure 2, I_2 is given for several values f (equals I_1) as a function of the velocity parameter n. The upper part of figure 2 represents the velocity profiles for different values of n.

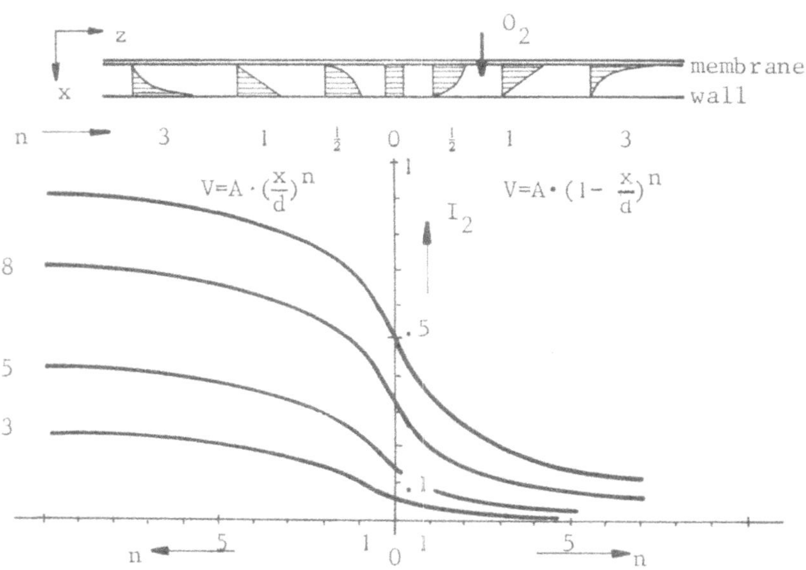

Figure 2 The variation of the flow moment with the velocity parameter for various values of the fractional saturation change.

It can easily be seen that the greater the flow along the membrane the better the oxygenation. There is a great change in the saturated flow moment for values of $n \leq 2$. This is also the region where such velocity profiles are encountered in existing membrane oxygenators. Plugflow is represented by $n=0$, nearly parabolic flow by $n=\frac{1}{2}$, shearflow by $n=1$, and nearly couette flow by $n=2$. In the development of an oxygenator the therm I_2 can be helpful in choosing an appropriate velocity profile for the device.

The general A F model presented here depends on situations where only one side of the flow channel is permeable to oxygen. For the case of membranes on both sides of the channel, eq. 23 and 24 and the equations in tabel I are still applicable. With symmetrical flow in such a channel, the penetration depth q now varies between 0 and $\frac{1}{2}$. The problem of membranes on both sides and an asymmetric flow profile in the channel can be solved by utilizing the one membrane equations presented here and through the use of the appropriate velocity profiles one has to preform two calculations to determine the penetration depths q_1^* and q_2^* at either side of the membranes. The modelling of the two membrane channels by two one membrane channel is valid as long as $q_1^*+q_2^* \leq 1$. The blood is fully saturated when $q_1^*+q_2^*=1$. Similarly to figure 2 (when $I_3 . M=0$) I_2 as a function of n is given in figure 3 for $q_1^*+q_2^*=1$ (f=1). Comparison of figures 2 and 3 shows that a channel with membranes on both sides reduces the flow moment three to four times compared to the one membrane channel for the case $I_1=f=1$. For the region $n \leq 2$ the influence of the velocity profile on I_2 is not very significant. This is contrary to the behaviour shown in figure 2.

CONCLUSIONS

Derivation of A F equations from the generalised A F model (equations 23 and 24) for a given flow-oxygenation situation, reduces the question to the resolution of three simple integral formulas. The defined flow moment can be used to quantify the mean influence of the velocity profile on the dimensionless length of a flow channel.

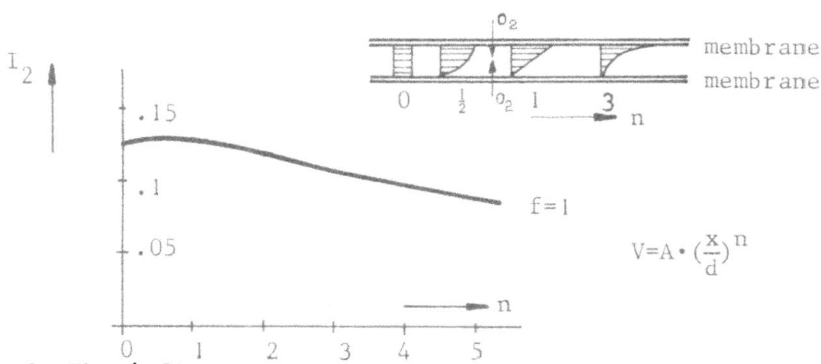

Figure 3. The influence of the flow parameter on the flow moment for the two membrane channels with an asymmetric velocity profile.

NOTATION

A = constant
α_m = solubility coeff. of O_2 in the membrane material
α_v = solubility coeff. of O_2 in blood plasma
C_g = O_2 concentration
C_i = initial oxygen concentration
C_{om} = O_2 concentration in the membrane at the blood interface
C_{ov} = O_2 concentration in the blood at the membrane interface
C = O_2 concentration
d = channel height
d_m = membrane thickness
D_m = diffusion coeff. of oxygen in membrane
D_v = diffusion coeff. of oxygen in blood
h = max O_2 binding capacity
L = lenght of the flow channel
n = velocity parameter
$\emptyset_v$ = blood flow rate
p = distance from the origin to the A F
P_g = constant partial pressure in the gas side
P_i = initial uniform partial pressure in the blood
P_o = partial pressure at the blood membrane interface
q^* = dimensionless distance from the origin to the A F
r = radius
R = inner radius of the tube
S = oxygen saturation
$\bar{S}$ = average oxygen saturation
S_i = initial oxygen saturation
$\bar{V}$ = mean velocity
V_z = local velocity
x = depth in the channel
z = distance along the flow channel

REFERENCES

1. Buckles, R.G., Merrill, E.W., and E.R. Gilliland, AIChE J., 14:703 (1968)
2. Dorson, W.J. Jr., Larsen, K.G., Elgas, R.J., and M.E. Voorhees, Trans. A.S.A.I.O., 17:309 (1971)
3. Dorson, W.J. Jr., in: Blood Oxygenation, D. Hershey, ed., Plenum Press, NY(1970) p 355-372
4. Lightfoot, E.N., AIChE J., 14,669 (1968)
5. Overcash, M.R., Ph. D. Thesis, University of Minnesota (1972)
6. Spaan, J.A.E., Pflügers Arch., 342, 289 (1973)

ACKNOWLEDGEMENTS

This work was partially supported by a grant from Stiftung Volkswagenwerk. Discussion with Dr. Pieter Stroeve about this paper is appreciated.

A THEORETICAL MODEL OF THE RESPIRATORY FUNCTION OF BLOOD

J.H. Meldon and L. Garby

Department of Physiology, Odense University

Odense, Denmark

The physiology and pathophysiology of oxygen transport as mediated by changes in erythrocyte acid-base status and organic phosphate content have been subjects of intense research activity in recent years. These endeavors have been inspired by the discovery of the dramatic effect of changes in red cell 2,3 diphosphoglycerate (DPG) concentration upon hemoglobin oxygen affinity (3,4), and such clinical observations as the inverse relationship between the amounts of DPG and hemoglobin in the blood of anemic patients (5,9). However, in the face of insufficient as well as conflicting data, the significance of changes in the oxygen affinity of hemoglobin as an adaptive mechanism for the maintenance of sufficient oxygen supply remains a matter of speculation (see, for example, the reviews of Bellingham, Rørth, and Woodson in ref. 6).

A theoretical evaluation of the relative importances of various factors which effect the delivery of oxygen to tissue requires a model of the gas transport system which includes not only the blood, but also the lungs and respiring tissue. We have developed such a model and solved the equations which describe its dynamic behavior using numerical methods and digital computation. An outline of our model is presented here along with results from an examination of the means by which a requisite amount of oxygen is supplied in cases of anemia.

CONCEPTION OF THE MODEL

The physiological hemoglobin ligands which most strongly effect the protein's affinity are DPG plus protons and carbon dioxide, with the effect of the latter mediated largely by its influence upon pH (for a review of the biochemistry, see ref. 10). At rest, average blood pCO_2 is effectively determined by conditions in the lungs, while pH is a function of pCO_2 as well as the base excess of the blood, which is itself a function of pCO_2 (15). The DPG level is apparently strongly dependent upon red blood cell (RBC) pH (7), although oxyhemoglobin concentration has been proposed as an additional factor (1).

It seems, therefore, safe to say that the *in vivo* oxygen affinity of hemoglobin is strongly dependent on alveolar carbon dioxide tension. This motivates inclusion of the lungs in our model, but for present purposes it is assumed that lung function can be represented by steady-state arterial pO_2 and pCO_2 values. Thus, no effort is made to analyze for the separate contributions of atmospheric gas tension, breathing rate, and gas phase-to-RBC diffusional resistances to the determination of these arterial tensions. Instead, the composition of blood leaving the lungs is calculated from the gas tensions and a knowledge of the kinetics and equilibria of the chemical reactions and RBC-plasma redistributions which occur during gas exchange.

The uptake of O_2 and release of CO_2 in the lungs, and the reverse process in the systemic capillaries involve an array of flows and reactions, the most important of which are illustrated in Fig. 1. All the chemical reactions shown are quite rapid and the same is generally believed to be true of alveolar-plasma-RBC gas tension equilibrations and the HCO_3^- - Cl^- (Hamburger) shift. (Relevant kinetic data and their sources are listed in ref. 8.) However, not included in the figure is the uncatalyzed plasma CO_2 hydrolysis-H_2CO_3 dehydrolysis reaction, the half-time of which is an order of magnitude greater than the normal lung and systemic capillary transit times of approximately one second. Consequently, RBC and plasma pH do not approach electrochemical equilibrium until 10 to 20 seconds beyond the capillaries.

Kinetic considerations dictate, therefore, that there is no single relationship (namely, that which would prevail at chemical equilibrium) amongst end-capillary pO_2, pCO_2, and pH values. The possible implications of this

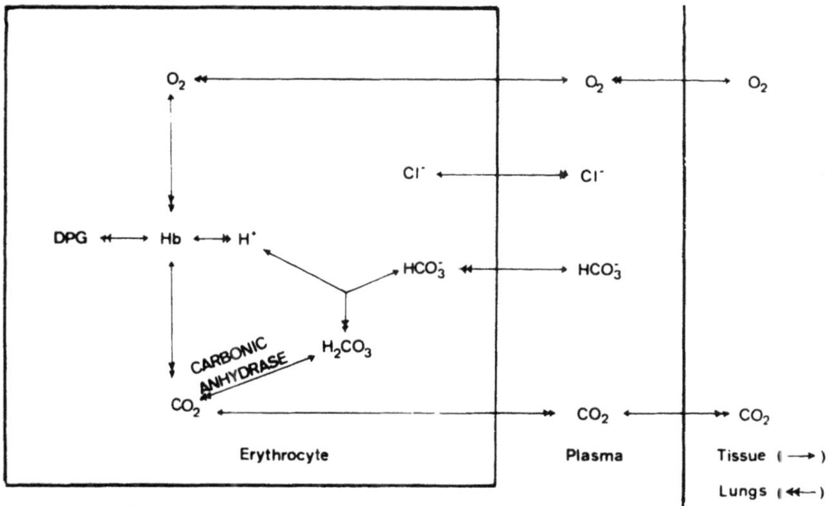

Fig. 1: Diagram of important reactions and flows.

fact regarding both the average pH of the circulating blood and the amount of CO_2 which can be unloaded at alveolar pCO_2 are examined in our model, which is based on simplification of the blood circuit to the closed loop illustrated in Fig. 2a.

The composition of blood leaving the lungs and entering the arteries is calculated from alveolar pO_2 and pCO_2 and an educated guess for RBC pH, assuming the complete equilibration of all RBC-plasma distributions and reactions with the exception of plasma CO_2-H_2CO_3 interaction. The extent of the latter reaction during lung transit is assumed to be negligible, and plasma pH is therefore set equal to end-venous. Thermodynamic equilibrium is approached as the blood flows through the arterial system.

The circulating blood flows from the arteries to the small gas-exchanging vessels, modelled here by an isolated skeletal muscle capillary (Fig. 2b). The vessel is assumed to supply O_2 to and remove CO_2 (in equal amount) from a tissue volume of cylindrical cross-section, the radius of which varies along the length of the capillary as a function of blood pO_2 according to the Krogh-Erlang relation (11). The pO_2 value at the tissue's radial extremity is assumed to be 30 mm Hg, representative of conditions at rest. The volume of tissue is constrained to equal that of a right-circular cylinder of diameter equivalent to spacing between active capillaries under resting conditions (set here at 87μm, inclusive of capillary diameter=10μm).

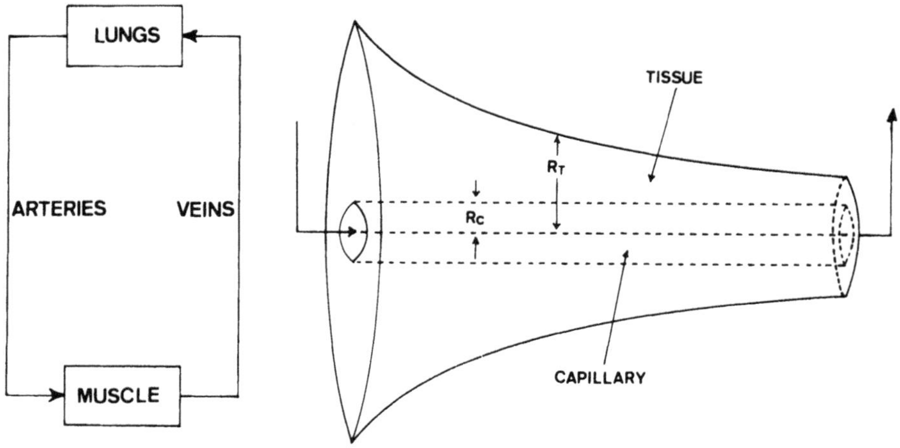

Fig. 2: a) Closed loop model of blood circuit. b) Sketch of assumed capillary and tissue geometries.

This in effect determines capillary blood velocity, since flowrates higher or lower than the correct value result in respectively higher or lower amounts of supplied tissue, and allows for a comparison of different O_2-Hb affinities as they effect the required velocity. Arterial and venous transit times are taken to be proportional to that in the capillary, and are calculated on the basis of standard values of 20 and 40 sec, respectively, at rest with normal hematocrit (=45), RBC DPG (=5 mM), and arterial gas tensions (pO_2=90 mm Hg, pCO_2=40 mm Hg).

As with the lung capillaries, the blood leaving muscle capillaries is in a state of disequilibrium which relaxes along the length of the veins. End venous conditions are then used to calculated the composition of blood leaving the lungs, which must match with those originally calculated for the entrances of the arteries.

MATHEMATICAL ANALYSIS

For present purposes it is assumed that one can safely neglect diffusion along the length of the capillaries in blood and tissue, radial concentration variations within the plasma and RBC, changes in RBC volume, and dissolved O_2 in comparison with that bound to hemoglobin. Furthermore, the transfer of base between blood and tissue in response to changes in arterial pCO_2 (15) will not be considered.

The equations describing blood composition changes with position along the muscle capillary then reduce to:

$$u \frac{dC^e}{dx} = -\left(r_{sv} J^{ep} + \rho^e \right)$$

$$u \frac{dC^p}{dx} = \left(\frac{h}{1 - h}\right) r_{sv} J^{ep} + \frac{2J^{tp}}{R_c(1 - h)} - \rho^p$$

where u is blood velocity, C^e is erythrocyte concentration of a given component, x is distance along the length of the capillary, r_{sv} is the ratio of erythrocyte surface to volume (e.g., in cm^{-1}), J^{ep} is flux from RBC to plasma, ρ^e is rate of consumption by reaction in erythrocyte, C^p and ρ^p are corresponding plasma quantities, h is the fractional hematocrit or percent corpuscular volume (PCV) divided by 100, J^{tp} is flux from tissue to plasma, and R_c is capillary radius, all in consistent units (e.g., fluxes in moles/cm^2/sec).

The rate of RBC-plasma HCO_3^- - Cl^- exchange is calculated from plasma and RBC HCO_3^- concentrations, the local Donnan potential and the Goldman equation. Changes in pH are constrained to satisfy conditions of electroneutrality in erythrocyte and plasma and the conservation of chloride. The same set of relations describe changes in the arteries and veins (with dt replacing dx/u), with tissue-plasma fluxes now vanishing. The complete set of equations was solved by numerical methods, using an IBM 360 computer which converged to steady-state solutions following between 10 and 100 seconds of computer time (depending on hematocrit). Sources of the necessary blood and tissue physicochemical data and preliminary results from an earlier version of the model which included only isolated capillary and tissue are given in ref. 14. A detailed description of our analysis is forthcoming (13).

STUDY OF ANEMIA

The model was used to simulate the conditions in anemic individuals, i.e. patients with subnormal hematocrits. For purposes of comparison, the recently published data of Lichtman et al. (12) from patients with hypoproliferative anemia was most convenient in views of their measurements of DPG concentration, venous pH and pCO_2, and *in vivo* p_{50} in addition to hemoglobin concentration.

Table I: Steady-state results, DPG=7 mM, PCV=25, at rest.

	Artery		Capillary	Vein
	Lung Output	Cap Input	Cap Output	Lung Input
Time (sec)	0.0	11.6	12.3	35.5
Sat (%)	97.7	97.7	74.6	74.6
pO_2 (mm Hg)	90.0	89.6	42.3	42.2
pCO_2 (mm Hg)	31.1	31.2	36.8	35.5
pH, plasma	7.462	7.475	7.474	7.462
pH, RBC	7.222	7.219	7.208	7.209
R_T (m)		63.7	34.5	
p_{50} (mm Hg)		27.5	28.7	

What they observed were the alkalosis, hyperventilation (low pCO_2), and elevated DPG typical of anemic individuals. We therefore started with a programmed linear dependence of end-lung pCO_2 upon PCV (pCO_2=40 at PCV=45, pCO_2= 20 at PCV=22.5), while maintaining arterial pO_2 at 90. The PCV was varied between 10 and 70, with a DPG ranging from 1 to 9 mM in the erythrocytes.

Table I lists resulting blood composition parameters in the beginning and end of the arteries and veins for the particular case of a PCV of 25 and DPG of 7 mM, which is illustrative of the type of profile found in all runs. As indicated earlier, the major plasma pH changes occur in the arteries and veins. Non-equilibrium within the lungs does not amount to a significant effect upon CO_2 unloading in this case, although pCO_2 decreases from 36.8 to 35.5 mm Hg within the veins. In the capillary, the increase in pCO_2 and decrease in erythrocyte pH promote a 1.2 mm Hg increase in *in vivo* p_{50}, a modest decrease in affinity which enhances oxygen release to a small extent.

Figure 3 is a plot of calculated capillary velocity, normalized by the value of 0.041 cm/sec obtained at normal DPG and hematocrit, as a function of the latter two variables. The effect of increasing DPG can be seen to be quite large, and amounts to a 50% decrease in flowrate, for a DPG increase from 3 to 7 mM at PCV=25. The actual DPG level for a given hematocrit can be predicted on the assumption that it is determined by the time-averaged erythrocyte pH. Thus Fig. 4a relates the latter quantity to DPG and PCV, and includes a linear fit of the data of Astrup et al. (2), who measured DPG levels in erythrocytes stored for long periods of time at various pH levels. Data points for the plot of DPG vs. PCV in Fig. 4b are taken from the intersections of the experimental line with the theoretical curves of Fig. 4a. As can be seen, there is reasonable

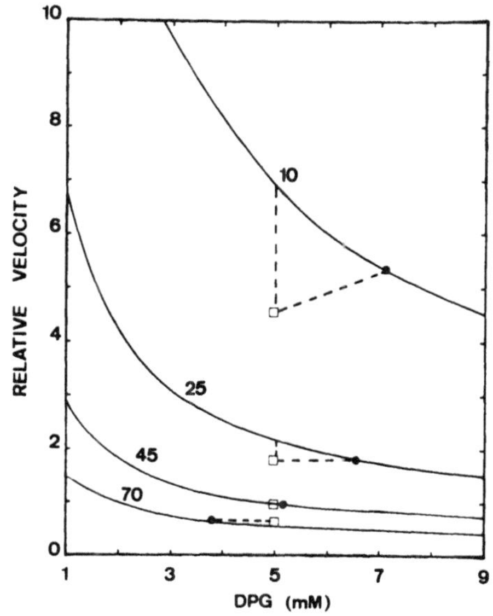

Fig. 3: Calculated normalized velocity vs. DPG concentration at four PCV levels. Solid circles are data points taken from Fig. 4b; hollow squares are calculated for arterial pCO_2=constant at 40 mm Hg.

agreement with the regression line for the experimental data of Lichtman et al.

Returning to Fig. 3, the DPG-PCV combinations of Fig. 4b have been plotted as solid circles, and compared with numerical results at the various hematocrits obtained with DPG held at 5 mM, and with normal arterial pCO_2 (hollow squares). It can be observed that the net effect of hyperventilation in anemia is predicted to be a somewhat increased workload on the heart (as reflected by capillary velocity), in comparison with the situation for normal pCO_2. Still, the increased DPG levels of Fig. 4b compensate significantly for the adverse effect of alkalosis upon O_2-Hb affinity. This is in essential agreement with the observation by Lichtman et al. that blood alkalosis and the accumulation of DPG cancel each other's effects.

CONCLUSIONS

The model of the respiratory function of blood as outlined here is judged to be a powerful tool for the evaluation of the potential effects of changes in blood as well as tissue parameters upon the supply of oxygen to tissue. The erythrocyte-plasma disequilibria in lung and systemic

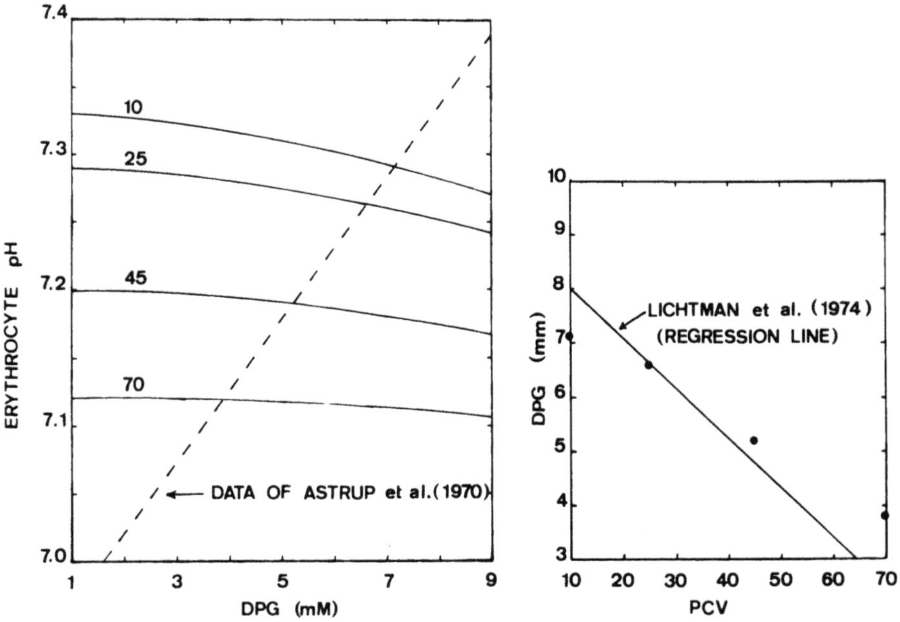

Fig. 4: a) Calculated time-averaged RBC pH vs. DPG concentration and PCV, and comparison with _in vitro_ pH-DPG data. b) DPG-PCV data obtained experimentally from anemic patients, and compared with values predicted from the intersections in Fig. 4a (plotted as solid circles).

capillaries which is a consequence of the slowness of plasma CO_2 hydrolysis are not significant in terms of the delivery of oxygen to tissue, but result in slightly lower unloading of CO_2 in the lungs compared to that which might occur at full equilibration. However, the effects might be of greater interest when relating pH values measured by _in vivo_ sampling to actual values prevailing within the capillaries.

The physiological importances of hyperventilation and elevated DPG levels in anemia cannot as yet be clarified. If anything, it appears that increased DPG is a compensatory mechanism to restore proper O_2-Hb affinity in alkalosis, while the purpose for an alkalosis is not obvious.

REFERENCES

1) Asakura, T., Saito, Y., Minakami, S. and H. Yoshikawa (1966). _J. Biochem. Tokyo 59_, 524.

2) Astrup, P., Rørth, M. and C. Thorshauge (1970). Scand. J. Clin. Lab. Invest. 26, 47.

3) Benesch, R. and R.E. Benesch (1967). Biochem. Biophys. Res. Comm. 26, 162.

4) Chanutin, A. and R.R. Curnish (1967). Arch. Biochem. Biophys. 121, 96.

5) Eaton, J.W. and G.J. Brewer (1968). Proc. Nat. Sci. USA 61, 756.

6) L. Garby (ed.) (1974). Clinics in Hematology 3, 575-720.

7) Guest, G.M. and S. Rapoport (1939). Am. J. Dis. Child 58, 1072.

8) Hill, E.P., Power G.G. and L.D. Longo (1973). Am. J. Physiology 224, 904.

9) M. Hjelm (1969). Försvarsmedicin 5, 219.

10) Kilmartin, J.V. and L. Rossi-Bernardi (1973). Physiol. Rev. 53, 836.

11) A. Krogh (1919). J. Physiol. London 52, 409.

12) Lichtman, M.A., Murphy, M.S., Whitbeck, A.A. and E.A. Kearney (1974). Brit. J. Hæmat. 27, 439.

13) J.H. Meldon, manuscript in preparation.

14) Meldon, J.H. and L. Garby (1975). Acta Med. Scand. Suppl. 578, in press.

15) Shaw, L.A. and A.C. Messer (1932). Am. J. Physiol. 100, 122.

16) J.H.M. was supported by Nat. Heart and Lung Institute (USA) Postdoctoral Fellowship 5 F02 HL54901-02.

SOME MODEL RESULTS ON HEMOGLOBIN KINETICS AND ITS RELATIONSHIP TO OXYGEN TRANSPORT IN BLOOD

John E. Fletcher

National Institutes of Health, LAS, DCRT

Bldg. 12A, Rm 2041, Bethesda, Md. 20014

Introduction: In attempting the difficult process of constructing a mathematical model to represent transport of oxygen within the microcirculation, numerous simplifying assumptions are made to reduce the geometrical and physicochemical relationships to a mathematically tractable form. Any simplification which reduces the model's mathematical complexity carries with it the implicit requirement that this simplification is, in some sense, justified. There is, of course, a continuing need to reexamine the assumptions and the modeling process with each improvement in experimental data and/or change in the geometrical concepts of the microcirculation.

It is the purpose of the results presented here to critique a mathematical description of the oxygen-hemoglobin kinetics, and to quantitate, for the Krogh cylinder model, the effects of neglecting the dissociation velocity of oxygen bound to the hemoglobin of the red cells. As a natural extension of this examination, we also evaluate the possible effect and contribution of the position, or "shift", of the oxygen dissociation curve and its relationship to oxygen transport. The Krogh model concept of microcirculatory geometry, shown in Fig. 1, is well known and need not be developed here. See (1) and (2) for a detailed development.

A mathematical model which includes convective transport, oxygen-hemoglobin kinetics, capillary wall effects, and tissue space diffusion and consumption of oxygen has been given for this geometric model, (2), (3). It is described by the following:

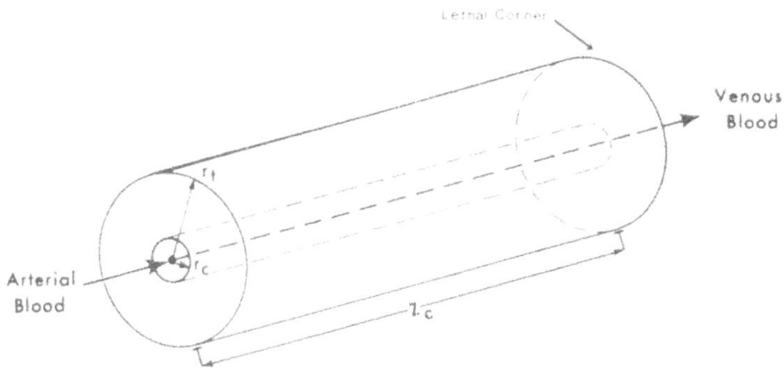

Figure 1. The Krogh cylinder model of microcirculation.

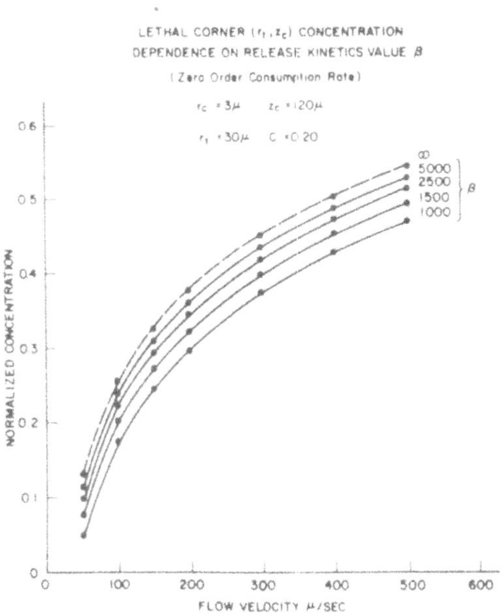

Figure 2. Lethal corner concentration as a function of release velocity parameter β.

In the Tissue,

(1) $$\frac{\partial U}{\partial t} = \frac{1}{r}\frac{\partial}{\partial r}\left(rD_r\frac{\partial U}{\partial r} \right) + \frac{\partial}{\partial z}\left(D_z\frac{\partial U}{\partial z} \right) - Q(u),$$ with

(2) $$D_z\frac{\partial U}{\partial z}(r,0,t) = D_z\frac{\partial U}{\partial z}(r,z_c,t) = 0,$$ and

(3) $$D_r\frac{\partial U}{\partial r}(r_t,z,t) = 0.$$

At the Capillary-Tissue Interface,

(4a) $$\alpha(z)[W(z,t) - U(r_c,z,t)] = -S_tD_r\frac{\partial U}{\partial r}(r_c,z,t),$$

for $\alpha(z)$ finite, and if $\alpha(z)$ is infinite then

(4b) $$W(z,t) = U(r_c,z,t).$$

Within the Capillary,

(5) $$\eta(H)\left[\frac{\partial H}{\partial t} + v(t)\frac{\partial H}{\partial z}\right] = -X(H)[H(z,t) - W(z,t)];$$

(6) $$\frac{\partial W}{\partial t} + v(t)\frac{\partial W}{\partial z} = \rho\frac{2}{r_c}D_r\frac{\partial U}{\partial r}(r_c,z,t) + CX(H)[H(z,t) - W(z,t)],$$

where $\rho = S_t/S_b$, and S represents the solubility.

In these equations, $U(r,z,t)$ represents the tissue PO_2, $W(z,t)$ is the nonequilibrium plasma PO_2, and $H(z,t)$ is the equilibrium PO_2, each normalized to arterial values. The coefficient functions $X(H)$ and $\eta(H)$ are data which characterize the particular oxygen-hemoglobin kinetics. The data of Staub, et. al., (4) was used in the determination of normal values for $X(H)$. The oxygen dissociation function $\psi(H)$ where $d\psi/dH = \eta(H)$ was determined from the data of Severinghaus et. al., (5). For details of this development, see references (2) and (3).

Many authors simplify models similar to the one shown here by making the kinetic equilibrium assumption $H(z,t) = W(z,t)$. By a direct substitution of equation (6) into (5) and using this assumption, a model which neglects the release velocity of oxyhemoglobin is derived:

The Rapid Kinetics Model,

(7) $$\frac{\partial H}{\partial t} + v(t)\frac{\partial H}{\partial z} = \rho\frac{2}{r_c}\frac{D_r}{[1 + C\eta(H)]}\frac{\partial U}{\partial r}(r_c,z,t).$$

Of interest is a comparison of solutions for the model equations (1) through (4) coupled with (5) and (6), and solutions for the model (1) through (4) coupled with (7). The results at the Krogh Cylinder lethal corner are shown in Fig. 2 as a function of capillary flow velocity with release rate $X(H) = \beta$ as a parameter.

The limiting value $\beta = \infty$ corresponds to the solution for the model (1) through (4) coupled with (7), (i.e., the rapid kinetics model), and the other curves represent solutions of the model (1) through (4) coupled with (5) and (6). Clearly the rapid kinetics solution forms an upper bound for the other solutions, and they are monotone increasing with values of the parameter β .

The value of β found for normal blood is approximately 5000, and we may conclude that neglecting the velocity of dissociation introduces an error of only 2% to 3% over most of the flow range. However, if the hemoglobin kinetics are abnormal, (resulting in reduced values of β) then the error in neglecting the release velocity may go as high as 10%. This suggests that in model studies of blood kinetics containing abnormal hemoglobin, the dissociation velocity of oxygen may become a significant factor, and should be considered in the model equations.

Whenever conditions are such that the dissociation velocity can be neglected, equation (7) represents the capillary transport and supply of oxygen to the tissue cylinder. This equation can be used to give some insight into the effect of the shift in the position of the oxygen-hemoglobin dissociation curve and its relation to the oxygen transfer rate into tissue. The terms on the right in equation (7) represent the rate at which oxygen is crossing the capillary wall. The coefficient

$$\rho \frac{2}{r_c} \frac{D_r}{[1 + C\eta(H)]}$$

is effectively a transfer parameter, and the derivative in the denominator of this expression is the slope of the oxygen dissociation curve. This suggests that the oxygen transfer rate into tissue may be modified by both the <u>position</u> of the dissociation curve, and by its slope. At high values of PO_2, $d\psi/dt = \eta(H) \approx 0$, and the transfer rate is limited only by diffusion.

As the plasma PO_2 values decrease along the capillary length, $\eta(H)$ increases monotonically and thus has the effect of reducing the transfer rate into tissue. In other words, the dissociation curve "unloading rate, $\eta(H)$" tends to limit the transfer rate at lowered capillary PO_2 values.

It has been suggested (6), (7), (8), (9), and (10) that a rightward shift of the oxygen dissociation curve due to 2,3 DPG, pH, or other effects, results in better conditions for oxygen delivery to tissue during lowered arterial PO_2 values. Numerical experiments designed to examine this effect were conducted with the family of oxygen dissociation curves shown in Fig. 3. The solid curve was obtained for the normal data of Severinghaus et. al., at pH 7.4, 2,3 DPG concentration of 14.6 mM/gHb, and a P_{50} point of 26.7mmHg. The shifted curves were obtained from patient data provided the author by Dr. Claude Lenfant, NHLI, N.I.H. The leftward shifted curve corresponds to a decreased 2,3 DPG concentration to 8.1 mM/gHb, the data are corrected to a pH 7.4, and the P_{50} point is 21.5 mmHg. The rightward shifted curve

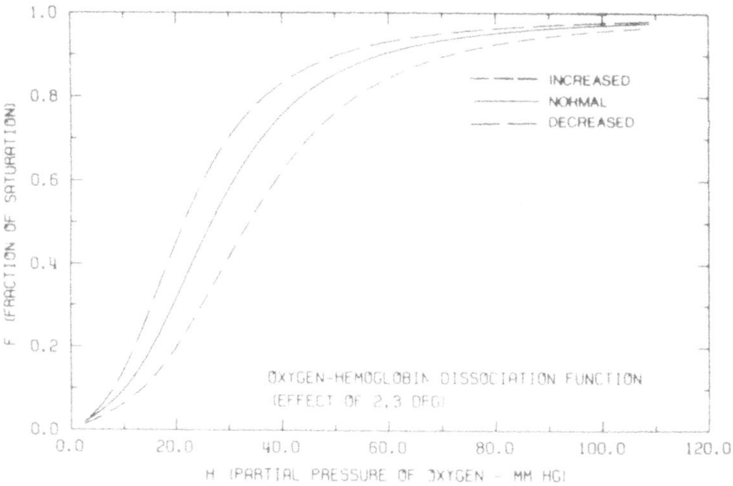

Figure 3. A family of oxygen-hemoglobin dissociation curves.

corresponds to an increase in 2,3 DPG concentration to 23.5 mM/gHb, it also was corrected to pH 7.4, resulting in a P_{50} point of 33.8mmHg.

For fixed tissue cylinder parameters, the venous PO_2 values were computed as a function of arterial PO_2 for each of the dissociation curves. The computations were terminated when lethal corner values dropped to the critical level of 1 mmHg. The venous PO_2 values as a function of arterial PO_2 are shown in Fig. 4.

At arterial pressures above 25 mmHg the rightward shift of the curve always results in a higher venous PO_2 for a given average arterial PO_2. That is, a smaller pressure drop from arterial to venous conditions is required for the supply of a given region under fixed conditions with the rightward shift of the curve. A better contrast of the shift effect is seen if we compare the computed extraction range on the normal curve at 95 mmHg with that of the rightward shifted curve at 55 mmHg. This is one aspect of aclimatization from sea level conditions to those at approximately 10,000 ft altitude. These model results are shown in Fig. 5. Under defined "normal" conditions (i.e., 95 mmHg on the normal curve) the extraction range is over a pressure drop of 67 mmHg. In contrast, at adapted conditions (i.e., 55 mmHg on the rightward shifted curve), the extraction range is over a pressure drop of only 27 mmHg. The shifted curve clearly supplies the required amount of oxygen over a much smaller pressure drop. This, of course, is the desired effect. The cost is a lower oxygen reserve in the venous blood, i.e., only a 37.2% reserve as compared to a 53.8% reserve at the normal sea level conditions.

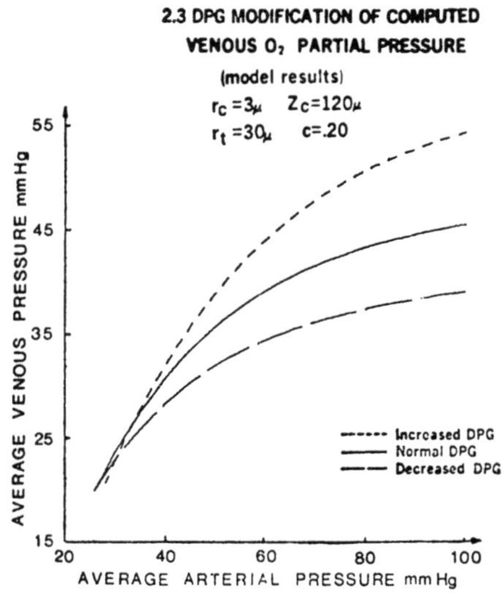

Figure 4. Venous PO_2 as a function of arterial PO_2 at fixed tissue conditions.

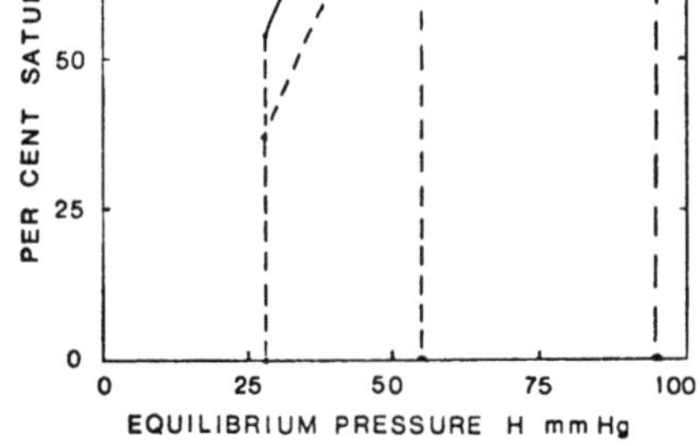

Figure 5. A comparison of oxygen extraction at normal and at altitude conditions, (see text).

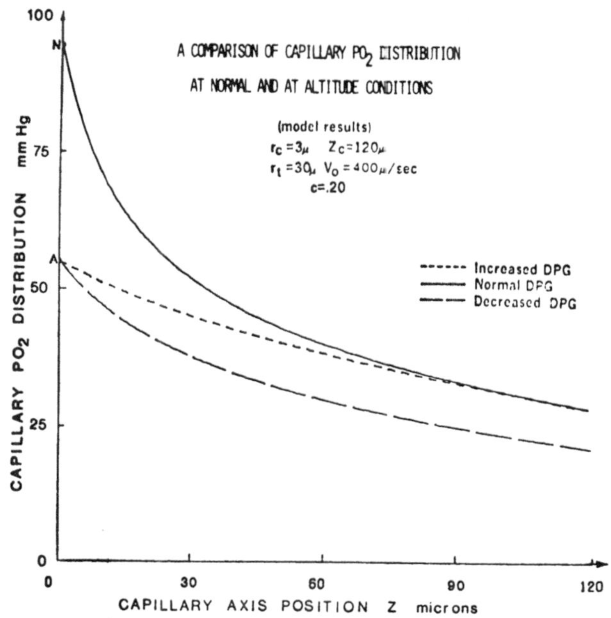

Figure 6. A comparison of capillary PO_2 distribution at normal and at altitude conditions.

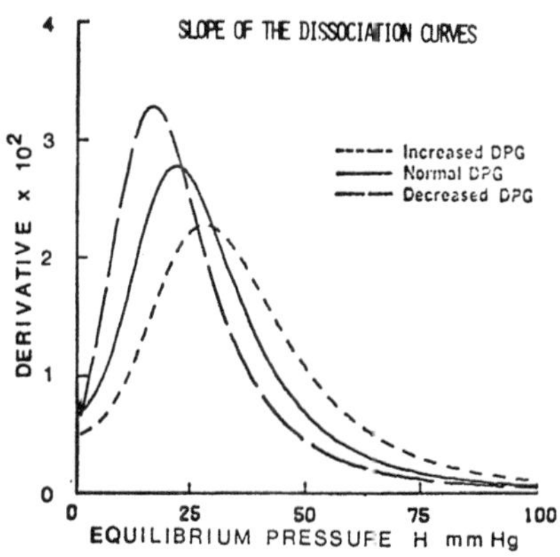

Figure 7. A comparison of oxygen dissociation curve slopes over the pressure range 0 - 100 mm Hg.

There are other compensating mechanisms which improve this latter figure, but they were not examined here. The question is, "How is this effect accomplished?" The mechanism seems to be the increase in the slope of the dissociation curve with the rightward position shift. That is, the PO_2 "unloading" rate is modified.

Fig. 6 shows the PO_2 distribution along the capillary wall for three conditions. The normal curve at a PO_2 of 95 mmHg permits an excess of oxygen to accumulate near the entrance region of the capillary, whereas the shifted curve at 55 mmHg induces an almost linear decrease of PO_2 values along the capillary. The leftward shift, for an arterial PO_2 of 55 mmHg, results in a much lower pressure distribution than for the rightward shifted curve.

Summary and Discussion: The results presented here have shown that the assumption of kinetic equilibrium in capillary transport models is justified under normal conditions. The computations shown were carried out for only the Krogh model, but the qualitative results should apply more generally since the nature of the blood kinetics are independent of model geometry. However, if systems involving abnormal hemoglobin are being modeled, the nonequilibrium kinetics should be considered. The model results presented here indicate that the shift in the oxygen-hemoglobin dissociation curve adjusts oxygen transport to tissue by modifying the unloading rate from hemoglobin which in turn alters the transfer rate into tissue. The compensatory effect is to elevate venous pressure to near normal conditions in adapting to lowered arterial conditions. The results presented here suggest that venous conditions might be more significant in regulating microcirculatory function than arterial conditions, and thus autoregulatory or adaptive sensors might be located in the venous side of the microcirculation rather than the arterial side.

With the rightward shift of the dissociation curve, the slope of the dissociation curve, shown in Fig. 7, is shifted downward and to the right, and the point of maximum slope varies linearly with 2,3 DPG concentration. We note that the peak derivative in each case occurs near the point of intersection with next shifted curve and corresponds to a value near the P_{50} point on the dissociation curves themselves. This suggests that a description of the dissociation curves in terms of the PO_2 yielding the maximum slope rather than the P_{50} point is perhaps a more meaningful parameter. Again, the computed results are for the Krogh model, but the qualitative results should be similar for other model geometries.

References

1. A. Krogh, "The Number and Distribution of Capillaries in Muscles with Calculations of the Oxygen Pressure Head Necessary for Supplying the Tissue," J. Physiol., 52(1919), 409-415.

2. J. Fletcher, "Distributed Parameter Modeling of the Micro-circulation, "in Systems Analysis of Biomedical Transport (D. Reneau, ed.) Marcel Dekker, Inc. New York, (To be published first quarter 1975).

3. J. Fletcher, "A Model Describing the Unsteady Transport of Substrate to Tissue from the Microcirculation," SIAM J. Appl. Math., Vol. 29, No. 2, September 1975.

4. N. Staub, J. Bishop, and R. Forster, "Velocity of of O_2 Uptake by Human Red Blood Cells," J. Appl. Physiol., 16 No. 2 (1961), 511-516.

5. F. Roughton, and J. Severinghaus, "Accurate Determination of O_2 Dissociation Curve of Human Blood above 98.7% Saturation with Data on O_2 Solubility in Unmodified Human Blood From 0° to 37° C," J. Appl. Physiol., 35 no. 6 (1973), 861-869.

6. C. Finch and C. Lenfant, "Oxygen Transport in Man," New England Jour. of Med., 268, (1972), 407-415.

7. C. Lenfant and K. Sullivan, "Adaptation to High Altitude," New England Jour. of Med., 284, (1971), 1298-1309.

8. L. Moore, G. Brewer, F. Oelshlegel, and A. Rose, "Pharmacological Stimulation of Red Blood Cell Metabolism for High Altitude Preadaptation," in Oxygen Transport to Tissue, Pharmacology, Mathematical Studies, and Neonatology, (D. Bruley and H. Bicher eds.), Vol. 37B, Plenum Press, New York, 1973, 693-698.
9. C. Bauer, "Influence of 2,3 DPG and Hydrogen Ions on the Kinetics of the Oxygen Hemoglobin Reaction," in Alfred Benzon Symposium IV, proceedings, Oxygen Affinity of Hemoglobin and Red Cell Acid Base Status, (M. Rorth and P. Astrup, eds.), Munksgaard, Copenhagen, 1972, 511-517.

10. R. Forster, "Influence of 2,3 DPG on the Velocity of Oxygen Uptake and Delivery by Red Blood Cells," in Alfred Benzon Symposium IV, proceedings, Oxygen Affinity of Hemoglobin and Red Cell Acid Base Status, (M. Rorth and P. Astrup, eds.), Munksgaard, Copenhagen, 1972, 518-524.

THE MECHANICAL BASIS FOR FICK'S LAW AND ITS GENERALIZATIONS

E. L. Roetman
Department of Mathematics

and

R. E. Barr
Department of Opthalmology

University of Missouri
Columbia, Missouri 65201, U.S.A.

In 1855 Fick [1] wrote about the problem of diffusion of one fluid species through another. After a rather long discussion of the basis for such diffusion in terms of molecular motion and the difficulties of careful analysis based on molecular theory, Fick proposed, by analogy to heat flow, that the concentration satisfies the differential equation

$$\frac{\partial c}{\partial t} = D\nabla^2 c \ .$$

Today we recognize that part of Fick's argument was a conservation of mass statement and the remaining gave a constitutive relation connecting the mass flux to the concentration. In this context, one may write Fick's law as

$$\frac{\partial c}{\partial t} + \text{div } \underline{J} = 0 \qquad (2)$$

$$\underline{J} = -D(\text{grad } c) \qquad (3)$$

where $\underline{J}$ is the flux vector.

There are many objections to Fick's law including the infinite signal time and inextendability to several components. If equation (1) is an accurate model of the system, then, since it is a parabolic partial differential equation, a disturbance will propagate with infinite signal speed. That is, a change in the environment at one point will instantly effect a change in concentration everywhere to some degree. The development of the above equations do not easily extend to cases with more than two components such as oxygen and carbon dioxide in saline.

Fick refers to earlier authors who considered the problem without conclusion and admits that he too would not bring the discussion to a definitive conclusion. It seems, however, that no essentially new ideas were brought to the subject until the C. Eckart, 1940 [2], paper which approached the problem as one of fluid mixtures within the context of fluid dynamics. There followed a series of papers: Truesdell, 1957, 1962, Adkins, 1960, 1963 and thereafter a mini-avalanche, see Gurtin, 1971 [3] for references. This continuum approach for a two-component mixture starts with mass and momentum balance equations for each component of the fluid where $\rho_i, \underline{v}_i, \underline{f}_i, \underset{\sim}{T}_i, \underline{S}_i$ (i=1,2) are the densities, field velocities, body forces, such as gravity, internal fluid stresses and the fluid component interactive forces respectively:

mass balance

$$\frac{\partial}{\partial t} \rho_i + \operatorname{div}(\rho_i \underline{v}_i) = 0 \tag{4}$$

momentum balance

$$\rho_i \left(\frac{\partial}{\partial t} \underline{v}_i + \underline{v}_i \cdot \nabla \underline{v}_i\right) = \rho_i \underline{f}_i + \operatorname{div} \underset{\sim}{T}_i + \underline{S}_i \tag{5}$$

Define mixture parameters: density $\rho = \rho_1 + \rho_2$, concentrations $c_i = \rho_i/\rho$ (i=1,2), mean velocity $\underline{v} = c_i \underline{v}_1 + c_2 \underline{v}_2$, and diffusion velocities $\underline{u}_i = \underline{v}_i - \underline{v}$; assume constitutive relations $\underset{\sim}{T}_i = p_i \underset{\sim}{E}$, p_i is the partial pressure where $p_i = p_i(c_i)$, and $\underline{S}_i = \sigma_i \rho_i \mathcal{J}^{-1}(\underline{v}_2 - \underline{v}_1)$ $(\sigma_1 = +1, \sigma_2 = -1)$; and assume further that it is characteristic of the system that $\underline{v}$ is negligible, ρ is constant and that the body forces $\underline{f}_i$ are negligible. The equations (4) and (5) then yield for $i = 1,2$

$$\frac{\partial}{\partial t} c_i + \operatorname{div}(c_i \underline{u}_i) = 0 \tag{6}$$

$$c_i \left(\frac{\partial}{\partial t} \underline{u}_i + \underline{u}_i \cdot \nabla \underline{u}_i\right) = -\rho^{-1} \operatorname{grad} p_i + \sigma_i c_i \mathcal{J}^{-1} (\underline{u}_2 - \underline{u}_1) \tag{7}$$

Consider the first component as the solvent, the second the solute and assume that the mixture is very dilute. That is, $c_1 >> c_2$. Then $\rho \simeq \rho_1$, and, since $\underline{v} = 0$, $\underline{u}_1 = c_2\underline{u}_2$. Since c_2 is so small, $\underline{u}_1$ is taken to be negligible. Finally, assume that $\underline{u}_2$ is so small that the convective terms can be ignored (this is the usual linearization assumption in fluid flow). Then

$$c_2 \frac{\partial}{\partial t} \underline{u}_2 = \frac{\partial}{\partial t} (c_2\underline{u}_2) - \underline{u}_2 \frac{\partial}{\partial t} c_2 .$$

Equation (6) gives

$$c_2 \frac{\partial}{\partial t} \underline{u}_2 = \frac{\partial}{\partial t} (c_2\underline{u}_2) + \underline{u}_2(\nabla \cdot (c_2\underline{u}_2))$$

$$\simeq \frac{\partial}{\partial t} (c_2\underline{u}_2) .$$

One can then write equations (6) and (7) in the form

$$\frac{\partial}{\partial t} c_2 + \text{div } (c_2\underline{u}_2) = 0 \tag{8}$$

$$\frac{\partial}{\partial t} (c_2\underline{u}_2) = \frac{-p'_2(c_2)}{\rho} (\text{grad } c_2) - c_2\vartheta^{-1}\underline{u}_2 \tag{9}$$

Since only the subscript 2 appears, one can ignore the subscripts. To facilitate comparison with equations (2) and (3), set $\underline{J} = c\underline{u}$ in (8) and (9), write $D = \dfrac{\vartheta p'(c)}{\rho}$ and collect terms to obtain

$$\frac{\partial}{\partial t} c + \text{div } \underline{J} = 0 \tag{10}$$

$$\frac{\rho D}{p'(c)} \frac{\partial}{\partial t} \underline{J} + \underline{J} = -D(\text{grad } c) \tag{11}$$

If one ignores the first term in (11), then (2) and (3) are recovered exactly. If the partial pressure is related to the concentration according to Henry's law, $p = kc$, the divergence of (11) with substitution from (10) produces, as a first generalization of Fick's law, the equation

$$\frac{\rho D}{k} \frac{\partial^2}{\partial t^2} c + \frac{\partial}{\partial t} c = D \nabla^2 c. \tag{12}$$

The many simplifying assumptions that were made to obtain (12) provide a framework in which to interpret the applicability of Fick's law. If p does not follow Henry's law or if $\mathcal{J}$ depends upon c one obtains a nonlinear equation similar to (12), while if some other assumption is violated one obtains a more general system of equations that must be solved for c and $\underline{u}$ simultaneously, including for example convective mass transfer. The approach can clearly be extended to multi-component mixtures, with corresponding complications, ofcourse.

Equation (12) is a damped wave equation or Telegrapher's Equation. It provides for a finite signal time and other wave equation properties as well as properties associated with a parabolic equation [4], [5]. Let $s = (k/\rho)^{1/2}$, $\alpha = D/k$. The transient solution to the equation (12) with $c(x,0) = f(x)$ and $\frac{\partial c}{\partial t}(x,0) = 0$ is

$$c(x,t) = \frac{1}{2}\exp(-t/\alpha)\ \{f(x+st) + f(x-st)\}$$

$$+\int_{-\infty}^{\infty} f(z)\ K(x,t;z;\alpha)\,dz$$

where

$$K(x,t;z;\alpha) = \frac{-tJ'_0(\{[z-(x+st)][z-(x-st)]\}^{1/2})}{4\alpha\{[z-(x+st)][z-(x-st)]\}^{1/2}},$$

if $x - st \leq z \leq x + st$

0 otherwise.

One sees that s is the transient signal velocity and α is the reciprocal of the logarithmic decrement. Define the transient decay time as that required for the exponential factor $\exp(-t/\alpha)$ to decay from 1 to 0.1. Then

$$\tau = -2\alpha\log(.1) = 4.6\ \alpha\ . \tag{15}$$

In order to get some feel for the significance of these terms, consider the problem of oxygen diffusion through water whose geometry is such that the problem reduces to a one space variable problem. That is, consider the concentration changes in the x direction only. As parameters take

$$D = 2.17 \times 10^{-5}\ cm^2\ sec^{-1},\ [6],\ k = 3.72 \times 10^{-3}\ gm(sec^2 cm)^{-1}\ [7],$$

and $\rho = 1$ gm cm^{-3}.

Then

$$s = .61 \text{ mm sec}^{-1}$$

$$\alpha = .58 \times 10^{-3} \text{ sec}$$

$$\tau = 2.7 \times 10^{-3} \text{ sec}$$

The distance traveled by a transient front before the decay factor drops to 0.1 is

$$\tau s = 1.7 \times 10^{-3} \text{ mm} .$$

The above discussion illustrates that the transient wave effects are within measurable time and distance limits in biological systems. In particular, we note that the development suggests that the propagation speed is dependent on k but independent of D. This may then provide a means for independent determination of k. Periodic systems also have special properties including "cut off" frequencies that may be useful in biological application. We hope to report on this aspect at a future time.

References

[1] A. Fick. Ueber Diffusion. Ann. Physik 94(1855) 59-86.

[2] C. Eckart. The thermodynamics of irreversible Processes II. Fluid Mixtures. Phys. Rev. 58(1940) 269-275.

[3] M. Gurtin. On the thermodynamics of chemically reacting fluid mixtures. Arch. Rational Mech. Anal. 43(1971) 198-212.

[4] V. Smirnov. A course of Higher Analysis, vol. II. Pergamon: Oxford, 1964.

[5] W. Fulks and R. Guenther. Damped wave equations and the heat equation. Czech. Math. 21(96) (1971) 683-695.

[6] P. Altman and D. Dittmer, editors. Respiration and Circulation. Federation of American Societies for Experimental Biology: Bethesda, Maryland, 1971.

[7] Standard Methods for Examination of Water by American Public Health Association. Reported in: Beckman Instructions 1223-B, June 1964, Beckman Instruments Inc.

A STOCHASTIC MODEL FOR THE TRANSPORT OF OXYGEN TO BRAIN TISSUE

Duane F. Bruley, Dept. of ChE, Tulane Univ., New Orleans, La., U.S.A.; Lynn J. Groome, Dept. of ChE, Clemson Univ., Clemson, S.C., U.S.A.; Haim Bicher, Dept. of Pharmacology, Med. School of Arkansas, Little Rock, Ark., U.S.A.; and Melvin H. Knisely, Dept. of Anatomy, Med. Univ. of S.C., Charleston, S.C., U.S.A.

ABSTRACT

Material balances around a small, but finite volume element have formed the basis for previous mathematical models describing the transport of oxygen in the brain microcirculation. Seeking a model which would be both simple and versatile, a stochastic model was proposed based on the assumption that oxygenation of the brain can be described quantitatively by simulating the activity of only one erythrocyte and the oxygen molecules surrounding it. Compared with existing deterministic models, the capillary space-average oxygen partial pressure profiles were in close agreement. Tissue tensions were decidedly different.

SCOPE

Mathematical modeling has long played an integral role in the study of biological systems. These models, together with their ensuing equations, have provided explanations for well-known processes, as well as predicting yet-to-be proven phenomena.

To date, the models developed for simulating the transfer of oxygen from blood to other living tissues have been deterministic, i.e., based on macroscopic material balances. In an effort to obtain a simple and versatile model, this study was undertaken to develop a stochastic model capable of predicting oxygen tensions in capillaries and surrounding tissue.

Random walk techniques can be used in two distinct ways, the first being simply the solution of differential equations.

Solutions obtained in this way may be computationally simpler than their corresponding analytical or numerical solution. Halberg, Bruley and Knisely (4) and Hunt, Bruley, and Knisely (6) used approaches similar to this in their Monte Carlo solutions of coupled, non-linear, partial differential equations describing the transfer of oxygen in the capillaries and tissue of the human brain.

The second method is the direct simulation of the actual physical process using discrete entities such as molecules. Bugliarello and Hsiao (1) took this route in simulating convective diffusion in the axial plasmatic gaps of capillaries. For this study, this approach was used to model the oxygenation of the brain microcirculation.

MODELING OF THE MICROCIRCULATION

Based on the "Krogh tissue cylinder" Reneau, Bruley and Knisely (10, 11) presented a coupled set of non-linear partial differential equations describing the transport of oxygen in the brain microcirculation. In deriving the equations it was assumed that (1) equilibrium exists between the dissolved oxygen and hemoglobin, i.e., the oxygen dissociation curve[1] serves as a reaction curve, (2) resistance at the capillary-tissue interface is negligible, and (3) blood and tissue are homogeneous phases.

As is evident from the set of coupled equations, predicting oxygen levels is a formidible task, even under steady-state conditions. To simplify this, while at the same time affording a more basic model, the following stochastic model has been developed. This model does not involve solving the deterministic model, but instead is based on the assumption that oxygenation of the brain can be described by simulating the activity of only one erythrocyte and the oxygen molecules which surround it.

Treatment of the Capillary

Oxygen is transferred in the capillary by bulk flow and molecular diffusion, with gradients in both the axial and radial directions. The simulation procedure consists of displacing each oxygen molecule a distance $v_x \Delta t$ and then using three Gaussianly distributed random numbers to determine the final position. In the three-dimensional case the net displacements during the time interval Δt are:

$$x = x' + \phi_x{}^b\ (R_n) + v_x \Delta t\ , \qquad (1)$$

$$y = y' + \phi_y{}^b\ (R_n)\ , \qquad (2)$$

$$z = z' + \phi_z^b (R_n) \quad , \tag{3}$$

and, for the erythrocyte,

$$x_e = x'_e + v_x \, \Delta t, \tag{4}$$

where it has been assumed that bulk flow is in the x-direction only. In the case of three-dimensional flow, i.e., bolus flow, the velocity field required as an input to the convective step can be determined by a numerical solution of the Navier Stokes equations.

At the capillary entrance the number of oxygen molecules η_o, surrounding the erythrocyte is determined and is chosen as the basis: η_o molecule exert a partial pressure P_B within a volume V_B. Erythrocytes are biconcave discs approximately 8 microns in diameter, with the rim of the disc being thicker (2 microns) than the center (1 micron) (7). The effective volume V_B was chosen based on a cylindrical length of 1 micron, the thickness of an erythrocyte at its center. The effect of the erythrocyte volume on the movement of oxygen was assumed negligible. Since the solubility is defined as

$$S_o^b = \frac{C_o^b}{P_o^b} \tag{9}$$

where C_o^b and P_o^b are the concentration of oxygen in the blood and the partial pressure of dissolved oxygen in the blood, respectively, a pseudo-solubility is calculated as

---

[1] Several empirical relations have been developed relating equilibrium values of the fractional saturation of hemoglobin with oxygen to oxygen partial pressures in the plasma. The following expression was used in this study since it is the most accurate to date (8); It was fitted to the momograph by Grote (14).

$$\Psi = \frac{\theta^3 + b - 1}{\theta^4 + b - 1} \tag{5}$$

where

$$\theta = \frac{1 + aP_o}{aP_o} \tag{6}$$

and a and b are functions of the carbon dioxide partial pressures,

$$a = a_o + a_1 P_c + a_2 P_c^2 \tag{7}$$

and

$$b = b_o + b_1 P_c + 1 \tag{8}$$

$$S_o^{\,b} = \frac{\eta_o/V_B}{P_B} \tag{10}$$

Under normal conditions P_B is 95 mmHg.

Once the convective step is completed, the number of oxygen molecules η_o within the volume V_B surrounding the erythrocyte is determined. Since the oxygen carried on an erythrocyte is chemically bound to the hemoglobin, the fractional saturation Ψ can be thought of as the ratio of the number of hemoglobin sites filled (N_f) to the total number of hemoglobin sites available at saturation (N_s). Thus,

$$\Psi = \frac{N_f}{N_s} \tag{11}$$

and the change in Ψ is a direct measure of the number of oxygen molecules released by the erythrocyte,

$$N_r = -N_s \cdot \Delta\Psi \quad , \tag{12}$$

where N_r is the change in the number of oxygen molecules bound to the erythrocyte for some change $\Delta\Psi$ in the fractional saturation of the erythrocyte.

Assuming equilibrium to exist between the oxygen dissolved in the plasma and the oxygen bound to the erythrocyte, the following relations must be observed:

$$P_o = \frac{(\eta + Nr)\ /V_B}{S_o^{\,b}} \tag{13}$$

$$\Psi = \frac{\theta^3 + b\text{-}1}{\theta^4 + b\text{-}1} \tag{5}$$

where θ is given by equation (6), and

$$N_r = -N_s\ (\psi - \Psi_i), \tag{14}$$

where η is the number of oxygen molecules surrounding the erythrocyte <u>before</u> any oxygen is released by or absorbed onto the erythrocyte, and Ψi is the previous erythrocyte saturation value. From the above set of equations (equations 5, 13, and 14) the numbers of oxygen molecules released from the red blood cell can be determined. Since η, $S_o{}^b$, V_B, N_s, and Ψi are known, there are three equations and three unknowns (P, Ψ, and N_r). A modified Fibonacci search routine is used to converge on the partial pressure P. Once the oxygen tension is known, the fractional saturation can be found (equation 5) and the number of oxygen molecules released determined using equation 15. The positions of the released molecules are uniformly distributed within the volume V_B around the erythrocyte center.

Treatment of the Capillary-Tissue Interface

The deterministic model discussed earlier was developed with the assumption that oxygen diffused freely across the capillary wall. Since the capillary wall is approximately 0.5 microns thick (2), as compared with a capillary radius of 2.5 microns, membrane resistance may be significant. Permeability effects can be readily incorporated into the stochastic model in the following manner. Let P_m denote the capillary wall permeability such that

$$0 \leq P_m \leq 1 \tag{15}$$

where the lower limit ($P_m = 0$) represents a capillary wall of infinite permeability and the upper ($P_m = 1$) is a completely impermeable membrane. A uniformly distributed random number R_n between zero and one is generated and compared to P_m. If $R_n > P_m$, the particle is allowed to pass across the capillary wall into the tissue, otherwise it is reflected back into the capillary. To account for the finite thickness of the capillary wall, an inert region of approximately 0.5μ should be included.

Treatment of the Tissue

Oxygen travels in the tissue by molecular diffusion only, with gradients existing in both the radial and axial directions. As in the capillary, the diffusion process is governed by the Gaussian distribution function. For three-dimension, the net displacements during the time interval Δt are

$$x = x' + \delta_x{}^t\,(R_n) \quad , \tag{16}$$

$$y = y' + \delta_y{}^t\,(R_n) \quad , \tag{17}$$

and

$$z = z' + \delta_z{}^t\,(R_n) \quad , \tag{18}$$

Following movement by diffusion, the next step in the simulation is to determine if the molecule has been consumed by chemical reaction in the time interval Δt. Since previous investigators have assumed a constant oxygen consumption rate to be valid under normal conditions, several techniques were tried in simulating the zero-order reaction.

For a zero-order reaction the probability density was found to be (3)

$$P_x(t) = \frac{(kt)^{x_o - x}}{(x_o - x)!} e^{-kt} \tag{19}$$

and the expected number of molecules reacting in the time interval Δt is

$$E[N(\Delta t)] = k\Delta t, \tag{20}$$

where k is the zero-order rate constant. A tubular plug flow reactor was simulated by removing $k\Delta t$ molecules from the system for each stochastic step, and these results were then extended to the capillary-tissue system.

It is known (5) that, for a Markov pure-jump process, the waiting time τ until a particle reacts is exponentially distributed:

$$P(\tau \leq t) = 1 - e^{-\mu t}, \tag{21}$$

where $P(\tau \leq t)$ is the distribution function for τ. Using a set of exponentially distributed random numbers, τ was generated, and the particle was allowed to move until $t \geq \tau$, at which time it was deleted from the system.

Since the reaction mechanism within the tissue has not been positively established, it was decided to attempt the simulation assuming a first-order reaction. For a single particle, the probability of reaction is given by Wyman and Kosten (13) as

$$P_r = e^{-k\Delta t}. \tag{22}$$

In carrying out the simulation a uniformly distributed random number R_n is generated and compared to P_r. If $R_n > P_r$. the molecule is said to have reacted and is deleted from the system; otherwise the molecule continues its random walk.

RESULTS AND DISCUSSION

In comparing the results of the stochastic and deterministic models for predicting oxygen profiles in the microcirculation, it should be emphasized that although the two models are intended to simulate the same system, they are basically quite different and therefore exact agreement between the two is not to be expected.

Choosing a Basis. Ideally, a one-to-one correspondence between the number of oxygen molecules employed in the simulation and the actual number of oxygen molecules per red blood cell in vivo should exist, but rather than using such a large number of molecules, the following approach was taken. One hundred fifty moleucles were assumed to exhibit an oxygen partial pressure of 95 mmHg in a volume element of 19.6×10^{-12} ml of blood. A 'pseudo-solubility', valid for simulation purposes only, was then back-calculated. Various bases were tried, all of which gave similar results, but 150 molecules was chosen to allow for rapid computation time.

Determination of the Number of Active Hemoglobin Sites. Approximately 99% of the oxygen transported by the blood is carried as oxyhemoglobin. Thus, the number of hemoglobin sites available for binding with oxygen will significantly influence the oxygen profiles.

Under normal conditions, the venous oxygen tension has been experimentally determined to be approximately 34mmHg. Utilizing this information, a trial and error procedure (similar in concept to that used by Reneau, Bruley and Knisely (10) to determine the capillary length) was used to find the number of hemoglobin sites per erythrocyte which would yield this venous oxygen partial pressure under normal conditions. Values for the capillary radius and length, oxygen diffusivity and blood velocity, both for normal and pathological conditions, were those used by Reneau, Bruley and Knisely. Choosing as a basis 150 molecules/95 mmHg, 40000 hemoglobin sites were found to correspond with the venous oxygen tension of 34 mmHg. Experimental data on the number of active hemoglogin sites per normal erythrocyte was not available. However, a quick calculation can be made to determine if the number found by trial and error procedure is at least reasonable. Using equation 5, the fractional saturation of hemoglogin in equilibrium with oxygen dissolved in the plasma necessary for an oxygen partial pressure of 95 mmHg was calculated to be

$0.9668 \dfrac{cm^3 O_2}{cm^3 O_2 \text{ at saturation}}$. That is, 96.68% of the hemoglobin sites (38,672 of 40,000 sites) are filled. So, for a basis of 150 molecules/95 mmHg, approximately 99.6% of the oxygen entering the capillary is in the form of oxyhemoglobin. This is consistent with the known experimental observation.

The Capillary Model

Comparison of the Stochastic Model to the Deterministic Model. Numerous solutions of the deterministic model are available (2, 4, 6, 8, 10). In particular, comparisons will be made between the earlier results of Reneau, Bruley, and Knisely (10), McCracken, Bruley, Reneau, Bicher, and Knisely (8) more recent results, and those obtained in this study.

A comparison has been made of the stochastic results with those obtained by McCracken for the axial oxygen partial pressure profile under normal conditions. The stochastic model agrees closely with McCracken's numerical solution, particularly at the venous end of the capillary. This agreement at the venous end is not surprising since the number of hemoglobin sites was chosen so that the venous oxygen partial pressure would be 34 mmHg, the same as that calculated by McCracken.

The effect of decreased blood flow on the venous oxygen partial pressure was considered. The stochastic model is not quite as sensitive to changes in blood velocity as is the deterministic model.

Validity of the Capillary Model. The validity of any mathematical model can best be evaluated by the model's ability to predict experimental data. The amount of experimental data pertaining to oxygen profiles in the brain microcirculation is scarce, the only available to date being the effect of arterial oxygen partial pressure on the venous oxygen tension under normal conditions (a carbon dioxide partial pressure of 40 mmHg) and under hypocapnic conditions (a carbon dioxide partial pressure of 20 mmHg). Various arterial oxygen partial pressures were used as input data for the stochastic model and the resulting venous oxygen tensions were calculated and compared with the corresponding experimental values determined by Opitz and Schneider (9) and the numerical values obtained by Reneau, Bruley, and Knisely (10). For normal conditions, the venous oxygen partial pressures fall below the experimental values, with the maximum difference being approximately 13% for an arterial oxygen partial pressure of 40 mmHg.

Permeability Effects. The effects of the capillary wall permeability to oxygen on the axial oxygen partial pressure profile was determined. As expected, decreasing the permeability increased the oxygen partial pressure at any given axial position.

The Tissue Model

Most researchers are of the opinion that oxygen consumption occurs at a constant rate within the tissue. This being the case, the approach taken was to first simulate a tubular flow reactor with a zero-order reaction, and then extend the results to the tissue region. Since the reaction is assumed to be independent of the mode of transport, the results obtained from the tubular reactor simulation should be applicable to the tissue. Derivations of the probability distribution for a zero-order reaction, the expected number of molecules reacting in a time interval Δt for a zero-order reaction, and the waiting time for one molecule to be consumed are given elsewhere (3).

Two approaches in the zero-order simulation were taken. In the first approach, it was assumed that $k\Delta t$ molecules were consumed in each stochastic step, with each molecule being chosen at random from the volume element. Agreement between the stochastic and deterministic solutions is excellent, but the computation time made it impractical when applied to the tissue region; one hundred fifty minutes were required for less than 1/20 completion.

For a pure-jump Markov process the waiting time until a change occurs (in this case, particle consumption) is an exponentially distributed random variable. Using uniformly distributed random numbers between zero and one, waiting times were generated. For low rates of reaction, the results are in good agreement with the deterministic solution. However, as the reaction rate increases, the discrepancy between stochastic and deterministic becomes apparent. This discrepancy was attributed to an approximation made in deriving the mean number of molecules reacting per stochastic step (3).

CONCLUDING REMARKS

The work presented here was intended to develop a stochastic model which is simple and versatile, affording a more fundamental description of the oxygenation of the brain microcirculation while simultaneously avoiding the mathematical complexities inherent in the numerical solution of the deterministic model. The stochastic model as presented has one basic assumption: oxygen partial pressures can (and are) obtained through the simulation of only one erythrocyte and the oxygen molecules surrounding it. The model does agree well with existing deterministic results and available experimental data for capillary space-average oxygen tensions. Although more work is still required before adequate tissue results are available, the proposed stochastic model does have considerable potential in its extension to complex anatomical patterns and multicomponent systems.

ACKNOWLEDGMENT

Financial support for this work was provided by NIH grant 1 R01 NS 12009 01.

LITERATURE CITED

1. Bugliarello, G., and G. C. Hsiao, "Numerical Simulation of Three-Dimensional Flow in the Axial Plasmatic Gaps of Capillaries", Digest of the Seventh International Conference on Medical and Biological Engineering (1967).

2. Davis, E. J., D. O. Cooney and R. Chang, "Mass Transfer Between Capillary Blood and Tissues", to be published.

3. Groome, L. J., "The Random Walk as Applied to Stochastic Modeling of the Brain Microcirculation", unpublished Masters Thesis, Clemson University, Clemson, South Carolina, 1974.

4. Halberg, M. R., Bruley, D. F., and M. H. Knisely, "Simulation of Oxygen Transport in the Brain by Monte Carlo Methods", Simulation, Vol. 15, No. 5, pp. 206-212, November 1970.

5. Hoel, P. G., S. C. Port, and C. J. Stone, Introduction to Stochastic Processes, Houghton Mifflin Company, Boston, 1971.

6. Hunt, D. H., D. F. Bruley, H. I. Bicher and M. H. Knisely, "Oxygen Transport In the Brain Microcirculation by A Hybrid Computer Nonlinear Monte Carlo Method", Proceedings of Summer Computer Simulation Conferences, Montreal, Canada, July 1973.

7. Langely, L. L., I. R. Telford and J. B. Christenson, Dynamic Anatomy and Physiology, McGraw-Hill Book Company, 1969.

8. McCracken, T. A., Bruley, D. F. and M. H. Knisely, "A Systems Analysis for the Transport of Oxygen and the Simultaneous Transport of Oxygen, Carbon Dioxide and Glucose in the Capillaries and Tissues of the Human Brain" Proceedings of First Pacific Chemical Engineering Congress, Kyoto, Japan, pp. 137-143, October, 1972.

9. Opitz, E., and M. Schneider, "The Oxygen Supply of the Brain and the Mechanism of Deficiency Effects", Ergebnisse der Physiologie, biologischem, Chemie, und experimentallen Pharmakologie, 46, 126 (1950).

10. Reneau, D. D., D. F. Bruley and M. H. Knisely, "A Mathematical Simulation of Oxygen Release, Diffusion and Consumption in the Capillaries and Tissue of the Human Brain", in Chemical Engineering in Medicine and Biology, ed., by D. Hershey, Plenum Press, N. Y., 1967.

11. Reneau, D. D., D. F. Bruley, and M. H. Knisely, "A Digital Simulation of Transient Oxygen Transport in Capillary-Tissue Systems (Cerebral Grey Matter), "AIChE Journal, 15, 916, November, 1969.

12. Wyman, C. E., "Numerical Solution of Multidimensional and Non-linear Diffusion Problems", unpublished Ph.D. Dissertation, Princeton University, Princeton, New Jersey, 1971.

13. Wyman, C. E., and M. D. Kosten, "Stochastic Green's Function Method for Calculating the Concentration Profile of a Chemically Reactive Species", Chemical Engineering Computing, November (1971).

14. Grote, Jurgen. "Biological Problems of Gas Exchange in Human Organism" unpublished paper, Physiologisches Institute, Johannes Gutenberg -- Universitat, Mainz, West Germany, April, 1968.

MODELS FOR O_2 AND CO_2 TRANSFER IN MACROSCOPIC FLOW CHANNELS AND THEIR PHYSIOLOGICAL IMPLICATIONS

William J. Dorson, Jr. and Marc E. Voorhees

Chemical and Bio Engineering Department, Arizona State University, Tempe, Arizona 85281, U.S.A.

Membrane artificial lungs are capable of long term supplementation of the lung respiration processes. An increasing number of such commercial devices are becoming available for clinical use. Simultaneous with the development of practical units, a growing theoretical understanding has evolved of the convective-diffusive-reactive processes taking place in the macroscopic flow channels. Although the analytical progress had as its foundation the earlier physiology oriented investigations, recent advances in extracorporeal devices research have not been explored for their in vivo implications.

Basic differences exist between in vitro macroscopic and in vivo microscopic processes. An artificial lung has large blood volumes, long transfer channel lengths and blood residence times, and cross sectional channel dimensions which are orders of magnitude greater than red blood cell dimensions. Diffusion is a very rapid and effective means for transporting dissolved species within near capillary dimensions, but highly inefficient in macroscopic flow channels. In fact, the design of a membrane artificial lung with straight flow paths is limited, for O_2 transfer, by convective-diffusive transport within the blood stream. The long blood residence times in artificial lungs required to saturate hemoglobin also insures the validity of assuming local chemical equilibria. The large cross sectional dimensions makes the application of continuum differential balances feasible. Apparently, the dynamics of individual red cell motions in macroscopic flow channels do not contribute significantly to the transfer of O_2 or CO_2. Conversely, the capillary transport processes are better modeled with a bolus flow of individual red blood cells with, perhaps, a well mixed plasma zone separating the cells. The red cell transit times through systemic capillary beds are known to be shorter than those of the suspending plasma phase. These phenomena would be expected since the maximum red blood cell dimension is the same magnitude as the capillary diameter. Also, it is probable that the red blood cell and plasma phases are not in true equilibrium under all physiological conditions (6).

In the following development of equilibrium transport theory for macroscopic flow channels, the effect of multiple chemical species on O_2 and CO_2 transfer is considered. The differential balance which describes the variation of dilute specie concentrations in a single homogeneous and isotropic phase can be stated as

$$\sum_{i=1}^{n} \frac{\partial C_i}{\partial t} + \sum_{i=1}^{n} \operatorname{div}(\vec{v}C_i) = \sum_{i=1}^{m} \nabla \cdot D_i \nabla C_i \qquad (1)$$

where reaction terms between different species are cancelled by the summation operation. For O_2 and CO_2 in macroscopic flow channels at steady state, Equation 1 can be stated as

$$\text{Convective change of all content species} = \text{Flux change of major diffusing species} \qquad (2)$$

For flow in a tube with CO_2 or O_2 species in local equilibrium (3,4)

$$v_x \left(1 + \frac{\partial C_T}{\partial C_1}\right) \frac{\partial C_1}{\partial x} = \frac{D_1}{r} \frac{\partial}{\partial r} \left[\left(1 + \frac{D_2}{D_1} \frac{\partial C_2}{\partial C_1} + \cdots\right)\left(r \frac{\partial C_1}{\partial r}\right)\right] \qquad (3)$$

With the gross assumption that diffusion coefficient ratios (D_2/D_1, etc) and equilibrium slope relations between different diffusing species ($\partial C_2/\partial C_1$, etc) are constant, Equation 3 can be expressed as

$$v_x \frac{\partial C_1}{\partial x} = \frac{D_e}{rF} \frac{\partial}{\partial r} \left(r \frac{\partial C_1}{\partial r}\right) \qquad (4)$$

which is in the form of non-reactive convective-diffusive transport except for the ratio D_e/F(note: D_e/F generally $\leq D_1$ for O_2 and CO_2).

Excellent reviews exist of the more general aspects of theoretical models applied to macroscopic flow channels (2, 7, 8, 9). Equation 4 can be solved for specific boundary conditions. Of importance to artificial lung design is the conjugated boundary condition which requires the matching of O_2 or CO_2 fluxes at the permeable boundaries. A dimensionless resistance, γ, is thus developed which relates boundary resistances to transfer hindrance within the flow channel. This approach is also relevant to in vivo capillary transport problems, but heretofore not considered in detail. The solution of Equation 4 (and its equivalent in cartesian coordinates) can be represented as generalized dimensionless variables expressed as

$$\theta = \frac{\bar{P}-P_i}{P_g-P_i} \quad , \quad X^* = \frac{\pi N D_e x}{2QF} \quad , \quad Z^* = \frac{4WND_e z}{3aQF}$$

with the dimensionless boundary resistances given by

$$\gamma \text{ (cylindrical)} \quad = \alpha_1 D_e \sum_j \frac{\ln(R_{oj}/R_{ij})}{\alpha_j D_{ej}} \tag{5}$$

$$\gamma \text{ (cartesian, dual membrane channels)} = \frac{\alpha_1 D_e}{a} \sum_j \frac{\ell_j}{\alpha_j D_{ej}} \tag{6}$$

The resistances are defined, respectively, for axial flow in a cylinder bounded by j stagnant (pure solution-diffusion processes) but permeable membranes in series and flow in a straight semi-infinite channel bounded on both sides by j stagnant but permeable membranes in series (X^* and Z^* are the respective dimensionless axial coordinates). Solutions obtained by utilizing confluent hypergeometric functions (1) are shown on Figures 1 and 2.

Straight line approximations for the content or individual specie relations with dissolved O_2 and CO_2 between inlet and outlet conditions can be used in estimating F and D_e values. Both numerical (7) and advancing front (3,4) approaches have also been applied successfully to O_2 transport in macroscopic channels. Along with similar definitions of dimensionless boundary resistances, the governing cylindrical parameters are (3):

$$f = \frac{S-S_i}{1-S_i} \quad , \quad X^{**} = \left(\frac{P_g-P_i}{C_{bi}}\right)\left(\frac{\alpha_1 \pi N D_1 x}{4Q}\right)$$

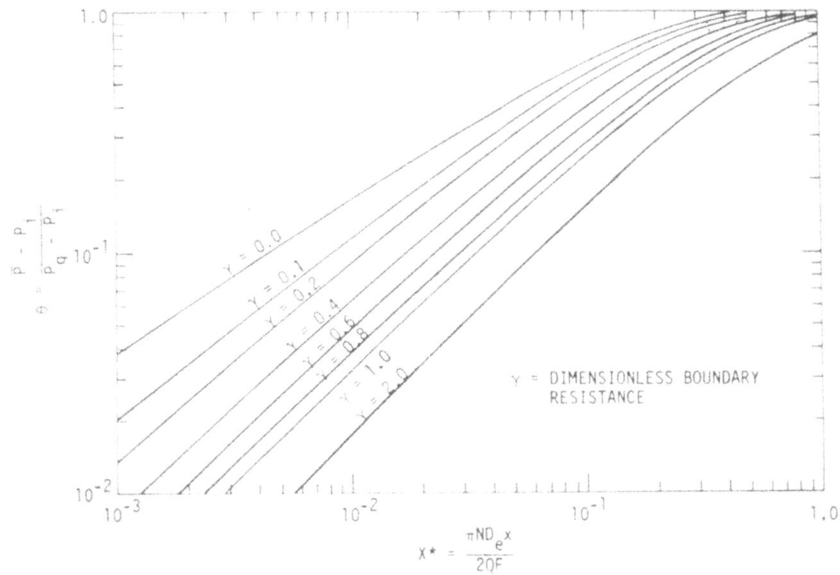

Figure 1. Dimensionless Partial Pressure Change with Axial Distance and Boundary Resistance for N Tubular Channels in Parallel

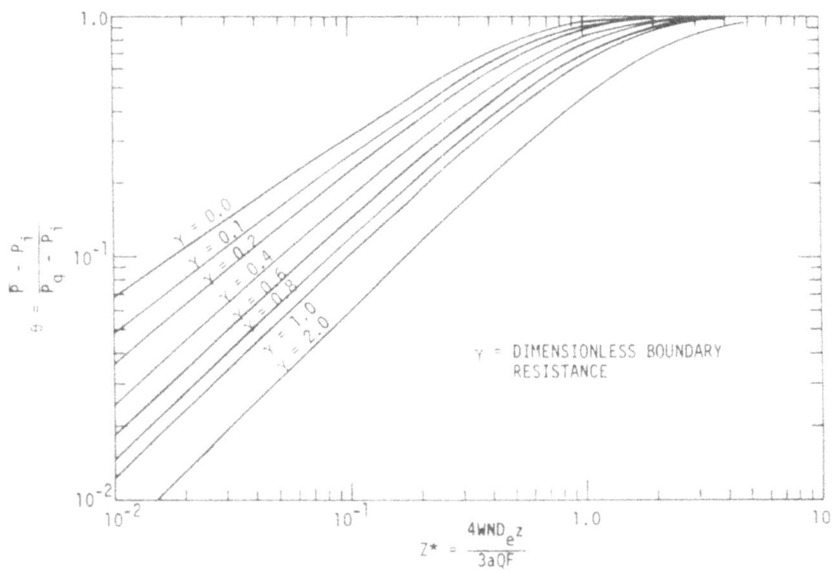

Figure 2. Dimensionless Partial Pressure Change with Axial Distance and Boundary Resistance for N Flat (Cartesian) Channels in Parallel

Both O_2 and CO_2 analytical methods have been verified for macroscopic channels by comparison with data (3,4,7).

Analyses of lung respiration have utilized a variety of alveolar-capillary blood transfer rates ranging from overall experimental values (6) to transport phenomena analogies (5). Neither of these approaches account for the combined physicochemical contributions to transport. The cylindrical geometry results outlined herein were used to deduce transfer efficiences in the lung. Without considering boundary resistances ($\gamma = 0$), both O_2 and CO_2 in lung capillaries were estimated to be rapidly in equilibrium with alveolar gas partial pressures. Based on the transfer concepts in this analysis, dissolved CO_2 would achieve equilibrium with alveolar gas concentrations much faster than O_2. This CO_2 equilibrium is calculated to occur in less than the initial 10% of the lung capillary transit time (8μ capillary diameter, 0.75 sec total transit time).

Perhaps of more significance is the ability to compute the relative transfer contributions of tissue separating the capillaries from the alveolar gas phase and the stagnant gas near the alveolar walls. With reference to Equation 5 the dimensionless resistances for CO_2 are estimated as

$$\gamma = \underset{\text{tissue}}{0.08} + \underset{\text{alveolar gas}}{0.0002}$$

For oxygen the relative tissue contribution would remain approximately the same but the alveolar gas resistance would be an order of magnitude lower. Thus, of the three series resistances to O_2 and CO_2 analyzed (blood, tissue, and stagnant alveolar gas), the convective-diffusive hindrance within the blood accounts for $\sim$ 90% of the total resistance ($\gamma \sim 0.1$). However, no appreciable difference between the alveolar gas and pulmonary artery tension can be attributed to these physical phenomena with normal lung functions. The analytical results are useful in assessing the validity of assumptions required in developing models for the lung respiration and in determining the effects of pathological conditions.

NOMENCLATURE

- a Half-channel height (dual permeable membranes)
- C_i Concentration of specie i
- C_1 Concentration of dissolved CO_2 or O_2
- C_2 Concentration of second diffusing species, etc.
- C_T Total content expressed as concentration
- C_{bi} Inlet concentration of unoxygenated hemoglobin
- D_i Diffusion coefficient of specie i
- D_1 Effective diffusion coefficient of dissolved O_2 or CO_2 in blood
- D_e Effective total diffusion coefficient in blood

D_{ej}	Effective total diffusion coefficient in phase j
j	Index for different boundary resistance phases
ℓ_j	Thickness of phase j boundary resistance
n	Index of each specie in total content
N	Number of parallel channels
m	Index for important diffusing species
$\underline{P}_i$	Inlet tension
$\overline{P}$	Average tension at x or z axial location
P_g	Gas phase partial pressure
Q	Total volumetric blood flow rate
r	Radial coordinate or position
R_{ij}	Inner radius of phase j
R_{oj}	Outer radius of phase j
S	Fractional saturation at x or z axial location
$\underline{S}_i$	Inlet fractional saturation
$\vec{v}$	Velocity vector
v_x	Axial velocity profile
W	Channel width
x	Axial coordinate or position (cylindrical geometry)
X^*	Dimensionless axial distance (cylindrical geometry)
X^{**}	Dimensionless axial distance, advancing front model
z	Axial coordinate or position (cartesian geometry)
Z^*	Dimensionless axial distance (cartesian geometry)
α_1	Solubility of dissolved specie
α_j	Solubility in phase j
γ	Dimensionless boundary phase resistance
θ	Dimensionless partial pressure function

REFERENCES

1. Davis, E.J., *Can. J. Chem. Eng.*, 51:562-572, 1973.
2. Dorson, W.J., Jr., in *Blood Oxygenation*, edited by D. Hershey, New York: Plenum Press, p. 355-372, 1970.
3. Dorson, W.J., Jr., K.G. Larsen, R.J. Elgas and M.E. Voorhees, *Trans. Amer. Soc. Artif. Int. Organs*, 17:309-315, 1971.
4. Dorson, W.J., Jr. and M. Voorhees, *Trans. Amer. Soc. Artif. Int. Organs*, 20:219-226, 1974.
5. Hills, B.A., *Gas Transfer in the Lung*, Cambridge, Great Britain: Cambridge University Press, 1974.
6. Hill, E.P., G.G. Power and L.D. Longo, *Am. J. Physiol.*, 224: 904-917, 1973.
7. Lightfoot, E.N. Jr., *Transport Phenomena and Living Systems*, New York: J. Wiley and Sons, Inc., 1974.
8. Spaeth, E.E., in *Blood Oxygenation*, edited by D. Hershey, New York: Plenum Press, p. 276-305, 1970.
9. Spaeth, E.E., in *CRC Critical Reviews in Bioengineering*, p. 383-417, 1973.

SUMMARY OF DISCUSSION - SESSION V:

MATHEMATICAL MODELS TO DESCRIBE OXYGEN TRANSPORT IN BLOOD AND TISSUE

Chairmen: W. Grunewald and D. D. Reneau

Following Dr. Oomens' presentation, Dr. Stroeve noted that it would be interesting to perform similar calculations for rectangular ducts. He recalled that Weizman (1973) reported anomalous oxygen uptake in this type of geometry. Dr. Stroeve suggested that perhaps Dr. Oomen's analysis may indicate what kind of flow would account for the high oxygen uptake.

Following Dr. Meldon's presentation, Dr. Siesjo asked how fast a compensatory changed occurred following a change in 2-3-DPG. Dr. Meldon stated that changes are reported to occur over a period of 12 hours to several days. Dr. Lubbers criticized the use of the Krogh cylinder as a representative geometric model, and Dr. Bruley questioned the assumption of zero axial diffusion. Dr. Meldon responded by stating that axial diffusion along a capillary should be small except at the arterial end or in the case of severe anemia coupled with inadequate flow. This degree of error was acceptable in their study.

Following Dr. Fletcher's presentation, Dr. Meldon asked if, under a given set of constant conditions, venous PO_2 could be read directly off a saturation curve without the necessity of numerical analysis. Dr. Fletcher responded that this was true if one assumes steady-state conditions, kinetic equilibrium everywhere, and neglects axial diffusion in the tissue. However, numerical analysis is necessary to solve implicit relationships.

Following Dr. Roetman's presentation, Dr. Meldon observed that Fick's Law is really proportional to activity gradients and not concentration gradients. Theoretical considerations, for certain conditions, can show diffusion against concentration gradients.

Dr. Roetman responded that there are scholarly publications opposing the irreversible thermodynamics approach.

Following Dr. Bruley's presentation, Dr. Fletcher asked if the stochastic technique was an improvement over the deterministic method. Dr. Bruley stated that possibly the stochastic method offered a computational time saving advantage with multicomponent systems and allowed the removal of fixed constraints such as geometries and complex histological patterns. However, extension of the model to unsteady-state might present formidable problems.

Oxygen Supply of the Central Nervous System I

CORRELATION BETWEEN THE REDOX STATE, ELECTRICAL ACTIVITY AND BLOOD FLOW IN CAT BRAIN CORTEX DURING HEMORRHAGIC SHOCK

A.G.B. Kovách, A. Eke, E. Dóra, L. Gyulai

Experimental Research Department, Semmelweis Medical University, Budapest, Hungary

Owing to its well developed autoregulatory mechanisms, total cerebral blood flow is stable over a wide range of mean arterial blood pressures and decreases significantly only when the perfusion pressure is below 50 mmHg.

It emerges from our earlier studies that, during the development of irreversible hemorrhagic shock, functional (1), hemodynamic (2,3) and metabolic (4,5,6) changes seriously affect the central nervous system. Spontaneous electrocortical activity and somatosensory evoked potentials disappeared during hypovolemia and did not return after retransfusion (7). Impairment of the central nervous system is not uniform in all regions. Uneven damage was indicated by electrical, metabolic and local blood flow studies (2,5,8).

In experiments carried out on baboons (8,9), anesthetized with Sernylan, regional CBF was recorded by two methods. Repeated measurements were taken by monitoring the cerebral clearance of ^{133}Xe and at different phases of the experiments, local blood flow was also determined by an autoradiographic technique employing ^{14}C-antipyrine.

^{133}Xe clearance measurements showed that CBF decreased significantly during hemorrhage and approximately doubled after reinfusion (Fig. 1).

The ^{14}C antipyrine autoradiographic studies are illustrated in Figure 2. On the left side of the picture is a coronal section autoradiogram obtained from a normal animal. The density of the print, i.e. the concentration of the radioactive tracer, is

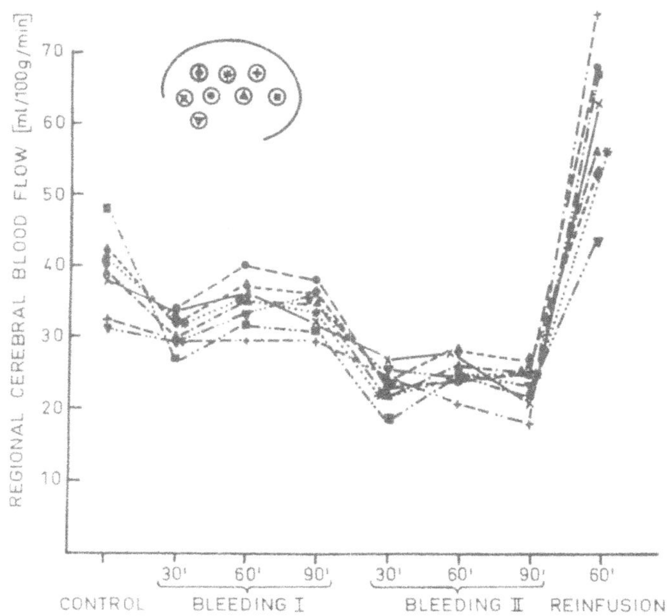

Figure 1: Cerebral blood flow measured by ^{133}Xe during hemorrhagic shock in baboon.

proportional to blood flow. The numbers on the Figure represent blood flow values in ml/100 g/min. The autoradiogram on the right was taken at the end of the second bleeding period. Besides a substantial reduction of CBF, patchy and circumscribed ischemic areas occurred in different brain regions. Areas deprived of circulation still existed after reinfusion even in neighborhoods of hyperperfused brain regions (8,9).

In order to increase our understanding of the effects of shock, in our next experiments we studied simultaneoulsy cortical redox state, blood flow and electrical activity.

Methods

Our experiments were performed on cats (2,5 - 3,5 kg) which were anesthetized with 60 mg/kg α-D glycochloralose, immobilized with 2-4 mg/kg flaxedil and artificially respired with a Harrard pump.

Respiration was adjusted to keep the arterial pCO_2 at 40 mmHg, and pO_2 above 100 mmHg. Cannulae were introduced into the femoral artery and vein and into the lingual artery. A T cannula was inserted into the abdominal aorta for the stabilization of arterial blood pressure.

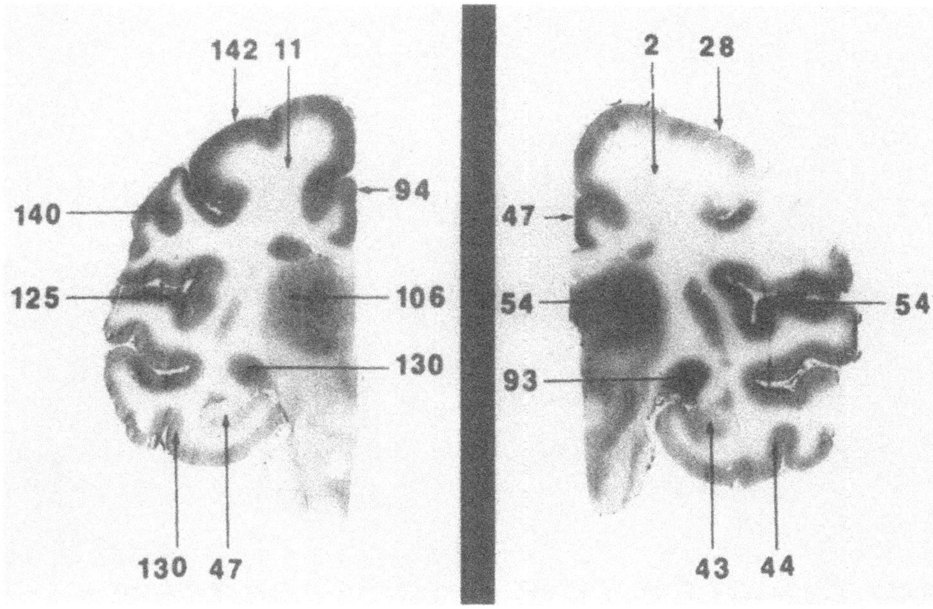

Figure 2: Regional cerebral blood flow measured by the ^{14}C antipyrine autoradiographic method. Left control, right during hemorrhagic hypovolemia (180 min) in baboon.

For microfluorometry a hole of 12 mm diamter was drilled in the parietal bone and the dura was removed. To prevent brain movement a thin glass window was fixed into the hole. In most of the experiments the anterior suprasylvian gyrus was studied by microfluorometry.

Hemorrhagic shock was induced by decreasing the arterial blood pressure by connecting the aortic cannula with a buffer system and bleeding to 35-40 mmHg. In one group of experiments the hypotension was maintained until 60-80% of the shed blood was spontaneously taken back into the animal from the buffer reservoir system. In other experiments the hypovolemia lasted until the EEG had been isoelectric for a period of 30-60 minutes and then all the blood remaining in the reservoir was reinfused.

The following parameters were recorded in the standardized experiments; mean arterial blood pressure, electrocorticogram, UV reflectance and NADH fluorescence reading. A correction was used according to Harbig _et al_. (10). A cortical field of 100 μ diameter was studied by the surface microfluorometry.

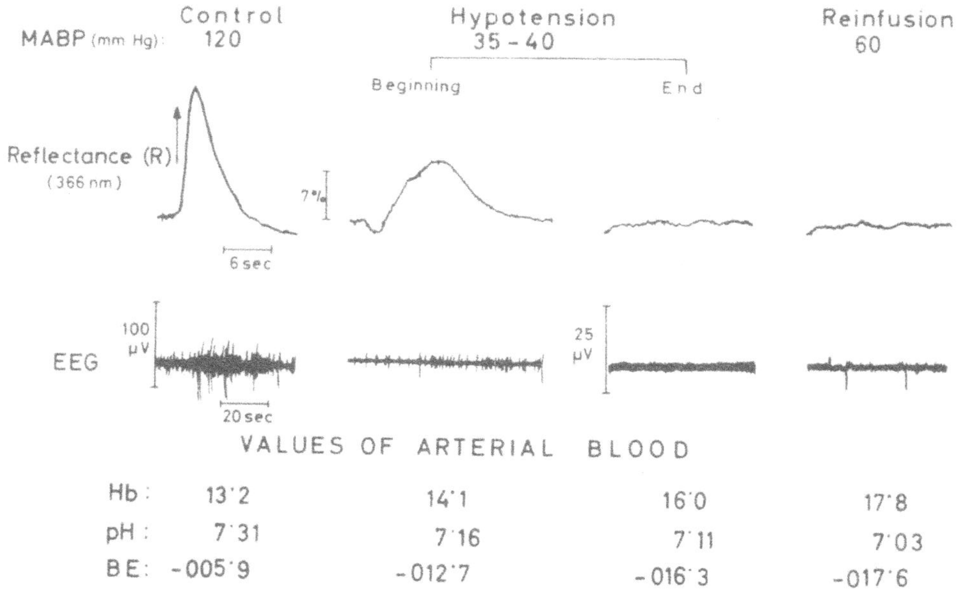

Figure 3: Saline flush induced cortical reflectance curves and electrocorticogram in control and hypovolemic shock.

Changes in blood flow were measured by analyzing the cortical reflectance curve induced by injecting 1 ml saline into the lingual artery. For blood flow estimation the appearance-time and decay-time of the reflectance curve was used. Electrical stimulation of the cortex was performed through two very thin silver plates. The following stimulation parameters were used: 10-20 V, 15-40 Hz, 0, 5-1,5 msec.

For EEG recording brass screws were fixed on both sides of the skull into the parietal and occipital bones. All parameters were recorded on a 8 channel Galileo-polygraph and part of the data was fed into a 4 channel Harvard tape recorder for further analysis.

The following tests were performed repeatedly before, during and after hemorrhage: (a) 1-2 min continuous direct cortical stimulation, (b) 1-1/2 min arterial anoxia, (c) cortical reflectance changes induced by injecting saline into the lingual artery.

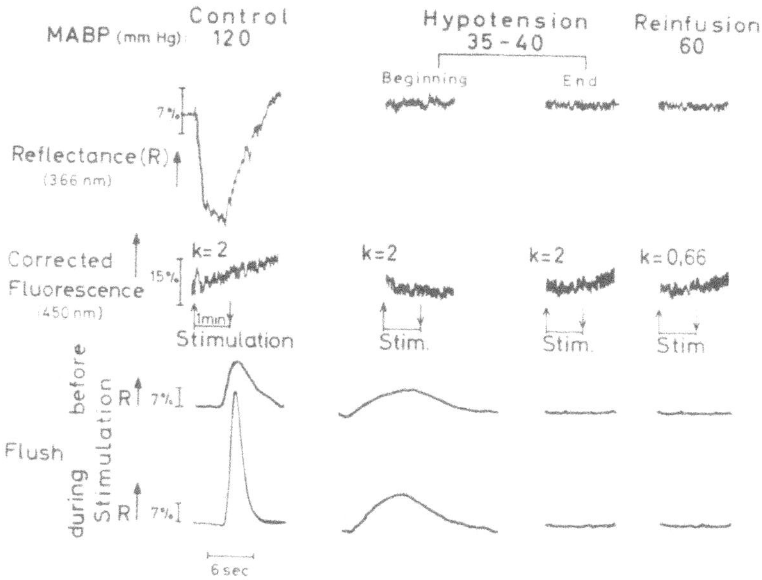

Figure 4: Cortical reflectance, corrected fluorescence and saline flush response changes after cortical stimulation in control and hemorrhagic shock cats.

Results

The results are demonstrated before and after hemorrhagic shock on original individual experimental records. Figure 3 shows the cortical reflectance curves and cortical electrical activity induced by saline flushes together with arterial blood acid-base values during (a) the control period, (b) hypotension, and (c) after reinfusion. Experiments are in progress in our laboratory to develop a method of measuring blood flow on the basis of reflectance changes induced by saline injection. We have found that the reflectance curve after saline flush is very characteristic for the actual cortical blood flow.

It is clear that the variation in the duration of the reflectance change and EEG pattern are correlated. In the control period the reflectance changes lasted 12 sec, at the beginning of the hypotension it was 24 sec, while at the end of hypotension and after reinfusion the saline bolus did not reach the illuminated cortical field. This suggests a complete absence of blood flow in the part of the brain cortex under observation.

Parallel with the reflectance changes the electrical activity was much diminished at the beginning of the hypotension and became isoelectric in the next two periods. The arterial blood acid-base values show the changes demonstrated earlier, namely pH decreased and BE increased both during the bleeding period and after reinfusion.

In Figure 4 the cortical reflectance and corrected fluorescence changes induced by direct cortical stimulation are demonstrated. The third curve from the top is the flush-response before and the fourth curve is during direct cortical stimulation. The cortical reflectance decreases by 17% due to stimulation in the control period, which indicates a massive vasodilatation. The corrected fluorescence trace did not show substantial change during cortical stimulation. Comparison of the flush responses before and during cortical stimulation shows substantial differences with the acceleration of the decay being obvious. The decrease of the reflectance curve means an increase in the blood flow of the stimulated area. After the beginning of hemorrhagic hypotension cortical stimulation did not induce any increase in blood flow, since neither the basic reflectance curve nor the flush-responses were changed.

Figure 5 demonstrates the reflectance and corrected fluorescence changes during N_2 cycles. The correction values are shown under the corrected fluorescence curves. During the control period the N_2 cycle produced a 27-28% reflectance decrease and a 35% NAD reduction. Both at the end of the hypotension period and after reinfusion the N_2 induced anoxia was not accompanied by any further NAD reduction. In both cases the cortical reflectance was temporarily lower after the N_2 cycle than before. The k value was 2,0 during hypovolemia and after reinfusion it decreased to 0,66.

Discussion

Rosenthal and Jöbsis (11) have found NADH oxidation following direct cortical stimulation. Chance (12) considers this indication an increase of mitochondrial ATP-production. In our experiments mostly vascular responses were found after cortical stimulation and the changes in corrected fluorescence were inconsistent. A reasonable explanation of these differences is a transient change of the k-value during the stimulation. This idea has to be taken into consideration especially in cases when the k-value is 1,0 (11). In our present experiment the vascular response to cortical stimulation had already disappeared at the beginning of the hypotension. Maximal dilatation of the cortical vessels due to tissue acidosis is probably the most adequate explanation of these results.

In the later stage of hemorrhagic hypotension and even after reinfusion no additional NAD reduction was found after N_2 inhala-

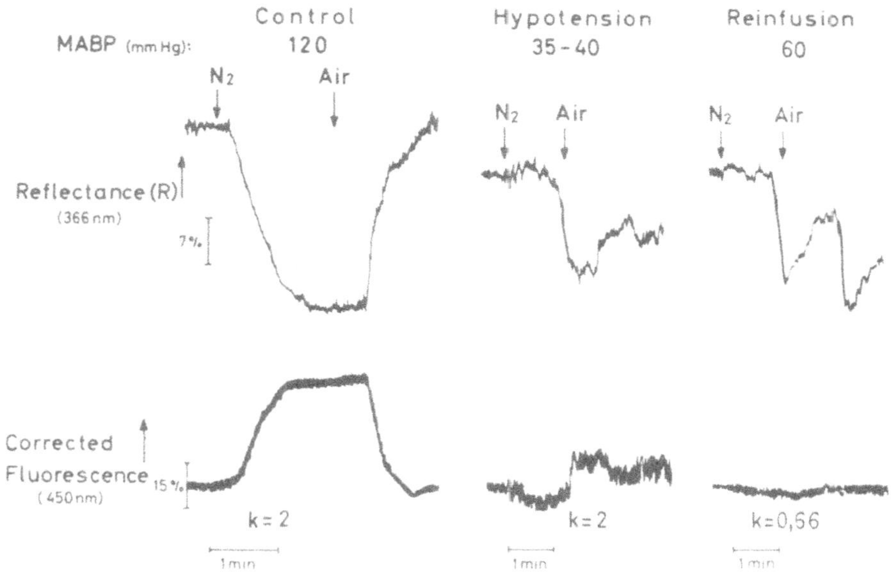

Figure 5: Cortical reflectance and corrected fluorescence changes during N_2 cycles in control and hemorrhagic shock cats.

tion. There was a good correlation between the loss of NAD reduction due to an N_2 cycle and the appearance of an isoelectric ECoG.

In conclusion we can suppose that during hemorrhagic hypotension in the cat the cerebral cortical tissue shows a continuous NAD-reduction, parallel with the isoelectric electrocorticographic reading.

After the irreversible shock phase developed, retransfusion did not bring back the reduced redox state to normal. Our experiments with direct cortical stimulation, N_2 cycles and saline flushes demonstrated that seriously diminished local blood flow is responsible for the NAD reduction. Histological studies with benzidine staining demonstrated sludged red cells in the cortical vessels. The development of blockage of the microcirculation was prevented by phenoxybenzamine pretreatment, which suggests the involvement of catecholamine metabolism in the cerebral microcirculatory impairment in hemorrhagic shock.

REFERENCES

1. Kovách, A.G.B.: The function of the central nervous system after haemorrhage. J.clin.Path.23.Suppl. 4. 202-212.1970.
2. Kovách, A.G.B., A. Mitsányi, E. Monos, I. Nyáry, A.Sulyok: Control of organ blood flow following hemorrhage. In: Neurohumoral and Metabolic Aspects of Injury. Ed. A.G.B. Kovách, H.B. Stoner, J.J. Spitzer. New York-London, Plenum Press, 1973. p.1-17. Advanc.Exp.Med.Biol.33.
3. Kovách, A.G.B.: Blood flow and metabolism in brain and in adipose tissue during hemorrhagic shock. In: Shock in Low- and High-Flow States. Ed.B.K.Forscher, R.C.Lillehei, S.S. Stubbs. Excerpta Med. Intern.Congr.Ser. 247.Amsterdam, p.65-76. 1972.
4. Kovách, A.G.B., A. Fonyó: Metabolic Responses to Injury in Cerebral Tissue. In: The Biochemical Response to Injury. Ed. H.B.Stoner, C.I. Threlfall. Blackwell Sci.Publ. Oxford. p. 129-161. 1960.
5. Kovách, A.G.B.: Importance of Nervous and Metabolic Changes in the Development of Irreversibility in Experimental Shock. Fed. Proc. 20. Suppl.9. 122-137. 1961.
6. Kovách, A.G.B.: Tissue blood flow and metabolism in control and phenoxybenzamine pretreated animals in experimental shock. In: Traumatic Shock. Ed. Gy.Szántó, V. Hönig, O. Székely. Akadémiai Kiadó, Budapest. p. 163-185. 1973.
7. Dóra, E., Kovách, A.G.B., Nyáry, I.: Hypothalamic and Cortical Evoked Potentials in Hemorrhagic Shock. In: Neurohumoral and Metabolic Aspects of Injury. Ed. A.G. B. Kovách, H. B. Stoner, J.J. Spitzer. New York-London, Plenum Press, 1973. p. 481-488. Advanc. Exp. Med. Biol. 33.
8. Reivich, M., A.G.B. Kovách, J.J.Spitzer, P. Sándor: Cerebral Blood Flow and Metabolism in Hemorrhagic Shock in Baboons. In: Neurohumoral and Metabolic Aspects of Injury. Ed. A.G.B. Kovách, H.B. Stoner, J.J. Spitzer. New York-London. Plenum Press, 1973. p. 19-26. Advanc.Exp.Med.Biol.33.
9. Nyáry, I., E. Dóra, P. Sándor, A.G.B.Kovách, M. Reivich: Cerebral Blood Flow and Metabolism in Hemorrhagic Shock in Baboon. 3rd Tbilisi Congress on Cerebral Circulation. Akadémiai Kiadó, Budapest, 1975.
10. Harbig, K., B. Chance, A.G.B. Kovách, M. Reivich:In vivo Measurement of Pyridine Nucleotide Fluorescence from the Cat Brain Cortex. Submitted to J. Appl. Physiol.1974.

11. Rosenthal, M., F.F. Jöbsis: Intracellular Redox Changes in Functioning Cerebral Cortex. II. Effects of Direct Cortical Stimulation. J. Neurophysiol. 34. 750-762. 1971.

12. Chance, B., B. Schöner, F. Schindler: The intracellular oxido-reduction state. In: Oxygen in Animal Organism. Ed. F. Dickens and E. Neil. New York, McMillan. p. 367. 1964.

This work was partially supported by NINDS-10939.

CORTICAL NADH, pO_2, ELECTRICAL ACTIVITY AND ARTERIAL BLOOD PRESSURE OSCILLATIONS IN HYPOXAEMIA[1]

E. Dóra, K. Olaffson[+], B. Chance[+], A.G.B. Kovách

Experimental Res.Department, Semmelweis Med.Univ. Budapest, Hungary and [+]Johnson Res. Foundation, Univ. of Pennsylvania, School of Med.,Philadelphia,Pa.

A large amount of work has been devoted to the description and analysis of blood pressure oscillation (1, 2, 3, 4, 5, 6, 13). However little is understood of the nature of the oscillator or what are the stimuli which unbalance the circulatory system.

We could not find any information on how the electrical activity, tissue oxygen tension and oxido-reduction state of the cells in the brain cortex alter when blood pressure oscillations occur.

Although it seems clear that hypoxia is the stimulus which is responsible in some way for the elicitation of the brain ischemic reflex and its associated oscillations, we could not find experimental proof for blood pressure waves being evoked by hypoxaemia.

Methods

The experiments were done on male Wistar rats (180-250 gr. body weight), anesthetized with i.p. injected nembutal (50 mg/kg). The animals were immobilized with 10 mg/kg Gallamine triethiodide and artificially respired. The femoral artery and vein and the trachea were cannulated. For fluorometry and tissue oxygen tension measurements the skull was opened carefully on both sides. Two brass screws were fixed bilaterally into the skull to record EEG. The following measurements were made routinely: arterial blood pressure; oxygen content of the inspired gas mixture; NADH fluo-

1. These studies were supported by the John A. Hartford Foundation and by NIH Grant P 01 NS 10, 939-01.

rescence and corrected fluorescence of the brain cortex (15), EEG. To avoid the influence of cortical blood flow changes in NADH measurements a correction method was used according to Harbig and Reivich (16, 17). In a few experiments oxygen availability of brain cortex was also measured with a 10 μ tip diameter Pt electrode. All the information was fed into a Bell and Howell recorder.

Results

In Fig. 1. a part of an oscillatory experiment is demonstrated. In Fig. 1A the beginning, in Fig. 1B the end of oscillations are shown. Oscillation was elicited by decreasing the oxygen content of inspired gas mixture from 30% to 6% as is marked by the arrow. As a consequence of hypoxia arterial blood pressure dropped from the initial 120 mmHg to 25 mmHg. Corrected fluorescence increased by 30% and reflectance changed moderately (10% increase) and EEG showed a slight decrease as compared to the control activity. Following these abrupt changes blood pressure started to increase. Oxido-reduction state of brain cortex shifted towards oxidation and the minimal value of NADH fluorescence and

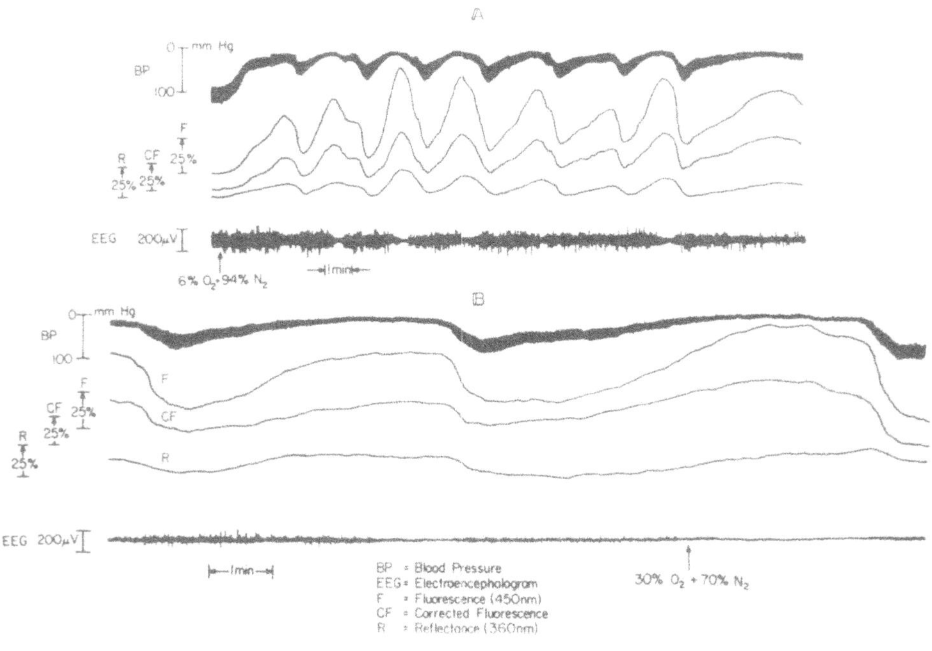

Figure 1.: In a typical experiment oscillations of arterial blood pressure (BP), EEG and fluorescence (F), corrected fluorescence (CF) and reflectance (R) of the rat brain cortex are shown.

the electrical activity were close to the control levels. It is interesting to note that the amplitudes of subsequent oscillations of reflectance and corrected fluorescence were not equal. First they increased then decreased and again increased. In Fig. 1B the waves as compared to Fig. 1A have slowed down. At the beginning one wave lasted for 2 min. but before oscillations stopped the waves had a periodicity of 5 min. The animal started to breath normal gas mixture at the time which is marked by the arrow but the recovery of the rat from hypoxia was very slow. Arterial blood pressure and corrected fluorescence and reflectance recovered almost completely 30 min. later but not the EEG. At this time activity had returned but it was considerably reduced as compared to the control. It is interesting to compare the anoxic reactions before and after oscillations.

In Fig. 2A following the disappearance of EEG, corrected fluorescence and reflectance plateaued at their maximal values. At the same time arterial blood pressure was 35 mmHg. In the recovery phase arterial blood pressure increased to 160 mmHg and reflectance declined to -60%. Following anoxia EEG was entirely restored within 40 sec, however it took 5 min for the initial values of arterial blood pressure and fluorescence and corrected fluorescence and reflectance to return. In Fig. 2B during pure nitrogen breathing corrected fluorescence increased by 50%, reflectance by 5% and the arterial blood pressure dropped from the starting value of 120 mmHg to 40 mmHg. All of the parameters recovered simultaneously, arterial blood pressure overshot, but no reflectance change accompanied this.

In a few oscillatory experiments cortical pO_2 was monitored as well as the usual parameters. In Fig. 3. the inspired oxygen was reduced from 25% to 10%. The cortical oxygen tension decreased from 32 mmHg to 3 mmHg, the corrected fluorescence increased to 30% and the EEG changed moderately. During the next blood pressure oscillation the corrected fluorescence reached 50%, the cortical oxygen tension was 0.5 mmHg and the EEG decreased near to isoelectric. Following this initial maximal oscillation both blood pressure and fluorescence underwent marked dampening which was most pronounced in the case of the reflectance oscillation. When the oscillation spontaneously stopped, the arterial blood pressure was 25 mmHg, the oxygen tension 2,5 mmHg, the EEG was slightly less than the control activity and the corrected fluorescence reached 31% with a reflectance -28%. The great reflectance decrease at the end of the hypoxic period might be due to a marked capillary dilatation in the brain cortex. This could account for the relatively well preserved EEG, while cortical oxygen tension is 2,5 mmHg, as well as for the increase of only 30% in corrected fluorescence.

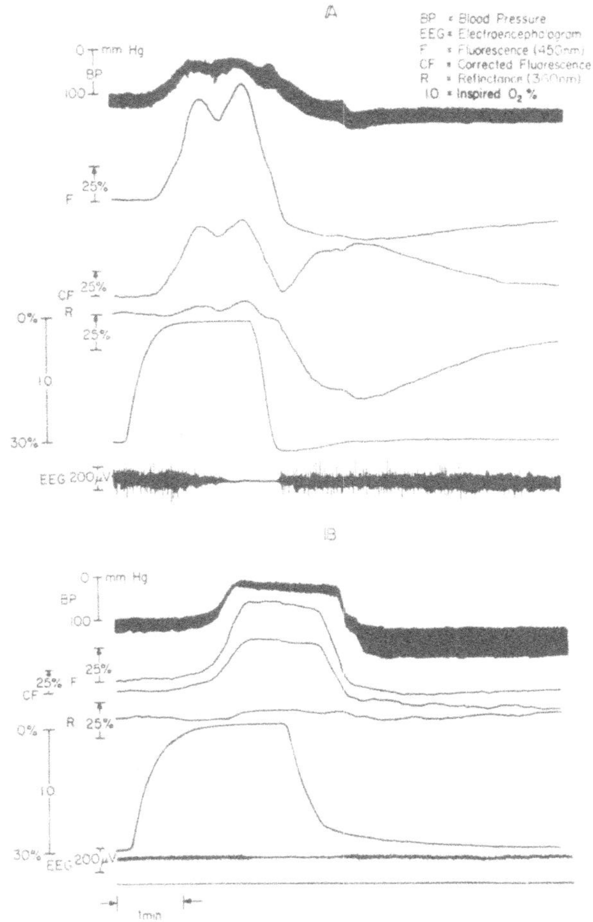

Figure 2.: Arterial blood pressure (BP), inspired O_2 (IO), EEG and fluorescence (F), corrected fluorescence (CF) and reflectance (R) measurements in the rat brain cortex in cycles of normoxia-anoxia-normoxia. 2A and 2B show results obtained on the same animal before and after hypoxic oscillations.

The number of oscillatory cycles differed from animal to animal, the largest number of waves was 25. In the table the results have been arranged according to the number of oscillations. A very obvious difference can be found between the two groups concerning the duration of one wave at the beginning of oscillations. There appears to be a good correlation between the number of waves and the starting frequency of oscillations. In both groups after an oscillatory period of 20 min - 2 hours the waves

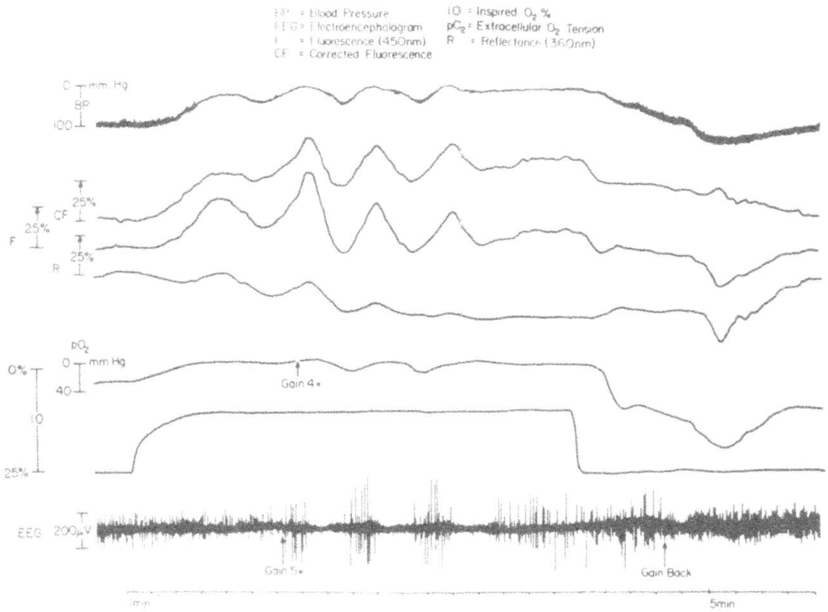

Figure 3.: In a single experiment oscillations of arterial blood pressure (BP), EEG, cortical fluorescence (F), corrected fluorescence (CF), reflectance (R) and tissue pO_2 are shown.

significantly slowed down and later stopped. Amplitudes of blood pressure, fluorescence, reflectance and corrected fluorescence waves as well as the minimal value of blood pressure during oscillations were nearly the same.

Discussion

Out of 50 hypoxic experiments oscillations appeared only in twelve cases. Therefore the question arises as to what is the reason that oscillations appear only occasionally. It seems that they can be elicited only by a certain degree of metabolic change. In our experiments the oscillations were strictly related to a certain inspired oxygen level. Increasing or decreasing the inspired oxygen concentration by 1-2% stopped the oscillation.

There was no detectable phase difference between the blood pressure and corrected fluorescence and reflectance waves. This might mean that the tissue NADH waves were governed by the blood pressure oscillations.

TABLE

Less than 8 waves

Exp.No.	Amplitudes of the oscillation of BP	EEG	CF	Duration of one wave at the beginning of the oscillation in sec.	Duration of one wave at the end of the oscillation in sec.	Number of waves
1	45	-	11	236,4	259,0	3
2	39	70	42	205,0	193,0	4
3	24	-	17,4	165,0	425,0	4
4	71	40	12,5	107,4	110,0	4
5	68	-	-	379,0	401,0	4
Mean	49,4	66,7	20,7	218,5 sec	277,0 sec	3,8

More than 8 waves

Exp.No.	BP	EEG	CF	Duration of one wave at the beginning of the oscillation in sec.	Duration of one wave at the end of the oscillation in sec.	Number of waves
6	40	-	21,2	110,0	356,2	10
7	60	60	36,5	151,6	283,7	15
8	42	60	28	180,0	555,8	9
9	26	10	29	199,0	393,7	8
10	-	-	16	78,9	195,8	21
11	54	60	30	107,4	268,4	20
12	41	81	24	154,7	331,6	8
Mean	43,8	54,2	26,4	140,2 sec	340,7 sec	13

Abbreviations: BP = Arterial blood pressure in mm Hg
EEG= Cortical electrical activity in % of control
CF = Corrected fluorescence in %

Chance et al. (12) have shown that in the transition from anoxia to normoxia the tissue NADH can oscillate in perfused heart. They found that the concentration minima and maxima correspond to the NADH maxima and minima. It might not be excluded that in our experiments the heart is the driving oscillator and the periodical heart contraction changes induce the oscillations. However the problem still remains, namely what drives the heart or the neurons of the medullary cardiovascular area. A great number of studies (7, 8, 9, 10, 11, 12, 14) show that the cytoplasmic and mitochondrial NADH (intact yeast cells, cell-free yeast and heart muscle extract) can oscillate in appropriate conditions. Therefore it is possible that in the case of hypoxic oscillation a metabolic oscillation is driving the heart or the medullary cardiovascular center.

REFERENCES

1. Barcroft, J., L.C. Khanna, Y. Nisimaru: J.Physiol.74.294. 1932.
2. Green, H.D., R.N. Lewis, N.D. Nickerson: Proc.Soc.Exper.Biol. Med. 53.228. 1943.
3. Guyton, A.C.: Amer. J. Physiol. 154. 45. 1948.
4. Sagawa, K., A.C. Guyton: Amer. J. Physiol. 200. 711. 1961.
5. Sagawa, K., A.E. Taylor, A.C. Guyton: Amer. J.Physiol. 201. 1164. 1961.
6. Sagawa, K., O. Carrier, A.C. Guyton: Amer. J.Physiol. 203. 141. 1962.
7. Chance, B., R.W. Estabrook, A. Ghosh: Proc. Nat. Acad. Sci. 51. 1244. 1964.
8. Chance, B., B. Hess, A. Betz: Biochem. Biophys. Res. Commun. 16. 182. 1964.
9. Chance, B., B. Stoner, S. Elsaesser: Proc. Nat. Acad. Sci. 52. 337. 1964.
10. Chance, B., A. Ghosh, J.J. Higgins, P.K. Maitra: Ann.N.Y.Acad. Sci. 115. 1010. 1964.
11. Chance, B., B. Schoener, S. Elsaesser: J. Biol. Chem. 240. 3170. 1965.
12. Chance, B., J. R. Williamson, D. Jamiesson, B. Schoener: Biochem. Zeitschrift. 341. 357. 1965.
13. Sawaga, K.: In: Physical Bases of Circulatory Transport. Analysis of the CNS Ischemic Feedback Regulation of the Circulation. (E.B. Reeve and A.C. Guyton, eds.) Saunders, Philadelphia, 1967. p. 129.
14. Ghosh, A.K., B. Chance, E.K. Pye: Arch. Biochem. 145. 319.1971.
15. Chance, B., V. Legallais, N. Graham, J. Sorge: In: International Symp. on Oxygen Transport to Tissue. (Abstracts). Eds.: M. H. Knisely, D.F. Bruley and H.I. Bicher. Charleston-Clemson, South Carolina, USA. 1973. p. 22.
16. Harbig, K., M. Reivich: Stroke. 4. 341. 1973.
17. Harbig, K., B. Chance, A.G.B. Kovách, M. Reivich: submitted to J. Appl. Physiol. 1975.

This work was partially supported by NINDS 10939.

THE EFFECT OF DECAPITATION ON THE OXIDATION-REDUCTION STATE OF NADH AND ECoG IN THE BRAIN OF THE AWAKE RAT

A. Mayevsky and B. Chance

Dept. of Life Sciences, Bar-Ilan University, Ramat-Gan, Israel, & Johnson Research Foundation, University of Pennsylvania, Philadelphia, Pennsylvania, U.S.A.

The effects of complete ischemia on brain energy metabolism have been studied in various animal preparation (1,2,3,4). One of the approaches on studying those effects is to convert the brain into a closed system, by decapitation, and after fixation of the tissue to measure changes in various metabolites such as glucose, lactate, ATP and creatine phosphate. The freezing procedure avoids most of the postmortem changes of brain metabolites levels, but the events of the first few seconds after decapitation are obscure.

The development of the surface fluorometry technique to measure oxidation-reduction state of NADH in the anesthetized and the awake rat (5,6,7) make possible the study of the effect of decapitation (a closed system) on NADH levels in the brain. In the present communication we describe the effects of decapitation on brain NADH fluorescence and electrical activity of the awake rat.

METHOD

The modified time-sharing fluorometer-reflectometer was used in all experiments. This fluorometer enables the measurement of NADH fluorescence (450 nm) and changes in intensity of reflected light at the excitation wavelength (366 nm) from the surface of brain cortex. The coupling between the fluorometer and the brain was done by a fused light guide (2 mm active diameter) made of quartz fibers (Schott Comp., Mainz, Germany). Figure 1 shows the experimental setup. Twelve male Wistar rats were used (180-220 gr.) and were anesthetized with Equi-thesin (Jensen-Salsbery Laboratories, U.S.A.) 0.5-0.6 ml injected intraperitoneally. The animal

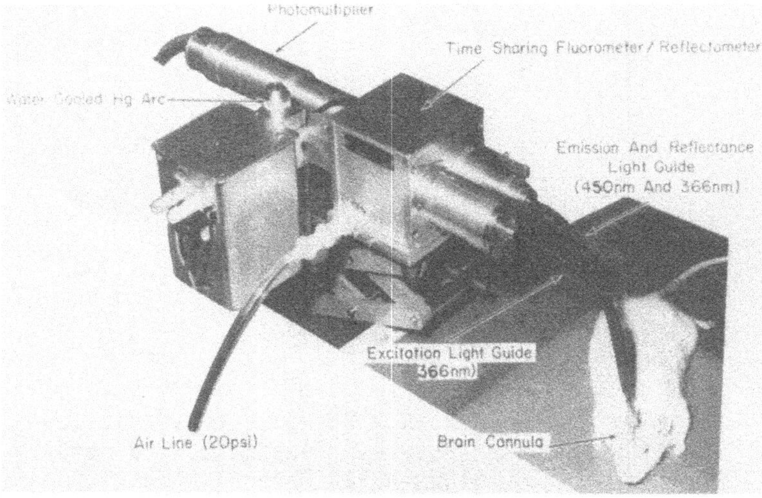

Fig. 1: An operated rat implanted with cannula connected to the time sharing fluorometer/reflectometer.

was mounted on a head holder for the operation time. The parietal bone was exposed and a hole (6 mm diameter) was drilled in the middle of the right side. Two stainless steel screws were implanted above each hemisphere for ECoG recording. A plexiglass cannula (light pipe holder) was screwed epidurally ($\sim$ 1 mm deep). The cannula and the screws were cemented to the skull using dental acrylic cement. Figure 2 shows the location of the cannula and the screws. The animal was connected to the fluorometer (30 min after operation) by inserting the common part of the light pipe into the cannula. This procedure avoids any type of movement artifact during the decapitation. Three to four hours after operation, when the animal was fully awake, decapitation was done using a guillotine (Stoelting Co.). Measurements of ECoG, NADH fluorescence and reflectance were taken during, as well as after, decapitation (10-15 minutes).

RESULTS AND DISCUSSION

The increase in NADH levels during N_2-O_2 breathing cycle was used as a test for the energetic state of the brain (8). All animals were exposed to N_2 for 1 min and the increase in NADH fluorescence under N_2 was 40-60% in comparison to the normoxic level, which has the same range as reported previously (7,8).

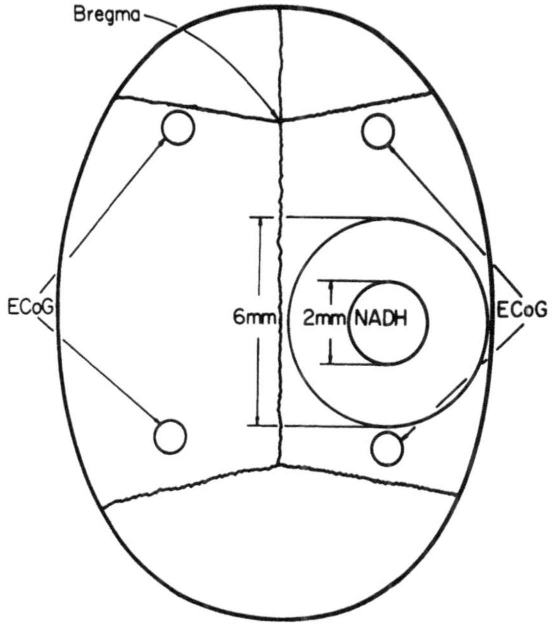

Fig. 2: Schematic presentation of the location of the cannula and the ECoG electrodes implanted above the brain.

Figure 3 shows a typical response of the awake brain to decapitation. The upper trace shows that the reflectance of 366 nm light increases immediately after decapitation by 20% and reached a plateau within 10 sec. In most animals this increase was smaller than 20% and in few even undetectable. Two minutes later a secondary increase in reflectance was recorded. This secondary increase in reflectance was recorded in 10 out of 12 animals. The second trace from the top shows the response of the 450 nm fluorescence. In this animal the maximum level of fluorescence was 130% above the normoxic level. The third trace shows the corrected fluorescence (the difference between the first and the second traces) response to decapitation. This correction technique was described earlier by others (9,10) and us (6,7) and the correction ratio in all experiments was 1:1. At the same time that the reflectance trace showed the secondary increase, the corrected fluorescence trace showed a transient decrease which returned to its maximum level within few minutes. The lower two traces show the ECoG response to decapitation. The right hemisphere was the same side from which the NADH fluorescence was measured. In most animals the ECoG traces showed a mechanical artifact when the decapitation was performed. In this animal the ECoG became flat within 10-15 seconds and the two hemispheres showed an identical response. Figure 4 shows the response of another animal to decapitation which is

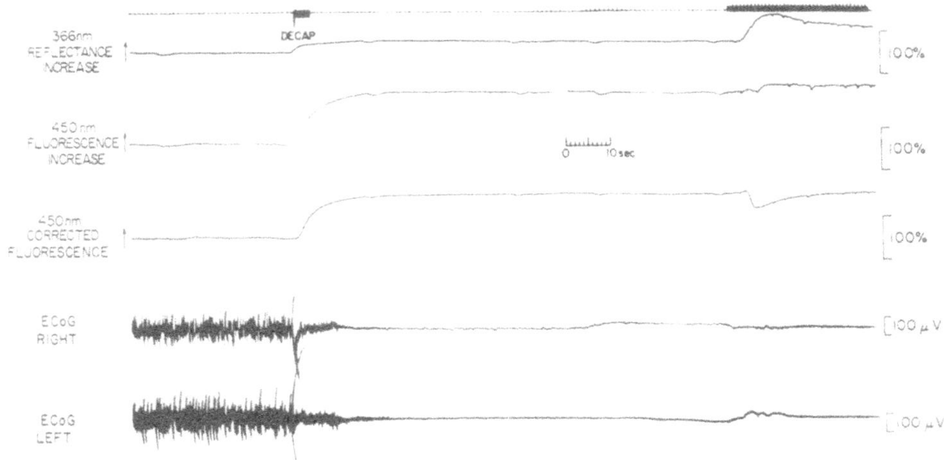

Fig. 3: The effects of decapitation on the oxidation reduction state of NADH and ECoG recorded from the cortex of the awake rat.

similar to the one shown in Figure 3.

In order to analyze the results obtained from all animals we defined a few parameters calculated from data obtained from experiments (Fig. 4).

- T_1 - Time when the ECoG amplitude was indistinguishable from the baseline level.
- T_2 - The time when corrected fluorescence reached its maximum level.
- T_3 - The time when corrected fluorescence reached 50% of the maximum level.
- T_4 - The time when the reflectance trace showed the secondary increase.

The calculation was done on data obtained from 12 rats. The means and their standard error were:

$T_1 = 12.5 \pm 0.9$ sec. $T_3 = 6.04 \pm 0.55$ sec.

$T_2 = 32.8 \pm 3.2$ " $T_4 = 66.3 \pm 9.5$ "

Changes in fluorescence intensity were calculated also. The maximum increase in corrected fluorescence (max ΔCF) at time T_2 was $81.6 \pm 6\%$ above the normoxic level measured before decapitation. The ΔCF at time T_1 was $65 \pm 6.3\%$ and by dividing the two values

$$\frac{\Delta CFT_1}{\Delta CF\ max} = 78.4 \pm 2.8$$

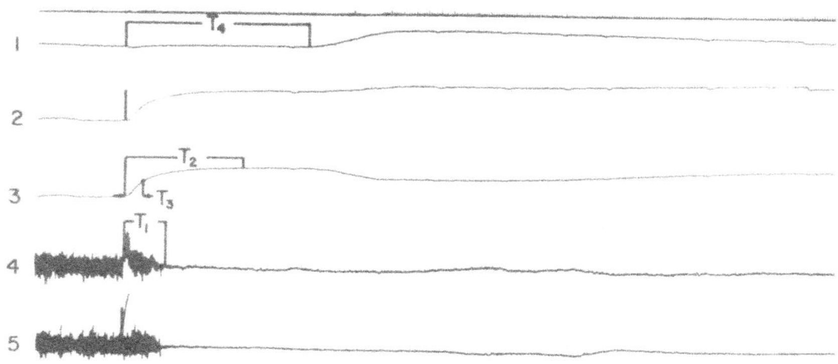

Fig. 4: Another example to show the effects of decapitation as in Fig. 3. The traces numbered 1-5 are the same and the parameters T_1-T_4 were calculated from the traces.

which means that the ECoG disappeared when NADH level reached about 80% of its maximum reduction. We measured also the time after decapitation when the corrected fluorescence started to increase, T_5, and the calculated value was 1.5 $\pm$ 0.14 sec. This value shows that the oxygen stores in the tissue are very small and as soon as the oxygen supply was interrupted the NADH level increased.

The results presented in this preliminary presentation show that when the brain is transferred to a closed system by decapitation one can study the correlation between electrical activity and the metabolic state of the brain. This approach was described by Swaab and Baer (3) and earlier by King et al. (11). They described the effects of decapitation on the ECoG activity and found that at 10 seconds the activity disappeared from cortical area and, in our finding, it is in the same range of time (12.5 seconds). The main advantage of our approach is that we can measure the NADH oxidation-reduction state in the decapitated brain continuously and correlate it to the electrical activity. The ECoG disappeared when the NADH was reduced to 80% from its maximum level and the same result was obtained when the animal was exposed to N_2 environment (7,8). We can assume that the rate of increase in NADH levels in the decapitated brain is dependent on the oxygen store in the tissue as well as the rate of consumption. This model will enable us to study the effects of various factors, such as anesthetics or hypoxia, on the rate of oxygen consumption in the decapitated brain.

ACKNOWLEDGMENT

This work was supported in part by NINDS 10939-02, the Research Committee, Bar-Ilan University, and the B. de Rothschild Foundation for the Advancement of Science in Israel.

REFERENCES

1. Lowry, O.H., Passonneau, J.V., Hasselberger, F.X., and Schulz, D.W., J. Biol. Chem. 239, 18-30 (1964).
2. Folbergrova, J., Lowry, O.H., Passonneau, J.V., J. Neurochem. 17, 1155-1162 (1970).
3. Swaab, D.F. and Baer, K., J. Neurochem. 19, 2843-2853 (1972)
4. Gercken, G., and Preuss, H., J. Neurochem. 16, 761-767 (1969)
5. Chance, B., Cohen, P., Jöbsis, F.F., and Schoener, B., Science, 137, 499-508 (1962)
6. Chance, B., Oshino T. Sugano, and Mayevsky, A., in H.I. Bicher and B.F. Bruley (eds.) Int. Symp. on Oxygen Transport to Tissue, Advanc. Exp. Med. Biol. Plenum Press, New York, 1973, pp 277-292.
7. Mayevsky, A., and Chance, B., Ibid, pp. 239-244 (1973)
8. Mayevsky, A., Chance, B., Brain Res. 1975 (in press)
9. Jöbsis, F.F., O'Connor, M., Vitale, A., and Verman, H., J. Neurophysiol. 34, 735-749 (1971)
10. Harbig, K., and Rievich, M., Stroke 4, 341 (Abstract VI-43) 1973)
11. King, L.J., Schoepele, G.M., Lowry, O.H., Passonneau, J.V., and Wilson, S., J. Neurochem. 14, 613-618 (1967)

CEREBRAL OXYGEN SUPPLY IN BRAIN EDEMA AND DURING VENTRICULO-CISTERNAL PERFUSION

J. Grote, R. Schubert, A. Fenske and J. Brantzen

Departments of Applied Physiology and Neurosurgery, University of Mainz, 65 Mainz

Numerous brain injuries and brain tumors lead to edema in brain tissue which can have consequences for the oxygen supply to the damaged tissue as well as to adjacent tissue areas. In studies made of the blood flow and oxygen supply in perifocal edematous tissue of brain tumors and lesions in patients undergoing various brain operations a direct relationship between the regional blood flow and the water content could be demonstrated (3). As the water content of the tissue increased, the blood flow through it diminished. In many cases, the reduction of the blood flow in the brain tissue induced an insufficient oxygen supply. In the tissue samples under investigation, the CrP and ATP concentrations were diminished in comparison to normal brain tissue. At the same time a marked rise in the lactate concentration and the lactate-pyruvate ratio was determined. The studies in patients were the starting point for further animal experiments.

CEREBRAL OXYGEN SUPPLY IN BRAIN EDEMA

In cats the influence of localized edema on blood flow and oxygen supply of the brain tissue was investigated.

METHODS

The experiments were performed on a total of 26 cats weighting 2.1 - 4.9 kg. Twenty-four hours after the creation of a cryolesion in the right frontal brain after KLATZO (5, 6) the regional blood flow and the concentrations of various metabolites were determined in the area of the lesion, in the immediately adjacent area, and in the remote parts of the damaged hemisphere (Fig. 1). The extent of the edema could be visualised by i. v. injection of 2 % Evans blue (1 ml/kg b.w.). The data of the undamaged hemisphere served as control values.

All experimental animals were anesthetized with sodium pentobarbital (Nembutal, 30 mg/kg b.w.). After tracheotomy and complete relaxation (Imbretil, 1.6 - 2.0 mg initially and 0.2 - 0.3 mg/30 min), the cats were artificially ventilated so that the regular controlled respiratory gas partial pressures and the pH of the arterial blood lay within the norm. The arterial blood pressure, the blood pressure in the sinus system and the cisternal fluid pressure were continually measured after cannulation of the a. fem., the sup. sag. sinus and the cisterna magna. The body temperature was kept in normal ranges. Following a bilateral craniotomy leaving the dura intact and a catheterization of both lingual arteries for tracer injection, the regional cerebral blood flow (rCBF) could be measured using the Kr^{85}-clearance technique.

At the end of the experiment the concentrations of CrP, ATP, lactate and pyruvate were enzymatically determined in tissue samples which were removed from the investigated brain areas after freezing the brain with liquid nitrogen (11). The necrotic zone in the area of the lesion was carefully separated and excluded from consideration. In the majority of cases the single probe consisted of cortical tissue and a small layer of white matter. The water content of the tissue was determined by drying to a constant weight at 105° C.

RESULTS AND DISCUSSION

The results are summarized in Table 1. Under normoxic, normocapnic conditions regional blood flow in the area of the lesion (L) as well as in immediately adjacent areas (A) and in the remoter areas (R) of the damaged hemisphere was markedly decreased in comparison to the control data of the undamaged hemisphere (C). The water content of the tissue in the area of the lesion and in the immediately adjacent tissue zone was increased (Fig. 1). The control data for the water content of the undamaged hemisphere are smaller than comparable values for the normal cortical tissue (1) because the investigated probes contained parts of white matter.

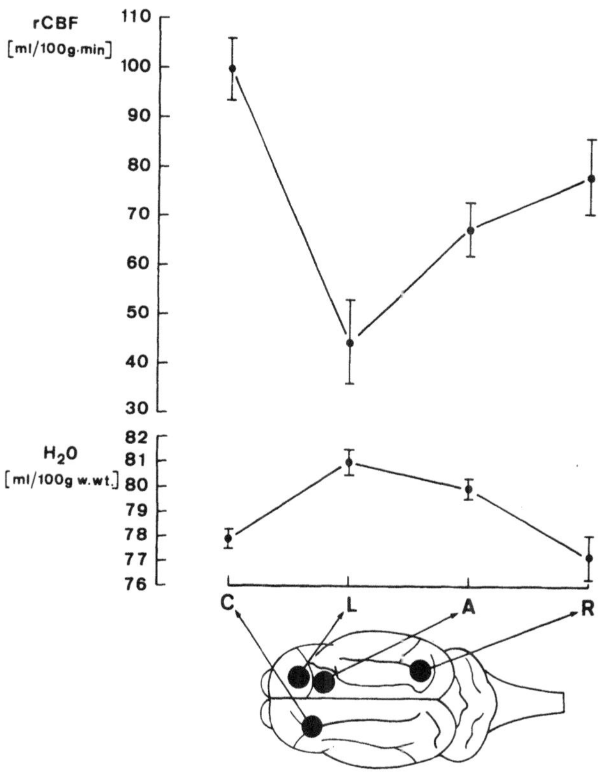

Fig. 1. Regional blood flow and local water content in the area of the lesion (L), in adjacent (A) and remote (R) areas of the damaged hemisphere and in the undamaged hemisphere (C).

Simultaneously, as can be seen from Fig. 2, the lactate concentration and the lactate-pyruvate ratio in the lesion and in the immediately adjacent brain tissue was increased. In the specific damaged areas, additionally,

Table 1. Regional blood flow, metabolite and water content in cerebral tissue of the lesion area (L), adjacent (A) and remote (R) areas of the injured hemisphere and of the contralateral hemisphere (C).

$\bar{x} \pm s_{\bar{x}}$ are given, total number of measurements indicated in parenthesis. rCBF expressed as ml/100 g per min, metabolite concentrations expressed as μmoles/gram wet weight, water content expressed as ml/100 grams wet weight.

	C		L		A		R	
rCBF	99.7 ± 6.4	(24)	44.2 ± 9.1	(9)	67.8 ± 5.4	(26)	84.1 ± 9.0	(11)
Water	77.9 ± 0.4	(25)	81.0 ± 0.5	(10)	80.0 ± 0.4	(23)	77.2 ± 0.9	(10)
Lactate	2.40 ± 0.44	(9)	5.58 ± 0.81	(8)	5.75 ± 0.93	(11)	3.12 ± 0.64	(9)
Pyruvate	0.10 ± 0.02	(11)	0.20 ± 0.02	(8)	0.23 ± 0.03	(11)	0.18 ± 0.04	(9)
Lact./Pyr.	21.4 ± 3.4	(6)	27.9 ± 2.5	(8)	26.1 ± 2.8	(11)	18.1 ± 3.3	(7)
CrP	4.32 ± 0.29	(8)	2.81 ± 0.25	(8)	4.19 ± 0.45	(8)	4.09 ± 0.27	(8)
ATP	2.32 ± 0.19	(7)	1.62 ± 0.12	(8)	2.49 ± 0.33	(8)	2.39 ± 0.19	(8)

the CrP and ATP concentrations were decreased. The findings can be interpreted to be the direct result of insufficient tissue oxygen supply which resulted from diminishment of the regional blood flow after increase of tissue water content. They are in substantial agreement with the experimental results of FREI et. al. (2). The mean perfusion pressure in all instances lay within the norm. The blood flow regulation in the edematous tissue zones was impaired or suspended. After progressive decrease in arterial oxygen tension at normocapnia and normal arterial blood pressure, there were no, or at most, very slight changes in rCBF while regulation was normal in the unaffected brain tissue (4).

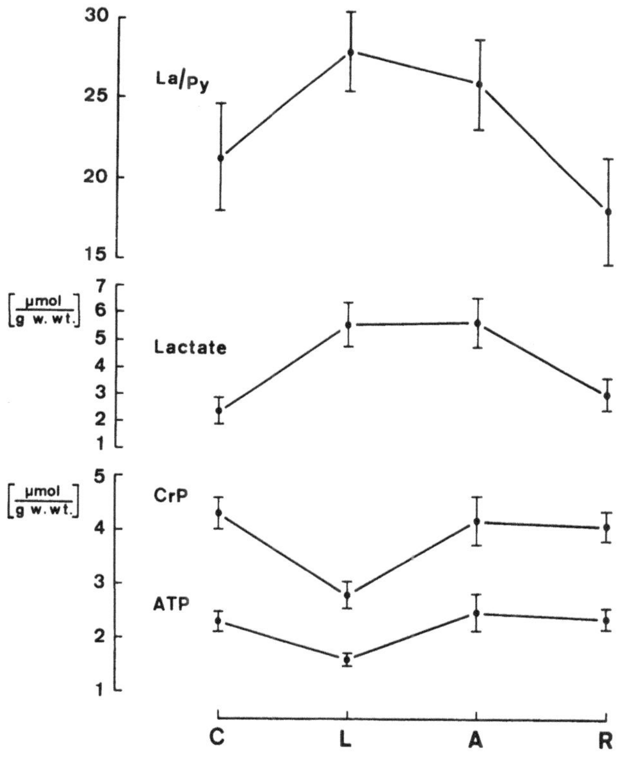

Fig. 2. Local brain tissue concentrations of lactate, CrP and ATP and the lactate-pyruvate ratio in the area of the lesion (L), in adjacent (A) and remote (R) areas of the damaged hemisphere and in the undamaged hemisphere (C).

CEREBRAL OXYGEN SUPPLY DURING VETRICULO-CISTERNAL PERFUSION

A therapeutic influencing of brain edema is limited, due in part to the specific characteristics of the blood brain barrier. In order to circumvent this barrier, it has been attempted to influence the brain edema from the liquor side (7). A ventricular perfusion appears to be an alternative approach of drug application.

The mentioned brain model seems to us to be sufficient to carry out such investigations. The prerequisites for the investigations are the development of a suitable perfusion technique as well as the proof that the perfusion of the venticular system in normal brain is without deleterious consequences for the cerebral oxygen supply. In the first series of experiments we tried to fulfill these prerequisites. The aim of the study was to investigate whether a ventriculo-cisternal perfusion with artificial liquor of different CO_2 tensions may influence brain water content and cerebral blood flow.

METHODS

Under experimental conditions which correspond closely with the described investigations, a ventriculo-cisternal perfusion was accomplished on cats (n = 17) after stereo-operative insertion of a cannule into the right lateral ventricle and cannulation of the cisterna magna. Ventriculo-cisternal perfusion was performed under pressure control using an artificial cerebro-spinal fluid (CSF) according to MERLIS (8). The artificial CSF was equilibrated with gas mixtures containing 4 % and 8 % CO_2 and approx. 15 % O_2 corresponding to a PCO_2 of 30 and 55 mmHg and a PO_2 of about 90 to 100 mmHg respectively . The perfusion period was extended to 4 hours, the flow rate was 1.2 - 1.6 ml/min.

During the experiments the arterial blood pressure, the blood pressure in the sinus system, as well as the pressure in the right lateral ventricule and in the cisterna magna were continuously measured. The animals were normoventilated.

Regional blood flow of the cortex was determined in the frontal lobe using the Kr^{85}-clearance method. The regional blood flow primarily of the white matter was determined by the Xe^{133}-clearance technique with the scintillation probe being placed over the occipital lobe. Simultaneously with the flow measurements, the respiratory gas partial pressure values and the pH of the arterial blood, the mixed cerebral venous blood and the blood of the sup. sag. sinus as well as of the artificial CSF - both influx and efflux - were determined. Based on the measured data we were able to calculate the regional oxygen uptake rate of the brain tissue.

RESULTS AND DISCUSSION

Fig. 3 summarizes the results of experiments on 10 cats relating to the influence of ventriculo-cisternal perfusion on regional blood flow and regional oxygen uptake of brain areas primarily containing white matter.

During the control period under normoxic, normocapnic conditions the mean values for rCBF, CVR and $CMRO_2$ measured 20.0 ± 1.2 ml/100 g min, 6.6 ± 0.3 mmHg 100 g min/ml and 2.2 ± 0.2 ml/100 g min respectively. The respiratory gas partial pressure values and the pH of the CSF were $P_LO_2 = 59.3 \pm 2.8$ mmHg, $P_LCO_2 = 32.6 \pm 2.3$ mmHg and pH $= 7.431 \pm 0.025$. The blood flow values as well as the oxygen uptake rates which were measured before commenzing perfusion correspond to normal values; they lie between the values for the total brain and those for the white matter.

The 1.5 hour long perfusion of the ventricular system with artificial liquor having a CO_2 tension of 30 and 55 mmHg respectively led to no change in oxygen supply conditions in the investigated brain tissue. At the end of the perfusion period using artificial CSF with $PCO_2 = 30$ mmHg the mean values of the determined parameters were: rCBF $= 18.6 \pm 1.6$ ml/100 g min, CVR $= 7.0 \pm 0.7$ mmHg 100 g min/ml and $rCMRO_2 = 2.5 \pm 0.2$ ml/100 g min. The comparable data of subsequent ventricular perfusion with artificial CSF of $PCO_2 = 55$ mmHg were: rCBF $= 17.2 \pm 1.8$ ml/100 g min, CVR $= 7.1 \pm 0.6$ mmHg 100 g min/ml and $rCMRO_2 = 2.3 \pm 0.3$ ml/100 g min.

During the whole experiment PO_2, PCO_2 and pH of the arterial blood remained in normal range. The corresponding mean values for the gas partial pressures and pH in the cerebral venous blood were as follows:

1. control period: P_vO_2 = 36.4 mmHg, P_vCO_2 = 42.8 mmHg, pH = 7.357,
2. during ventriculo-cisternal perfusion (PCO_2 of artificial CSF = 30 mmHg): P_vO_2 = 33.7 mmHg, P_vCO_2 = 45.1 mmHg, pH_v = 7.360,
3. during ventriculo-cisternal perfusion (PCO_2 of artificial CSF = 55 mmHg): P_vO_2 = 30.0 mmHg, P_vCO_2 = 47.9 mmHg, pH_v = 7.334.

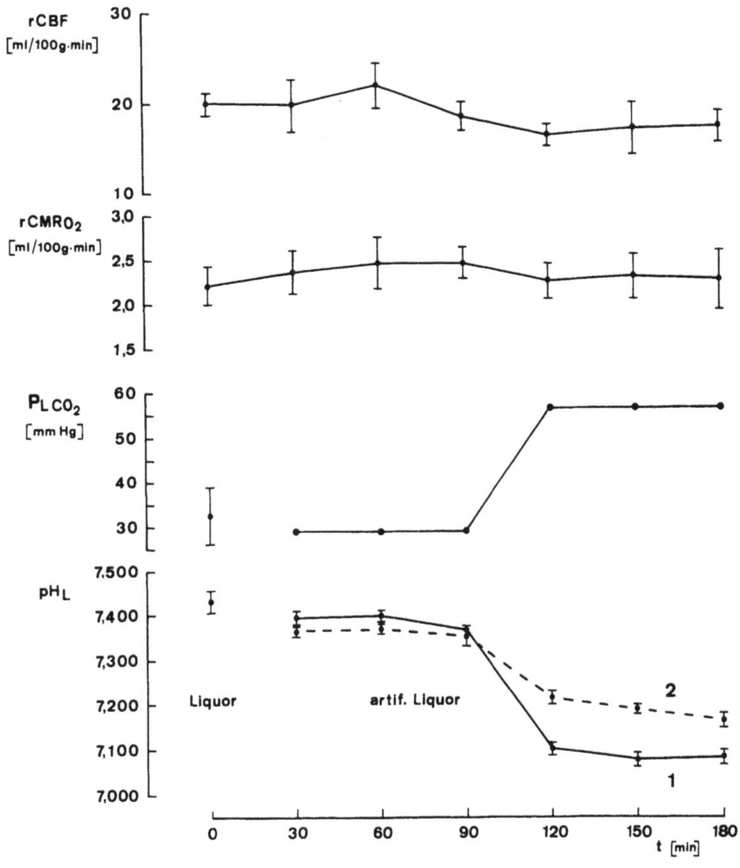

Fig. 3. Regional blood flow and regional oxygen uptake in brain areas containing primarily white matter during ventriculo-cisternal perfusion.
1. Artificial CSF, influx.
2. Artificial CSF, efflux.

The mean pH in the inflowing artificial CSF was a) 7.385 and b) 7.089 respectively. The water content of the grey and white matter of tissue probes taken at the end of the experiment from the corresponding brain areas of the right and left hemisphere lay in normal range (grey matter 79.6 and 79.7 ml/1oo g w. wt., white matter 68.8 and 68.5 ml/100 g w. wt.). The intracranial pressure did not exceed 6.5 mmHg during the experimental duration, the cerebral perfusion pressure was in normal range.

Following SIESJÖ et al. (12) who found changes in CBF when pH and (HCO_3^-) in artificial CSF were varied, we would have expected an increase of blood flow in cerebral tissue during ventriculo-cisternal perfusion with artificial liquor at PCO_2 = 55 mmHg. In our experiments the expected change did not occur and this corresponds to the findings of POSNER et al. (10) and PANNIER et al. (9). PANNIER an coworkers observed regional blood flow changes in the nucleus caudatus (heat clearance technique) but no detectable changes in hemispheric blood flow (X^{133}-clearance technique) when altering the acid-base composition in the cerebral ventricles.

The investigations of the influence of a ventriculo-cisternal perfusion on regional blood flow and regional oxygen uptake in the cortex of the frontal lobe of 7 cats led to comparable results. In these experiments the perfusion of the sinus system with artificial CSF with an adjusted PCO_2 of 30 mmHg had no demonstrable influence on the blood flow and oxygen uptake rate of the brain cortex. Both values remained within the normal range during the 1.5 hour perfusion.

The mean values for rCBF, CVR and $CMRO_2$ measured in the control period were 104.6 $\pm$ 5.6 ml/100 g min, 1.4 $\pm$ 0.1 mmHg 100 g min/ml and 8.3 $\pm$ 0.9 ml/100 g min. After the 90 minute long ventriculo-cisternal perfusion the following mean values for the three investigated parameters could be measured: rCBF = 87.8 ml/100 g min, CVR = 1.4 $\pm$ 0.1 mmHg 100 g min/ml an $rCMRO_2$ = 8.1 $\pm$ 1.8 ml/100 g min (Fig. 4).

In both series of investigations, the autoregulation as well as the CO_2 response of the cerebral blood flow were normal at the end of each individual experiment. An increase of mean arterial blood pressure of approx. 40 mmHg had no influence on the regional blood flow in the cerebral cortex, the rCBF changes after hyperventilation correspond to normal behaviour.

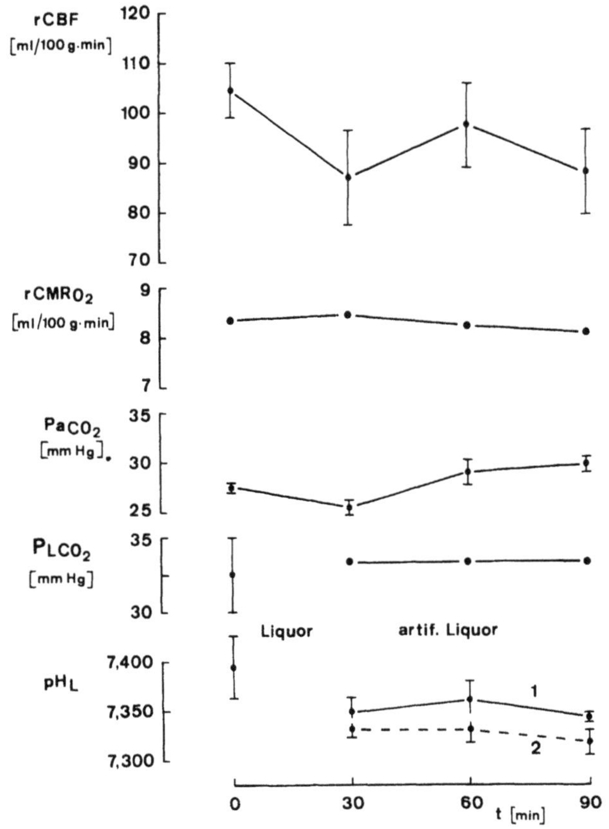

Fig. 4. Regional blood flow and regional oxygen uptake in the cerebral cortex during ventriculo-cisternal perfusion.
1. Artificial CSF, influx.
2. Artificial CSF, efflux.

It could be shown from both investigation series that a ventriculo-cisternal perfusion with high flow rates using artificial CSF with PCO_2 adjusted to normal values is without influence on the cerebral blood flow and cerebral oxygen supply. The perfusion model employed appears to us to be well suited to systematic investigations of the therapeutic influence of brain edema through liquor perfusion.

ACKNOWLEDGEMENT

This investigation was supported by a grant from the Deutsche Forschungsgemeinschaft.

REFERENCES

1. Bartko, D., H.J. Reulen, H. Koch and K. Schürmann: Effect of dexamethasone on the early edema following occlusion of the middle cerebral artery in cats. In: Steroids and Brain Edema, pp. 127 - 137. H.J. Reulen and K. Schürmann, eds. Berlin, Heidelberg, New York: Springer 1972
2. Frei, H.J., Th. Wallenfang, W. Pöll, H.J. Reulen, R. Schubert and M. Brock: Regional cerebral blood flow and regional metabolism in cold induced oedema. Acta Neurochir. 29, 15-28 (1973)
3. Grote, J., H. Kreuscher, H.J. Reulen, P. Vaupel and H. Günther: Respiratory gas transport in brain under normal and pathological conditions. In: Advances in Chemistry Series, 118, Chemical Engineering in Medicine, pp. 35-46. Washington: American Chemical Society 1973
4. Grote, J., R. Schubert, W. Schaaf, H.J. Reulen and Th. Wallenfang: The influence of brain edema on regional cerebral blood flow and regional vascular reactivity. Pflügers Arch. 343, R 28 (1973)
5. Klatzo, J., A. Piraux and E. Laskowski: The relationship between edema, blood brain barrier and tissue elements in local brain injury.
6. Klatzo, J., H. Wisniewski, O. Steinwall and E. Streicher: Dynamics of cold injury edema. In: Brain Edema, pp. 554-563. J. Klatzo and F. Seitelberger, eds. Wien, New York: Springer 1967
7. Matsen, F.A. III and C.R. West: Supracortical fluid: a monitor of albumin exchange in normal and injured brain. Amer. J. Physiol. 222, 532-539 (1972)
8. Merlis, J.K.: The effect of changes in the calcium content of the cerebrospinal fluid on spinal reflex activity in the dog. Amer. J. Physiol. 131, 67-72 (1940)
9. Pannier, J.L., J. Weyne, G. Demeester and I. Leusen: Influence of changes in the acid-base composition of the ventricular system on cerebral blood flow in cats. Pflügers Arch. 333, 337-351 (1972)
10. Posner, J.B., F. Plum and D. Zee: Ventriculocisternal pH and cerebral blood flow. Arch. Neurol. (Chic.) 20, 664-667 (1969)

11. Reulen, H.J., F. Medzihradsky, R. Enzenbach, F. Marguth and W. Brendel: Electrolytes, fluids and energy metabolism in cerebral edema in man. Arch. Neurol. 21, 517-525 (1969)

12. Siesjö, B.K., A. Kjällquist, U. Ponten and N. Zwetnow: Extracellular pH in the brain and cerebral blood flow. In: Cerebral Circulation, pp. 93-98. W. Luyendijk, ed. Progress in Brain Research, vol. 30. Amsterdam, London, New York: Elsevier 1968

TISSUE RESPONSES TO HYPOXIA, SHOCK AND STROKE

Ian A. Silver

University of Bristol, Department of Pathology

The Medical School, Bristol BS8 1TD, England

INTRODUCTION

Tissue hypoxia may occur in tissues either naturally or experimentally in association with arterial hypoxaemia, hypovolaemic shock and so-called endotoxic shock, together with acute ischaemia caused by thrombosis, or some other form of vascular occlusion. In an attempt to distinguish between the results of hypoxia at the cellular level produced by these different causes, a comparison has been made between the response of liver on the one hand, and the cerebral cortex on the other. Both these organs are susceptible to tissue hypoxia and prolonged hypoxia of either organ will ultimately be fatal. Investigations were carried out by using microprobes sensitive to oxygen, pH and other ions and also with an optical probe which gave measurements of the intracellular redox state as judged by pyridine nucleotide fluorescence (Chance et al 1962). There have been a number of papers on the effects of hypoxia on ionic movements in brain (see Bito and Myers 1972; Dora and Zeuthen 1975) and there have been preliminary observations of the changes in liver which occur during shock as compared to hypoxia (Silver 1973; Sinagowitz et al 1973; Kessler et al 1973, 1975). In view of the possible importance of changes in ionic balance both on local metabolism and in terms of possible systemic effects, this investigation has been mainly concentrated on extracellular ionic changes occurring during hypoxic episodes, while a small number of intracellular measurements have been made where feasible.

MATERIALS AND METHODS

The experiments were carried out using white Wistar rats of between 250 and 350 gms. The animals were anaesthetised with a variety of agents including pentobarbitone, urethane and halothane, in order to see whether different anaesthetic agents produced marked changes in tissue responses. Blood pressure was recorded from the femoral artery and chlorided silver electrodes were fixed in the skull to monitor cortical EEG. Holes were drilled over the cortex in the cingulate, temporal and frontal regions. The dura mater was removed and the various kinds of electrodes were inserted under stereotaxic guidance.

Electrodes were of several types. Those principally used were needle type oxygen electrodes (Silver 1965); all glass pH and sodium electrodes (Hinke 1959; Thomas 1970) and potassium and chloride ion exchanger probes (Zeuthen, Hiam and Silver 1974). On some occasions multi-barrelled electrodes were used which were sensitive to oxygen and to ions, usually potassium and chloride (Silver 1975).

Redox measurements of pyridine nucleotide were made by the method of Chance et al 1962 using an Ultrapak microscope (Zeiss) with a 0.2 mm spot with an exciting wavelength of 366 nm; the fluorescence was measured at 456 nm.

Experiments on liver were carried out using the caudate lobe which can be easily immobilised compared with the other lobes. Multiple electrode arrays were used in order to determine whether or not a change in ion concentration or hypoxia was uniform throughout the organ under study.

Hypoxia was induced (1) by allowing the animals to breathe a graded mixture of oxygen and nitrogen containing either 5%, 2.5% or 0% oxygen in nitrogen, (2) by inducing hypovolaemia by bleeding the animal through an arterial cannula over a period of 1 hour until the arterial blood pressure was 30 mmHg. This pressure was maintained by the withdrawal or infusion of blood. The animal's temperature was monitored and kept constant at 38 °C.

Endotoxic shock was induced by peritoneal injection of 6 mg of E. coli endotoxin (Difco)/100 gm body weight.

Local acute ischaemia was produced in rat brain by drilling a hole at the junction of the frontal and temporal bones to expose the lateral branch of the middle cerebral artery. This artery or one of its branches to the cortex was then compressed from the outside either by direct pressure or by ligation. Permanent occlusion was obtained with a cautery.

In a few experiments in collaboration with Dr. Reivich and Dr. Greenberg, a cat 'stroke' model was used in which the middle cerebral artery was clamped behind the orbit.

In the case of the liver, gross ischaemia could be produced by ligating the hepatic artery where it left the coeliac but it was usually found more convenient to apply local pressure to the liver in the vicinity of the electrode and to take measurements in the compressed region.

RESULTS

1. Effects of arterial hypoxia

(a) Brain

The effect of hypoxia on the brain with regard to ion movements was the same as that already described by Zeuthen et al (1974), and by Dora and Zeuthen (1975). There was a two stage increase in extracellular potassium concentration. In the first stage it began immediately after the drastic fall in oxygen tension from resting levels to zero. There was a small increase in potassium activity of between 2 and 5 mV, together with a similar small decrease of the DC potential. After 2 or 3 minutes this stage passed abruptly into a 'depolarization' phase when there was a rapid and large increase in the extracellular potassium, which over a period of another 2 to 5 minutes produced a 10-fold change in potassium activity. At the same time there was a marked decrease in the DC potential.

Preliminary observations with a Hinke type pH electrode indicated that at this stage the extracellular hydrogen ion concentration rose abruptly. Prior to the massive change in potassium concentration little or no change in pH could be detected. Recovery after 6 minutes of severe acute arterial hypoxia was rare. In some animals spontaneous respiration could still be restarted at this stage, but in none did the cortical EEG reappear, and neither did the pH or the potassium return to normal. In contrast to this, oxygen tension frequently rose up above the original level and stayed elevated.

(b) Liver

Arterial hypoxaemia had little effect on the ion or pH status of liver during the short period which caused severe changes in the brain. The only change was a rapid reduction in the PO_2 to zero, together with a slight lowering of pH. These changes are similar to those reported by Silver (1973) and Kessler et al (1975).

2. Hypoxia induced by hypovolaemia

(a) Brain

In animals which had been bled to 30 mmHg mean arterial pressure and maintained at this pressure until all the shed blood had been returned to the animal, it was found that in general the PO_2 in the brain fell progressively during initial bleeding, then stabilised, and finally declined to zero. A feature of the PO_2 in 'shocked' brain was that different areas showed marked variation in mean readings and response to O_2 breathing. Some areas appeared to be totally anoxic whereas others were merely mildly hypoxic. As the animal deteriorated to the stage of complete irreversibility the brain PO_2 gradually became uniformly depressed until most areas showed zero. Even when the blood volume was artificially expanded by the injection of dextran or saline, these areas usually failed to show any increase in PO_2. On the other hand, the areas still showing a positive reading frequently responded temporarily after injections.

Ionic changes in the brains of animals in hypovolaemic shock developed very slowly over several hours. During the initial period of bleeding there was little or no change and during the first hour or so after the blood pressure was held at 30 mmHg there was still no change. However when the pressure had to be maintained by returning the shed blood, and the blood pressure continued to fall, there was a slowly developing but continuous change in both the DC and in the extracellular pK. Coincidentally the extracellular pH decreased and terminally there was a drastic release of potassium and a large change of DC similar to that seen in late acute hypoxia; the pH fell about 0.5 unit. As with the PO_2 changes in pK during shock were not uniform over the surface of the brain, whereas in arterial hypoxia it was usual to find the same changes occurring in the different parts of the cortex simultaneously. In some animals there were sudden changes of pK during late shock with a cyclical pattern which suggested the occurrence of a 'spreading depression' type of phenomenon.

(b) Liver

In contrast to the brain, the liver showed early changes during the development of haemorrhagic shock, and indeed falls of PO_2 to zero were obvious in many sites early in the 'bleeding' phase. This condition was followed by a small increase in extracellular pK^+ together with a small change in pH. On some occasions with a 'Thomas' type of electrode it was possible to make measurements of intracellular pH for a period of about 30 seconds. The electrode response was rather slow and it is probable that the true intracellular pH was not registered. Another difficulty in making measurements in the liver is that it is almost impossible to keep an electrode in a natural extracellular space so that the tip of the probe was usually located in an area of damage. When true shock developed, the pH of the liver fell progressively to a value of 6.6 or less.

3. Endotoxic shock

In animals which had been injected with endotoxin there was at first little or no change in the blood pressure and none in ionic activity or PO_2 in either brain or liver. After about half to one hour depending on the individual animal, the blood pressure began to fall but conditions in the brain remained relatively constant, whereas the liver changes were similar to those in haemorrhagic shock. There was a progressive fall in PO_2 but there was also a much more obvious change in the potassium activity and in the pH. Whereas in haemorrhagic shock the pH and pK changed only very slowly, in endotoxic shock the change was larger and earlier. In the later stages of endotoxic shock the brain showed a fall in PO_2 together with marked extracellular pK shifts. These appeared to be uniform over the surface of the cortex rather than patchy as was the case with haemorrhagic shock.

4. Acute ischaemia

(a) In the brain during 'stroke' simulation the effect was similar both with regard to oxygen and to potassium activity to that of acute hypoxia although rather more rapid. The main difference between the stroke situation and the hypoxaemia was that the pH change appeared to coincide with the potassium leakage. Unfortunately our pH electrodes were not of sufficiently rapid response to give satisfactory time correlation of these events. In the rat brain acute ischaemia lasting for 4 minutes produced changes in pK, DC, PO_2 and pH which were almost indistinguishable from those seen after about 5 minutes of arterial hypoxia. Nevertheless, the condition could be reversed if the pressure on the blood vessel was released and perfusion restarted. This produced a period of hyperaemia with elevated PO_2 and a shift to above normal of the DC levels. Potassium activity very rapidly returned to normal unless the ischaemia had been too prolonged in which case the potassium activity remained high inspite of the increased PO_2. pH returned to normal, but no further cellular activity could be detected in the previously ischaemic regions.

(b) In the liver local or generalised ischaemia produced effects similar to those in hypovolaemic shock. There was a rapid fall to zero in the PO_2 which was accompanied some minutes later by small but progressive increases in extracellular pK, parallelled by a decrease in pH. If the circulation was allowed to return while the pH was still above 6.6, conditions appeared to return to normal. Electron microscopy of areas of liver in which the pH had been allowed to drop below 6.6 showed disruption of mitochondria.

A feature of the liver in endotoxic shock was that the endotoxin was at first localised in the Kupfer cells and later spread to the liver parenchyma. This could be demonstrated by staining liver tissue with fluorescent anti-endotoxin.

Tables 1 - 3 show changes of PO_2 and ion concentrations in different organs under different regimes.

TABLE 1

ARTERIAL HYPOXIA

	Time	0	30 sec.	5 min.
Brain	PO_2	22 ± 12.5 mmHg	3.8 ± 2.3	0
	K^+	3.0 ± 0.01 mM	3.1 ± 0.04	27.3 ± 1.3
	Na^+	143 ± 8.0 mM	-	-
	Cl^-	127.3 ± 6.1 mM	-	-
	pH	7.39 ± 0.04	7.39 ± 0.04	7.05 ± 0.21
Liver	PO_2	18.6 ± 10.1 mmHg	2.7 ± 1.8	0
	K^+	3.2 ± 0.07 mM	3.2 ± 0.08	3.5 ± 0.31
	pH	7.33 ± 0.10	7.33 ± 0.10	7.25 ± 0.03

TABLE 2

ACUTE ISCHAEMIA

	Time	0	30 sec.	4 min.
Brain	PO_2	22 ± 12.5 mmHg	2.1 ± 1.0	0
	K^+	3.0 ± 0.01 mM	3.3 ± 0.1	28.5 ± 2.2
	pH	7.39 ± 0.04	7.37 ± 0.03	7.0 ± 0.18
Liver	PO_2	18.6 ± 10.1 mmHg	1.7 ± 1.1	0
	K^+	3.2 ± 0.07 mM	3.3 ± 0.10	3.4 ± 0.12
	pH	7.33 ± 0.10	7.33 ± 0.10	7.32 ± 0.12

TABLE 3

HYPOVOLAEMIC SHOCK

	Time	0 Haemorrhage ---------->	1hr. 30 mmHg BP --------->	4 hour
Brain	PO_2	22 ± 12.5 mmHg	12.1 ± 6.1	8.3 ± 7.5
	K^+	3.0 ± 0.01 mM	4.3 ± 1.1	17.9 ± 5.3
	pH	7.33 ± 0.10	7.31 ± 0.18	6.8 ± 0.21
Liver	PO_2	18.6 ± 10.1 mmHg	2.4 ± 2.0	0
	K^+	3.2 ± 0.07 mM	4.3 ± 0.12 mM	9.7 ± 3.1
	pH	7.33 ± 0.10	7.12 ± 0.13	6.7 ± 0.32

DISCUSSION

The changes in oxygen tension and in ion activity reported in this study correlate reasonably well with changes in organs which have been reported by other workers (Mela et al 1975; Höper et al 1975; Kessler et al 1975). The most obvious feature is the difference between the sensitivity of the brain to arterial hypoxia as compared with the liver, and on the other hand the resistance of the brain presumably due to vascular homeostatic mechanisms during hypovolaemia and endotoxic shock. The liver resists pure short term hypoxia well provided that the circulation is maintained, whereas it is extremely sensitive to interference with its normal circulation.

It appears from the preliminary measurements of pH that while changes in extracellular potassium activity may be more obvious, it could be that these are a reflection of the increased hydrogen ion concentration intracellularly due to anaerobic respiration and the accumulation of lactate. If the cell can survive only as long as it can produce energy to drive the sodium pump and if this is oxygen dependant, as indeed it is in the central nervous system, then the ability to maintain cell membrane potentials will be limited by the store of energy rich phosphates. If however a cell can maintain its membrane potential and recharge its energy rich phosphate stores by anaerobic metabolism, some other mechanism must be postulated for the death of cells in hypoxic conditions. It seems reasonable to suppose that the accumulation of hydrogen ions can be tolerated only as long as they are removed either by an external sink, e.g. blood flow, or while they can be accommodated by a local intracellular buffering system (Kaasik et al 1970). It would seem that both in the brain and in the liver that the disruption of normal cellular activity may be forecast by a knowledge of the pH changes. The figure of pH 6.6 to 6.7 would appear to be critical for most cells. Exceptions to this may be the dormant fibroblast, the macrophage and the voluntary muscle cell.

The non-homogeneous nature of the changes that occur during haemorrhagic shock both in the brain and in the liver are of some interest. If the hypoxic areas represent regions either where there have been micro-emboli or vascular spasm, there is the possibility that they may act as loci from which metabolites of hypoxia spread out and damage neighbouring cells. In the brain it may seem surprising that damage to small regions by micro-thrombi or some other cause, does not always lead to a spreading depression type of effect (Leao 1947) since damage to cortical cells normally releases potassium which may result in a wave of depolarization spreading across the cortex (Vyskocil et al 1972; Lehmenkühler et al 1975). It is possible that such small waves do arise but it also seems likely that where the development of cerebral ischaemia is slow the potassium concentrations may never rise rapidly enough during cell death to trigger off the characteristic wave of spreading depression.

A problem which still has to be examined very carefully is that of how the extracellular potassium concentrations, and indeed concentrations of sodium and chloride, change during the predepolarization phase. It seems likely that these changes are caused by shifts of water from the extracellular to the intra-cellular space and this could be tested by measuring the DC or AC impedance across the brain at different points in different stages of hypoxia. Although this has been done in the past, no regular study has been under pathological conditions, and there is still considerable argument between morphologists (Van Harreveld 1971) as to the size of the extracellular space in the cortex. The size of this space is of considerable relevance when one is considering the importance or otherwise of the ionic shifts that have been described.

REFERENCES

Bito, L.Z. and Myers, R.E. (1972) J. Physiol. 221, 349.

Chance, B., Cohen, P., Jöbsis, F. and Schoener, B. (1962) Science, 137, 499.

Dora, E. and Zeuthen, T. (1975) In 'Ion Selective and Enzyme Electrodes' Eds. Kessler, M. et al. Urban and Schwarzenberg, Munich.

Hinke, J.A.M. (1959) Nature (London), 184, 1257.

Höper, J., Kessler, M. and Simon, W. (1975) In 'Ion Selective and Enzyme Electrodes' Eds. Kessler, M. et al. Urban and Schwarzenberg, Munich.

Kaasik, A.E., Nilsson, L. and Siesjo, B.K. (1970) Acta Physiol. Scand. 78, 433.

Kessler, M., Gornaudt, L., Thermann, M., Lang, H., Brand, K. and Wessel, W. (1973) In 'Oxygen Supply' Eds. Kessler, M. et al. Urban and Schwarzenberg, Munich.

Kessler, M., Höper, J., Starlinger, H. and Krumme, B. (1975) In 'Ion Selective and Enzyme Electrodes" Eds. Kessler, M. et al. Urban and Schwarzenberg, Munich.

Leao, A.A.P. (1947) J. Neurophysiol. 10, 409.

Lehmenkühler, A., Speckmann, E-J. and Caspers, H. (1975) In 'Ion Selective and Enzyme Electrodes' Eds. Kessler, M. et al. Urban and Schwarzenberg, Munich.

Mela, L., Goodwin, C.W. and Miller, L.D. (1975) In 'Ion Selective and Enzyme Electrodes' Eds. Kessler, M. et al. Urban and Schwarzenberg, Munich.

Silver, I.A. (1965) Med. Electron. Biol. Engn. 3, 377.

Silver, I.A. (1973) In 'The Biology of the Fibroblast' Eds. Kulonen, K. and Pikkarainen, J. Academic Press, London.

Silver, I.A. (1975) In 'Ion Selective and Enzyme Electrodes' Eds. Kessler, M. et al. Urban and Schwarzenberg, Munich.

Sinagowitz, E., Rahmer, H., Rink, R., Görnandt, L. and Kessler, M. (1973) Advances in Exp. Med. Biol. 37A, 505.

Thomas, R.C. (1970) J. Physiol. Lond. 210, 82P.

Van Harreveld, A. (1971) In 'The Structure and Function of Nervous Tissue' Vol. IV, 447. Academic Press, London.

Vyskocil, F., Kriz, N. and Bures, J. (1972) Brain. Res. 39, 255.

Zeuthen, T., Hiam, R.C. and Silver, I.A. (1974) In 'Ion Selective Microelectrodes' Eds. Berman, H. and Hebert, N. Plenum Press, N.Y.

CEREBRAL OXYGENATION IN ARTERIAL HYPOXIA

Bo K. Siesjö, Lars Borgström, Halldór Jóhannsson, Bengt Nilsson, Karin Norberg and Björn Quistorff

Brain Research Laboratory, E-Blocket, University of Lund, Lund, Sweden.

Pronounced increases in CBF occur in arterial hypoxia (see, for example Kety and Schmidt 1948, Cohen et al. 1967). The mechanisms of this hyperemia have never been clarified but it has been postulated that a decreased extracellular pH is responsible. The following evidence has been quoted in favour of this hypothesis. First, pronounced increases in CBF are observed in hypercapnia and hypoxia, conditions that are associated with cerebral acidosis. Second, in hypoxic hypoxia CBF increases when arterial P_{O_2} is reduced below about 50 mm Hg (Courtice 1941, McDowall 1966, Kogure et al. 1970) and, at this degree of hypoxia, there is also accumulation of lactic acid in the tissue (Gurdjian et al. 1944, Siesjö and Nilsson 1971). Third, it has been reported that induced hypoglycemia, by limiting the supply of glucose for cerebral glycolysis, prevents the increase in CBF which otherwise occurs in hypoxia (Kogure et al. 1970).

The evidence cited is far from conclusive and recent results, which will be briefly summarized, indicate that other factors than the cerebral extracellular pH is responsible for the CBF increase in hypoxia. Most of these results have been reported from our laboratory, and for original data and further discussion, the reader is referred to the articles quoted.

General methodology.

The experiments were carried out in rats that were exposed to hypoxic hypoxia (reduction of Pa_{O_2} to minimal values of 20 mm Hg) or to isovolemic, anemic hypoxia (reduction of hemoglobin content to minimally 3 g per 100 ml). Hypoglycemia was induced by administration of insulin (2-4 I.U. per kg of body weight) 2-3 hrs prior to induction of hypoxia. Animals anaesthetized with 70% N_2O were used for studies of anemic hypoxia and of hypoxic hypoxia of 45 sec duration, or longer. Hypoxic hypoxia of short duration (10 or 20 sec) was studied in unanaesthetized animals. Cerebral energy metabolism was evaluated from the cortical tissue contents of glycolytic and citric acid cycle intermediates, and of organic phosphates, after freezing the tissue in situ. Both the freezing technique (Pontén et al. 1973) and the analytical techniques (Folbergrová et al. 1974, Norberg and Siesjö 1975 a and b) have been described previously. For freezing the tissue in unanaesthetized animals the tissue was "freeze-clampled" according to Quistorff (see Norberg et al. 1975). Cerebral (cortical) blood flow (CBF) was measured according to Kety and Schmidt (1948), using the ^{133}Xenon desaturation technique previously described from the laboratory (Norberg and Siesjö 1974). Cerebral metabolic rate for oxygen (CMR_{O_2}) was calculated from the CBF and the arteriovenous difference in oxygen content (AVD_{O_2}). For non-steady state situations, changes in CBF were derived from AVD_{O_2}, or from continuous measurements of venous outflow from the cannulated retroglenoid veins (see Nilsson 1974). In some experiments the regional CBF was estimated using the technique of Landau et al. (1955, see also Reivich et al. 1969) as adopted to ^{14}C-ethanol and a 30 sec infusion period (Eklöf et al. 1974).

Results and discussion.

1. Anemic hypoxia. Results obtained with anemic hypoxia can be summarized as follows (see Jóhannsson and Siesjö 1974, 1975, Borgström et al. 1975). When the hemoglobin content was reduced from 15 to 12 and 9 g $\cdot$ (100 ml)$^{-1}$, CBF increased significantly. At 6 and 3 g $\cdot$ (100 ml)$^{-1}$, CBF increased to about 250 and 500 per cent of normal, respectively. CMR_{O_2}, cerebral venous P_{O_2} and cerebral venous saturation remained unchanged. At a hemoglobin content of 3 g $\cdot$ (100 ml)$^{-1}$, there was a small increase in the lactate content of the tissue but no other metabolic changes, suggestive of tissue hypoxia.

There has been some discussion whether or not the reduced viscosity in anemic hypoxia contributes to the increase in CBF (Häggendal and Norbäck 1966, Paulson et al. 1973). The results quoted here demonstrate that the increase in CBF occurring in moderate anemia must, at least partly, be due to reduced viscosity. However, when the hemoglobin content is reduced to 6 g $\cdot$ (100 ml)$^{-1}$, or lower, the increase in CBF is far in excess of what could be due to viscosity changes. By itself, this finding suggests that tissue hypoxia contribute. However, since venous

P_{O_2} and oxygen saturation are upheld, and since metabolic changes in the tissue are discrete, it is questionable if true tissue hypoxia is present. Thus, the mechanisms eliciting an increased CBF in anemic hypoxia remain undefined.

2. Hypoxic hypoxia. Results on hypoxic hypoxia have been described (Jóhannsson and Siesjö 1974, 1975, Borgström et al. 1975, Norberg and Siesjö 1975 a and b, Nilsson et al. 1975) and can be summarized as follows.

When the Pa_{O_2} was reduced in steps from 140 to 50 mm Hg there was a small, gradual increase in CBF. With further reduction in Pa_{O_2}, i.e. to values below 50 mm Hg, there was a steep increase in CBF which, at Pa_{O_2} values of 20-25 mm Hg, reached values of about 500 per cent of normal. At all Pa_{O_2} values studied, CMR_{O_2} remained constant. It has previously been shown that the energy state of the brain, as this can be evaluated from the tissue concentrations of ATP, ADP and AMP, remains essentially unaltered at even very low arterial P_{O_2} values (see e.g. Bachelard et al. 1974). It has recently been postulated that hypoxia is accompanied by a reduction in cerebral energy requirements, and that this may contribute to prevent energy failure (Duffy et al. 1972). However, since CMR_{O_2} remains constant the increase in CBF seems to provide the sole mechanism preventing a disruption of cerebral energy state.

In steady state hypoxia there is a rough correlation between the increase in CBF, and the severity of lactic acidosis in the tissue (see above). However, such a correlation does not exist in non-steady state hypoxia. Thus, when the Pa_{O_2} is abruptly reduced to about 25 mm Hg the maximal CBF response is obtained within 2 min (Borgströme et al. 1975) although very little lactic acid accumulates during this period (Norberg and Siesjö 1975 a). In fact, since the Pa_{CO_2} rapidly falls following induction of hypoxia, it can be calculated that no net acidosis develops in the first 2 min. Thus, there is a precipitous increase in CBF in spite of the fact that a transient alkalosis seems to develop (see Siesjö et al. 1975). Additional results were obtained in unanaesthetized animals exposed to about 6% O_2 (Norberg et al. 1975). There was no increase in the lactate concentration at 10 sec, a small accumulation at 20 sec and an increase by about 1.5 $\mu mol \cdot g^{-1}$ at 60 sec. However, since Pa_{CO_2} fell by almost 10 mm Hg, no net acidosis could have developed. In order to study the increase in CBF under similar conditions, rapid hypoxia was induced by switching between two respirators and CBF was estimated by measuring the venous outflow from the brain (Nilsson et al. 1975). The results showed that CBF increased at 10 sec and reached a maximal value at 30-40 sec.

The results quoted make it doubtful if the increase in CBF during hypoxia is at all related to extracellular acidosis. A similar conclusion has been reached by Ponte and Purves (1974) who conclude that the hyperemia is elicited reflexly from carotid body chemoreceptors.

3. Hypoxic hypoxia in hypoglycemic animals. Since the results reported by Kogure et al. (1970) seemed to provide a compelling argument for a coupling between lactic acidosis and increase in flow, these experiments were repeated. Six animals were made hypoglycemic by means of insulin. At the time of induction of hypoxia the blood glucose concentrations varied between 2.03 and 2.47 $\mu mol \cdot g^{-1}$, and all had a slow wave pattern in the EEG. The arterial P_{O_2} was then decreased to about 25 mm Hg at constant ventilation and arteriovenous differences in oxygen content were determined at 2 and 5 min. Since AVD_{O_2} was determined also before hypoxia was induced, the change in CBF could be derived from the AVD_{O_2}, assuming constant CMR_{O_2}.

The results are shown in the table. At 2 and 5 min, the blood pressure was similar to that recorded in the prehypoxic period and, since the mean Pa_{CO_2} had decreased by 3 and 5 mm Hg, respectively, neither increase in blood pressure nor hypercapnia could have contributed to the increase in CBF (to 490 and 333 per cent of normal, respectively).

In the experiments quoted, the induction of hypoxia caused a further, rapid fall in blood glucose concentration and several animals developed an isoelectric EEG during prolongation of the hypoxia. Thus, there can be no doubt that the animals were profoundly hypoglycemic (see Lewis et al. 1974). In order to verify that CBF increased, i.e. that the assumption of a constant CMR_{O_2} was valid, hypoxia was induced in three additional, hypoglycemic animals, and regional CBF was estimated from the uptake of ^{14}C-ethanol. At 2 min of hypoxia these showed increases in CBF to about 300 per cent of normal. Since the ^{14}C-ethanol method tends to underestimate CBF at high flow values (see Eklöf et al. 1974) the results are in close agreement with those obtained with the AVD_{O_2} method.

In conclusion, the results obtained do not support the hypothesis of a coupling of lactic acidosis and increase in CBF during hypoxia. It must be concluded that other mechanisms than acidosis are responsible for the homeostatic increase in CBF. These mechanisms may well involve a neurogenic control of the cerebral resistance vessels.

TABLE. Influence of insulin-induced hypoglycemia upon CBF response to hypoxia.

Exp. group	MABP mm Hg	Pa_{O_2} mm Hg	$[T_{O_2}]_a$ ml · (100 ml)$^{-1}$	$[AVD]_{O_2}$ ml · (100 ml)$^{-1}$	CBF %
Control (normoxia)	150 ±5	104 ±6	23.70 ±0.21	9.44 ±0.72	100
Hypoxia 2 min	150 ±2	25.6 ±0.9	7.49 ±0.33	2.14 ±0.27	487 ±83
Hypoxia 5 min	150 ±3	25.0 ±1.1	7.80 ±0.50	3.25 ±0.56	329 ±52

Prior to induction of hypoxia the blood glucose contents were 2.03-2.49 $\mu mol \cdot g^{-1}$. The table includes data for mean arterial blood pressure (MABP), arterial oxygen content ($[T_{O_2}]_a$), arteriovenous difference in oxygen content (AVD_{O_2}), and changes in CBF calculated on the assumption of constant CMR_{O_2}. Means ± S.E.M. n = 6 in all groups.

Acknowledgements. Mrs Lena Barnekow provided excellent technical assistance. The projects were supported by funds from the Swedish Medical Research Council (Projects No. 14X-263 and 14X-2179), from the Swedish Tercentenary Fund, and from U.S. PHS Grant No. R01 NSO 7838-05 from NIH.

References.

1. Bachelard, H.S., L.D. Lewis, U. Pontén and B.K. Siesjö, Mechanisms activating glycolysis in the brain in arterial hypoxia. J. Neurochem. 1974. 22. 395-401.

2. Borgström, L., H. Jóhannsson and B.K. Siesjö, The influence of acute normovolemic anemia on cerebral blood flow and oxygen consumption of anaesthetized rats. Acta physiol. scand. 1975. In press.

3. Borgström, L., H. Jóhannsson and B.K. Siesjö, The relationship between arterial P_{O_2} and cerebral blood flow in hypoxic hypoxia. Acta physiol. scand. 1975. In press.

4. Cohen, P.J., S.C. Alexander, T.C. Smith, M. Reivich and H. Wollman, Effects of hypoxia and normocarbia on cerebral blood flow and metabolism in conscious man. J. appl. Physiol. 1967. 23. 183-189.

5. Courtice, F.C., The effect of oxygen lack on the cerebral circulation. J. Physiol. 1941. 100. 198-211.

6. Duffy, T.E., S.R. Nelson and O.H. Lowry, Cerebral carbohydrate metabolism during acute hypoxia and recovery. J. Neurochem. 1972. 19. 959-977.

7. Eklöf, B., N.A. Lassen, L. Nilsson, K. Norberg, B.K. Siesjö and P. Torlöf, Regional cerebral blood flow in the rat measured by the tissue sampling technique; a criticial evaluation using four indicators C^{14}-antipyrine, C^{14}-ethanol, H^3-water and $Xenon^{133}$. Acta physiol. scand. 1974. 91. 1-10.

8. Folbergrová, J., B. Ljunggren, K. Norberg and B.K. Siesjö, Influence of complete ischemia on glycolytic metabolites, citric acid cycle intermediates, and associated amino acids in the rat cerebral cortex. Brain Res. 1974. 80. 265-279.

9. Gurdjian, E.S., W.E. Stone and J. E. Webster, Cerebral metabolism in hypoxia. Arch. Neurol. Psychiat. 1944. 51. 472-477.

10. Häggendal, E. and B. Norbäck, Effect of blood viscosity on cerebral blood flow. Acta chir. scand. 1966. Suppl. 364. 13-22.

11. Jóhannsson, H. and B.K. Siesjö, Blood flow and oxygen consumption in the rat brain in dilutional anemia. Acta physiol. scand. 1974. 91. 136-138.

12. Jóhannsson, H. and B.K. Siesjö, Cerebral blood flow and oxygen consumption in the rat in hypoxic hypoxia. Acta physiol. scand. 1975. In press.

13. Kety, S.S. and C.F. Schmidt, The effects of altered arterial tensions of carbon dioxide and oxygen on cerebral oxygen consumption of normal young men. J. clin. Invest. 1948. 27. 484-492.

14. Kogure, K., P. Scheinberg, O.M. Reinmuth, M. Fujishima and R. Busto, Mechanisms of cerebral vasodilatation in hypoxia. J. appl. Physiol. 1970. 29. 223-229.

15. Landau, W.M., W.H. Freygang, Jr., L.P. Rowland, L. Sokoloff and S.S. Kety, The local circulation of the living brain; values in unanesthetized and anesthetized cat. Trans. Amer. neurol. Ass. 1955. 80. 125-129.

16. Lewis, L.D., B. Ljunggren, R.A. Ratcheson and B.K. Siesjö, Cerebral energy state in insulin-induced hypoglycemia, related to blood glucose and to EEG. J. Neurochem. 1974. 23. 673-679.

17. McDowall, D.G., Interrelationships between blood oxygen tension and cerebral blood flow. In: Oxygen Measurements in Blood and Tissues, ed. J.P. Payne and D.W. Hill. pp. 205-214. Churchill, London 1966.

18. Nilsson, B., Measurement of overall blood flow and oxygen consumption in the rat brain. Acta physiol. scand. 1974. 92. 142-144.

19. Nilsson, B., K. Norberg, C.-H. Nordström and B.K. Siesjö, Influence of hypercapnia and hypoxia on CBF in rats. 7th Intern. Symp. on Cerebral Circulation and Metabolism, Aviemore, Scotland. Submitted for publication.

20. Norberg, K. and B.K. Siesjö, Quantitative measurement of blood flow and oxygen consumption in the rat brain. Acta physiol. scand. 1974. 91. 154-164.

21. Norberg, K. and B.K. Siesjö, Cerebral metabolism in hypoxic hypoxia. I. Pattern of activation of glycolysis; a re-evaluation. Brain Res. 1975. In press.

22. Norberg, K. and B.K. Siesjö, Cerebral metabolism in hypoxic hypoxia. II. Citric acid cycle intermediates and associated amino acids. Brain Res. 1975. In press.

23. Norberg, K., B. Quistorff and B.K. Siesjö, Effects of short-term hypoxia on energy metabolism in the cerebral cortex of unanaesthetized and anaesthetized rats. Brain Res. Submitted for publication.

24. Paulson, O.B., H.H. Parving, J. Olesen and E. Skinhøj, Influence of carbon monoxide and of hemodilution on cerebral blood flow and blood gases in man. J. appl. Physiol. 1973. 35. No. 1. 111-116.

25. Ponte, J. and M.J. Purves, The role of the carotid body chemoreceptors and carotid sinus baroreceptors in the control of cerebral blood vessels. J. Physiol. (Lond.) 1974. 237. 315-340.

26. Pontén, U., R.A. Ratcheson, L.G. Salford and B.K. Siesjö, Optimal freezing conditions for cerebral metabolism in rats. J. Neurochem. 1973. 21. 1127-1138.

27. Reivich, M., J. Jehle, L. Sokoloff and S.S. Kety, Measurements of regional cerebral blood flow with antipyrine ^{14}C in awake cats. J. appl. Physiol. 1969. 27. 296-300.

28. Siesjö, B.K. and L. Nilsson, The influence of arterial hypoxemia upon labile phosphates and upon extracellular and intracellular lactate and pyruvate concentration in the rat brain. Scand. J. Clin. Lab. Invest. 1971. 27. 83-96.

THEORETICAL AND EXPERIMENTAL ASPECTS OF BRAIN TISSUE OXYGENATION DYNAMICS

William J. Dorson, Jr. and Beuford A. Bogue

Department of Chemical and Bio Engineering, Arizona State University, Tempe, Arizona 85281, U.S.A. and Department of Chemical Engineering, University of Virginia, Charlottesville, Virginia, U.S.A.

This investigation concerns the brain tissue response to variations in carotid artery pO_2. A theoretical model was developed and several experimental methods employed to produce dynamic arterial pO_2 changes in intubated cats, outlined as follows:

Method	Experiments
Changes in Inspired O_2	Hyperoxic Step Changes (air → 95% O_2-5% CO_2) Hypoxic Step Changes (air → N_2, or O_2-CO_2 mixtures → N_2) Oscillating Changes $\leq$ 0.1 Hz (air → N_2, or O_2-CO_2 mixtures → N_2)
Blood Exchange System	Hypoxic Changes Oscillating Changes $\leq$ 1.0 Hz Pseudo-Random Noise Changes

All animals were anesthetized and placed on respirator control. The blood exchange system involved cannulation of both common carotid arteries and jugular veins. A computer controlled pump exchanged equal amounts of venous and arterial blood in an otherwise open flow assembly (3,4). All other vessels leading to the brain and peripheral regions were clamped.

Continuous measurements were made (and recorded) of carotid artery pO_2*, cerebral cortex tissue pO_2* (normally intracellular),

---

* Model 721 Oxygen Microelectrode, Transidyne General Corporation, Ann Arbor, Michigan, U.S.A.

and venous pO_2*, total common carotid artery blood flow rate (E.M. in-line probe), arterial blood pressure, temperature, EKG, EEG, and cellular action potentials using the tissue pO_2 electrode and a modification** of the technique of Kunke, et.al. (8). Serial arterial and venous blood samples were withdrawn for Hb, Hct, pO_2, pH, and oxygen saturation. In addition to determining total brain O_2 reaction rate and base excess, the serial samples were also used to provide an in-vivo calibration check of venous and arterial pO_2 electrodes.

The cats were heparinized and anesthetized (sodium pentobarbital) throughout the experiments. Exposed brain tissue was covered with heated paraffin oil to prevent O_2 diffusion from the surrounding atmosphere. The tissue electrode was mounted into a microdrive capable of continuous and repeatable increments of 2.5 micron step insertions into the cerebral cortex. This probe was generally moved in a linear direction until both measurable pO_2 and action potentials were simultaneously observed. Both the total cat weight and excised brain weight were determined (2.7 to 6.7 Kg and 22.0 to 31.5 gm ranges respectively). Attempts were made to study each response with different arterial pCO_2 levels as obtained by respirator control.

A theoretical model was developed in accord with known geometric and transfer properties of brain tissue (4,6). The mathematical representation of the brain (see Figure 7, ref. 6) contains three capillary compartments (V_2, V_3, V_4), two interstitial fluid regions (V_6, V_7), two intracellular components (V_8, V_9), a mixing region between the arterial measurement site and capillary entrance (V_1) along with a pure delay time, Δt_1, and a mixing region between the capillary exit and venous measurement site (V_5) along with a pure delay time Δt_2. Numerical solution techniques allowed variations in the flow rate, delay times, and cellular metabolism. With experimental data input, this model was used to calculate the following linearized passive transfer coefficients:

$$K_1' = K_1A_{26} = K_1A_{47} = 2K_1A_{36} = 2K_1A_{37}$$

and

$$K_2' = K_2A_{68} = K_2A_{79}$$

Cellular metabolism in the brain is a complex entity, and several simplified approaches were investigated in this study (M_8 and

* Model 721 Oxygen Microelectrode, Transidyne General Corporation, Ann Arbor, Michigan, U.S.A.

** Model MPA-8 Differential Millivolt Headstate, Transidyne General Corporation, Ann Arbor, Michigan, U.S.A.

M_9 in Figure 7, ref. 6) including: constant (but different) metabolic rates, cellular metabolism proportional to action potential frequency, calculated metabolism from A-V pO_2 measurements ($\Delta t_1 = \Delta t_2 = 0$), and an elementary kinetic theory. The latter kinetic theory was developed by restricting the 22 metabolic steps listed by Chance (5) to the rate limiting (slowest) reactions given below (4).

$$\text{GLUCOSE} \xrightarrow{k_1} 2\ \text{PYRUVATE} \tag{1}$$

$$\text{PYRUVATE} + \text{DPH} \underset{k_3}{\overset{k_2}{\rightleftarrows}} \text{LACTATE} + \text{DPN} \tag{2}$$

$$\text{PYRUVATE} + 4\ \text{DIN} \xrightarrow{k_4} \text{DIH} \tag{3}$$

$$4\ \text{DIH} + 3O_2 \xrightarrow{k_5} 4\ \text{DIN} + 3CO_2 + 3\ H_2O \tag{4}$$

This metabolic scheme is in a primative unbalanced form with the correct stoichiometry accounted for in the calculation of reaction rates and rate constants. The multitude of intermediate species are assumed to be in equilibrium with products and reactants in Equations 1 through 4.

The experimental values for glucose and oxygen consumption and lactate and pyruvate production from Sacks (10) and Gottstein (7) were tested with Equations 1 through 4 and the latter rates chosen for subsequent calculations. The concentrations of DPH and DPN were assumed constant, glucose, lactate and pyruvate normal concentrations taken from Tower (11), and loss of lactate and pyruvate to capillary blood assumed to be proportional to their tissue concentrations. The kinetics were initially assumed to be elementary in the remaining time varying species and the kinetic rate constants derived from the referenced steady-state rates and concentrations along with the lactate conversion rate from Chance (5). This latter kinetic rate was needed to independently solve for the kinetic rate constants since transport of lactate and pyruvate between the cells and capillary blood was incorporated into the calculations. Over the brief time periods for a specific dynamic experiment it was normally assumed that tissue glucose levels remained at the pre-test values.

RESULTS

Due to the extensive surgical procedures and complex instrumentation the physiological condition of the cat was highly variable at the beginning of each test series. Also, as a given experiment continued, the animal's condition would deteriorate. This was especially true following a severe anoxic period. Tests involving extended hypoxemia were generally postponed during the better preparations. However, a method was developed to correlate dynamic tissue responses with the varying physiological states.

Vital signs and action potentials were monitored during these experiments, but the single correlating factor in determining the dynamic response was an estimate of the net cellular O_2 consumption, M_C. Serial blood samples along with the measured blood flow rate and excised brain weight were converted to a normalized brain O_2 reaction rate. Extra free acids built up as the animal's condition deteriorated (measured as negative base excess based on pH and pCO_2). On the assumption that this was primarily due to lactic acid and that all compartments were in equilibrium with this increased level, the metabolic equations were solved for changes in the O_2 reaction rate as a function of lactic acid concentration. The results are shown on Figure 1. The total brain O_2 reaction rate was corrected

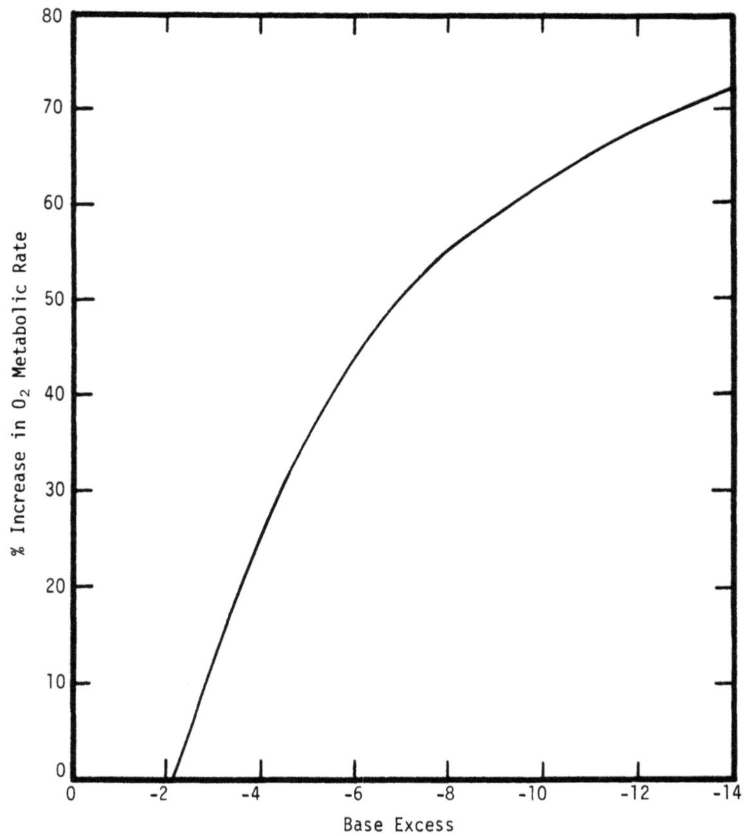

Figure 1. Calculated Increase in the O_2 Consumption Rate due to Lactic Acid.

using this graph to establish a net cellular O_2 consumption, M_C, associated with the glucose reaction in brain tissue. Thus, four definitions of the animal's physiological state evolved as a function of M_C.

Animal Condition	M_C(ml O_2/100 gm Brain Weight/min)
Good (G)	$\geq$ 6.0
Depressed Signs (DS)	4.0 - 5.9
Reversible Pathological Condition (RPC)	2.0 - 3.9
Irreversible Pathological Condition (IPC)	$\leq$ 1.9

Observed and derived responses were highly correlated with the above four categories of oxygen metabolism in 324 separate test periods accomplished with 76 different cats.

The comparative characteristics of the dynamic response to changing arterial pO_2 for a cat in good condition are summarized as:

1. high pre-test carotid flow rate exceeding 100 ml/min-100 gms brain weight (normally $\sim$ 150 ml/min-100 gms but dependent on pCO_2).
2. rapid adjustment of carotid blood flow rate to changing arterial pO_2, usually in less than 10 to 20 sec.
3. well oxygenated brain tissue before each test with cellular pO_2 values variable but between 23 and 71 mm Hg in the majority of animals.
4. rapid autoregulation of tissue pO_2 in response to arterial pO_2 changes, minimizing the deviation from pre-test conditions.
5. low pre-test ratios of arterial blood pressure to arterial flow (2-4 mm Hg/ml/min).
6. little or no blood pressure variation during rapid arterial flow response to changing arterial pO_2.
7. very high calculated compartmental transfer coefficients, K_1' and K_2', of 50 to 70 ml/sec before and during a hypoxic test period with a moderate increase within this range during induced anoxia.

In contrast to the physiologic behavior of cats in good condition, even the defined depressed state resulted in a decrease of the transfer coefficients (K_1' and K_2') calculated from the experimental data to between 12 and 15 ml/sec prior to the test period and between 15 and 23 during induced anoxia. This decrease in the calculated transfer coefficients continued, following the defined animal's condition, to 1 ml/sec for the IPC. Also, larger arterial pressure responses and directly associated blood flow rate changes along with greater variations in tissue pO_2 were observed during arterial pO_2 anoxia tests in the DS and RPC. Neither blood pressure nor blood flow rate would respond significantly to arterial pO_2

changes in the IPC resulting in large tissue pO_2 variations.

Since the blood exchange system resulted not only in varying arterial pO_2 but also pCO_2 and metabolites, inspired oxygen changes were used to compare dynamic responses between the two methods. No significant differences were observed for either hypoxic step changes or oscillating arterial pO_2 tests up to the 0.1 Hz inspired O_2 variation limit. Observed responses to both test methods were correlated by the animal's condition (G to IPC).

Specific test results follow to illustrate these, as well as other, conclusions. Test indexing contains first a two digit cat number followed by the magnetic tape location (3 to 4 digits). Hyperoxic respirator step changes (air to 95% O_2-5%CO_2) of 60 sec duration doubled carotid artery pO_2 (70 to 140 mm Hg) with a cat in good condition, but the tissue pO_2 only rose from 29 to 32 mm Hg with no significant blood pressure or flow change (arterial pCO_2 $\sim$ 25 mm Hg). Large blood pressure and flow changes were only observed in the IPC with a pCO_2 of 70 mm Hg. Percent changes in tissue pO_2 increased as the animal's condition deteriorated.

A variety of responses were observed during hypoxic step changes, but the salient features are shown first with a cat in good condition on Figure 2 followed by a cat in depressed condition on Figure 3.

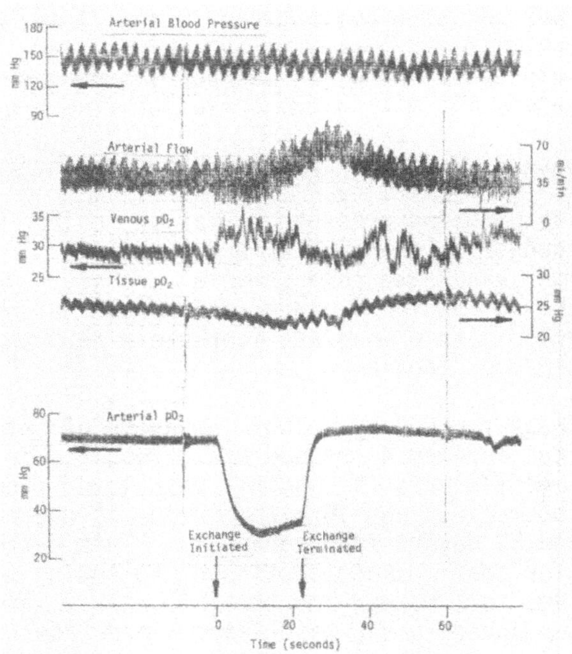

Figure 2. Observed Response to Control Induced Hypoxic Step Change (pCO_2 $\sim$ 25 mm Hg, Test 51-1548, Good Condition)

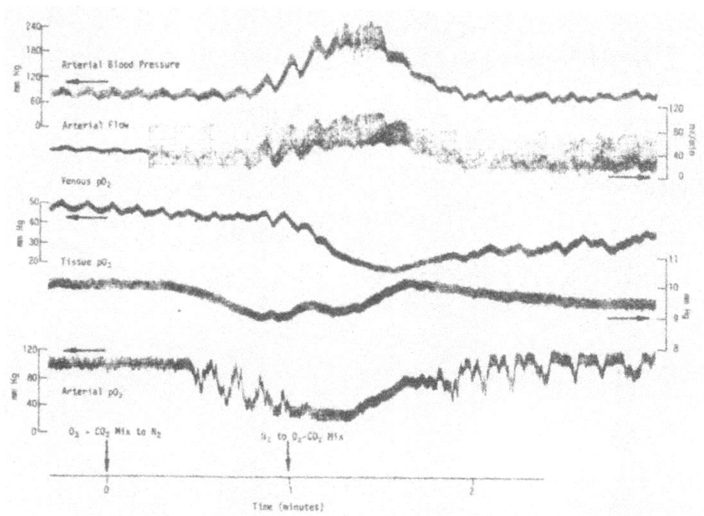

Figure 3. Observed Response to Respirator Induced Hypoxic Step Change ($pCO_2 \sim 70$ mm Hg, Test 69-1386, DS)

In all experiments elevated arterial pCO_2 resulted in increased arterial flow rate with no observed differences in tissue behavior within the scope of these tests. However, the relative number of test periods with cats in good condition was small (36/324) and this similarity between pCO_2 and flow behavior may only apply to deteriorated physiological conditions.

Tissue pO_2 autoregulation is again demonstrated by the response to oscillating arterial pO_2. The behavior of a cat in good condition is shown on Figure 4. In contrast, limited local stasis is shown on Figure 5 with a cat in RPC. Note that the induced oscillations dominate over a natural tissue instability during the test duration. These natural tissue oscillations could be temporarily eliminated by increasing the frequency of arterial pO_2 changes (0.08 Hz) and augmented with an induced frequency (≥ 0.1 Hz) the same as the natural tissue oscillation. Tissue pO_2 instabilities of two types were observed: 1. high frequency (≥ 0.1 Hz) oscillations corresponding to simultaneous flow and pressure variations, and 2. low frequency (<0.1 Hz) oscillations with no appreciable fluctuations in flow or blood pressure. Figure 5 is an example of the first type where oscillating tissue pO_2 values could exceed pre-test values. All natural tissue instabilities were associated with deteriorating animal conditions. For the better animal conditions within these categories the increase in oscillating tissue pO_2 shown on Figure 5 was simultaneously associated with a dynamic flow resistance decrease compared to pre-test values (ratio of blood pressure amplitude to arterial flow amplitude less than either

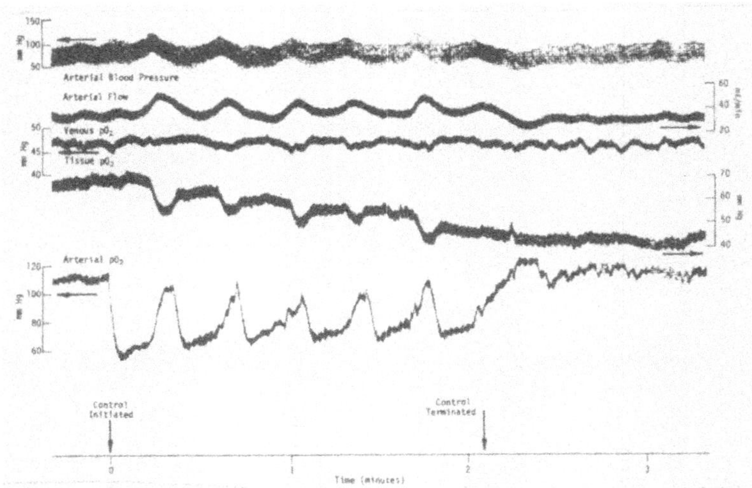

Figure 4. Observed Response to 0.05 Hz Control Induced Oscillations ($pCO_2 \sim 40$ mm Hg, Test 68-237, Good Condition)

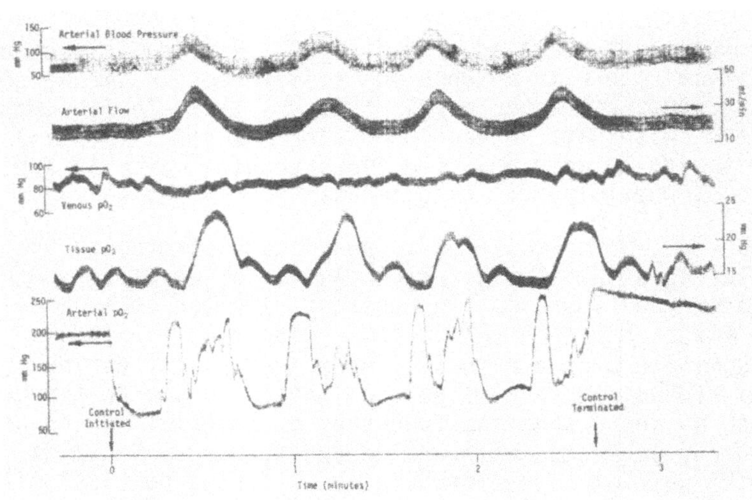

Figure 5. Observed Response to 0.025 Hz Control Induced Oscillations ($pCO_2 \sim 40$ mm Hg, Test 68-775, RPC)

the oscillating mean ratio or pre-test ratio). Conversely, a decrease in the oscillating tissue pO_2 values compared with pre-test levels was associated with both a more deteriorated animal condition and an increase in the pressure-flow amplitude compared to the pre-test ratio of pressure to flow.

Natural instabilities of the first type associated with blood pressure and flow oscillations could also be interrupted but not eliminated by short term anoxia. The lower frequency instabilities unrelated to blood pressure and flow could be induced or eliminated by changing the average level of arterial pO_2. Even when interrupted by induced arterial anoxic oscillations, they would return and sustain themselves. These were assumed to be metabolic in nature, and again, were not observed with animals in good condition.

The effect of transport coefficients on the predicted steady-state values of tissue pO_2 are shown on Figure 6 (parametric blood flow variation) and Figure 7 (parametric arterial pO_2 variation). Tissue pO_2 is shown to be highly sensitive to both arterial blood flow and pO_2 while little variation is observed with transfer coefficients exceeding 20 to 30 ml/sec. Tissue pO_2 is also highly sensitive to the level of cellular metabolism. Average values used to calculate these results are: brain weight = 25 gms, Hb = 12 gm%, Hct = 36 and pH = 7.25. The theoretical dynamic response was calculated with arterial and venous mixing volumes of 10 ml respectively (V_1 and V_5) in the form of Bode graphs. The response was sensitive to the level of arterial flow rate and to arterial pO_2. Changes in the transport coefficients above 15 ml/sec only affect the dynamic

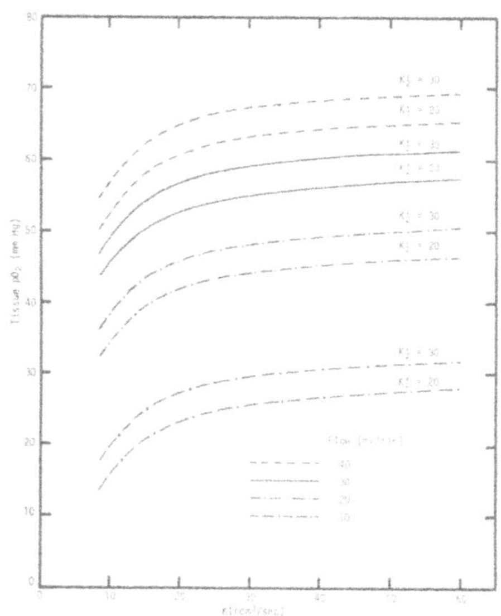

Figure 6. Predicted Steady State Tissue pO_2 (M_C = 3.4 ml O_2/100 gm/min, Arterial pO_2 = 70 mm Hg)

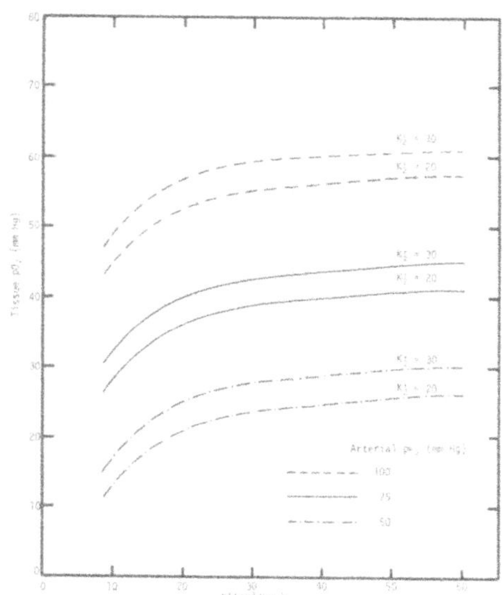

Figure 7. Predicted Steady State Tissue pO_2 (M_C = 3.4 ml O_2/100 gm/min, Flow Rate = 30 ml/min)

response slightly above 0.3 Hz while the level of metabolism primarily affects response below 0.08 Hz. This theoretical result would allow a separation of these two effects (metabolism versus transfer coefficients) during a single pseudo-random noise experiment.

The compartment model transfer coefficients were derived from experimental data in two ways. Steady-state data, such as pre-test values, could be used with the arbitrary assumption that $K_1' = K_2'$. During oscillating tests either the mean data values could be used in a similar manner or a sophisticated computer program utilized to derive independent values for K_1' and K_2' based on optimization techniques. The two calculation methods compared favorably, especially with deteriorating physiological conditions. For a cat in good condition the pre-test calculation yielded $K_1' = K_2' = 60$ ml/sec while the subsequent mean oscillating values resulted in $K_1' = K_2' = 70$ ml/sec and the optimum coefficients during the oscillations were $K_1' = 54.4$ and $K_2' = 75.1$ ml/sec (test 68-237). The magnitude of these coefficients would neither be highly accurate nor affect the dynamic response, but they emphasize an O_2 transport mechanism operating with maximum efficiency.

The theoretical model was evaluated in several ways. With a known arterial pO_2 time function, the theoretical cross-correlation could be calculated and compared to the same function obtained from the averaged experimental data (6). Good agreement demonstrated that the theoretical compartment model is adequate in describing the dynamic response of brain tissue to rapid changes in arterial pO_2. Theoretical predictions could also be compared directly with the time varying data. Using the observed arterial pO_2 as input to the model, the effects of three flow rate functions could be determined during the induced transients. The three functions were: constant flow rate equal to the pre-test value, a variable flow rate dependent on known steady-state responses to pO_2, pCO_2, and arterial pressure (4), and the measured total carotid flow rate during the test period. In all cases (step changes and oscillations) the use of the experimental flow rate resulted in a more stable predicted tissue pO_2 response closer to the data than either of the other two flow functions.

Using both the experimental arterial pO_2 and flow functions as input to the model, the effects of different cellular metabolic concepts could be determined. These results are shown on Figure 8 for a step change. The theoretical predictions with the kinetic theory developed herein were closest to the observed data for both step and oscillating arterial pO_2 variations. However, the theoretical model still does not contain all aspects of the complex autoregulation of tissue pO_2 when an animal is in good condition. Arbitrary changes in metabolite concentrations, reaction rate orders, and kinetic rate constants were parametrically investigated but failed to improve the comparison of theory with data.

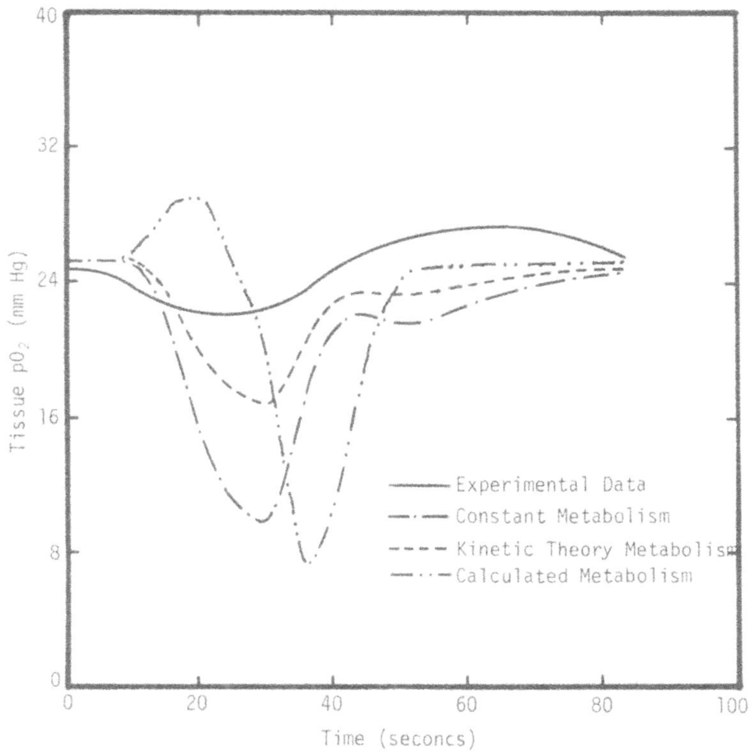

Figure 8. Predicted and Observed Tissue pO_2 with Different Metabolic Concepts ($pCO_2 \sim 25$ mm Hg, Test 51-1548, Good Condition)

In former studies of tissue response to step changes in respirator O_2 concentrations, significant depression of cellular pO_2 was followed by a large overshoot in pO_2 after the termination of induced hypoxia (1,2). This behavior was often observed in this study when the physiological condition had deteriorated. This overshoot had been attributed to a delayed flow rate response of $\sim$ 80 sec (9). With an animal in good condition the observed flow responses were invariably much faster than this estimate. Even in the distressed state the only flow delay times of this order were with simultaneous respirator pCO_2 variations (O_2-CO_2 mixture to N_2 and return to O_2-CO_2).

The brain is highly inhomogeneous whereas arterial and venous measurements correspond to total or integrated brain behavior. Improved experiments should incorporate continuous O_2 saturation as well as regional blood flow measurements. There was a direct relation of tissue pO_2 response with different flow-pressure behavior which should also be explored. Pseudo-random noise oscillations in arterial pO_2 were also accomplished and the results will be presented elsewhere.

These studies were supported by Arizona State University.

NOMENCLATURE (see references 4 and 6)

DIH Intramitochondrial reduced diphosphopyridine nucleotide
DIN Intramitochondrial diphosphopyridine nucleotide
DPH Extramitochondrial reduced diphosphopyridine nucleotide
DPN Extramitochondrial diphosphopyridine nucleotide
k_1-k_5 Kinetic reaction rate constants
K_1' Normalized capillary to extracellular fluid transfer rate
K_2' Normalized extracellular to intracellular transfer rate
M_c Corrected cellular O_2 metabolic rate

REFERENCES

1. Bicher, H.I. and M.H. Knisely, *J. Appl. Physiol.*, 28: 387-390, 1970.
2. Bicher, H.I., in *Oxygen Transport to Tissue: Instrumentation, Methods, and Physiology*, edited by H.I. Bicher and D.F. Bruley, New York: Plenum Press, Vol. 37A, p. 215-222, 1973.
3. Bogue, B.A. and W.J. Dorson, Jr., in *Oxygen Transport to Tissue: Pharmacology, Mathematical Studies, and Neonatology*, edited by D.F. Bruley and H.I. Bicher, New York: Plenum Press, Vol. 37B, p. 903-909, 1973.
4. Bogue, B.A., "Feline brain tissue pO_2 response to step and oscillating arterial pO_2 changes," Ph.D. thesis, Arizona State University, 1974.
5. Chance, B., D. Garfinkel, J. Higgins and B. Hess, *J. Biol. Chem.*, 235: 2426-2439, 1960.
6. Dorson, W.J. and B.A. Bogue, in *Oxygen Transport to Tissue: Instrumentation, Methods and Physiology*, edited by H.I. Bicher and D.F. Bruley, New York: Plenum Press, Vol. 37A, p. 251-259, 1973.
7. Gottstein, U., A. Bernsmeirer and J. Sedlmeyer, *Klin. Wschr.* 41: 943-948, 1963.
8. Kunke, S., W. Erdmann and H. Metzger, *J. Appl. Physiol.*, 32: 436-438, 1972.
9. Reneau, D.D. Jr., H.I. Bicher, D.F. Bruley and M.H. Knisely, in *Blood Oxygenation*, edited by D. Hershey, New York: Plenum Press, p. 175-200, 1970.
10. Sacks, W., in *Handbook of Neurochemistry*, edited by A. Lajtha, New York: Plenum Press, Vol. 1, p. 301-324, 1969.
11. Tower, D.B., in *Handbook of Physiology, Neurophysiology*, edited by W.F. Hamilton and P. Dow, Baltimore, Md.: Williams and Wilkins, Vol. 3, p. 1793-1813, 1960.

SUMMARY OF DISCUSSION - SESSION VI:

OXYGEN SUPPLY OF THE CENTRAL NERVOUS SYSTEM I

Chairmen: B. K. Siesjö and I. A. Silver

In connection with the communication of Kovách *et al.*, Jöbsis raised the question about the significance of small changes in NADH fluorescence and Lübbers wondered why fluorescence did not return to baseline after saline flushing. Kovách agreed that, in view of the difficulties of correcting for blood volume changes, small changes in fluorescence should be interpreted with caution. He said that baseline was usually, but not always, reached after flushing. Siesjö wondered if the changes in fluorescence and PO_2 were most marked in the classical boundary zones between the distribution territories of the major arteries but Kovách said that this was not always the case.

Discussions of the communication by Dorá *et al.* centered around the genesis of the oscillations, and the situations in which they occur. Siesjö remarked that blood pressure oscillations occur in animals anaesthetized with barbiturates, but not with nitrous oxide, and suggested that they reflected a cardiotoxic effect of the anaesthetic used. Dorá remarked, however, that oscillations also occur in cats anaesthetized with chloralose and had observed such oscillations in the absence of blood pressure changes. Mayevsky added that they could be observed in unanaesthetized animals exposed to 5% O_2. The discussion that followed did not shed light on the genesis of the oscillations.

Mayevsky's measurements of NADH fluorescence and ECoG following decapitation, stimulated a discussion of oxygen stores and of metabolic rate in the brain. Siesjö remarked that Kety had calculated that, for human brain, the oxygen stores would suffice for 6-7 sec. of oxidative metabolism but that any such calculation is critically dependent on the metabolic rate and on the volume of blood that can unload oxygen. In the rat, assuming a capillary volume of 0.5% of tissue volume, the oxygen content would suffice for only about 1 sec. Lübbers emphasized the difficulty of drawing conclusions from changes in NADH fluorescence since changes observed depend on blood volume and saturation of hemoglobin, and Bicher was sceptical about the validity of metabolic rates measured after decapitation. On the whole, though, the measurements of Mayevsky and Chance add valuable information on the rapidity of metabolic changes following sudden ischemia, that is complementary to results previously obtained with the "closed system" method of Lowry and collaborators (1964) and the clinical observations of Rossen et al (1943).

Following Grote's communication, it was remarked that changes in PCO_2 of perfusion fluid should not change tissue PCO_2 (see Pappenheimer et al 1965) and it was asked if the HCO_3^- concentration had been changed. This had not yet been done. It was also asked how white matter flow could be obtained. Grote was of the opinion that the position of the detector over the occipital lobe ensured that mainly white matter flow was obtained. The uncertainty of the actual flow measured undoubtedly makes it somewhat difficult to evaluate the quantitative significance of the CMR_{O_2} values. It was also asked if ventriculocisternal perfusion could be expected to change ECF composition in cortical areas and Grote agreed that long periods of perfusion were needed to achieve this. It was also questioned if perfusion pressure can be measured in edematous tissue without methods for measuring tissue pressure. Grote remarked that tissue pressure must be taken into account.

In connection with the communication by Silver, Beran agreed that there should be qualitative differences in tissue PO_2 of brain and liver in response to the noxious stimuli (there is such a difference between brain and kidney), but wondered if the differences were statistically significant. Silver remarked that they were. It was asked why ECF pH was so high. Siesjö mentioned that, in rats, CSF HCO_3^- is around 27 mmol/l and the pH therefore should exceed 7.4. He asked if changes in ECF $[K^+]$ or $[H^+]$ were seen with inhalation of 5% O_2. Silver replied that any such changes were very small. The results of Silver thus support the hypothesis that changes in $[H^+]$ or $[K^+]$ are not responsible for the vasodilatation observed in hypoxia.

The paper given by Siesjö stimulated an intense discussion of the mechanisms of CBF increase in hypoxia. It was remarked from the floor that so many previous results had demonstrated a coupling between acidosis and hyperemia. Siesjö remarked that there were several other situations in which no coupling is apparent (barbiturate anaesthesia, hypoglycemia, amphetamine administration) and stressed the results obtained by Ponte and Purves (1974) on the reflex control of CBF in hypoxia. Nemoto wondered if changes in ATP, ADP or AMP were sufficiently sensitive to disclose disturbances in cerebral function and suggested that EEG might be better, and Dorá wondered about NAD reduction. Siesjö remarked that changes in EEG and NADH/NAD^+ ratios occur at PO_2 values that are not associated with changes in organic phosphates. The latter are useful in revealing a degree of hypoxia that threatens to damage neurons. Siesjö also remarked that some functional changes may reflect a disturbed transmitter metabolism rather than overt energy failure. Bicher pointed out that when studying mechanisms of increase in flow, rapid methods must be used. Siesjö answered that this had been done by measurements of outflow from the retroglenoid veins (Nilsson et al 1975). The results showed that with rapid induction of hypoxia CBF increased after only 10 sec.

Following Dorson's paper, Nemoto remarked that no mathematical model had yet taken into account that the intercapillary distances can change by recruitment. Dorson remarked that he had plans for doing that now, when hemodynamic data were available.

The last communication in the session, read by Leniger-Follert, stimulated discussion on a possible local control of oxygen tension. Two possible mechanisms were discussed: increase in blood flow and variation in metabolic rate. It was stressed that the results showed that local PO_2 always decreased to zero when nitrogen gas was administered, irrespective of the original level. These results are thus at variance with those previously reported by Bicher. Silver reported that he had some evidence for local control of blood flow. Thus, when PO_2 is measured at the neuronal cell surface, and the cell is "driven" by a stimulus, there is a fall in PO_2, followed by a rise to normal level. When the cell stops firing there is a rise in PO_2 followed by a return to normal level. The half times for these responses are about 1.5 sec. However the PO_2 does not change if electrodes are placed more than 0.75 mm from the cell recording site. This suggests a very localized control mechanism. Honig urged that we do not equate local mechanisms with metabolic ones since adrenergic and non-adrenergic mechanisms exist that can be affected by hypoxia.

The results of Leniger-Follert are compatible with the view that there are local "O_2 sensors" that can induce either increase in flow or reduction in oxygen consumption. Since the results reported by Siesjö _et al._ demonstrate that CMR_{O2} is upheld in even relatively pronounced hypoxia any decrease in oxygen consumption by cells must be local and compensated by increased rates at other sites. At the present time, it is not quite clear how flow rates obtained from local hydrogen clearance relates to nutritive flow and further measurements seem required to evaluate the interesting hypothesis of regulation of metabolism at the microvascular level.

REFERENCES

Rossen, R., Kabat, N. and Anderson, J.P. Arch. Neurol. Psychiat. (1943), 50, 510-528.

Pappenheimer, J.R., Fencl, V., Heisey, S.R. and Held. D. Am. J. Physiol. (1965), 208(3), 436-450.

Lowry, O.H., Passonneau, J.V. J. biol. Chem. (1964), 239, 31-42.

Oxygen Supply
of the Central Nervous System II

LOCAL TISSUE Po_2 AND MICROFLOW OF THE BRAIN CORTEX UNDER VARYING ARTERIAL OXYGEN PRESSURE

E. Leniger-Follert, W. Wrabetz and D. W. Lübbers

Max-Planck-Institut für Systemphysiologie, 46 Dortmund
GFR

In the last few years contradictory results of the influence of reduced arterial oxygen supply on the Po_2 of the brain cortex have been reported by different authors. As this could be caused by methodological factors, we investigated this problem systematically in a broader range of arterial oxygen supply. We measured local tissue oxygen pressure (Po_2) with a platinum multiwire surface electrode simultaneously on up to eight adjacent sites of the cortical surface, and with a platinum needle electrode in the deeper layers of the cortex.

Methods. The experiments were performed on 19 adult cats weighing 2.0 to 2.5 kg. The animals were anaesthetized with Nembutal[R] (25 - 30 mg/kg) i. p., relaxed with Flaxedil[R] and ventilated with a Starling pump. Arterial blood pressure and endtidal CO_2 contents were registered continuously and were in the normal range. Rectal temperature was kept constant at 38 °C by a heating pad. Arterial pH, hematocrit and hemoglobin contents were determined at intervals and ranged at the normal level. Arterial Po_2 was measured polarographically. In six animal experiments blood glucose was also determined. None of the animals was in a hypoglycemic state.

After trepanation of the right calvarium a small piece of the dura mater was removed and a Po_2 multiwire surface electrode according to Kessler and Lübbers (1966) was placed on the surface of the gyrus suprasylvius of the cat. The electrode had been modified to make it light and suitable for measurements on the moving cortex. It contained eight 15-µm platinum wires separately connected to the measuring device and was covered with a 12-µm cellophane layer and a 12-µm Teflon layer. The separate connection of the Pt wires allowed individual polarographic measurements of local tissue Po_2 simultaneously on eight adjacent sites of the superficial layers of the brain cortex.

In addition to the Po_2 measurements on the surface of the brain, local Po_2 was measured in deeper layers of the cortex with a new platinum needle electrode of a tip diameter of 1 - 2 μm according to Baumgärtl und Lübbers (1974). The reference electrode was sputtered onto the shaft of the glass and consisted of Ag/AgCl. Thus, the reference electrode was very close to the measuring electrode.

In six experiments microflow was registered continuously in addition to the oxygen measurements. Microflow was qualitatively recorded according to Lübbers und Stosseck (1970) by local generation of hydrogen and by recording the hydrogen partial pressure. We performed the measurements by using an element with 4 different platinum wires each of them with a diameter of 100 μm. Our experiments included the record of tissue Po_2 at first under air respiration and constant experimental conditions. Then the animals were ventilated with various mixtures of oxygen and nitrogen consisting of increased oxygen contents of 100, 60 and 40 %, and decreased oxygen contents of 10, 5, 2, and 0 %. Each reaction was repeated several times.

The following results were obtained:

1. When the arterial Po_2 was suddenly increased from 100 to 200 or 300 Torr or to higher values by ventilating the cats with 40, 60, or even 100 vol % O_2 instead of normal air, different reactions of local tissue Po_2 occurred simultaneously on adjacent sites. On some sites local tissue Po_2 remained constant or increased but little or even decreased, while on other ones it rose proportionally to the oxygen contents of the gas mixture. In some cases, local Po_2 first increased and subsequently dropped down to the initial value or even below it, although the supply with high oxygen mixtures was continued. As a rule, return to air respiration reestablished the initial values. When the reaction was repeated several times, local tissue Po_2 mostly showed the same behaviour as before.

Figure 1 shows an example for this different behaviour of Po_2. Local Po_2 was simultaneously recorded on seven adjacent sites during respiration with 40 vol % O_2. In total, about one third of 93 sites measured in the superficial layers showed a proportional increase in tissue Po_2 after sudden increase in arterial Po_2, whereas with two thirds no or only little effect on local tissue Po_2 was observed.

Po_2 measurements performed with patinum needle electrodes in the deeper layers of the brain cortex showed in principle the same discriminating behaviour as noticed in the superficial layers.

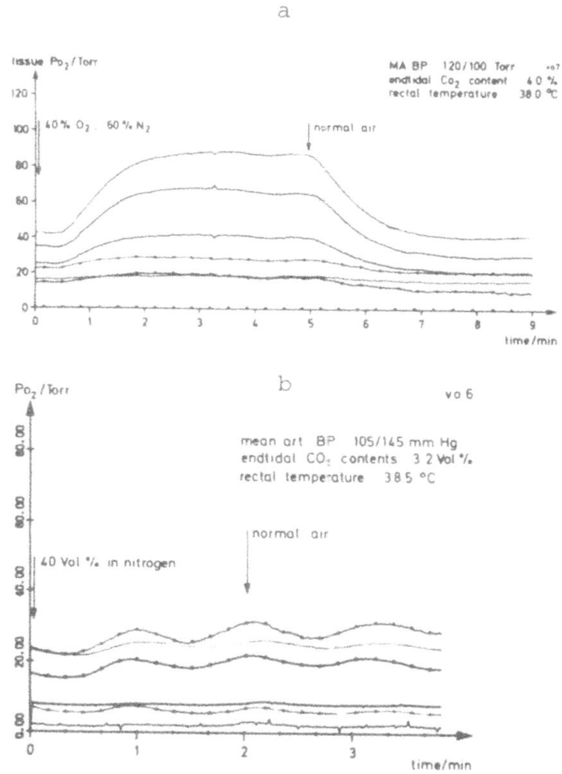

Figure 1
Original record of local tissue Po_2 measured simultaneously on seven sites of the gyrus suprasylvius with a platinum multiwire surface electrode during exposure to 40 vol % O_2.
a) Different reactions of local Po_2 to increase in arterial Po_2. Po_2 increases considerably on some sites, on other ones it remains constant.
b) Local Po_2 does not change on all sites measured.

Whalen (1975) reported an increase in 22 out of 29 locations measured with needle electrodes in the cortex during respiration with 100 vol % O_2.

2. In contrast to the very different reactions of local Po_2 to increased arterial oxygen supply the response of local tissue Po_2 to reduced arterial supply was found to be uniform. Local Po_2 decreased on all sites during a few seconds regardless of the level of the initial Po_2.

Fig. 2a shows the response of Po_2 to respiration with 10 vol % O_2 recorded on seven sites. A new steady state was established which lay, as a rule, above 0 Torr. Return to respiration with

a

b

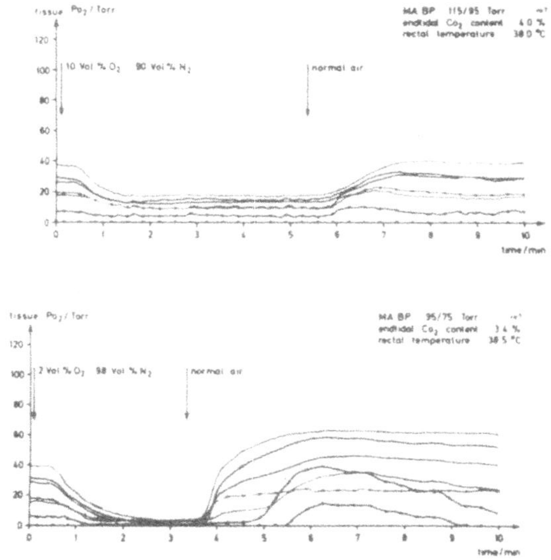

Figure 2

Local tissue Po_2 recorded during reduced supply of arterial oxygen

a) Exposure to 10 vol % O_2 effects a drop in tissue Po_2 on all sites. A new steady state lying above 0 Torr is reached. After return to air respiration only slight overshoots occur.

b) During respiration with 2 vol % O_2 all tissue Po_2 values drop down to 0 Torr. Return to air respiration causes strong overshoot on all sites measured.

notmal air mostly yielded no overshoot of Po_2 or only small ones in a few cases.

Fig. 2b shows the response of tissue Po_2 to administration of 2 vol % O_2. It is to be seen that the different initial values start decreasing within 20 to 30 seconds and then all of them drop down to 0 Torr without any plateau. During air respiration a strong overshoot is observed on all sites with different time constants. After some minutes the Po_2 values gradually drop again to the initial values. This same behaviour was also seen during respiration with nitrogen. If nitrogen was respired for longer than 40 seconds, the tissue Po_2 always reached 0 Torr.

Fig. 3 shows the decrease of Po_2 during respiration with nitrogen measured with a platinum needle electrode in the deeper layers of the cortex. Simultaneous measurements of microflow on four different sites conducted in addition to the Po_2 registration

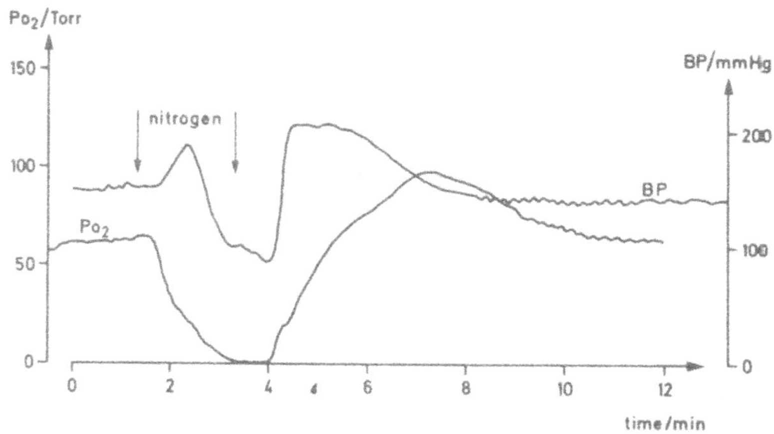

Figure 3
Tissue Po_2 of the grey matter (cat) measured with platinum needle electrodes
During exposure to nitrogen local Po_2 drops down to 0 Torr

during reduced arterial Po_2 revealed that microflow in the grey matter does not behave uniformly during anoxia. Exposure to 5, 2 or 0 vol % O_2 produced a strong increase in microflow in most cases which was maintained for some time after return to air respiration. Then the microflow gradually reached the initial level recorded before anoxia. However, on other sites we regularly found simultaneous decreases in microflow. When tissue anoxia was repeated, this decrease of microflow was always seen at the same site as in the preceding reaction. This different behaviour of microflow during anoxia is shown in Figure 4.

The results show that local tissue Pp_2 reacts quite uniformly to reduced arterial oxygen supply. Local Po_2 decreases in each case. In our systematical investigations of more than 100 measurements recorded at different sites of the brain we never saw the behaviour described by Bicher (1973, 1974). He found that respiration with nitrogen first lowered tissue Po_2 slightly after a latency of at least thirty seconds, and that then the Po_2 level remained constant even though arterial Po_2 approached 0 Torr. We found in agreement with other authors that local tissue Po_2 decreased in each case rapidly down to 0 Torr, if the arterial oxygen supply was strongly reduced. Furthermore, we found a redistribution of microflow during tissue anoxia. We assume that this redistribution is caused by local metabolism in such a way that in areas with high metabolism microflow strongly increases, whereas in other areas with less metabolism microflow can even decrease.

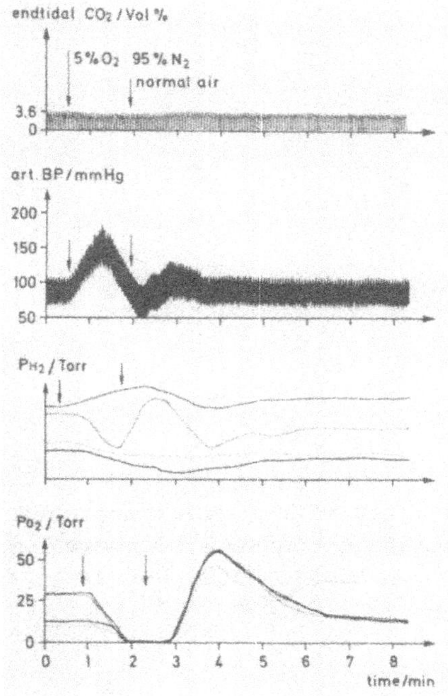

Figure 4
Local Po_2 and microflow recorded during respiration with 5 vol % O_2
Po_2 decreases uniformly, whereas microflow (pH_2) reacts differently. Mostly, microflow increases, but decreases in one case. (Increase in pH_2 means decrease in microflow, decrease in pH_2 means increase in microflow.)

In contrast to the uniform reaction of local tissue Po_2 to reduced arterial oxygen supply, the response of Po_2 to increases in arterial oxygen pressure is very different on adjacent sites of the tissue. This response is independent of the absolute level of the initial Po_2. The results support the assumption of a local Po_2 regulation. We have experimental evidence that local changes in microflow are responsible for that different behaviour. Further experiments are necessary to clarify the question of whether also oxygen consumption changes during increased arterial oxygen pressure. Until now it is not sufficiently clarified whether or not local oxygen receptors play a rôle in the Po_2 regulation described. Further attempts will be made to understand this problem.

References

1. Baumgärtl, H., Lübbers, D. W. (1974) Unpublished results.

2. Bicher, H. I.: Autoregulation of oxygen supply to brain tissue. In: Oxygen Transport to Tissue, eds. H. I. Bicher and D. F. Bruley, 215 - 222, Adv. Exp. Med. Biol. 37A, Plenum Press, New York 1973

3. Bicher, H. I.: Brain oxygen autoregulation. A protective reflex to hypoxia? Microvasc. Res. 8, 291 - 313 (1974)

4. Erdman, W., Kunke, St., Krell, W.: Tissue Po_2 and cell function. An experimental study with multimicroelectrodes in the rat brain. In: Oxygen Supply. Theoretical and Practical Aspects of Oxygen Supply and Microcirculation of Tissue, eds. M. Kessler, D. F. Bruley, L. C. Clark Jr., D. W. Lübbers, I. A. Silver, J. Strauss, 169 - 174, Urban & Schwarzenberg, München - Berlin - Wien 1973

5. Kessler, M., Lübbers, D. W.: Aufbau und Anwendungsmöglichkeiten verschiedener Po_2-Elektroden. Pflügers Arch. ges. Physiol. 291, R 82 (1966)

6. Leniger-Follert, E., Lübbers, D. W.: Regulation of local tissue Po_2 in the grey matter of the cat. Proc. 3rd Tbilisi Symp. on Brain Blood Supply, June 5 - 7, 1974, 34 - 35 Metsnierka Publ. Tbilisi 1974

7. Lübbers, D. W., Stosseck, K.: Quantitative Bestimmung der lokalen Durchblutung durch elektrochemisch im Gewebe erzeugten Wasserstoff. Naturwiss. 57, 311 - 312 (1970)

8. Lübbers, D. W., Leniger-Follert, E.: Oxygen supply to the cells of the brain during various functional states. Alfred Benzon Symp. VIII: On the Working Brain, Copenhagen, May 26 - 30, 1974

9. Nair, P., Whalen, W. J., Buerk, D.: Po_2 of cat cerebral cortex. Response to breathing N_2 and 100 % O_2. Microvasc. Res. 9, 158 - 165 (1975)

10. Silver, I. A.: Brain oxygen tension and cellular activity in oxygen supply. In: Oxygen Supply. Theoretical and Practical Aspects of Oxygen Supply and Microcirculation of Tissue. Eds. M. Kessler, D. F. Bruley, L. C. Clark Jr., D. W. Lübbers, I. A. Silver, J. Strauss, 186 - 188, Urban & Schwarzenberg, München - Berlin - Wien 1973

11. Stosseck, K., Lübbers, D. W., Cottin, N.: Determination of local blood flow (microflow) by electrochemically generated hydrogen. Pflügers Arch. 348, 225 - 238 (1974)

AN ANALYSIS OF ION DISTRIBUTION IN BRAIN FOLLOWING ANOXIA

D. Reneau[1], T. Zeuthen[2], E. Dóra[3], I. Silver[2]

[1]Department of Biomedical Engineering
Louisiana Tech University
Ruston, Louisiana 71270 USA

[2]Department of Comparative Pathology
Bristol University
Bristol, England

[3]Department of Physiology
Semmelweis University
Budapest, Hungary

INTRODUCTION:

Experimental measurements of changes in the extracellular ion concentrations of rat brain cortex have been made with ultramicroelectrodes (1). During extended anoxia of several minutes duration, the changes in ionic concentrations may be characterized by the following statements:

(1) Changes occurred in two phases: A preanoxic depolarization phase and an anoxic depolarization phase.

(2) The preanoxic depolarization phase was characterized by small increases in extracellular Na^+, K^+, Cl^- concentrations and usually a slight decrease in brain DC potential.

(3) The anoxic depolarization phase was characterized by very rapid increases in extracellular K^+, simultaneous decreases in Na^+ and Cl^-, and rapid decreases in DC potential.

The general purpose of this paper is to present the development and solution of a mathematical framework for analyzing ionic transport between extracellular and intracellular regions during normal and abnormal conditions. Specific application will be given in an attempt to arrive at a reasonable explanation of ionic concentration changes that occur during the pre-anoxic depolarization phase and during the anoxic depolarization phase.

Mathematical Considerations

Mathematical description of ion transport between intracellular and extracellular environments was developed by viewing the intracellular and extracellular regions as two compartments separated by a selectively permeable membrane. The description is based on a method recently reported in the literature (2), and our adaptations (3) were applied in this work to conditions of total anoxia after cessation of capillary blood flow. The mathematical considerations attempt to describe the passive and active transport of ions, the passive transport of water due to osmolality changes, and changes in resting membrane potential. The development is summarized in the following paragraphs.

Exchange of ions between compartments are assumed to be governed by concentration gradients, voltage gradients and active transport. From the Nernst-Planck equations, it can be shown that passive diffusion across a membrane due to electro-chemical gradients can be described by the equation;

$$J_i = \frac{E_m F}{RT} P_i Z_i \frac{C_{i,I}\, e^{Z_i E_m F/RT} - C_{i,E}}{1.0 - e^{Z_i E_m F/RT}}$$

Where i refers to a specific ion species, J_i is ion flux, P_i is permeability, Z_i is ion valance, E_m is resting membrane potential, F is the Faraday constant, R is the universal gas constant, T is absolute temperature, $C_{i,I}$ is intracellular ion concentration and $C_{i,E}$ is extracellular ion concentration.

The flux of water across the membrane is given as

$$J_{H_2O} = P_{H_2O} \;(OSMI - OSME)$$

Where, P_{H_2O} is the hydraulic permeability, OSMI , OSME is the intra and extracellular osmolarity respectively.

Active fluxes of potassium and sodium ions are related to to extracellular potassium concentration and intracellular sodium concentration. The method of calculation is outlined in the literature (2) as follows:

$$J_i \text{ Active} = J_{i,o} \frac{A}{Ao}$$

where ,

$i = Na^+, K^+$

$A = A_K A_{Na}$

$$A_K = 1.5 \left[1.0 - \left(\frac{C_{K,E} + 2.5}{2.5}\right) e^{\left(-0.45C_{K,E}\right)}\right]$$

$$A_{Na} = 5.7 \left[1.0 - e^{\left(-0.35 C_{Na,I}\right)}\right]$$

The flux $J_{i,o}$ is equal to the passive flux of i at steady-state.

Transient intracellular changes are calculated as,

$$\frac{dN_{i,I}}{dt} = (J_i \text{ passive} + J_i \text{ active}) A$$

$$V_i = \frac{N_{H_2O,I} \cdot MW_{H_2O}}{p_{H_2O}}$$

$$C_{i,I} = \frac{N_{i,I}}{V_I}$$

where, N_i is moles of i, MW is molecular weight, V_I is intracellular volume, and A is membrane area; and,

$i = K^+, Na^+, Cl^-, H_2O$ but only K^+ and Na^+ are to be considered as actively transported.

Transient extracellular changes are calculated as,

$$\frac{dN_{i,E}}{dt} = \frac{dN_{i,I}}{dt}$$

$$V_E = \frac{N_{H_2O}\ MW_{H_2O}}{\rho_{H_2O}}$$

$$C_{i,E} = \frac{N_{i,E}}{V_E}$$

It has been suggested that changes in resting membrane potential can be determined by transient ionic fluxes as follows (2),

$$\frac{dE}{dt} = \frac{dQ}{C}$$

where Q is charge and C is membrane capacitance

$$dQ = F\sum_i,\ Z_i\ (J_{i\ passive} + J_{i\ Active})$$

Consequently, the above equations can be solved simultaneously and values predicted as a function of time in both the intracellular and extracellular compartments.

SOLUTION TECHNIQUES

The ion transport equations outlined here were solved on an IBM 360 Computer using numerical techniques available with the CSMP simulation language. Ion concentrations and resting membrane potentials were predicted as a function of time following a specified departure from steady-state. Care was taken in selection of integration time increments to insure stability and checks were always made for the maintenance of electroneutrality.

DISCUSSION OF RESULTS

The ion transport model was standardized with literature values (2) and checked for accuracy by simulating known experimental responses to known changes. A "trend" analysis was conducted by simulating variable changes and searching for most probable causes.

Preanoxic Depolarization Phase. A most probable cause for the preanoxic depolarization phase was predicted to be a function of water shifts from extracellular regions to intracellular regions during the initial phases of intracellular anaerobic glycolysis. As products of anaerobic glycolysis initially accumulate in the intracellular region, the osmolality balance is changed and water is transported from extracellular spaces to intracellular spaces. As ion concentrations change due to volume (water) changes, ion transport occurs across the membrane, and a small depolarization occurs. However, the initial effect on ion concentration is dominated by water exchange.

For instance, a theoretical simulation of these conditions indicates that at the end of the preanoxic depolarization time period the extracellular volume has decreased 20%, all extra-ceullular concentrations have increased, and the membrane has depolarized 2.2 mv. The depolarization is due to ion exchange across the membrane, but extracellular increases in ion concentration is predominantly the result of a decreasing extracellular volume.

Anoxic-Depolarization Phase. The theoretical analysis demonstrates that trends similar to the experimentally measured anoxic depolarization phase can occur from a failure of the active transport process. Following a theoretical failure of the active transport process, the extracellular concentrations of sodium and chloride rapidly decrease, potassium increases, and the cell quickly depolarizes.

The assumption of active transport failure during anoxic depolarization is a reasonable assumption. ATP during anoxia could lead to active transport failure as a result of insufficient energy; or a decrease in pH as a result of increasing quantities of lactic acid may destroy the active mechanism.

CONCLUDING COMMENTS

The theoretical results presented herein are given as a trend analysis, and are used to establish areas of most probable cause for explanation of the experimental results. The solution techniques have been carefully examined, regional electroneutrality has been maintained at all times, and a multivariable search conducted. Experiments must now be designed to test the hypotheses.

This work was supported in part by NIH Grant NS-08802 and the Frost Foundation of Shreveport, Louisiana.

References

(1) Zeuthen, T., and E. Dora: Brain Metabolism and Ion Movements in Brain Cortex of the Rat During Anoxia, Proceedings of the International Workshop on Ion Selective Electrodes, Ulm, Germany (In Press).

(2) Brace, R. A., and D. K. Anderson: J. Applied Physiol., 35, 90-94, 1973.

(3) Reneau, D. D.: A Mathematical Analysis of Simultaneous Transport Phenomena in the Microcirculation, Proceedings of the International Workshop on Ion Selective Electrodes, Ulm, Germany (In Press).

COMPARISON OF OXYGEN TENSION IN THE SPINAL CORD AND GLOBUS PALLIDUS DURING HYPERBARIC OXYGEN EXPOSURE OF RATS UNDER PENTOBARBITAL ANESTHESIA

Robert W. Ogilvie, J. Douglas Balentine, and Richard C. Hunt

Departments of Anatomy and Pathology
Medical University of South Carolina
Charleston, South Carolina, U.S.A.

INTRODUCTION

Lesions in the brain and spinal cord have been produced by exposing rats to hyperbaric oxygen. Complete or partial necrosis of nuclear groups with damage to myelin, axons and glia have been produced consistently in the globus pallidus and spinal cord gray matter of unanesthetized rats after intermittent exposures to 100% oxygen at 60 P.S.I.G. (Pounds per Square Inch by the Guage).[1,2] Pentobarbital anesthesia has been found to protect the globus pallidus from the necrotic lesions of hyperbaric oxygen, but it potentiates lesions of the spinal cord.[3] In exploration of the causal mechanism of these lesions, we have previously reported direct measurements of oxygen tensions in the globus pallidus of rats anesthetized with pentobarbital and compressed to 60 P.S.I.G. with 100% oxygen.[4] Oxygen tensions up to 475 mmHg were recorded within five minutes after achieving a pressure of 60 P.S.I.G. The oxygen tensions then fell to an average value of 60 mmHg within 45 minutes.

The purpose of the present study was to obtain measurements of oxygen tensions in the brain and spinal cord during hyperbaria so that oxygen tensions in a pentobarbital protected area (globus pallidus) could be compared with oxygen tensions in an unprotected area (spinal cord gray). In order to limit the variables, simultaneous measurements as well as independent measurements of oxygen tensions in the globus pallidus and spinal cord gray were taken during a one hour exposure to hyperbaric oxygen.

MATERIALS AND METHODS

The experiments were carried out in adult female Sprague Dawley rats, weighing 150-230 grams. Each rat was anesthetized with sodium pentobarbital (40 mg/kg). The trachea was cannulated and respiratory rate and depth were monitored either clinically or by measuring the differential temperature during inspiration and expiration using a small 24 gauge thermistor temperature probe placed in the trachea cannula. EKG and EEG were monitored and recorded. Cup electrodes fixed to both forelimbs and the left hindlimb were used for EKG. Electrodes for monitoring EEG consisted of 1 mm D. stainless steel screws put into the skull. The reference EEG electrode was over the nasal cavity and the active EEG electrode over the parieto-occipital region.

The spinal cord was prepared for oxygen measurements first by performing a laminectomy overlying the lumbosacral enlargement. The dura mater was removed over the area selected for oxygen measurements. Then the rat was stabilized in a head and body stereotaxic apparatus. The brain was then prepared by removing the skin, fascia and bone over the left frontal area.

The external referenced electrodes used for measuring oxygen were platinum wire glass insulated with tip between 5 and 10 microns. The electrodes and current amplifiers used are commercially available from the Transidyne General Corporation, Ann Arbor, Michigan, USA. The electrodes were calibrated before and after the experiment by measuring the current obtained when they were immersed in a constant temperature saline bath equilibrated with nitrogen (zero % oxygen), compressed air (21% oxygen) and 100% oxygen. The electrodes were calibrated between 29-36°C, corresponding to temperatures equal to the rectal temperatures of rats following anesthesia. If the electrode calibration values at the beginning and end of an experiment failed to agree within 5%, that experiment was not included in the series.

Electrode placement coordinates for the globus pallidus were 7 mm caudal to the frontal suture, 3 mm lateral to the midsaggital suture, and 5 mm deep into the brain. The coordinates for the anteromedial horn gray were 1 mm lateral to the dorsal median septum and 1.5 mm deep into the spinal cord. A reference electrode for each oxygen electrode was placed into nearby muscle tissue. In order to check the actual placement of each electrode at the end of the experiment the oxygen electrodes were removed and replaced, using the same coordinates, by a 25 gauge spinal needle filled with trypan blue, inserted to a depth 1 mm less in the brain and 0.5 mm less in the spinal cord. After the needle was removed leaving a marker, the brain and spinal cord were removed, fixed in formalin and later coronally sliced to locate the track. The site of the electrode tip was determined by measuring from the surface along the stained track to the total depth that the oxygen electrode had been placed. In all experiments reported here the electrodes were found to be placed in the globus pallidus and spinal cord anteromedial horn gray.

Recordings of oxygen tensions, EKG, EEG and respiration rates were made using two Model 7PA Grass Polygraphs. Fast recordings (5 mm/sec. to 100 mm/sec.) of all measurements were made on one polygraph while slow recordings (2.5 mm/min.) were made of the oxygen tensions of the brain and spinal cord on the other polygraph. Even though it is not claimed in these experiments that the oxygen tensions are absolute, the partial pressure of oxygen was calculated using the average barometric pressure and average calibration temperature (for determining the water vapor pressure) so that the values are considered to be near actual tissue oxygen tensions. The polygraph recording needle was set so that a full scale excursion corresponded to the oxygen tension in saline equilibrated with 100% oxygen at 34°C at ambient pressure. This is equivalent to a partial pressure of oxygen equal to 720 mmHg.

The exposure of the rat to hyperbaric oxygen was carried out in the following manner. A Bethlehem #1836H small animal hyperbaric chamber was utilized for all exposures. Each rat was placed into the chamber and baseline recordings obtained. The chamber was then flushed with oxygen (usually 10 minutes) until the gas measured from an outflow valve was determined to be 99.5-100% oxygen by a Servomex oxygen meter. Compression to 60 P.S.I.G. was by 4 increments of 15 P.S.I.G. each over a 3 to 4 minute period. Compression at 60 P.S.I.G. was maintained for one hour. The chamber was ventilated to insure that there was no build-up of carbon dioxide. At the end of one hour, decompression was staged in decrements over 8 minutes. Following decompression the rat was sacrificed with an overdose of pentobarbital or by flushing the chamber with nitrogen. When EEG and EKG were flat, the rat was considered dead. The chamber was then ventilated and recompressed with 100% oxygen to 60 P.S.I.G. Continuous recording of oxygen was maintained through each of these steps in order to determine what portion, if any, of the oxygen values obtained in the living rat were due to passive diffusion.

Oxygen tension determinations in the spinal cord gray and globus pallidus were made in 7 rats. In 4 of 7 rats the determinations in the brain and spinal cord were made simultaneously.

RESULTS AND DISCUSSION

The average respiratory rate for the animals used in this study at ambient pressure breathing air was 49 breaths per minute. The respiration rate slowed from the precompression value to an average of 39 breaths per minute soon after compression. Thirty minutes after compression (while still under 60 P.S.I.G.) the respiration rates rose to values approaching or above (61 breaths/minute) the rates at ambient pressure breathing air. In the remaining animals the respiratory rate increased slightly (about 5 breaths per minute) after compression.

The EEG channel on the polygraph was calibrated the same for all rats (0.5 cm - 200 microvolts) and therefore was used as an index of comparative levels of anesthesia as judged by the electrical activity. The rats used in these experiments ranged from deep to light anesthetic levels. Deep anesthesia was accompanied by low voltage EEG spikes and a 28/minute respiratory rate at the beginning of compression. Light anesthesia was characterized by high voltage EEG activity including many large spikes and a precompression respiratory rate of 80/minute. No seizure activity was observed in the EEG tracings or clinically in any of the rats.

The heart rate remained steady or decreased by as much as 100 beats per minute during the exposure to hyperbaric oxygen. The control (precompression) heart rates ranged from 300-480 beats per minute and the EKG was normal throughout each experiment.

A typical slow tracing of oxygen tensions measured in the brain and spinal cord before, during and immediately following the period of compression is shown in Figure 1. The response to oxygen flushing at ambient pressure was more pronounced in the spinal cord. During the compression period the spinal cord oxygen tension increased at a more rapid rate (220 mmHg/min.) than in the globus pallidus (28 mmHg/min.) The rise and fall of oxygen tension was at a steady rate in all cases (Fig.1) except that shown in the tracing illustrated in Figure 2. During the recompression after the animals were presumed dead by nitrogen or pentobarbital there was a slight rise in oxygen tension in the spinal cord in two rats which took about 8 minutes to develop 100 mmHg. The animal represented in Figure 2 was one of the two rats and as shown there is a transient lag in the rate of fall of oxygen tension in the spinal cord as evidenced by the quasi plateau. In the remaining rats no postmortem rise in oxygen tensions occurred in the spinal cord or globus pallidus as previously reported.[4,5] The slowing in the fall of oxygen levels in the spinal cord in 2 of the 7 animals may be due to some direct diffusion of oxygen into the spinal cord.

The values of oxygen tension at selected time intervals before, during, and after exposure were read off the tracings. These oxygen values were averaged and a composite plot of two curves obtained as shown in Figure 3. As determined by calculating the standard error of the mean for each point plotted, the average peak value of spinal cord oxygen tension was higher than that of the globus pallidus.

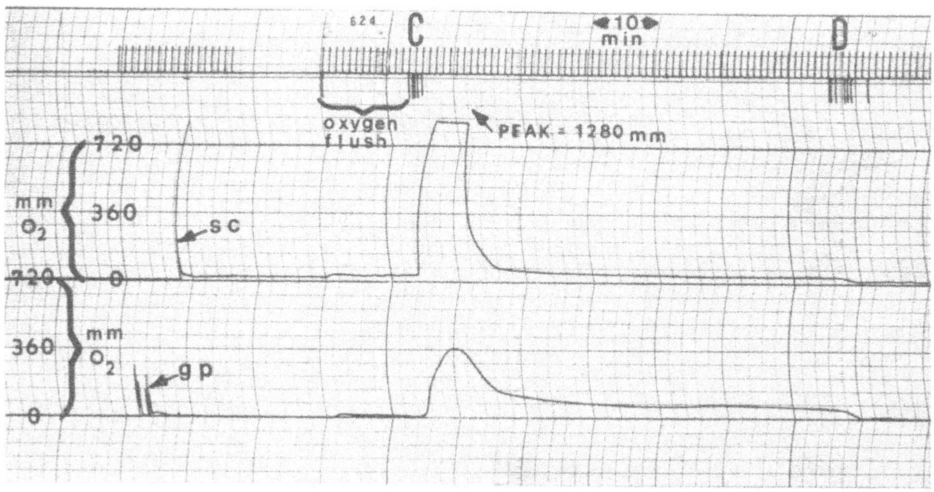

Figure 1. A photograph of a polygraph tracing of oxygen tensions in the spinal cord gray matter (top tracing) and globus pallidus (bottom tracing) during a one hour exposure to 100% oxygen at 60 P.S.I.G. Note the electrode insertion artifacts at gp and sc.
C = compression D = decompression

The spinal cord oxygen tension reached a lower value sooner than did the globus pallidus and tended to maintain a lower level until just prior to decompression. However, the total quantity of oxygen values throughout the one hour exposure was greater in the spinal cord than in the globus pallidus. The areas under the two curves from the beginning of compression to 30 minutes after compression were determined by cutting the areas out of the oxygen tracings for each rat and weighing the polygraph paper on a Mettler balance to determine the mass. The mass of the area under the spinal cord curve was found to be 1.36 times greater than the mass of the area under the globus pallidus curve. This is proportional to the quantity of available oxygen during the 30 minute period. Even though the oxygen level measured in the globus pallidus after 10 minutes of compression tended to remain above the level recorded in the spinal cord, a check of the standard error of the means of the two determinations during this period shows this not to be significant.

The findings in this study indicate that during hyperbaric oxygen exposure the oxygen tensions in the spinal cord and globus pallidus are significantly elevated. These data support the interpretation that necrotic lesions resulting in these areas of the central nervous system following hyperbaric oxygenation are the consequence of excessive tissue oxygenation. The qualitative differences in in the oxygen tension curves as the function of

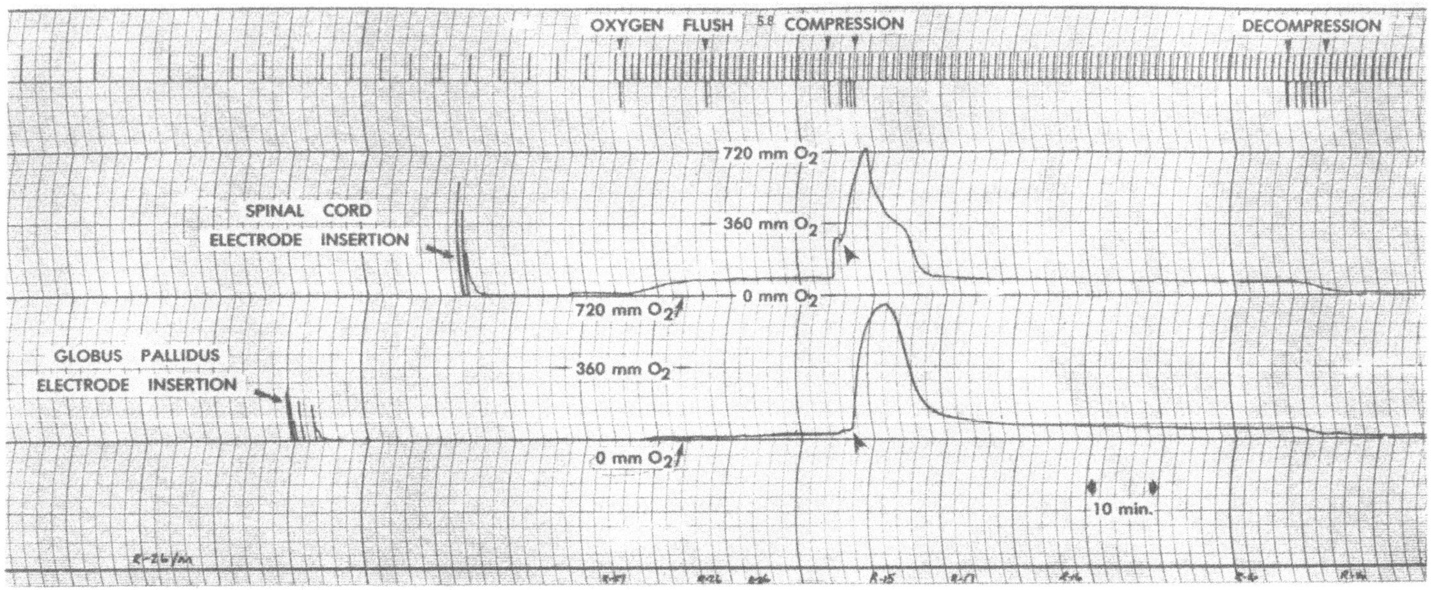

Figure 2. Photograph of a polygraph tracing of oxygen tensions obtained simultaneously from the globus pallidus and spinal cord anteromedial horn gray before, during, and immediately after 1 hour of compression at 60 P.S.I.G. with 100 percent O_2. In this experiment a short interruption occurred in the compression process which resulted in a temporary lag in the rise of oxygen tension in the chamber, in the brain, and in the spinal cord. By comparing the notch (arrows) in each of the tracings it becomes obvious how much more rapid the oxygen tension was rising in the spinal cord.

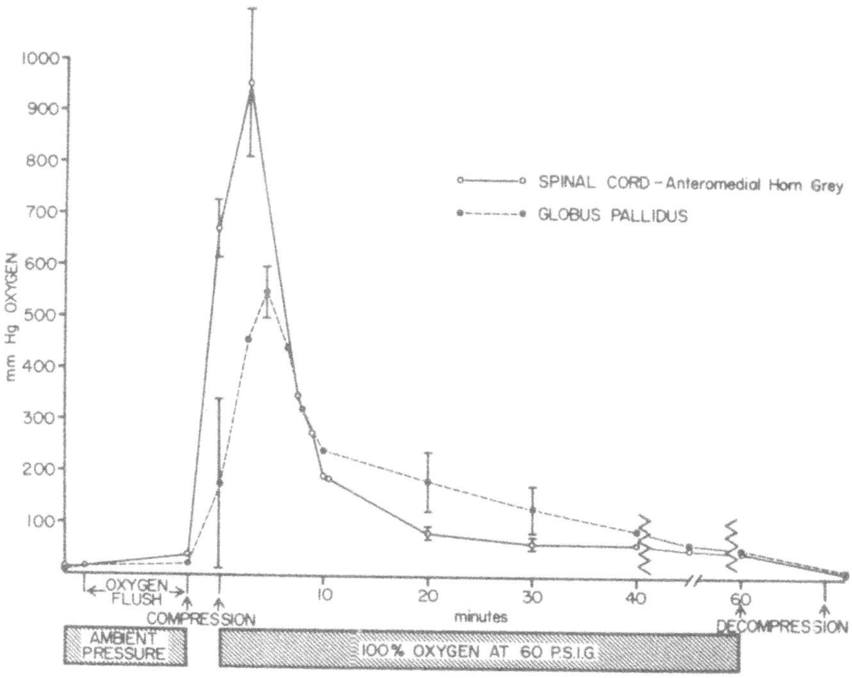

Figure 3. Plots of the means of oxygen tensions in the globus pallidus and spinal cord anteromedial horn gray of six rats just before, during 1 hour at 60 P.S.I.G. of 100 percent O_2, and immediately after decompression.

pentobarbital anesthesia, which tends to protect the forebrain from the development of necrotic lesions, were less apparent when the measurements were made simultaneously in the same animal than they were when these values were obtained independently, as previously reported.[4,5] Although the curves look more or less the same when measured simultaneously, they were not identical and some crucial observations were recorded. For instance, consistently in the spinal cord, there is an earlier and explosive rise in oxygen tension, whereas the globus pallidus recording suggests that blood flow regulating mechanisms are constantly working to limit the rise in tissue oxygen tension. These characteristics of the oxygen tension responses in the spinal cord indicate that a greater quantity of oxygen is present overall for the hour's duration in the spinal cord than in the globus pallidus. Therefore, it is probable that the greater overall quantity of oxygen tension in the spinal cord and not the qualitative characteristics of the curve may be responsible for the fact that the spinal cord gray is not protected by pentobarbital anesthesia from oxygen induced necrosis.

The differences in the rates at which oxygen tensions rise and fall during hyperbaric oxygenation in two areas of the central nervous system that are susceptible to oxygen induced cellular injury, underscores the correlation of pathological and physiological events and suggests that perhaps both qualitative and quantitative differences in oxygen tension values within different areas of the central nervous system during hyperbaric oxygen exposure may occur in other areas of the brain and spinal cord. They also suggest that the areas of the central nervous system not susceptible to the toxic effects of oxygen may show different responses. Further studies are in progress to elucidate the possible differential oxygen tension values obtained in areas of the brain and spinal cord susceptible and non-susceptible to lesions when the organism is subjected to hyperbaric oxygen.

REFERENCES

1. Balentine, J. D. Central necrosis of the spinal cord induced by hyperbaric oxygen exposure. J. Neurosurg. (In Press).

2. Balentine, J. D. and B. B. Gutsche. Central nervous system lesions in rats exposed to oxygen at high pressure. Amer. J. Path. 48: 107-127 (1966).

3. Balentine, J. D. and B. B. Gutsche. Influence of pentobarbital anesthesia on the distribution of central nervous system lesions in rats exposed to oxygen at high pressure, in Brown, I. E. (ed.): Proceedings of the Third International Conference on Hyperbaric Medicine, Washington: National Academy of Sciences, 1966, pp. 145-150.

4. Ogilvie, R. W. and J. D. Balentine. Oxygen tensions in the deep grey matter of rats exposed to hyperbaric oxygen, in Bicher, H. and D. Bruley, (eds.): Oxygen Transport to Tissue. Advances in Experimental Medicine and Biology, Vol. 37A: 299-304, 1973, Plenum Press, New York.

5. Ogilvie, R. W. and J. D. Balentine. Oxygen tension in the grey matter of the spinal cord during exposure to hyperbaric oxygen at 5 atmospheres. J. Neurosurg. (In Press).

AUTONOMIC AND PHARMACOLOGICAL CONTROL OF OXYGEN AUTOREGULATION MECHANISMS IN BRAIN TISSUE

Bicher, H.I., Marvin, P., Hunt, D. and Bruley, D.F.*

Dept. Pharmacol., Univ. Ark. Med. Center, Little Rock, Arkansas, USA and *Dept. Chem. Engin., Tulane Univ., New Orleans, Louisiana, USA

In previous publications (1,3) we have described a precisely controlled autoregulatory mechanism to maintain a constant brain TpO_2 level. This includes a theoretical "tissue oxygen sensor" able to simultaneously regulate cerebral blood flow and tissue O_2 consumption through reflex inhibition-excitation of generalized neuronal activity; it is defined by four criteria in the physiological compensatory response elicited by a short period of anoxic anoxia: 1) short "reoxygenation time" (RT, the time required for TpO_2 to return to the pre-anoxic level), 2) increase in cerebral blood flow, 3) presence of an "overshoot" (period after reoxygenation during which TpO_2 is higher than baseline, and 4) a period of "anoxic silence" in neuronal activity.

All four responses can be suppressed by the α-adrenergic blocking agent, phenoxybenzamine. In the present experiments other autonomically active agents were tested. Also, a fifth autoregulation criteria, the small or non-existing rise in brain TpO_2 during normoatmospheric O_2 breathing, was added as an additional test.

MATERIALS AND METHODS

The experiments were performed on 55 cats anesthetized with sodium pentobarbital and under positive-pressure breathing. Femoral artery blood pressure and carotid artery blood flow were recorded on a Beckman Offner, type RB, Dynograph using standard transducers. Blood and tissue pO_2, as well as the electrical activity of single cortical neurons were determined using our ultra microelectrodes as described below and recorded on the Beckman

Dynograph. The different respiratory mixtures tested were administered through the artificial respiration pump, and all solutions were injected into the cannulated femoral vein.

Experimental Procedures

Measurement of tissue pO_2 with oxygen ultramicroelectrode. The oxygen cathode basically consists of a very finely drawn (2 µm diam.) tungsten shaft which has a thin film overcoating of platinum, covered with two layers of an oxygen-impervious resin, Seran F 310 (supplied by Dow Chemicals, Midland, Michigan), leaving an exposed length of tip of approximately 2 µm. Gold is then electrochemically deposited at the tip, which is afterward coated with Rhoplex (Rohm and Haas, Philadelphia, Pa.). This probe has been used as an "external reference" oxygen microelectrode as described in previous papers (2,4,6). The oxygen microelectrodes used in the present work were supplied by Transidyne General Corporation, Ann Arbor, Michigan, according to our specifications. The electronic circuitry to measure the polarographic current was provided by a model 1200 Chemical Microsensor System (Transidyne General Corporation, Ann Arbor, Michigan), and the results were recorded on a Beckman Offner type RB Dynograph (Beckman Instruments, Palo Alto, California). The procedure for electrode calibration was the same as previously described (6). Cortical reoxygenation times were determined as previously described (2). This procedure involves the determination of the time necessary to reach back baseline oxygen levels after a short period of anoxic anoxia and seems to be a good indication of the ability of the circulation to transport oxygen to tissue.

In several experiments a platinum-irridium Teflon coated wire, 120 µm diameter was used as O_2 electrode. Although the calibration is not as reliable to determine actual TpO_2 values, it was found that in determining transients (RT and overshoot) the obtained values correlated well with those obtained using microelectrodes.

Blood pO_2. Blood pO_2 was recorded using a polarographic catheter electrode as previously described (5) manufactured by Mediscience Technology Corporation, Cherry Hill, New Jersey, according to our specifications.

Blood pressure. Blood pressure was measured from a cannulated femoral artery using a Statham transducer.

Measurement of indications of flow and rates of changes in flow. Measurement of indications of flow and rates of changes in flow were made with the use of an electromagnetic flowmeter, model 202 (Carolina Medical Electronics, King, North Carolina). The probe or electromagnetic cuff was placed around a carotid artery and recordings were made continuously.

Operation. Observations were made on over 55 cats. The animals were anesthetized with sodium pentobarbital. The head of the animal was fixed in a David Kopf model 1730 stereotaxic instrument. The surface of the brain was exposed through a small hole drilled through the periosteum. The electrode was fixed in a micromanipulator (David Kopf model 1760) and lowered into the surface of the brain. The hole in the periosteum was resealed with Agar after electrode positioning. Micromovements of the electrode within brain tissue were achieved using a David Kopf model 1707B hydraulic microdrive. Measurements were made only in the upper 3 mm of brain prefrontal cortex.

Materials

Those drugs used in the series were obtained from the following sources: atropine, Merck, Rahway, N.J.; propranolol, Ayerst Laboratories, N.Y.; Isuprel, Sterling-Winthrop Research Institute, Nensslaer, N.Y.; Bemegride, Abbott, North Chicago, Ill.; tolazoline, CIBA, Summit, N.J.; dibenamine, Smith, Kline, and French, Philadelphia, Pa.; and phenoxybenzamine, Smith, Kline, and French, Philadelphia, Pa.

RESULTS

O_2 Breathing

Upon respiration of pure O_2 for 5-7 minutes, arterial pO_2 rises to about 600 mm Hg. TpO_2 changes are very limited. In most electrode locations there is a small increase (averaging +26% of original value) or no change. In other locations there is a small decrease.

The infusion of phenoxybenzamine, 30 mg/Kg over a period of 30 minutes while breathing O_2 induced a further increase in TpO_2 in 8 out of 9 animals. The mean increase was 67% above pre-infusion levels (see Fig. 1).

Breathing 5% CO_2 - 95% O_2 caused a large increase of 210% in 10 animals; however, after phenoxybenzamine infusion this effect was smaller (average 143% in 4 of 18 tests) or reversed (average fall of 48% in 12 or 18 tests.) (See Fig. 2)

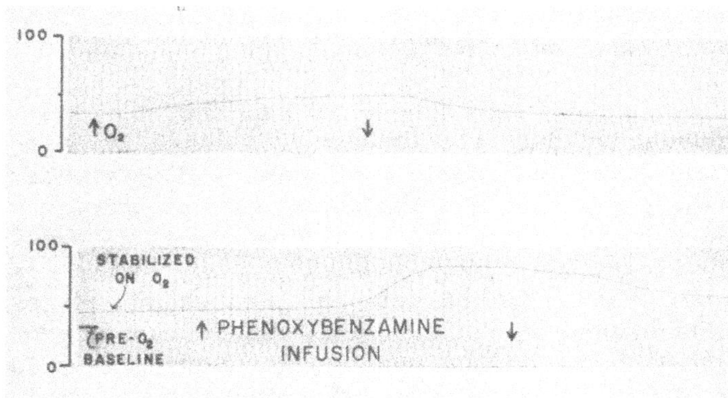

Figure 1: BRAIN TpO_2 UNDER O_2 BREATHING. Note small rise when changing from air to oxygen breathing (upper tracing). Marked additional TpO_2 rise when phenoxybenzamine is infused (lower tracing). Time scale, 1 square = 10 seconds.

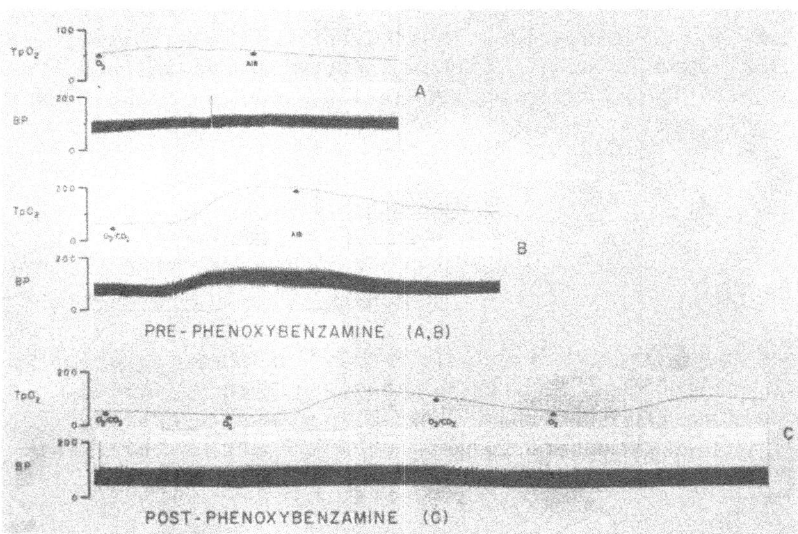

Figure 2: EFFECT OF PHENOXYBENZAMINE AND CO_2 ON BRAIN TpO_2. Trace A: Small TpO_2 rise during O_2 breathing. Trace B: Large increase in TpO_2 caused by 95% O_2 - 5% CO_2 breathing. Trace C: After phenoxybenzamine infusion, O_2 breathing rise in TpO_2 is larger than the pre-infusion effect. Contrariwise 95% O_2 - 5% CO_2 causes a fall in TpO_2. Time scale: 10 seconds between time marks (chart center).

Drug Effects

Several agents known to act on autonomic nervous systems or to increase cerebral metabolism and blood flow were investigated. The effects on reoxygenation time and cerebral blood flow are summarized in Table 1. All α-adrenergic blocking agents (tolazoline, dibenamine and phenoxybenzamine) did prolong the RT and abolish the "overshoot," as previously reported for phenoxybenzamine (1). The other drugs tested were devoid of such action.

TABLE 1: AVERAGE PERCENT CHANGE ABOVE (+) OR BELOW (-) CONTROL RESPONSES TO N_2 BREATHING FOR 50 SECONDS

DRUG	REOXYGENATION TIME	CAROTID FLOW
Atropine (2 mg/Kg)	+21%	- 7%
Propranolol (4 mg/Kg)	+34%	-25%
Isuprel Infusion (2 mg/min, 1 hr.)	-47%	-15%
Bemegride Infusion (100 μg/min, 0.5 hr.)	+ 4%	+66%
Tolazoline (300 mg)	+95%	-100% (to zero)
Dibenamine (200 mg)	+48%	-79%
Phenoxybenzamine (200 mg)	+98%	-95%
No drug, after 2.5 hrs.	-19%	+92%

DISCUSSION

In previous papers (1,3) we have established four criteria used to identify the oxygen autoregulation mechanism in brain tissue, following a short period of anoxic anoxia:

(1) Short "reoxygenation time."
(2) Increase in cerebral blood flow.
(3) Presence of an "overshoot."
(4) Presence of a period of electrical silence paralleling the period of TpO_2 depression.

After administration of phenoxybenzamine in increasing doses, the response to anoxic anoxia was fundamentally changed as follows:

(a) On the TpO_2 record, the "reoxygenation time" is much longer, and the "overshoot" disappears.
(b) The increase in carotid artery blood flow was no longer present.
(c) The "anoxic silence" of cortical neurons was no longer present. Prolongation of the anoxic period for more than 5 minutes does not reduce the rate of neuronal firing.

Therefore, it can be assumed that the adrenolytic agent blocks or reverses all four parameter changes used as evidence for the O_2 autoregulation mechanism.

The experiments hereby reported suggest that a fifth autoregulation criteria should be adopted, namely the limited rise in brain TpO_2 during pure O_2 breathing, even under high blood pO_2 tensions (7). Phenoxybenzamine seems to block this regulation mechanism when infused for a prolonged period of time, although to a limited degree.

The presence of an α-adrenergic mechanism involved in brain O_2 autoregulation seems to be confirmed by the fact that the 3 α-blocking agents tested, (phenoxybenzamine, dibenamine, and tolazoline) did prolong the RT, abolish the overshoot and suppress the increase in carotid blood flow induced by hypoxia. All other agents tested failed to do so.

There seems to be an effect of α-adrenolytic drugs in blocking the effect of CO_2 on brain TpO_2 levels. Additional experiments are currently being conducted to elucidate the mechanism of this interaction.

SUMMARY

The effect of several agents active on autonomic nervous

system functions was tested on brain oxygen autoregulation parameters.

It was found that atropine, propranolol and isproterenol had no influence on the measured parameters. Phenoxybenzamine, tolazoline and dibenamine all suppress autoregulation.

In an additional experimental series, a phenoxybenzamine infusion was given during O_2 breathing. The infusion induced a marked rise in TpO_2. It is concluded that an α-adrenergic mechanism is part of the autoregulation process, and its pharmacological blockade could be used to raise TpO_2 levels in brain with O_2 breathing at normal atmospheric pressure. Also, the increase in brain TpO_2 induced by 95% O_2 - 5% CO_2 breathing seems to be blocked by α-adrenolytic drugs.

REFERENCES

1. Bicher, H.I. Brain autoregulation: A protective reflex to hypoxia. Microvascular Research, 8:291-313, 1974.

2. Bicher, H.I., Bruley, D.F., Reneau, D.D. and Knisely, M.H. Effect of microcirculation changes on brain tissue oxygenation. J. Physiol., 217:689-707, 1971.

3. Bicher, H.I. Reneau, D.D., Bruley, D.F. and Knisely, M.H. Brain oxygen supply and neuronal activity under normal and hypoglycemic conditions. Am. J. Physiol., 224: 275-282, 1973.

4. Bicher, H.I., Reneau, D.D., and Knisely, M.H. Brain tissue oxygenation as determined with a new ultramicro oxygen electrode. In: Blood Oxygenation, (D. Hershey, ed.). pp. 201-207, Plenum Press, New York, 1970.

5. Bicher, H.I., Rubin, J.W. and Adams, R.J. Clinical use of a new intra-arterial catheter electrode system. In: Oxygen Transport to Tissue: Instrumentation, Methods, and Physiology. (H.I. Bicher, and D.F. Bruley, eds.), pp. 107-113, Plenum Press, New York, 1973.

6. Bicher, H.I. and Knisely, M.H. Brain tissue reoxygenation, demonstrated with a new ultramicro oxygen electrode. J. Appl. Physiol., 28:387-390, 1970.

7. Lubbers, D.W. Personal communication.

EFFECTS OF SO-CALLED "CEREBRAL BLOOD FLOW INCREASING" DRUGS ON TISSUE-OXYGENATION OF THE BRAIN

Wilhelm Erdmann, Wolfgang Braun, James H. Halsey, Stefan Kunke and Wilfred Nix

Departments of Anesthesiology and Neurology

University of Alabama in Birmingham

Besides the physiological decrease of cerebral blood flow in aged individuals caused secondarily by proceeding physiological cell death (Puppe, 1971, Puppe-Erdmann, 1973) and decrease of oxygen demand, there may exist a pathological decrease of cerebral blood flow primarily induced by the so-called "arteriosclerosis" of the vessel wall leading to hypoxic death of cells.

To prevent relative hypoxia of the brain, above all in elderly patients, many drugs have been used in clinical medicine. Very little is known regarding the action and effect of these drugs, however, and studies on their differential effects, especially in those areas which are the most sensitive to lack in oxygen supply, have not been possible with the hitherto used macrophysiological* methods. The limitation of these methods is that they are insensitive to potential inhomogeneities of local oxygen consumption and flow distribution. Thus, an increase of macrophysiologically measured CBF does not at the same time mean that capillary perfusion and oxygen supply to every microarea is also increased.

By means of modern microphysiological methods for measurement of PO_2, action potential, capillary perfusion and pH in the inter-

*Macrophysiological methods are methods applied for integrating measurements over areas above the microphysiological level. Cerebral microphysiology can be arbitrarily defined as anything concerning the physiology of those vascular segments within the cranium whose vessels are less than 100 μ in diameter and of the dependent tissue areas corresponding to the definition of cerebral microcirculation by Rosenblum, 1975.

capillary tissue, however, it is now possible to register in comparative animal studies directly the effects of drugs in those areas which are to be affected by the treatment. Previous studies on intravenous anesthetic drugs (Erdmann and Kunke, 1973) revealed new aspects of how drugs can influence the microcirculation and tissue oxygenation either by 1) decreasing or increasing tissue perfusion, 2) decreasing or increasing oxygen consumption, or 3) directly interfering with the autoregulatory PO_2-rhythms of the microarea, perhaps a sign of rhythmic perfusion changes.

In the following study the two most common drugs for treatment of supposed failure in oxygen supply of the brain tissue have been examined:

a) Xantinol nicotinate (Complanim(R)) a synthetically produced substance consisting of a water soluable compound of nicotinic acid and a substituted base of Xanthine. The acting substances are nicotinic acid and Theophylline.

b) Raubasin (Lamuron(R)) a weak indol base closely related to the rauwolfia alkaloid serpentin.

Methods:

The experiments were performed with platinized gold microelectrodes described in previous publications (Erdmann, Kunke and Krell, 1971). In a first series, experiments were performed in the parietal cortex of 40 white Albino rats of the Wistar tribe (1½ years of age; weight 250-300 gr.). The rats were initially anesthetized with Na-pentobarbital (30-40 mg/kg body weight) intraperitoneally and tracheotomized. Analgesia was maintained by N_2O-O_2 (7.9:2.1) led through a T-shaped cannula inserted into the trachea. The rat was fixed in a stereotactic holder inside a screened cubicle (Siemens, Erlangen, Germany, B 83100). The microelectrodes are driven into the parietal cortex through holes drilled into the skull cap of less than 1 mm in diameter by means of a micromanipulator. Information was led to an H_2-PO_2-AP-amplifier which was driven by two 12-volt batteries (Erdmann, 1973)(fig. 1). The output signals were led to light emitting diodes which transmit information through the space between the two cages to a light receiving phototransistor. There existed no galvanic connection between the inside and the outside of the shielded chamber. Relative tissue perfusion measurements were performed with H_2-clearance after equilibration of the tissue with inhaled H_2 instead of N_2O (Heidenreich, Erdmann, Metzger and Thews, 1970).

Arterial blood pressure was continuously recorded by Statham elements connected to a DC-Wheatstone bridge. The signal was transmitted from inside the cage to the outside via light transmission as described above. Inspiratory oxygen concentration was kept constant by continuous control via IBC oxygen analyzer (International

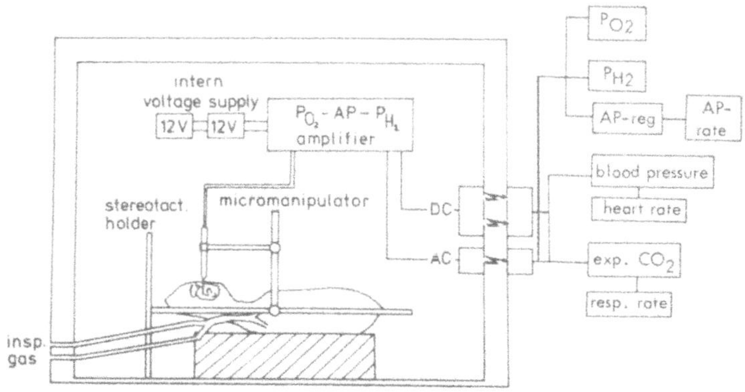

Figure 1: Schematic of the experimental set-up

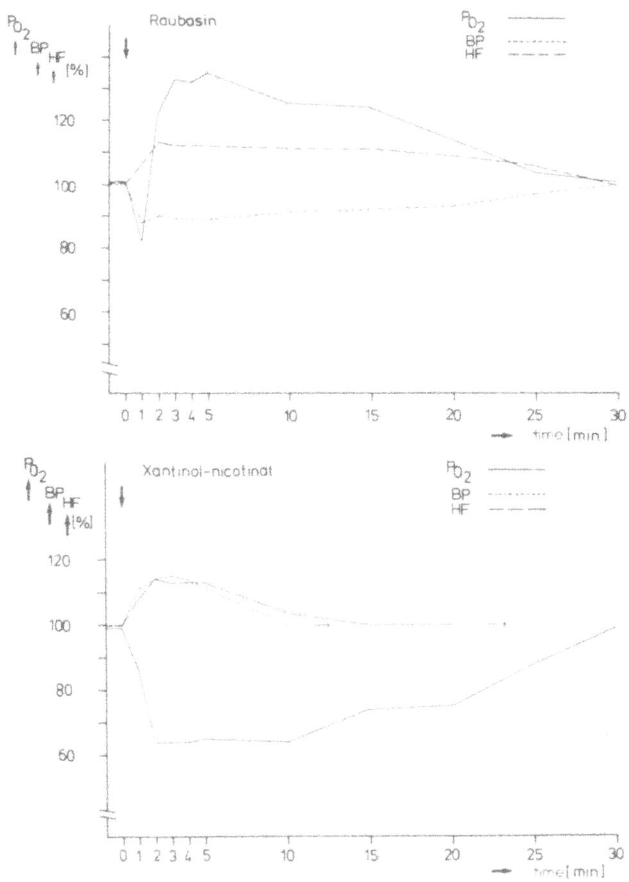

Figure 2. a/b: Changes of tissue PO_2, heart rate (HF) and blood pressure (BP) after application of Raubasin and Xantinolnicotinate

Biophysics Corporation, California) and expiratory CO_2 by an infra-ultra-red-adsorption spectrometer (URAS), Hartmann & Braun, Frankfurt/Main. Heart-rate and respiration rate were analyzed by frequency conversion from expiratory CO_2 changes and blood pressure.

After registration of steady state initial values (not before 30 minutes after application of the barbiturate), the drugs to be tested were injected intravenously in a dosage of 5 mg/kg body weight for Xantinol-nicotinate and 0.15 mg/kg body weight for Raubasin with an injection time of not less than 5 seconds.

Similar studies were also performed in three monkeys (Macca speciosa). The monkeys had undergone surgical opening of the skull cap with implantation of a screw with a 0.8 cm hole some weeks before measurement. For the measurements the awake monkeys were put into a monkey chair. Cannulas were inserted into an arm vein and into the arteria radialis; the plastic cover over the hole of the skull cap screw was removed and the microelectrodes were driven into the cortex of the fully awake and not-premedicated animal. For this purpose the electrodes were fixed to a microdrive inserted into the hole of the skull cap screw (Wells Micromanipulator, Set 457). After registration of the initial values for 15 minutes, the drugs were injected in a dosage corresponding to the above. Blood pressure and heart rate were continuously controlled and arterial blood gases in 1 minute intervals by an JL-microblood gas analyzer (Instrumentation Laboratory, Inc., Boston, Mass., U.S.A.).

<u>Results</u>:

<u>Xantinol-nicotinate</u> has been tested in 15 adult rats and 3 monkeys. After intravenous application of Xantinol-nicotinate, the PO_2 in the rat cortex decreased to a value 40% below the initial value. The decrease developed with a time delay of 30 seconds. Despite the decrease of the PO_2, systolic and diastolic blood pressure and heart rate increased by 10 to 15 per cent. While blood pressure and heart rate normalized very quickly, the PO_2 depression was maintained for more than 30 minutes, although a slow, continuous recovery of the PO_2 began 2 minutes after the injection. The changes of the tissue PO_2 after Xantinol-nicotinate were statistically significant (fig. 2a).

In five rats, H_2-clearance was performed after application of Xantinol-nicotinate. The H_2-clearance was unchanged in two experiments, in one experiment slightly increased and in 2 further experiments slightly longer. The changes remained within the control range (fig. 3a).

In the 3 monkeys Xantinol-nicotinate proved to depress the cortical PO_2 slightly. The change was less than in the rats. The recovery time was about the same (fig. 4), whereas arterial blood gases did not change.

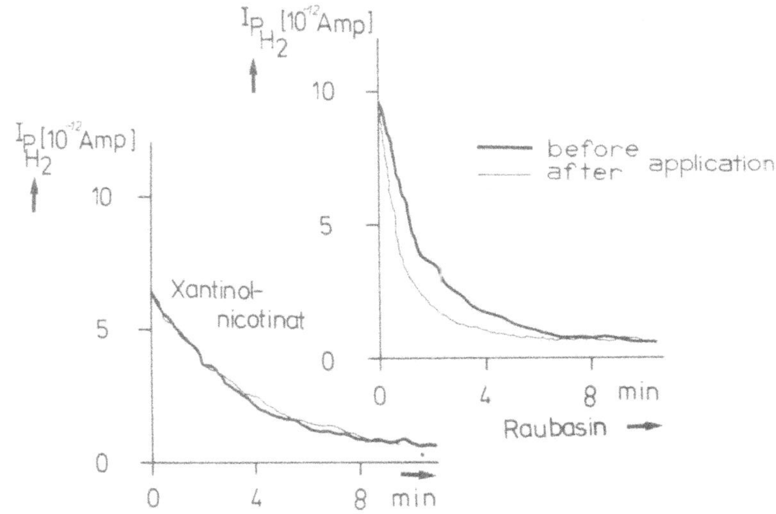

Figure 3. a/b: Changes of H_2-Clearance after application of Xantinolnicotinate and Raubasin

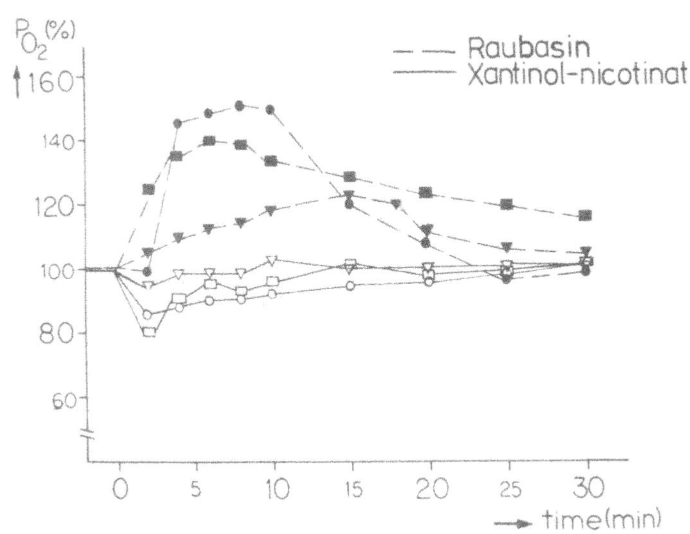

Figure 4: Changes of Tissue-PO_2 after application of Raubasin and Xantinolnicotinate in the parietal cortex of 3 monkey experiments

Raubasin was tested for its effect of the oxygen supply of the tissue in 15 rats and for its effect on tissue perfusion in 5 additional rats. After injection of Raubasin the PO_2 showed a brief decrease, recovered 2 minutes after the application and reached a value 25% above the initial value 1 minute later. This significantly increased tissue PO_2 value remained high over 15 minutes and then slowly decreased to reach the initial value 30 minutes after the application. The blood pressure did not show corresponding changes, fell down to 10% below the initial, and recovered only 25 minutes after application. Heart frequency showed an opposite effect with an increase of about 15%. In the mean the PO_2 increase after Raubasin reached its maximal value with 30-40% above the initial value between the 3rd and 5th minute after application. The above-described effects were highly significant (fig. 2b).

As with Xantinol-nicotinate, also for Raubasin, H_2-clearance curves were registered in 5 animals. In all 5 animals the time constant of clearance was significantly shortened which proved an increase of tissue perfusion (fig. 3b).

In all 3 monkey experiments, Raubasin increased tissue oxygenation decisively with a subsequent long-lasting slowly decreasing slope (fig. 4). No significant blood gas changes were seen.

Discussion:

The described results have been obtained in a series of rat studies with control studies in several monkeys to prove that the achieved data are transferable to the primate. The experiments reveal significant effects on the tissue PO_2. In the cortex the statistically achieved results in rats could be proved by control studies in monkeys.

Xantinol-nicotinate does not increase but reduces the PO_2 in the intercapillary tissue. This happens without a significant change in microperfusion. Also there were no changes of blood pressure which could explain this effect. Our results coincide with those described by Kuemmerle, et.al. (1973) who did not see a significant increase of cerebral circulation, except peripheral. The effect on the skin is known for nicotinate acid. The theophillin component, however, should lead to a decrease of cerebral circulation due to its vessel resistance increasing effect. This effect, however, seems not to be relevant in the combination with nicotinate. The reason for the decrease in tissue PO_2 in response to Xantinol-nicotinate may be an increase in local O_2 consumption as shown by Brenner, et.al. (1972).

Raubasin induced an increase of tissue perfusion simultaneously with a corresponding increase of tissue PO_2. The transient depression of PO_2 may be due to the depression of the blood pressure which was not immediately compensated for by autoregulation. In the second minute there is perceived the increase of tissue perfusion directly produced by Raubasin. A similar effect of Raubasin on total cerebral blood flow has been demonstrated in previous experiments (references in: Braun, 1975). The depression of the blood pressure could be due to the sympatholytic effect of reduction of tissue catecholamines, according to Kuschinsky (1970) and Kuemmerle (1973).

These experimental findings demonstrate that the effect of substances which should change the supply of autoregulated brain tissue is very unpredictable. Xantinol-nicotinate seems to increase metabolic rate (Brenner, et.al., 1972) and therefore oxygen consumption, without a corresponding increase of tissue-perfusion. A relative hypoxia of intercapillary tissue PO_2 is the consequence. Raubasin seems not to affect tissue-metabolism significantly but induces an increase in tissue-perfusion and thus a relative increase of tissue-oxygenation.

REFERENCES

Braun, W.: Vergleichende Untersuchungen zum interkapillaeren corticalen Sauerstoff druckverhalten nach Gabe von Xantinol-nicotinat und Delta-Yohimbin, Messungen in vivo unter Vervendung von Gold-Mikroelektroden. Med. Diss., Mainz, 1975.

Brenner, G. and Brenner, H.: Ueber die Einwirkung von Xantinol-nicotinat auf den Stoffwechsel des Gehims. Tierexperimentelle Untersuchungen ueber die Beeinflussung der Glucose-C^{14}-Permeation und der Pyridin-und Adenin-Nucleotide. Arzneimittelforschung (Drug. Res.) 22, 754-759, 1972.

Erdmann, W.: Pathophysiologie der Sauerstoffversorgung des Gehirns bei Mononarkosen mit intravenous applizierbaren Anaesthetika. Med. Habil., Mainz, 1973.

Erdmann, W., Kunke, S., Krell, W.: Tissue-PO_2 and Cell Function. An experimental study with Multimicroelectrodes in the Rat Brain. In: Oxygen Supply. Eds. Kessler, et.al. Urban & Schwarzenberg, München-Berlin-Wien, 1973.

Erdmann, W. and Kunke, S.: Changes of oxygen supply to the tissue following intravenous application of anaesthetic drugs. In: Oxygen Transport to Tissue. Eds. Bicher, H. I. and Bruley, D. F. Plenum Publishing Company, New York, 1973.

Heidenreich, J., Erdmann, W., Metzger, H. and Thews, G.: Local Hydrogen-Clearance and PO_2-Measurements in Micro-Areas of the Rat Brain. Experientia 26, 257-259, 1970.

Kuemmerle, H. P., Garrett, E. R., Spitzy, K. H.: Klinische Pharmakologie und Pharmakotherapie. Urban & Schwarzenberg, München-Berlin-Wien, 1973.

Kuschinsky, G.: Taschenbuch der moderness Arzneibehandlung und angewandten Pharmakologie. Georg Thieme Verlag, Stuttgart, 1970.

Puppe-Erdmann, B.: Mikrofluometrische Bestimmungen der Acridin Orange-Bindungskapazitaet von Leber-parenchym- und Nierentubuluszellkernen in Abhaengig Keit vom Lebensalter. Med. Diss., Mainz, 1973.

Puppe, K. P.: Bindungskapazitaet der Acridin Orange in Abhaengigkeit rom Lebensalter bei GroB-und Kleinhirnzellen der Meerschweinchen. Med. Diss., Mainz, 1971.

SUMMARY OF DISCUSSION – SESSION VII: OXYGEN SUPPLY OF THE CENTRAL NERVOUS SYSTEM

Chairmen: A.G.B. Kovach and H. I. Bicher

Paper of Drs. Reneau et al.

Meldon: Is electroneutrality maintained?
Reneau: Yes.

Lubbers: Can you predict the effect of H^+ transport?
Reneau: We are incorporating this into our studies.

Metzger: What is the connection between action potential and anaerobic glycolysis?
Reneau: We are predicting changes in a resting membrane potential, not action potentials.

Siesjo: Does your model consider an electrogenic Na-K pump?
Reneau: Yes, the Na^+/K^+ ratio is 1.6.
Siesjo: Does your model distinguish between glia cells and nerve cells?
Reneau: Not at present. However, the model is general and applicable to different types of cells provided data is available.

Bicher: Can the K^+ leak be any other than energy breakdown.
Reneau: Perhaps. Total membrane disintegration would be one example.

Paper of Drs. Ogilvie et al.

Nemoto: How many animals were used to establish the pattern of neuropathological change observed as a result of high oxygen pressure?

Ogilvie: Dr. Ballentine, I think, tabulated the data from a total of about 80 rats. It is different from the pattern of damage observed from anoxia which has cortical neuropathology. I do not think that there really is a particular pattern for ischemic anoxic brain damage. We have now subjected numerous monkeys to ischemic anoxia and there is quite a large variability in the areas damaged from monkey to monkey. In some, severe cortical damage is observed with variable basal ganglia and midbrain damage. On the other hand, in some, little cortical damage is found.

Jobsis: Did you make stepwise compressions holding at each step and correlating the rise in TpO_2?

Ogilvie: We have not done a series of experiments to show this. However, this was done in at least one animal as I recall. The rises in pO_2 were similar to the rapid compression except they were less. Each elevation began to decline toward baseline in the manner seen in rapid compression to 60 P.S.I.G.

Rink: May values in the spinal cord be due to diffusion?

Ogilvie: Certainly not the initial rise and peaking of pO_2 to high values, because postmortem pO_2 elevations did not begin until 4 minutes after compression was accomplished, and these values only reached their peaks in 8 minutes. These postmortem elevations occurred in two of the severe animals studied and only in the spinal cord. In these two rats the beginning of a quasi plateau on the falling on the pO_2 in the spinal cord was at about 8 minutes after compression which correlates in time with the maximum elevation of pO_2 in these animals during postmortem compression at 60 P.S.I.G. with pure oxygen. No quasi plateau in the falling slope of spinal cord pO_2 was observed in the other 5 animals.

Tannick: How dependent is neurological damage on exposure time and pressure? Some patients are exposed to 3 atmospheres during such procedures as radiotherapy and oxygenation of gas gangrene.

Ogilvie: There is much variation in the susceptibility of animals and man to toxicity with oxygen at high pressure. It is of interest to note that J. D. Balentine has produced central necrosis of the spinal cord in rats exposed to 3 atmospheres of pure oxygen continuously for five hours. R. E. Whalen reported oxygen toxicity in two of ten human subjects breathing pure oxygen at 3.4 atmospheres. One developed the symptoms of anxiety, mild nausea and paresthesias of the lips followed by a grand mal seizure in 24 minutes while the other developed symptoms within 14 minutes.

Lubbers: Where was the reference electrode?
Ogilvie: Between the periosteum and muscle.
Lubbers: The reference should be in brain tissue to avoid influence of D.C. Potentials.

Paper of Drs. Bicher et al.

Lubbers: I would like to make the following points: 1) We have discussed the problem of calling the prescribed reactions "pO_2 autoregulation" several times and agreed on the important points. As I remember, our results differ only in the respect that we report that we reach "zero pO_2" during anoxia whereas you are not sure of it. Nevertheless, I prefer to call these reactions just "local pO_2 regulations" in a more descriptive manner, since we do not know how some of these reactions are brought about. 2) You showed a simple scheme of a possible local O_2 regulation. After our experiments, the scheme must be more complex, since we found a quick reaction, which should take place in the arterial part of the system and a slower reaction which is possibly caused by secondary processes of the tissue. The quick regulation can be abolished by tissue anoxia, and is re-established shortly after return to a sufficient arterial oxygen tension, whereas the slower reaction should have two parts. One is directly influenced by the arterial pO_2, whereas the other one is influenced by the state of tissue oxygenation. This local signal is distributed in the tissue and may reach the regulatory vessel by diffusion or probably the capillary itself is involved in the transmission process.

Bicher: 1) As you pointed out, Professor Lubbers, we agree on most of the important points in our conception of the processes controlling the levels of TpO_2 in tissue. As for the semantic question, probably calling this process local pO_2 regulation will avoid further misunderstandings. As for the question if TpO_2 falls to zero within a few seconds after N_2 breathing, we prove it one way or the other. 2) The idea that the "overshoot" phase may depend on a slower, perhaps metabolic process is appealing, and certainly deserves elucidation in the future. As for the location of the tissue pO_2 receptor the matter is certainly open to speculation at this time. The "receptor" could be an anatomical unit, a physicochemical process or perhaps a synaptic membrane mechanism.

Siesjo: I was a bit worried by two things. First, when you give drugs that alter the "recovery" of pO_2, many of them seem to decrease blood pressure appreciably. Wouldn't that by itself alter the recovery? Second, in general, wouldn't you expect that the recovery is influenced by such factors as the blood pressure that will determine the rate of perfusion after hypoxia? In other words, there must be mechanisms operating outside the tissue that determine pO_2 in the tissue, especially if this has been exposed to hypoxia.

Bicher: Your two points seem to center around the effect of lowering blood pressure on reoxygenation times. We have shown that when blood pressure is lowered by other means (e.g. ganglion blocking agents) the reoxygenation time is not altered.

Honig: Two factors may introduce some degree of non-specificity into results with anti-adrenergic agents: 1) Blood pressure falls, which may induce vasodilation in cerebral levels. This would decrease the extent to which flow can be further increased (law of initial value). 2) Anti-adrenergic drugs influence Ca^{++} responsiveness to any baramotor stimulus. We should keep in mind, that neural and metabolic mechanisms may co-exist. As Prof. Lubbers has just suggested, a rapidly acting mechanism, presumably neural may be followed by a slower, longer lasting, presumably metabolic mechanism.

Bicher: Very good comment, Carl. It certainly may be so. We are just trying to point out that there is an organ regulation of TpO_2, and that there is a neural mechanism that certainly does not exclude a metabolic or a systemic cardiovascular function working in the same direction. As for the changes in systemic blood pressure, I have answered that to Dr. Siesjo.

Kovach: Have you measured the blood and tissue pCO_2 after phenoxybenzamine administration?

Bicher: We have monitored the blood pCO_2 after phenoxybenzamine, and found it unchanged. We did not measure tissue pCO_2.

Dora: How has the cortical electrical activity changed after giving such a big amount (50 mg/Kg) of dibenzyline.

Bicher: We understand that this drug has some local anesthetic effect. The EEG rhythm sometimes slowed followed the dibenzyline injection.

Oxygen Supply of Different Organs

OXYGEN SUPPLY TO THE OPEN RABBIT CORNEA

R.E. Barr, V.G. Murphy, E.L. Roetman and M.B. Hennessey

Departments of Ophthalmology & Mathematics
and The Dalton Research Center
University of Missouri
Columbia, Missouri 65201 U.S.A.

INTRODUCTION. The cornea is composed of three principal cellular layers, the epithelium, stroma and endothelium. Each layer requires oxygen in sufficient amount for aerobic metabolism to occur at some minimum level if normal corneal transparency is to be maintained over any extended time period. It has been well established that the surrounding limbal circulation supplies little, if any, oxygen to the central portion of the cornea. Thus, oxygen must be supplied from the atmosphere, in the case of an open eye, and/or the aqueous humor in the anterior chamber.

The cornea lends itself to a simple mathematical model, as a first approximation, in describing oxygen diffusion through it.[1] This model is that of a plane sheet, infinite in two dimensions, to which is applied the standard diffusion equation based on Fick's law. With this model, two parameters must be considered in deriving an oxygen tension profile through the cornea, the oxygen consumption rate, Q, and oxygen permeability, Dk (the product of corneal oxygen diffusivity, D, and Henry's law constant, k). Ideally, these parameters must be known for each corneal layer.

For more than a decade, work, both experimental and theoretical, by Dr. Irving Fatt with collaborators and students at the University of California, Berkeley has dealt with the problem of oxygen diffusion through the cornea. Based on sketchy data from earlier experiments,[2,3] an oxygen tension profile was calculated[1] for the cornea using a three compartment model, where each compartment represented one of the three principal corneal layers. The result of this calculation for the open eye is shown in Fig. 1, curve A. Recently, more detailed and sophisticated ex-

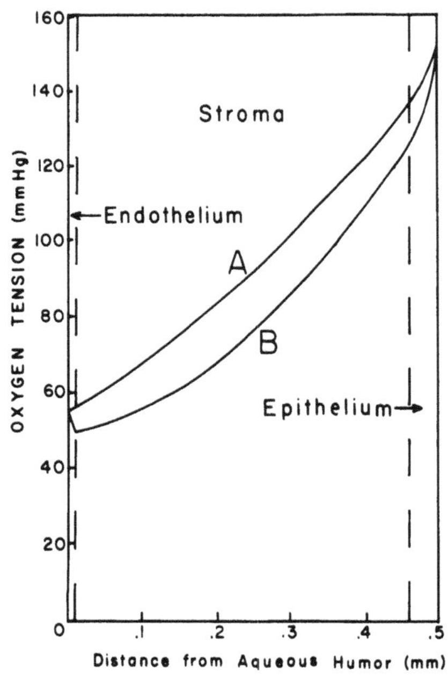

Figure 1. Oxygen tension profiles through the human cornea. Curve A is from reference 1 and curve B is from reference 6.

periments[4,5] and the ensuing theoretical analysis[6] have produced the oxygen tension profile indicated by curve B of Fig. 1.

There is one significant difference between the two curves shown in Fig. 1. Curve A implies oxygen into the endothelium is supplied by the air at the corneal surface, whereas, curve B implies oxygen into the endothelium is supplied by the aqueous humor of the anterior chamber. Since the endothelium is of paramount importance in maintaining normal corneal hydration, and hence transparency,[7,8] it is of interest to properly understand how endothelial aerobic metabolism is affected by wearing contact lenses, by closing eyelids for extended periods and by other conditions that drastically change the oxygen tension at the anterior corneal surface. The initial step in developing this understanding is to know where oxygen for the endothelium comes from under normal open eye conditions.

It would seem that curve B of Fig. 1 would represent a reasonable physiological situation whereby oxygen to the endothelium is not markedly affected by environmental conditions at the anterior surface of the cornea. However, recent work in our laboratory and a careful analysis of Freeman's[4] experimental data tend to contradict the situation depicted by curve B.

METHODS AND RESULTS. The data we have collected are the results of three sets of experiments. The first two sets of experiments involved measuring oxygen tension changes in the anterior chamber aqueous humor under in vivo conditions. The third set of experiments made use of an in vitro simulation of normal corneal conditions, whereby oxygen tension gradients were measured in an agar mold behind the cornea.

In all experiments a platinum (70%)-iridium (30%) oxygen microelectrode was employed to detect oxygen tension levels. The measuring electrode was polarized at -0.7 volts with respect to a Ag-AgCl reference electrode. Electrodes for the in vivo experiments were pre-poisoned in aqueous humor before calibration.

All experiments made use of rabbit corneas. The rabbits were New Zealand white rabbits weighing between two and three kilograms. For the in vivo experiments rabbits were anesthetized with

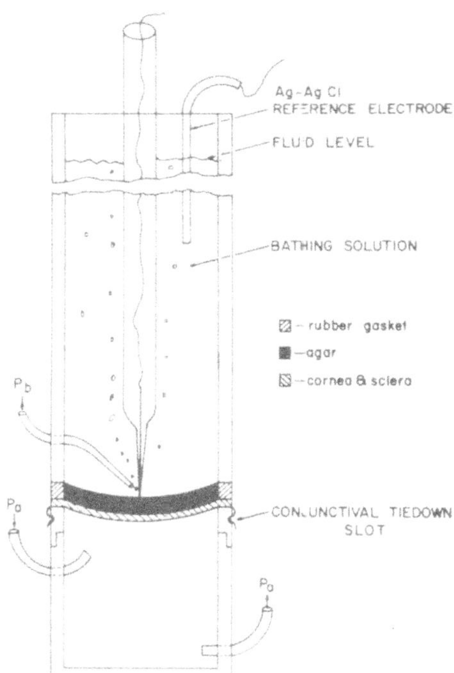

Figure 2. In vitro test chamber for determining oxygen flux directions through the cornea.

sodium pentabarbital, administered through an ear vein cannula, 20 mg/kg initially, followed by maintenance doses every 10 to 15 minutes thereafter. The rabbits' heads were rigidly fixed in a stereotaxic headholder, eyelids were retracted with hemostats and an electrode, mounted on a micromanipulator, was inserted into the anterior chamber at a point about one millimeter behind the limbus from the direction of the lateral canthus. The electrode tip was positioned close to the anatomical axis of the eye.

In the *in vitro* experiments, corneas with a scleral rim were carefully extracted from eyes of rabbits terminated by an overdose of Nembutal. The cornea was placed on a preset sterile agar mold and its thickness measured using an electrode mounted to a micromanipulator. The cornea and agar mold were then mounted in a chamber, as diagrammed in Fig. 2. The top chamber was filled with a Krebs bicarbonate Ringer's solution adjusted to pH of 7.4. The height of the column produced a pressure of about 12 mmHg at the cornea. A pointed oxygen microelectrode was inserted down the column and into the agar mold. The Ringer's solution was equilibrated at various oxygen pressures while the chamber below the cornea was continuously flushed with moist air. The chamber was surrounded by a waterjacket which was maintained at 36°C.

The first set of experiments was conducted on *in vivo* corneas. The experimental protocol was one of measuring oxygen tension changes in the anterior chamber aqueous as environmental changes were made at the corneal surface. The changes that were made and the results obtained are shown in Table 1.[9]

Table 1. Changes in the oxygen tension of rabbit eye aqueous in relation to various environmental conditions at the surface of the cornea. Shown are mean values ± one standard deviation with range of measurements in parentheses.

Environmental Conditions	Absolute Values (mm Hg)
A. Normal open eye	32.1 ± 9.0 (22.0 - 48.0)
B. Contact lens	9.6 ± 4.5 (3.9 - 16.7)
C. Cellophane	9.0 ± 4.5 (4.2 - 16.1)
D. Closed lids	8.7 ± 4.5 (1.9 - 14.8)
E. Nitrogen	9.6 ± 2.9 (6.4 - 14.7)
F. Air	31.8 ± 2.3 (28.9 - 34.0)
G. Oxygen	138.0 ± 32.1 (86.7 - 176.6)

The second set of experiments utilized a similar *in vivo* experimental set up as in the first set of experiments. The protocol of these experiments was to hold the eyelids open with room air at the corneal surface and to record oxygen tension values at a number of positions along the anterior-posterior axis in the anterior chamber. Typical sets of data are shown in Fig. 3. and the results of the entire set of experiments is shown in Fig. 4.[10] It is a plot of oxygen tension versus distance behind the corneal surface. A least squares analysis yielded the regression line shown, which has the equation $y = -29.5x + 75.8$.

The third set of experiments utilized the *in vitro* system and corneal preparation described above. The protocol of these experiments was to vary the oxygen concentration in the Ringer's solution above the agar mold, while maintaining air flow at the epithelial surface of the cornea, and to measure the direction of oxygen flux through the agar mold. The object was to determine that value of oxygen tension in the Ringer's solution for which the oxygen flux in the agar was zero. The results of these experiments are shown in Table 2.

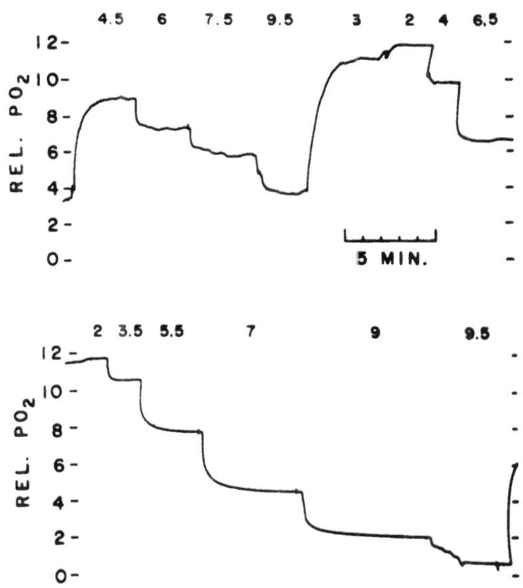

Figure 3. Illustrative sets of data showing oxygen gradients through the anterior chamber. The ordinate is relative pO_2 and the abscissa is time. Numbers at the top of each recording are electrode tip distances (in units of 0.25 mm) behind the corneal surface.

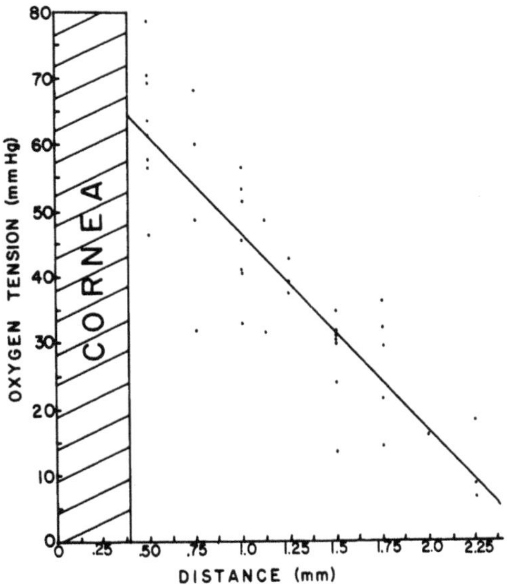

Figure 4. Oxygen tension in the anterior chamber aqueous versus distance behind the corneal surface. The regression line fits the equation $y = -29.5x + 75.8$.

DISCUSSION. Beginning with the first set of experiments, it appeared logical to infer that the only way the environmental changes could produce such a marked effect on aqueous oxygen tension was for oxygen to have been diffusing through the cornea into the aqueous humor under normal open eye conditions. This seemed to be true especially in view of the low pO_2 values obtained when oxygen was blocked from the corneal surface. But the data was not sufficient to draw a firm conclusion from it.

The establishment of an oxygen gradient through the aqueous humor of the anesthetized rabbit was serendipity in its initiation. Nevertheless, the existence of this gradient would be possible only if oxygen were diffusing through the cornea into the aqueous humor. However, it is known that barbituate anesthetics reduce blood flow to the uveal system and, therefore, it could be that in the normal state more oxygen is being supplied to the aqueous humor via the anterior uveal blood supply than is indicated by our data. In a few experiments this hypothesis was confirmed by allowing rabbits to partially arouse from a deep state of anesthesia while monitoring aqueous oxygen tension. As time after the last dose of anesthetic increased, so also did aqueous oxygen tension. Thus, the possibility existed that normal oxygen diffusion conditions through the cornea were not accurately re-

Table 2. Direction of oxygen flux across the endothelial surface for various values of oxygen tension in the Ringer's solution.

Oxygen Flux	Out of Cornea	Zero Net Flux	Into Cornea
Solution pO_2	95.9	102.5	106.8
S.D.	7.1	5.5	6.1
N	35	28	35

presented by conclusions drawn from the aqueous oxygen gradient data.

Although the main purpose for performing the in vitro set of experiments does not belong in this presentation, the results of that study are very pertinent and permit a final conclusion to be made concerning the source of oxygen for the cornea, especially the endothelium. It has been demonstrated mathematically that the direction of oxygen flux in the agar mold corresponds to the direction of oxygen flux at the endothelial-agar surface. In particular, when the net oxygen flux through the agar is zero, the net oxygen flux across the endothelial surface is zero. As shown in Table 2, the net oxygen flux through the agar, and hence across the endothelial-agar surface was zero at about 102 mmHg. The most important aspect of this value is that it is as high as or higher than normal arterial oxygen tension, therefore, it would be impossible for the blood to supply oxygen to the endothelium via the aqueous humor.

As a concluding comment of this discussion, it can be seen from part of Freeman's data,[4] that essentially the same oxygen tension level, c. 98 mmHg, was found for a zero oxygen flux condition at the endothelial surface under markedly different experimental conditions.

In summary, three sets of experiments have been performed which, together, lead to the concrete conclusion that all three principal layers of the cornea receive oxygen from the air under normal open eye conditions in rabbits.

REFERENCES

1. Fatt, I. and M. T. Bieber (1968), The Steady-State Distribution of Oxygen and Carbon-Dioxide in the In Vivo Cornea. I. The Open Eye in Air and the Closed Eye. Exp. Eye Res. 7:103-112.

2. Takahashi, G. H. and I. Fatt (1965), The Diffusion of Oxygen in the Cornea. Exp. Eye Res. 4:4-12.

3. Takahashi, G. H., I. Fatt, snd T. K. Goldstick (1966), Oxygen Consumption Rate of Tissue Measured by a Micropolarographic Method. J. Gen. Physiol. 50:317-335.

4. Freeman, R. D. (1972), Oxygen Consumption by the Component Layers of the Cornea. J. Physiol. 225:15-32.

5. Freeman, R. D. and I. Fatt (1972), Oxygen Permeability of the Limiting Layers of the Cornea. Biophys. J. 12:237-247.

6. Fatt, I., R. D. Freeman and D. Lin (1974), Oxygen Tension Distributions in the Cornea: A Re-examination. Exp. Eye Res. 18:357-365.

7. Maurice, D. M. (1972), The Location of the Fluid Pump in the Cornea. J. Physiol. 221:43-54.

8. Dikstein, S. and D. M. Maurice (1972). The Active Control of Corneal Hydration. Israel. J. Med. Sci. 8:1523-1530.

9. Barr, R. E. and I. A. Silver (1973), Effects of Corneal Environment on Oxygen Tension in the Anterior Chambers of Rabbits. Invest. Ophthal. 12:140-144.

10. Barr, R. E. and E. L. Roetman (1974), Oxygen Gradients in the Anterior Chamber of Rabbits. Invest. Ophthal. 13:386-389.

STUDIES ON RETINAL OXYGENATION

M. Tsacopoulos, R. Baker and S. Levy

Clinique Universitaire d'Ophtalmologie
Geneva, Switzerland.

Mammalian retina is partially vascularized. The capillaries, supplied by the central retinal artery, extend as deep as the inner nuclear layer, while the outer layers remain avascular. However, the photoreceptor's inner segment contains huge mitocondriae. This fact indicates intense oxidative activity at this level, and the oxygen used for this process presumably diffuses from choriocapillaries through the Bruch's membrane. This particular mode of oxygenation should determine a structured metabolism based on a combination of oxidative and anaerobic capacity.

There is no experimental data providing information about the oxygenation and respiration characteristics of the different retinal layers. This lack of knowledge is due, first to the complexity of accurate oxygen measurement in microareas and to the difficulty of successful introduction of Pt microelectrodes into the different retinal layers. This paper briefly describes the technique for making PO2 microelectrodes as well as the system permitting their introduction and advancement into the retina. A few examples will demonstrate the efficiency of these techniques.

METHODS

The system is described in detail in a previous paper (1). The PO2 microelectrodes are made following, in general, the technique of Baumgärtl and Lübbers (2) and Sinagowitz and Kessler (3). However, our technique of bevelling the microelectrode tip is different than theirs. We use an air-driven and air-supported steel plate (80 x 20 mm), rotating with adjustable speed (depending on the air flow) without wobble. The abrasive material (alumina 0.01 μm or 1 μm) is imbedded in a thin and absolutely regular layer of polyurethane (Desmophen 1100 Desmodur HL, Bayer, Germany). The microelectrode to be bevelled is mounted on a sort of record player arm and smoothly positioned on the abrasive surface of the rotating disc. The electrode tip's electrical resistance is continuously monitored and bevelling is interrupted when the desired resistance is obtained. Electrodes after bevelling have about 1 μm tip diameter and 3-5 MΩ electrical resistance.

Microelectrodes can be introduced into the intact miniature pig's eye after the animal has been stabilized with a head holder and an ocular fixation ring. A versatile system for the introduction and manipulation of the electrode consists generally of three coaxially oriented tube-like structures which interadapt in a telescopic fashion : an illuminator is threaded into the main body of a micromanipulator, the electrode, in turn, is threaded into the fiber optics illuminator. The whole central axis therefore moves in unison as the micromanipulator is positioned or advanced by a remotely-controlled hydraulic motion operating system. Two drive jacks, angularly attached to the main body, can move the central axis within a 38° conical plane around the vertical axis. Intravitreal and transretinal vertical movements (down to 2 μm) can be executed by coarse and fine controls respectively.

RESULTS

Figure 1 shows tissue PO2 measurement with the microelectrode placed in the preretinal vitreous and then again when it is in the inner vascularized retina. In the vitreous, the PO2 is lower than in the inner retina. When the microelectrode is advanced by steps of 50 μm (or less) from the inner retina toward the choroid, a remarkable drop of tissue PO2 is recorded.

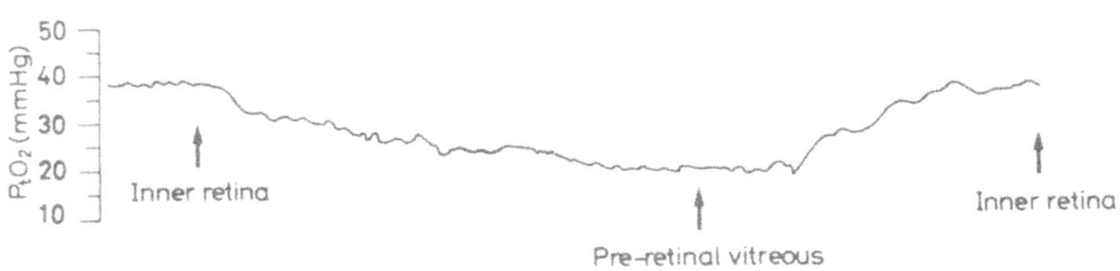

Fig. 1 : Tissue PO2 recording. For explanation, see text.

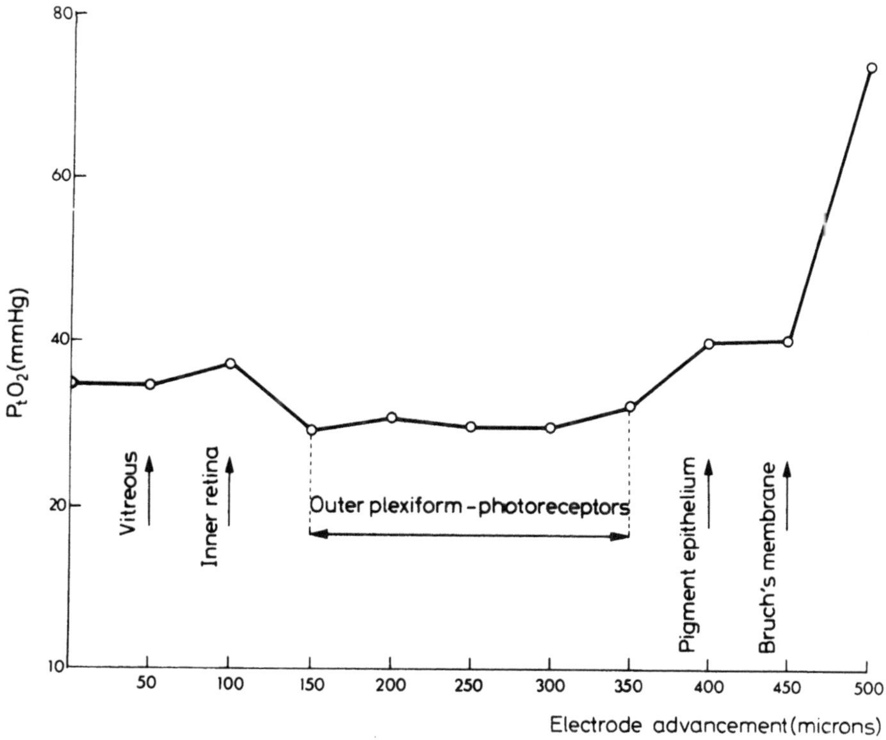

Fig. 2 : Retinal oxygenation profile. See also text.

The graph in figure 2 shows that from the outer plexiform layer to the photoreceptor's layer the tissue PO2 is lower than in the inner retina or pigment epithelium. When the microelectrode crosses the Bruch's membrane (essentially collagen tissue of 3-4 µm thickness), a dramatic increase of tissue PO2 is recorded. Bioelectrical evidence of crossing Bruch's membrane is provided by recording local electroretinogram (ERG) by the same Pt electrode. When the microelectrode was at the choroidal side of Bruch's membrane, the polarity of ERG was completely reversed (1).

Figure 3 shows an original transretinal PO2 tracing obtained by using a 2 µm tip microelectrode. After 250 µm advancement, the electrode crossed the Bruch's membrane followed by a noticeable increase of tissue PO2.

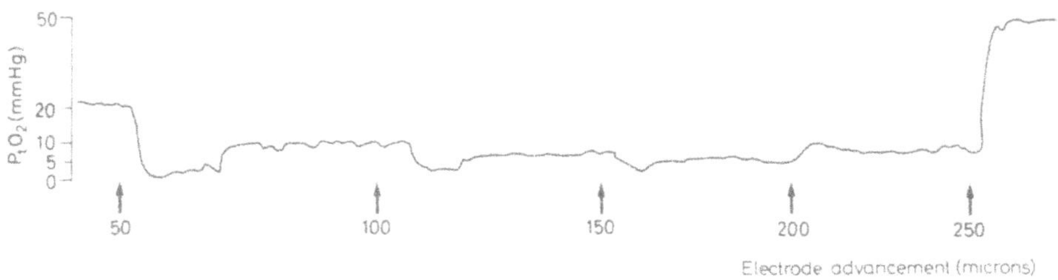

Fig. 3 : Example of transretinal PO2 recording using 2 μm tip Pt microelectrode.

DISCUSSION

The preliminary results presented here suggest that retinal oxygenation is not uniform but there are different oxygen fields. The identification of the microelectrode tip's position in the different retinal layers, in relationship to the tissue PO2 measurements, was uncertain in the experiments presented here. The shape of local retinal electrical activity in response to light is variable depending on the layer of the retina. Consequently the form of local ERG would help to identify the position of the measuring transretinal PO2 microelectrodes. Efforts to record simultaneously tissue PO2 and local ERG from the same electrodes (theoretically possible) have been unsuccessful in our laboratory, but the problem is now under extensive investigation.

The examples of transretinal PO2 recordings presented in this paper provide evidence that the system used to study the retinal oxygenation and metabolism is reliable and flexible. Further development should bring valuable information about retinal metabolism and function.

REFERENCES

1. Tsacopoulos, M., Baker, R., Levy, S. and J.L. Munoz - A versatile system for studying mammalian intraretinal metabolism and function in situ. Exp. Eye Res. 1975 (accepted for publication).

2. Baumgärtl, H. and D.W. Lübbers - Platinum needle electrode for polarographic measurement of oxygen and hydrogen. In Oxygen Supply (Eds. Kessler, M., Bruley, D.F., Clark, L.C., Lübbers, D.W., Silver, I.A. and Strauss, J.) Urban and Schwarzenberg, München 1973, pp. 130-136.

3. Sinagowitz, E. and Kessler, M. - Standardization of producing needle electrodes. In Oxygen Transport to Tissue (Eds. Bicher, H.I. and Bruley, D.F.) 37A, 23-27, Plenum Press, New York (1973).

A SYSTEM FOR IN VIVO MEASUREMENT OF OXYGEN IN INTRAOCULAR TISSUE

Robert W. Flower

The Applied Physics Laboratory and The Wilmer Ophthalmological Institute of The Johns Hopkins University and Hospital, Baltimore, Maryland, U.S.A.

INTRODUCTION

The sensory retina of the eye is unique in that it is nourished by the two separate circulations between which it lies--the retinal vasculature supplying the inner retinal layers and the choroidal vasculature supplying primarily the outer layers. The extremely high metabolic rate of retinal tissue makes it susceptible to ischemic damage when the retinal blood supply is segmentally or totally disrupted; the effect of interrupted choroidal blood supply is currently less well documented. Consequently, the relationship between individual contributions of the retinal and choroidal circulations to retinal oxygenation is fundamental to a thorough understanding of the physiology associated with ischemic eye disease. A number of investigators interested in intraocular oxygen distributions have applied the technique of polarographic oxygen measurements using microelectrodes[1,2,3...], and one has even coined the convenient term "ophthalmopolarography".[4]

Intraocular oxygen measurements with microelectrodes is particularly attractive since much of the intraocular tissue (vitreous and aqueous) is homogenous and nearly acellular making measurements in it closely approximate to those made in the normal saline generally used for electrode calibration.[5] Since the vitreous itself is almost metabolically inert, oxygen measurements made in preretinal vitreous probably closely reflect oxygen availability in the metabolically active retina whose blood supply is easily visualized and -- since the advent of laser photocoagulation -- can be somewhat manipulated. Optics of the eye readily permit observation of the inside of the globe, facilitating positioning of electrodes at least up to the vitreal-retinal interface. These attractions not withstanding, a number of problems are attendent upon performing ophthalmopolarography. Included among the more important ones are the fact that the complex interdependencies of tissue oxygenation, intraocular and blood pressures, and blood-flow dynamics are not easily kept in balance in an opened eye; presence of the electrode mass and oxygen utilization by it might produce local ischemia instead of simply detecting it, and precise electrode positioning very near or within the retina is difficult even using stereopsis.

This paper briefly describes a system developed to permit measurement of pO_2 in tissues of the intact primate eye under near-physiologic conditions and without destruction of the eye. (This last is important since it permits repeating measurements from the same eye at different times and allows for evaluation of blood-flow dynamics in the eye by standard angiographic technique following experimental procedures). The system developed as a conglomerate of methods most of which have been used individually with success in previous investigations and each of which offered the potential of overcoming some specific problem attendent upon intraocular oxygen measurement.

METHODS

As much of our work concerns the ocular effects of hyperbaric oxygenation, the equipment needed for conducting animal experiments at elevated pressures was mounted along with that for ophthalmopolarography inside a hyperbaric chamber. Methods for maintaining anesthesia, controlling respiration, and monitoring such physiological parameters as temperature, EKG, and intraocular and blood pressures while inside the chamber have been previously described.[6] The chamber provides excellent electrical shielding for polarographic measurements, and mounting the large chamber mass on isolation pads resulted in significant dampering out of building vibrations which would otherwise have caused excessive motion between the microelectrodes and the eye.

An anesthetized monkey is placed inside the hyperbaric chamber in a stereotaxic headholder which is mounted on gimbals in such a way that the monkey's body can be rotated in both horizontal and vertical planes using the pars plana of either eye as a center of rotation. A gas sterilized oxygen microelectrode, mounted in an electromechanical advancer,[7] enters the eye through a scleral puncture needle at the pars plana after the method of Brown;[8] thus, the combined motion provided by the electrode advancer and headholder allows positioning of the microelectrode in the eye using a spherical coordinate system which has the pars plana as its origin. A neutralizing contact lens placed on the cornea, permits direct visualization of the electrode tip through a telescope as long as it is in the clear vitreous; this contact lens also prevents dehydration of the cornea during experiments. Once in contact with the retina, location of the tip within the retina may be determined by local electroretinographic (LERG) activity--again after the method of Brown.[9]

At the end of an experimental session, the contact lens, microelectrode, scleral puncture needle, and reference electrode are removed from eye and the scleral flap and conjunctival opening are sutured closed. Antibiotics are administered topically and systemically. Following a recovery period of a week or two, the eye can be re-entered usually through the same openings; however, greater care must be exercised as loss of vitreous from the eye becomes more likely each time following the first entry.

The Oxygen Microelectrode

A glass insulated exposed Pt-tipped electrode (modified Model 721, Transidyne General Corp., Ann Arbor, Michigan) is used in conjunction with a small sterilized Ag/AgCl reference electrode placed under the conjunctiva. Scanning electron micrographs of a number of these electrodes indicate tip geometries to be fairly consistent. Exposed Pt tips of the microelectrodes are generally conical with rounded ends (axial length ≐ 10.5μm., base radius ≐ 3.3μm., end radius of curvature ≐ 1.2μm., and Pt surface area ≐ 170μm^2). Electrode surface areas calculated from the micrographs were compared to previously determined electrode impedances to provide a correlation by which future selection could be made of microelectrodes having dimensions within an acceptable range.[10]

The Electronic System

The flexible electronic system indicated in the block diagram of figure 1 consists of three major elements: A time-programmer, current monitor, and averaging digital voltmeter. Of these, only the current monitor is located inside of the hyperbaric chamber to minimize the lengths of leads to electrodes.

(1) Timer-programmer - The polarizing potential applied to microelectrode is a four-part sequence of stepwise potentials as indicated in figure 2 (top): First, the platinum electrode is made negative with respect to the Ag/AgCl reference electrode; then the electrode pair is shorted; next, the platinum electrode is made positive with respect to the reference electrode; and finally, the electrode pair is again shorted. The positive pulse is a "cleaning" pulse for the Pt tip, and the shorting

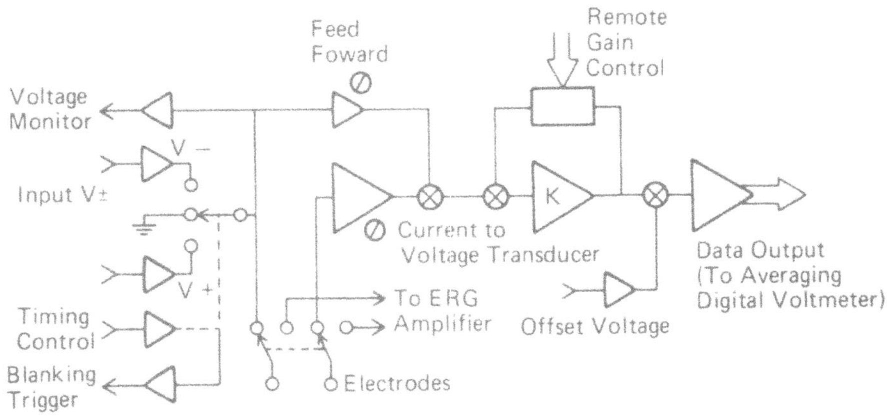

Fig. 1 Block Diagram of Electronic System

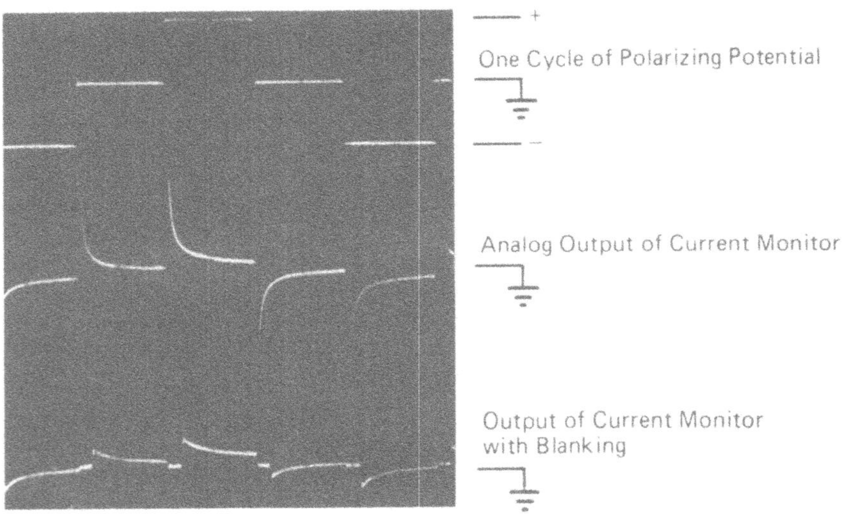

Fig. 2 Characteristic Electrical Signals

of the electrode pair after each polarizing pulse is to assure complete depolarization. The time length of each segment of the four-part sequence is independently variable (from .01 to 9.99 sec.), and the magnitudes of the positive and negative potentials are also independently variable (from 0 to 1.5 V.). This four-part sequence can be applied to the electrode pair continuously in a cyclic manner or it can be applied as a single cycle triggered to be in phase with an external signal such as the EKG.

(2) Current Monitor - The oxygen microelectrode and the Ag/AgCl reference electrode are connected by short leads to the current monitor which converts the current to an analog voltage output. In one mode of operation these leads are connected directly to the ERG preamplifier; in the other mode they are connected to the current monitoring circuitry. A polarizing potential derived from the timer-programmer is applied to the electrode pair, and the currents in the range of 10^{-9} to 10^{-6} amps can be detected. The frequency response of the current monitor is approximately d-c to 100K Hz.

When the polarizing potential is applied to the electrode circuit, there is initially a high current flow which falls off exponentially to a steady value (fig. 2, middle). The peak of this pulse can be as much as two orders of magnitude higher than the steady state value. As with the timer-programmer, the solid state circuitry of the current monitor was designed to provide very fast response times, with the high degree of accuracy and stability. The demand placed upon the operational amplifiers used in the circuitry is such that when operating at high amplification in order to record small changes in the range of steady current, the operational amplifiers must be protected from overload resulting from the initially high current flow following application of the polarizing potential. To accomplish this, a blanking period which momentarily "shuts off" the current monitor input can be programmed into the current monitor along with the polarizing potential initiated by the timer-programmer (fig. 2, bottom). With some electrodes fairly high residual currents were found to exist in calibration solutions equilibrated with N_2. When this occurred, residual current was subtracted from the current monitor output by means of a feed forward network (see figure 1) which generates a signal equal in magnitude but of opposite signs to the steady state input current and combines it with the original input current signal.

(3) Averaging Digital Voltmeter - This meter detects the analog voltage output of the current monitor, samples 100 microseconds of this voltage at any pre-selected time following application of the polarizing potential, and averages any given number of such samples.

Electrode Calibration

Electrodes are inserted through an O-ring sealed opening into a gas sterilizable plexiglas cell. The cell has a 2 ml. volume, contains an Ag/AgCl reference electrode identical to those used in the eye, and has valved entry and exit ports respectively located at the bottom and top. This calibration cell is jacketed by a second cell through which thermostatically controlled, heated water flows. (All calibrations are done at 37°C to avoid changes in electrode current resulting from a temperature differential between calibration solutions and the tissue.) The calibration cell is placed inside the hyperbaric chamber in place of the headholder, and sterile isotonic saline solutions equilibrated with humidified O_2 - N_2 gas mixtures at 37°C are sequentially introduced into the cell. Electrode calibration can be performed just prior to and immediately following each animal experiment.

RESULTS AND DISCUSSION

Of the many oxygen microelectrode configurations reported to date, the glass insulated, exposed Pt-tipped electroded seems best suited for intraocular use. It is relatively simple to construct, possesses a reasonable (but less than ideal) structural integrity, and its relatively sharp tip should penetrate the tissue layers with minimal drag and cellualr damage. Since the electrode is being used in O_2 fields which have the potential to change rather quickly, an exposed electrode tip provides better time resolution than a recessed or membrane covered electrode. In addition to making oxygen measurements, the exposed Pt tip can be used to record LERG activity which provides a good index of electrode depth in retinal tissue.[9] Since the sensory retina is approximately 300μm in thickness, the 10.5μm axial length of the electrode tip provides a reasonable spatial resolution both for oxygen measurements and LERG recordings.

Pulsatile operation of exposed oxygen electrodes with alternating potential has been employed by other investigators[11,12,13] primarily to reduce consumption of oxygen during measurements and to obviate "poisoning" of the electrode when working with proteinaceous media. In the present case, pulsatile operation also offers the advantage of making O_2 measurements between pressure pulsatile events in the eye so long as single, short pulses are used. Generally, the negative polarizing pulse as well as the positive and two shorting pulses are of 410 msec. duration with pulse amplitudes of 0.6V; electrode current can be sampled at any fixed time following application of the negative pulse. It has been shown that sampling exposed electrode current later than 200 msec. after application of the negative pulse tends to increase flow sensitivity;[13] however, since motion artifacts inside the eye are virtually negligible, this time limitation is not applicable.

A typical electrode current profile is shown in figure 3. The initial high current and rapid decay are thought to result from depletion of oxygen in the barrier layer (x) next to the electrode surface, and the steady state level of current is then limited by diffusion of oxygen into the barrier layer.[11,14] Calibration curves were made for various times along the current vs. time curves, and although all of the calibrations were repeatable and stable, those made along the rapid decay portion of the curve were not as linear as those made along the steady current part of the curve; and in agreement with earlier work,[11] the resolution of calibration curves was found to become greater as the time for measuring current after application of the polarization potential was increased.

In most biological applications of polarography, existence of the current transient resulting from application of polarization potential is undetected or ignored. Although the significance of such transient phenomena is not entirely clear, they very likely contain information about the electrode barrier layer and possibly the orientation of polar molecules within the electrostatic field of the electrode. In any event, the system described here should permit evaluation of the transient current phenomena as well as the more conventional oxygen measurements derived from steady state current flow.

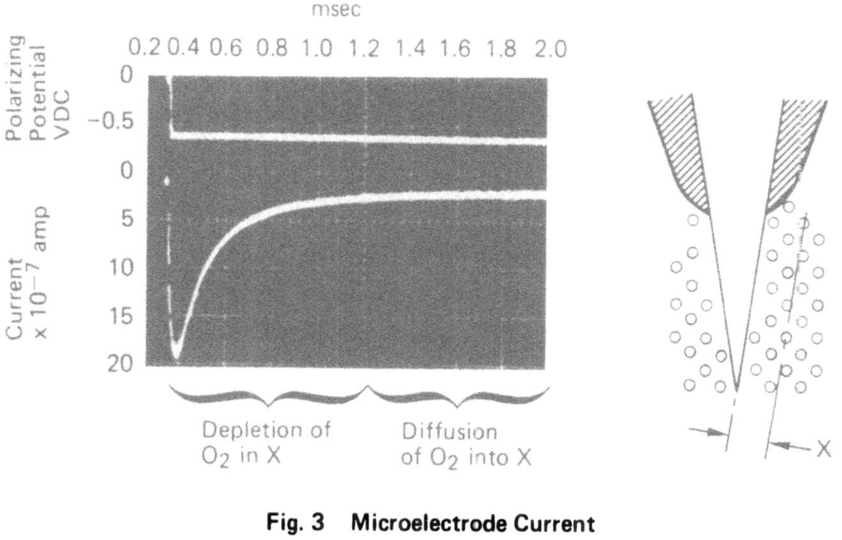

Fig. 3 Microelectrode Current

Acknowledgement: This work was supported by Grant EY-01008 of the National Eye Institute and was done at the Wilmer Institute with the cooperation of Dr. A. Patz.

REFERENCES

1. Briggs, D., Rodenhauser, J.-H.: Distribution and consumption of oxygen in the vitreous body of cats. In: Oxygen Supply, Kessler, M., Bruley, D.F., et al, 1971, University Park Press, p. 265.
2. Ernest, J. T.: In vivo measurement of optic disc oxygen tension, Invest. Ophthalmol. 12: 927, 1973.
3. Tsacopoulos, M., Baker, R., et al: The effect of arterial Pco_2 on inner-retinal oxygen availability in monkeys, Invest. Ophthalmol. 21: 449, 1973.
4. Jakovlev, A.A.: Die Untersuchung der Sauerstoff spannung in den Geweben und in Kammerwasser des Auges mit Hilfe der Polarographie, Albrecht v. Graefes Arch. klin. exp. Ophthal. 185: 108, 1972.
5. Alm, A., Bill, A.: The oxygen supply to the retina, I. Effects of changes in intraocular and arterial blood pressues, and in arterial Po_2 and Pco_2 on the oxygen tension in the vitreous body of the cat, Acta. Physiol. Scan. 84: 261, 1972.
6. Flower, R.W.: Construction of a versatile small-animal hyperbaric facility, J. Appl. Physiol. 27: 571, 1969.
7. Chubbuck, J.G.: An electromechanical micropositioner, IEEE Trans. Bio. Engr. (In press).
8. Brown, K.T.: Optical stimulator, microelectrode advancer, and associated equipment for intraretinal neurophysiology in closed mammalian eyes, J. Opt. Soc. Am. 54: 101, 1964.
9. Brown, K.T.: The electroretinogram: Its components and their origins, Vision Res. 8: 633, 1968.
10. Robinson, D.A.: The electrical properties of metal microelectrodes, Proc. IEEE, 56: 1065, 1968.
11. Olson, R.A., Brackett, F.S., et al: Oxygen tension measurement by a method of time selection using the static platinum electrode with alternating potential, J. Gen. Physiol. 32: 681, 1949.
12. Albanese, R.A., Chang, C.H., et al: Determination of the absolute oxygen tension in tissue by a new microelectrode technique. In: Hyperbaric Medicine, Brown, I.W., Cox, B.G., 1966, Publication 1404, Washington, NAS/NRC, p. 294.
13. Saulson, S.H.: High speed pulsatile operation of miniature oxygen electrodes. In: Oxygen Transport To Tissue, Bicher, H.I., Bruley, D.F., New York, 1973, Plenum Press, p. 29.
14. Longmuir, I.S.: Respiration rate of bacteria as a function of oxygen concentrations, Biochem. J. 57: 81, 1954.

THE O_2 SUPPLY OF THE ISOLATED CELL-FREE PERFUSED RAT KIDNEY

H. Franke and Ch. Weiss

Physiologisches Institut der Universität Kiel

2300 Kiel, Olshausenstr. 40/60 Germany

Compared to the organ in situ in all isolated cell-free perfused kidney preparations so far described tubular net sodium transport is considerably reduced (1, 2, 3, 4, 5). Since the active tubular transport of sodium is a basic function of the mammalian kidney a number of other dysfunctions of isolated kidneys may be caused by the reduced rate of sodium transport.

Three causal factors for the reduced net sodium transport are presently discussed: A lack of ADH and/or of aldosterone, an insufficient supply of renal substrates and an insufficient supply of O_2.

However, the addition of vasopressin and of aldosterone to the perfusion fluid of isolated kidneys in physiological and in higher concentrations exerts only small effects on net sodium transport and on the renal ability to concentrate (6, 7, 2, 8).

Raising the substrate concentrations above in situ values ROSS (9) and SCHURECK (10) reported increased rates of net sodium transport in the isolated kidney. The absolute values of net sodium transport and those of other renal functions remained, however, far below in situ values.

In the isolated rat kidney and in the isolated and the in situ dog kidney studies with the O_2-microelectrode not only revealed large pO_2-gradients in the renal cortex but also the presence of areas where the pO_2 lay below 2 - 3 Torr (11,12). It is reasonable to assume

that in these areas small decreases of the O_2-supply lead to hypoxia. Histological analysis supports this view. We observed two types of histological alterations: In Type I the cytoplasma in the proximal tubule is less dense, the mitochondri are swollen, the basal membrane ist thickened and a large number of resorption vacuoles is present (fig. 1).

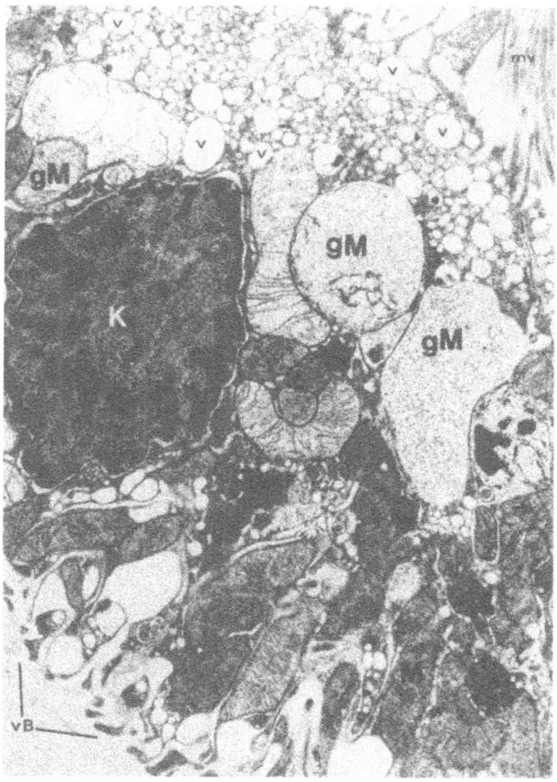

Fig. 1 Proximal tubule after 1 hr. perfusion with a medium containing hydroxy-ethyl starch. Extremely swollen mitochondria (gM). Thickened basal membrane (vB). Resorption vacuoles (v). Microvilli (mv). Mitochondria (M). Cell nucleus (K).

In type II the cytoplasma in the proximal tubule is extremely dense, cell organelles are hardly discernable. The microvilli are relatively well preserved. (fig. 2)

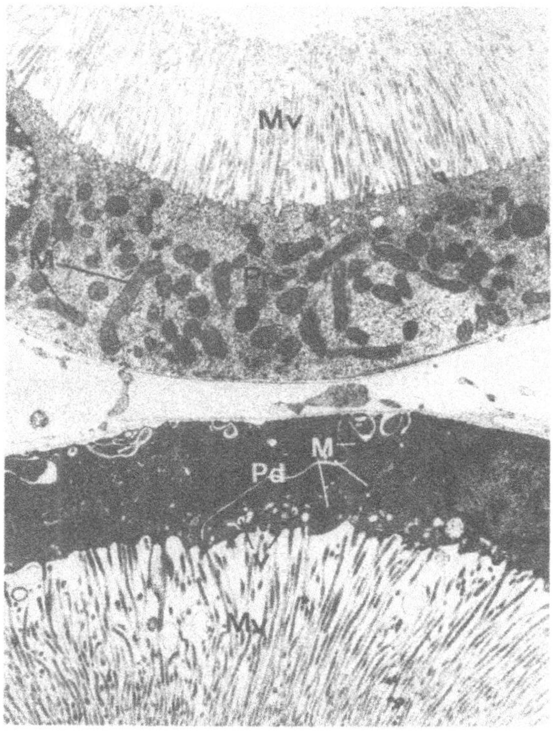

Fig. 2 Dense (Pd) and normal (Pn) proximal tubule after 60 min. perfusion with a medium containing hydroxy-ethyl starch. Microvilli (Mv). Mitochondria (M). Resorption vacuoles (v).

Both types of histological alterations have been described by several authors (13, 14) who interprete them as typical tissue reactions to hypoxia.

We observed a relationship between the abundance of these histological alterations (in the proximal tubules) and the remaining functional abilities of the isolated kidneys.

Under identical experimental conditions we perfused isolated rat kidneys either with a medium containing the gelatine derivate Haemaccel® (Behringwerke) or hydroxy-ethyl starch as colloidsosmotically active substances (tab. 1).

NaCl	118.0 mM	Na-pyruvate	2.0 mM
KCl	5.0 mM	Na-L-lactate	1.0 mM
$CaCl_2$	1.0 mM	Na-L-glutamate	0.5 mM
$MgCl_2$	0.3 mM	Na-acetate	2.0 mM
$NaHCO_3$	20.0 mM	Na-propionate	0.01 mM
Na_2HPO_4	0,84 mM	bovine albumin	2.0 g/l
KH_2PO_4	0.28 mM	insulin	4.0 i.u/l
urea	4.0 mM	^{14}C-inulin	10.0 uCi/l
D-glucose	5.0 mM		

+ (either haemaccel^R 35.0 g/l
or hydroxyethyl starch 60.0 g/l)

Table 1. Composition of the perfusion media

In the experiments with haemaccel net sodium transport lay at 75.4 uM/g x min. while in the hydroxy-ethyl starch experiments net sodium resorption amounted to 92.8 uM/g x min. Correspondingly, in the haemaccel kidneys 30 % of the proximal tubular cells showed alterations according to type I or type II while such histological changes occurred in only 15 % of these cells in the hydroxy-ethyl starch experiments (tab. 2).

	urine flow [ml/g x min]	U/P-Inulin	perfusion flow [ml/g x min]	glomerular filtration rate [ml/g x min]	Na-load [μMol/g x min]	Na-net transport [μMol/g x min]	fractional Na-reabsorption [%]	O_2-consumption [ml/g x min]	prox morph. alterations
Haemaccel n=24	0.17∓0.05	3.82∓1.22	16∓3.8	0.58∓0.17	93.2∓17.4	75.4∓16.2	80.9∓9.4	0.136∓0.02	>30%
Hydroxyethyl starch n=24	0.26∓0.08	3.43∓0.85	14∓2.1	0.85∓0.17	129∓18.4	92.8∓23.0	72.1∓12.1	0.16∓0.03	≈15%

Table 2 Functional data of isolated cell fre perfused rat kidneys. Upper column: Perfusion with haemaccel, lower column: perfusion with hydroxy-ethyl starch as colloid-osmotically active substance.

In the haemaccel experiments the perfusion rate, and thus the amount of O_2 supplied to the kidney per unit time exceeds that in the hydroxy-ethyl starch experiments. In spite of that the O_2-uptake in the hydroxy-ethyl starch experiments lies above the O_2 uptake in the haemaccel experiments. A different intrarenal distribution of the perfusing fluid with a relatively higher flow through the cortex in the hydroxy-ethyl starch experiments could explain this observation.

BOWMAN (7), LITTLE (15), ROSS (9) and TRIMBLE (16) obtained comparatively good functional data from isolated cell free perfused kidneys which were perfused with recirculating albumin containing media.

They measured perfusion rates as high as 35 ml/g x min. At such flow rates even cell free, i.e. oxygen carrier free media supply sufficient amounts of O_2.

In order to prove our contention that lack of O_2 is the main reason for the impaired function of isolated kidmeys we increased the O_2-capacity of the perfusion fluid by adding 7.9 vol. % of the fluorocarbon FC 43^R (3M Co).

75 ml FC 43^R (3M Co.) and 125 ml of a 20 % solution of the detergent Pluronic F 68^R (Wyandotte Chem. Corp.) in water were homogenized for 10 min. in a Ultraturrax homogenizer. The emulsion was further homogenized for 4 x 10 min. at a pressure of 500 atmospheres in a Gaulin homogenizer. Before the 5th homogenisation distilled water was added to a final volume of 960 ml. Subsequently the substances listed in table 1 were added with the exception of the colloidosmotically active substances. Measurement of the colloidosmotic pressure with a membrane osmometer showed that the presence of pluronic F 68^R and of the homoginzed FC 43^R provided the necessary colloidosmotic pressure of 25 Torr.

	urine flow [ml/g x min]	U/P-Inulin	perfusion flow [ml/g x min]	glomerular filtration rate [ml/g x min]	Na-load [µMol/g x min]	Na-net transport [µMol/g x min]	fractional Na-reabsorption [%]	O_2-consumption ml/g x min]
FC 43 n=30	0.25∓0.08	4.5∓1.32	18.8∓5.12	1.06∓0.24	168∓33	149∓32.4	88.5∓4.74	0.295∓0.03

Table 3 Functional data of rat kidneys perfused with emulsified fluorocarbon FC 43^R

Table 3 lists the measured functional parameters of an isolated kidney perfused with emulsified FC 43^R. At a tubular Na-load of 168 uM/g x min. 149 uM/g x min. were resorbed, corresponding to 88.5 % of the load. The O_2 consumption lay at 0.295 m/g x min., significantly higher than in all previous experiments.

Fig. 3 shows the relationship between net sodium resorption, tubular sodium load and percentage sodium resorption for fluorocarbon and for hydroxy-ethyl starch experiments. In the former at physiological tubular sodium loads of 150 uM/g x min. 93 % of the load were resorbed while in the latter at comparable loads only 72 % were resorbed.

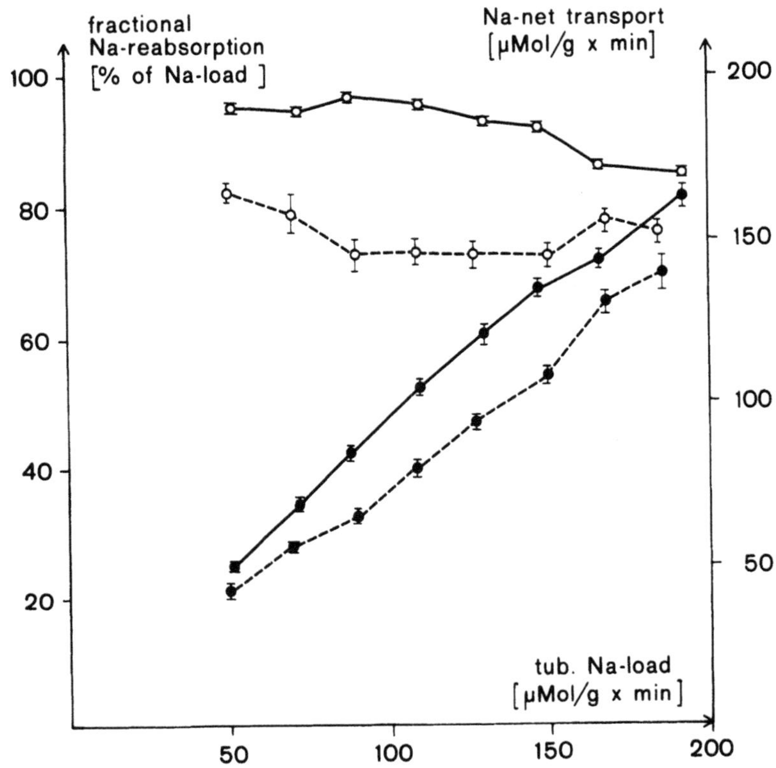

Fig. 3 Fractional Na-resorption (left ordinate), net sodium transport (right ordinate) versus tubular sodium load. Isolated rat kidneys perfused with a medium containing the fluorocarbon FC 43^R (solid lines), and kidneys perfused with hydroxy-ethyl starch as colloidosmotically active substance (broken lines). Full circle curves: net sodium transport. Open circle curves: fractional sodium resorption. Hydroxy-ethyl starch: n = 24. FC 43^R : n = 30.

The O_2 consumption of the fluorocarbon experiments is very high. However, extrapolation of the straight line relationship between net sodium resorption and suprabasal O_2-consumption from studies with haemaccel and hydroxy-ethyl starch containing media fits the O_2 uptake values of the FC 43^R experiments. Addition of the decoupling agent fluoryl-carbonyl-m-chloro-phenyl-hydrazine to haemaccel media doubled the O_2 uptake of isolated rat kidneys, thus speaking against a spontaneous decoupling in the FC 43 experiments.

The results presented support our contention that lack of O_2 is one of the main reasons for the dysfunction of isolated cell free perfused mammalian kidneys.

References

(1) Cuypers, Y., Nizet, A., Baerten, A.: Technique pour la perfusion de reins isolês de chien avec du sang heparinê. Arch. Inter. Physiol. Biochem. 72,245 (1964)

(2) Franke, H., Huland, H., Weiss, Ch., Unsicker, K.: Improved net sodium transport of the isolated rat kidney. Z.Ges. exp. Med. 156, 268 (1971)

(3) Huland, H., Seitz, H.J., Tarnowski, W., Weiss, Ch.: The fuels of respiration of the isolated perfused rat kidney. Life Sciences 14, 117 (1974)

(4) Schurek, H.J., Brecht, J.P., Lohfert, H., Hierholzer, K.: The basic requirements for the function of the isolated cell free perfused rat kidney. Pflügers Arch. (im Druck)

(5) Waugh, W.H., Kubo, T.: Development of an isolated perfused dog kidney with improved function. Amer. J. Physiol. 217, 277 (1969)

(6) Bahlmann, J., Giebisch, G., Ochwadt, B., Schöppe,W.: Micropuncture study of isolated perfused rat kidney. Amer. J. Physiol. 212, 77 (1967)

(7) Bowman, R.H., Maack, T.: Effect of albumine concentration and ADH on H_2O and electrolyte transport in perfused rat kidney. Amer. J. Physiol. 226, 426, (1974)

(8) Michael, U.F., Barenberg, R.L., Chavez, R., Vaamonde, C.A., Pappers, S.: Renal handling of sodium and water in the hypothyroid rat. Clearance and micropuncture studies. J. Clin. Invest. 51 1405 (1972)

(9) Ross, B.d., Epstein, F.H. and Leaf, A.: Sodium reabsorption in the perfused rat kidney. Amer. J. Physiol. 225, 1165 (1973)

(10) Schurek , H.J., Brecht, J.Pl, Brand, P., Lange, K., Kolbe, H., Keller, K.: Substrate action on transport and metabolism of the isolated perfused rat kidney (Action of pyruvate oxaloacetate, butyrate and succinate). In: Sympos. Biochem. aspects of renal function. Salzburg Ed. by M. Hohenegger, 110, Goldmann-Verlag München (1972)

(11) Leichtweiss, H.P., Lübbers, D.W., Weiss, Ch., Baumgärtl, H., Reschke, W.: The oxygen supply of the rat kidney measurements of intrarenal pO_2. Pflügers Arch. 309, 328 (1969)

(12) Baumgärtl., H., Leichtweiss, H.-P., Lübbers , D.W. Weiss, Ch., Huland, H.: The oxygen supply of the dog kidney: measurements of intrarenal pO_2. Microvasc. Res. 4, 247 (1972)

(13) Cain, H., Facecas, St.: Studien über die Folgen einer vorübergehenden experimentellen Nierenischaemie I. Die morphologischen Veränderungen des akuten Schadens und ihre funktionelle Bedeutung. Virchows. Arch. path. Anat. 336, 389, (1963)

(14) Thoenes, W.: Feinstrukturen des normalen und funktionsgestörten Nephrons. Verh. Dtsch. Ges. Path. 49. Tagung, 14 (1965)

(15) Little, J.R., Cohen,J.J.: Effect of albumine concentration on function of isolated perfused rat kidney. Amer. J. Physiol. 226, 512 (1974)

(16) Trimble, M.E., Bowman, R.H.: Na^+ and K^+ transport: effects of glucose, palmitate and -bromopalmitate. Amer. J. Physiol. 225, 1057 (1973)

EFFECT OF VASOPRESSORS AND HEMORRHAGE ON INTRARENAL OXYGENATION

Rex Baker, Anthony V. Beran, and Jose Strauss

Departments of Pediatrics
University of Miami School of Medicine
Miami, Florida, U.S.A.
California College of Medicine, U.C. Irvine
Irvine, California, U.S.A.

Hemorrhagic hypotension has been reported to be accompanied by liberation of catecholamines (1) and angiotensin (2). Aukland observed parallel blood flow decreases in cortex and outer medulla during hemorrhage and the injection of various vasopressor agents (3). From these data he suggested that vasopressors may be largely responsible for the increased renal vascular resistance of hemorrhagic hypotension. On the other hand, Rector et al. (4) observed intracortical blood flow redistribution during hemorrhage, but none during norepinephrine or angiotensin infusion. This suggested that the observed hemorrhagic intrarenal redistribution was due to factors other than humoral release of either norepinephrine or angiotensin. Grandchamp et al. (5) have suggested that the simultaneous action of both norepinephrine and local angiotensin are needed to produce the intrarenal blood flow redistribution of hemorrhagic hypotension.

Intrarenal oxygen availability (O_2a) values are determined in part by intrarenal blood flow distribution and in part by other factors such as hematocrit, temperature, pH, counter-current O_2 diffusion and oxygen consumption rate ($\dot{V}O_2$) (6,7). The latter is dependent on tubular sodium delivery and reabsorption (8). Munck et al. (9) noted that in dogs hemorrhagic hypotension of 49 mm Hg (mean arterial pressure) completely interrupted glomerular filtration. On the other hand, the glomerular filtration rate has been shown to fall only slightly during norepinephrine (10) and angiotensin (11) infusion and to remain unchanged in spite of ischemia during epinephrine infusion (12).

No study has been made of the comparative effects of vasopressors and hemorrhage on intrarenal oxygenation changes. This report will describe the intrarenal O_2a response differences between mild, gradually attained hemorrhagic hypotension, and single rapid bolus I.V. injections of norepinephrine, epinephrine and angiotensin. In addition, some of the probable causes of these response differences will be examined.

METHODS

Thirty four experiments were performed in 23 male New Zealand rabbits. These animals were implanted with O_2-sensitive bare-wire electrodes (Pt, active, negative, 175 μ diameter; Ag-AgCl, reference, positive, 500 μ diameter) at least two weeks prior to the experiments. The electrodes were placed in the cortex (C), outer medulla (OM), inner medulla (IM), and papilla (P) of the left kidney and an occluder was placed around the left renal artery (6). Electrode locations were confirmed by histological evaluation after the animal was sacrificed. Details of construction, calibration, selection and implantation of electrodes has been previously described (6,7,13).

On the day of the experiment the rabbit was loosely wrapped in a thin sheet and blindfolded (to prevent external visual stimuli) and the electrodes were connected to the polarographs to allow for stabilization. Jugular or ear vein and femoral artery catheterizations were performed under local anesthesia and a thermometer probe was placed in the deep subcutaneous tissue of the animal's back. The venous catheter was used for drug injection. The arterial catheter was connected to a Statham pressure transducer (model P23AA) which in turn was connected to an Offner strain-gauge preamplifier (model 9803) of a Beckman Dynograph (Type R). The arterial catheter was used for monitoring continuously central arterial pressure (CAP) and heart rate as well as for blood sampling, withdrawal, and reinfusion. Arterial blood PO_2, PCO_2 and pH were measured in a Radiometer Blood Micro System (model BMS-3b), and hematocrit in microtubes centrifuged for 5 min at 1,500 rpm. Body temperature was continuously monitored by a Yellow Springs Telethermometer (model 42 SC).

Following surgical preparation the animal was allowed to stabilize for 30 min to establish control values. It was then given a single rapid I.V. bolus injection of one of three vasopressor agents: Norepinephrine (Levophed (R), Winthrop Laboratories, 0.01-0.02 mg/kg b.w.); Epinephrine (Adrenalin (R), Parke-Davis and Co., 0.01-0.02 mg/kg b.w.); and Angiotensin (Hypertensin (R), CIBA, 0.0002 mg/kg b.w.).

After allowing one hour for recovery from the drug, the hemorrhagic shock phase of the experiment was begun. Shock was produced by withdrawing 10 ml blood volumes so that systolic CAP of 60 mm Hg was attained within 30-60 min. This systolic CAP was maintained for two hours while the shed blood was stored in cooled, capped, heparinized syringes. At the end of two hours, this blood was reinfused in no less than 30 min. Blood samples were taken before drug injection, and each 30 min during the control, shock and post-reinfusion phases of the experiment. Each animal served as its own control.

The response patterns of O_2a levels for each renal zone were followed after either a vasopressor agent injection or hemorrhagic shock production. The four stimuli were compared by noting O_2a levels at maximum response, maximum recovery and stabilization. Maximum recovery and stabilization of hemorrhagic experiments were those obtained after blood reinfusion.

RESULTS

Norepinephrine, epinephrine, angiotensin, and hemorrhagic shock all displayed a similar intrarenal O_2a response pattern in that all zones decreased, overshot and then stabilized. There were, however, differences between regarding the O_2a levels attained during each one of these responses.

All vasopressor agents caused a more marked decrease and overshoot in the outer than inner renal zones. Interzonally, O_2a response to epinephrine was the most marked and heterogeneous; to norepinephrine, it was the least marked and most homogeneous; to angiotensin, it was heterogeneous and successively smaller from outer to inner zones. The response to hemorrhage varied from that of the vasopressors in general since the inner rather than the outer zones showed slightly more marked O_2a decreases and overshoots. Stabilization took longer, and inner renal zone O_2a levels remained above control after hemorrhagic shock.

Administration of all vasopressors was accompanied by transient (<10 min) elevation in blood pressure and decrease in heart rate. Epinephrine had the most marked and angiotensin the least marked pressor and chronotropic effects. During hemorrhagic hypotension systolic CAP was maintained at 60 mm Hg. Tachycardia occurred during the initial part of the two hour shock. After restoration of the shed blood, both CAP and heart rate returned to values just under those of control.

DISCUSSION

Our data show intrarenal O_2a response pattern differences among the various vasopressors and hemorrhagic hypotension. The responses to all these stimuli can be partially attributed to an increased vascular resistance and a decreased total renal blood flow (3,4,5).

Hemorrhagic intrarenal blood flow redistribution alone does not supply information concerning the function and metabolism of the tissue itself. Intrarenal O_2a levels can significantly assist in providing this information. Due to the nature of the stimulus (single rapid bolus injection), the response to vasopressors principally reflected rapid vascular (blood flow) changes although they may have also influenced $\dot{V}O_2$ through sodium delivery and reabsorption changes.

The differences between O_2a response patterns of the vasopressors can be principally attributed to their various abilities to stimulate receptors, and to induce local angiotensin formation (14) at the renin-rich outer cortex (15). Norepinephrine is mainly an alpha-adrenergic stimulator. Epinephrine is a stronger alpha stimulator than norepinephrine and stimulates beta-adrenergic receptors as well (16). Both release renin either through direct stimulation of juxtaglomerular cells, intrarenal baroreceptors, the macula densa, or a combination of these mechanisms (10). Angiotensin has its own specific receptor sites which can be blocked by anti-angiotensin plasma, but not by the alpha blocker phentolamine (17). In addition it fails to release renin into the renal vein indicating a possible lack of local angiotensin formation (18).

The intrarenal O_2a response pattern of hemorrhagic hypotension varies from that of the vasopressors in general. The outer renal zones did not decrease or overshoot as markedly as the inner zones. Intrarenal blood flow redistribution data during hemorrhagic hypotension display the opposite trend (4,5) or a proportional blood flow decrease throughout the kidney (3).

The differences between intrarenal blood flow and O_2a changes caused by hemorrhage could be explained by $\dot{V}O_2$ changes. The inner renal zones are partially anaerobic (19) while the outer zones are principally areobic under normal conditions (20). Kramer and Deetjen (8) reported that $\dot{V}O_2$ in the mammalian kidney is related to sodium reabsorption rate. Munck (9) found that hemorrhage to a mean CAP of 40-60 mm Hg was capable of completely interrupting glomerular filtration. It is therefore likely that sodium delivery for reabsorption along the tubule in our shock experiments was low. The resultant decreased $\dot{V}O_2$ of the aerobic outer zones could have caused their higher oxygen availability than in the mainly anaerobic inner zones.

Glomerular Filtration Rate is unaffected by epinephrine infusion in spite of renal ischemia (12). It is only slightly decreased by norepinephrine (10) or angiotensin (11). Therefore a greater amount of sodium must be delivered to the proximal tubule following vasopressor injection than following hemorrhage. Alpha-adrenergic stimulation has been shown to increase proximal tubular sodium reabsorption (21) whereas angiotensin causes natriuresis in the dog

(11) and the rabbit (22).

In summary, differences in intrarenal O_2a levels were observed among various vasopressors and hemorrhagic shock. It was postulated that the rate of sodium delivery to and reabsorption by the tubuli together with intrarenal blood flow redistribution must play major roles in the O_2a level changes observed during the experiments reported here.

REFERENCES

1. Watts, D.T., and V. Westfall. Studies on peripheral blood catecholamine levels during hemorrhagic shock in dogs. Proc. Soc. Exptl. Biol. Med. 115: 601-604, 1964.

2. Scornik, O.A., and A.C. Paladini. Angiotensin blood levels in hemorrhagic hypotension and other related conditions. Am. J. Physiol. 206: 553-556, 1964.

3. Aukland, K. Kidney circulation during hemorrhagic hypotension. In: Microcirculation as Related to Shock, edited by D. Shepro, and G.P. Fulton. New York: Academic Press, 1968, p. 121-135.

4. Rector, J.B., J.H. Stein, W.H. Bay, R.W. Osgood, and T.F. Ferris. Effect of hemorrhage and vasopressor agents on distribution of renal blood flow. Am. J. Physiol. 222: 1125-1131, 1972.

5. Grandchamp, A., R. Veyrat, E. Rosset, J.R. Scherrer, and B. Truniger. Relationship between renin and intrarenal hemodynamics in hemorrhagic hypotension. J. Clin. Invest. 50: 970-978, 1971.

6. Strauss, J., A.V. Beran, C.T. Brown, and N. Katurich. Renal oxygenation under "normal" conditions. Am. J. Physiol. 215: 1482-1487, 1968.

7. Strauss, J., A.V. Beran, R. Baker, L. Boydston, and J.L. Reyes-Sanchez. Effect of hemorrhagic shock on renal oxygenation. Am. J. Physiol. 221: 1545-1550, 1971.

8. Kramer, K., and P. Deetjen. Oxygen consumption and sodium reabsorption in the mammalian kidney. In: Oxygen in the Animal Organism, edited by F. Dickens, and E. Neil. New York: Macmillan, 1964, p. 411-431.

9. Munck, O., N.A. Lassen, P. Deetjen, and K. Kramer. Evidence against renal hypoxia in acute haemorrhagic shock. Arch. Ges. Physiol. 274: 356-363, 1962.

10. Schrier, R.W. Effects of adrenergic nervous system and catecholamines on systemic and renal hemodynamics, sodium and water excretion and renin secretion. Kidney Internat. 6: 291-306, 1974.

11. Cannon, P.J., R.P. Ames, and J.H. Laragh. Indirect action of angiotensin infusion to inhibit renal tubular sodium reabsorption in dogs. Am. J. Physiol. 211: 1021-1030, 1966.

12. Bradley, S.E., and J.B. Coelho. Renal pharmacology of "shock" and its congeners. In: Drugs Affecting Kidney Function and Metabolism. Progress in Biochemical Pharmacology Vol. 7, edited by K.D.G. Edwards, and R. Paoletti. Basel: S. Karger, 1972, p. 1-58.

13. Strauss, J., A.V. Beran, and R. Baker. Fabrication of electrodes for continuous tissue O_2 monitoring. J. Appl. Physiol. 37: 988-990, 1974.

14. Granger, P., J.M. Rojo-Ortega, A. Gruener, H. Dahlheim, K. Thurau, R. Boucher, and J. Genest. On the intrarenal role of the renin angiotensin system. In: Control of Renin Secretion: Experimental Medicine and Biology, Vol. 17, edited by T.A. Assaykeen. New York: Plenum Press, 1972, p. 131-144.

15. Brown, J.J., D.L. Davies, A.F. Lever, R.A. Parker, and J.I.S. Robertson. The assay of renin in single glomeruli in the normal rabbit and the appearance of the juxtaglomerular apparatus. J. Physiol. 176: 418-428, 1965.

16. Innes, I.R., and M. Nickerson. Drugs acting on postganglionic adrenergic nerve endings and structures innervated by them (Sympathomimeteic drugs). In: The Pharmacological Basis of Therapeutics, edited by L.S. Goodman, and A. Gilman. The Mac millan Company, 1969, p. 477-520.

17. Hornych, H., M. Beaufils, and G. Richet. The effect of exogenous angiotensin on superficial and deep glomeruli in the rat kidney. Kidney Internat. 2: 336-343, 1972.

18. Wathen, R.L., W.S. Kingsbury, D.A. Stouder, E.G. Schneider, and H.H. Rostorfer. Effects of infusion of catecholamines and angiotensin II on renin release in anesthetized dogs. Am. J. Physiol. 209: 1012-1024, 1965.

19. Dell, R.B., and R.W. Winters. Lactate gradients in the kidney of the dog. Am. J. Physiol. 213: 301-307, 1967.

20. Strauss, J., A.V. Beran, N. Katurich, and C.T. Brown. Renal regional O_2 consumption under "normal" and hemorrhagic shock conditions. (Abstract). Am. Soc. Nephrol., Los Angeles, October 1967, p. 63.

21. Gill, J.R., and A.G.T. Casper. Effect of renal alpha-adrenergic stimulation on proximal tubular sodium reabsorption. Am. J. Physiol. 223: 1201-1205, 1972.

22. Lockett, M.F. Actions of adrenal, hypophysial and renal hormones on the renal excretion of water and electrolytes. In: Drugs Affecting Kidney Function and Metabolism. Progress in Biochemical Pharmacology, Vol. 7, edited by KDG Edwards and R. Paoletti. Basel: S. Karger, 1972, p. 94-145.

RENAL TISSUE OXYGENATION DURING HYPOXIC HYPOXIA

E. Sinagowitz, R. Baker*, J. Strauss*, and M.Kessler**
Urologische Universitätsklinik Freiburg,FRG,
*Department of Pediatrics, University of Miami, USA, **Max-Planck-Institut für Systemphysiologie Dortmund,FRG

In previous studies Kessler and coworkers demonstrated that in the dog liver a local redistribution of microcirculation is induced by breathing a 10 % oxygen gas mixture (1).
This paper will report on studies undertaken to determine wether or not a) there is a similar redistribution of microflow in the kidney; b) the intrarenal flow pattern among the various areas of the kidney is changed by hypoxic hypoxia.

MATERIAL AND METHODS

Fifteen rabbits (9 awake and 6 anesthetized) were exposed to a gas mixture containing 10 % oxygen for 15 or 30 min. This content corresponds to an altitude of 16.500 ft.
All animals were allowed to breath spontaneously.
Those anesthetized received pentobarbitale and were studied by means of the multiwire PO_2 surface electrode designed by Kessler and Lübbers (2,3). They also had an electromagnetic flowprobe (Micron) placed around the renal artery to monitor single kidney blood flow (SKBF).
The unanesthetized animals were wrapped in sheets and studied by means of the chronically implanted O_2 renal electrodes designed by Strauss and coworkers (4).
Each animal had a catheter placed in the femoral artery for monitoring of blood acid-base variables (Radiometer

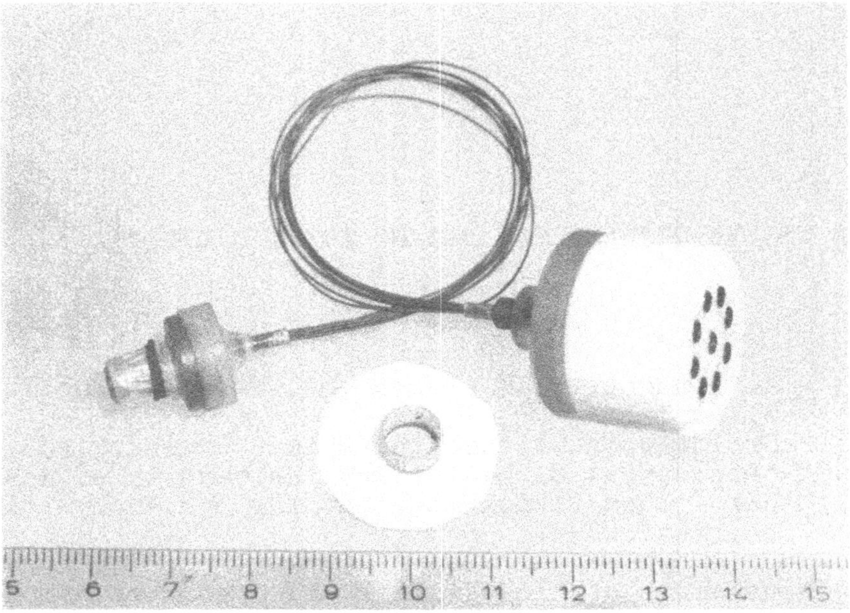

Fig. 1: Multiwire PO_2 electrode

Blood Micro System, Model BMS-3b) and mean arterial blood pressure (MAP)(Statham pressure transducer, P23AA, 0-750 mm Hg).

Fig. 1 presents the multiwire-surface electrode (2, 3). It is composed of the electrode head, the connecting wires, and the teflon-insulated plug. The electrode head contains 8 platinum wires, each one with a diameter of 15 µ and insulated in glass. This electrode makes possible to measure the real local tissue PO_2 simultaneously at different places on the surface of the kidney. By changing the electrode's position on the organ's surface a histogram can be obtained in a relatively short period of time.

Fig. 2 presents the chronically implanted electrodes (4). They are composed of: a) platinum electrodes (175 µ diameter) of adequate lengths for the rabbit's cortex (C), outer medulla (OM), inner medulla (IM), and papilla (P); b) Ag-AgCl anodes (500 µ diameter) one for each cathode, all implanted in the renal cortex; c) an occluder placed around the renal artery; a plug for connection to the recorder (Beckmann Dynograph, Type R).

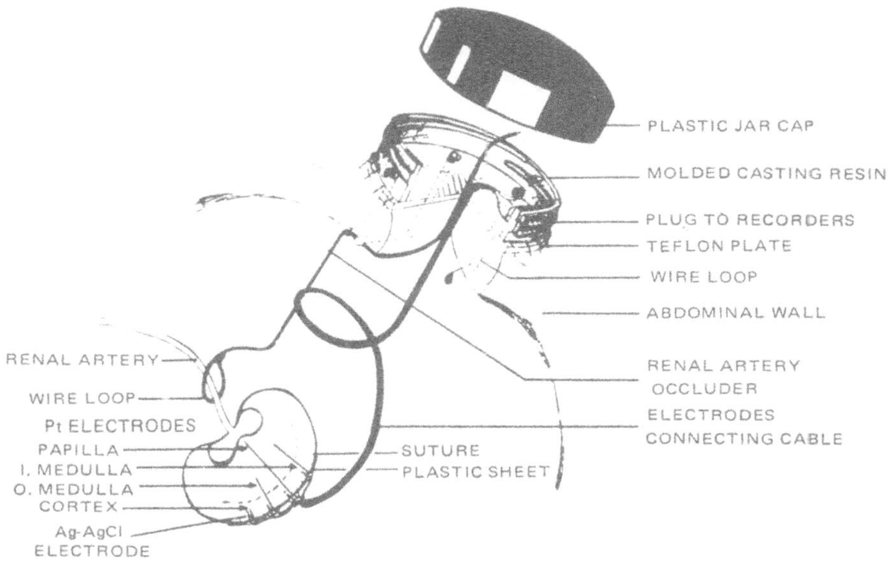

Fig. 2: Chronically implanted electrodes

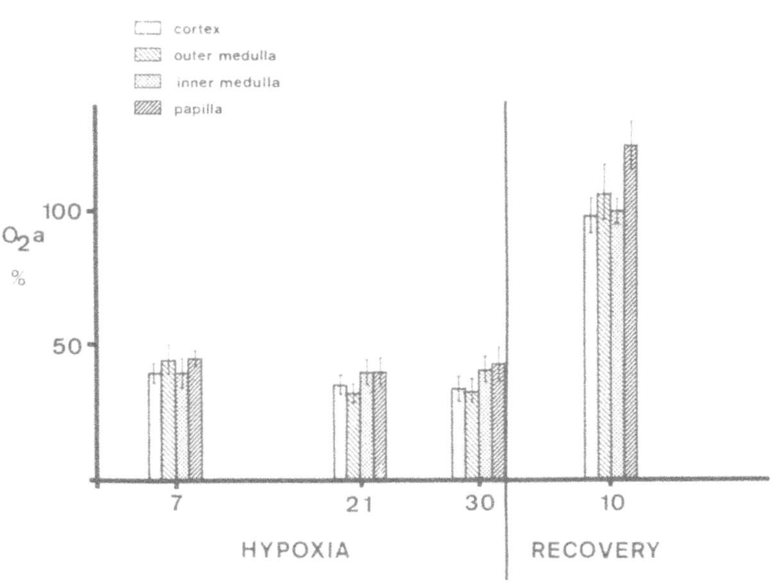

Fig. 3: O_2a in different areas of the kidney during a cycle of hypoxia and during recovery

RESULTS

Fig. 3 presents changes in O_2a during a hypoxic period of 3o min. and during recovery in unanesthetized animals. In the abscissa is the time, and in the ordinate is the O_2a in %. During hypoxia there was a rapid decrease and after hypoxia there was also a rapid return to control levels. During hypoxia the O_2a levels remained relatively stable in a range of 50 to 35 %. It is obvious that among the various renal areas there was no significant difference in O_2a.

Neither heart rate, MAP nor SKBF changed significantly. Reflecting the systemic respiratory alkalosis the extracellular pH increased by about half a pH-unit. This increase was nearly parallel to the compensatory hyperventilation of about 4o %.

Arterial oxygen tension decreased from about 100 mm Hg to 40 mm Hg at the end of either a 15 or a 30 min. hypoxic period. Venous PO_2 decreased from about 40 to about 25 mm Hg. The PO_2-histograms shifted to the left in both 15 and 30 min. hypoxic periods. At no time zero values were recorded. During recovery the histogram was nearly in the same position as in the control period. In all periods PO_2 of the renal vein blood was higher than the peak of the PO_2-distribution-curves.

Arterial and venous blood oxygen saturation and local oxygen saturation of capillaries were calculated using the hemoglobin dissociation curve (6). Since the local PO_2 gradient from the capillary to tissue is

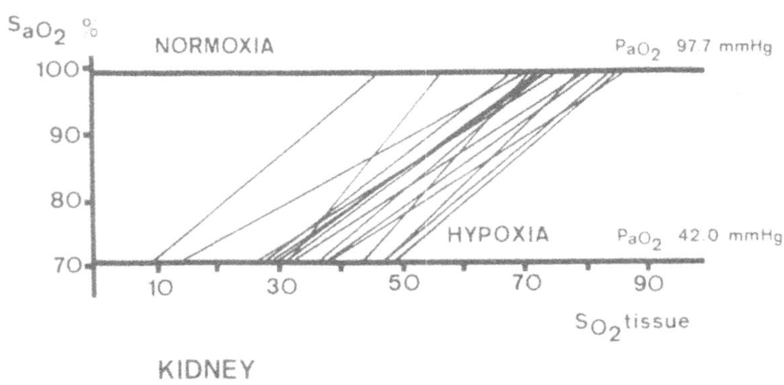

Fig. 4: Arterial and capillary oxygen saturation during normoxia and hypoxic hypoxia (10 % O_2)

not known, the real saturation of oxygen in tissue cannot be calculated. Therefore values of tissue oxygen saturation include a systematic error of about 10 %.

On the abscissa of fig. 4 is the calculated local oxygen saturation and on the ordinate is the calculated arterial O_2-saturation. During hypoxia the venous O_2-saturation decreased from 72 to 37 % (a difference of 35 %). The mean value of local tissue oxygenation decreased from 73 to 34 % (a difference of 39 %). Thus, the decrease of oxygen saturation of venous blood and of tissue decreased by similar percentages. There was also a nearly parallel shift of local oxygen saturation from higher to lower values.

During the hypoxic period renal blood flow was stopped by a short occlusion of the renal artery in awake animals. From the rapidly decreasing O_2a curve, the linear component was used to calculate the slope of O_2a (7). This was assumed to be an index of oxygen consumption. Factors influencing this slope as shifting oxygen dissociation curve by decreasing pH, flow and local PO_2 gradients were taken as a systematic error. Taking the control in each area as 100 % the so-called index of oxygen consumption decreased by about 5o % with exception of the papilla which decreased by only 3o %. After recovery the slope of O_2a returned to its control levels in cortex, outer and inner medulla, but increased in papilla to 140 %.

DISCUSSION

The rapid changes in O_2a during hypoxia and recovery support the interpretation that the chronically implanted electrodes reflect tissue oxygenation changes. Because of the electrode's relatively large diameter which is absolutely necessary for a stable implantation the signal is influenced by both the real local tissue PO_2 and flow. For this reason and the lack of an <u>in-situ</u> calibration only relative changes of tissue oxygen can be recorded. This is called oxygen availability: O_2a. The unlikely possibility that opposite changes of flow and PO_2 occured simultaneously cannot be excluded. The results suggest that all renal areas are affected similarly by hypoxic hypoxia.

The fact that the PO_2 of renal vein blood was higher than the peak of the PO_2 histograms seems to confirm previous statements regarding the lack of correlation between PO_2 of venous blood and the low values of tissue PO_2 appearing in the histograms (1, 8).

Because blood PO_2 along the capillaries decreases in a non-linear fashion, while oxygen saturation decreases linearly, blood and renal tissue oxygen saturations at normal and hypoxic PO_2 levels were compared as previously done in liver (1, 8). Tissue oxygen saturation of liver shifted in an overconvergent way from higher to lower values. This gave evidence for a compensatory redistribution of microcirculation. If in the kidney the same compensatory mechanism occured, a similar pattern should have occured. Namely the tissue oxygen saturation lines should have met at least in one narrow area. Since this did not happen (Fig. 4), it must be assumed that a period of hypoxic hypoxia with 10 % oxygen induces no significant changes of microcirculation in the renal cortex.

In previous experiments it was observed that during hypoxia on piglets there was an increased urine flow and increased urine/plasma ratio of sodium (9). This decreased tubular function (sodium reabsorption) could not be explained by circulatory changes neither in the previous nor in the present experiments. These findings suggest that the kidney diminished its tubular function very early. By decreasing its oxygen consumption the kidney seems to be able to preserve enough energy for its basic metabolism during hypoxic hypoxia. It seems logical to stipulate that an oxygen sensor may exist in renal tissue but no actual evidence exists in this regard. Further work should help clarify this important question.

CONCLUSION

No evidence was found to support the existence of changes in the intrarenal flow pattern among the different areas or of a compensatory redistribution of microcirculation in the renal cortex under hypoxia induced by breathing 10 % oxygen. It seems that under these conditions the kidney is able to preserve its basic metabolism by diminishing its oxygen consumption.

REFERENCES

1. Kessler, M., Lang, E., Sinagowitz, E., Rink, R., and Höper, J.: Homeostasis of oxygen supply in liver and kidney, in: Oxygen transport to tissue, ed. by Bicher, H.I. and Bruley, D.F., Advances in Experimental Medicine and Biology, Vol. 37 A, 351-360, Plenum Press, New York - London 1973

2. Kessler, M. and Lübbers, D.W.: Aufbau und Verwendungsmöglichkeiten verschiedener PO_2-Elektroden, Pflügers Arch. 291, R 82 (1966)

3. Kessler, M. and Grunewald, W.: Possibilities of measuring oxygen pressure fields in tissue by multiwire platinum electrodes, in: International Symposion on Oxygen Pressure Recording, Nijmegen 1968, Progr. Resp. Res. 3, 147 (Karger, Basel 1969)

4. Strauss, J., Beran, A.V., Brown, C.T., Katurich, N.: Renal oxygenation under "normal" conditions, Amer. J. Physiol. 215, 1482-1487 (1968)

5. Beran, A.V., Strauss, J., Brown, C.T., Katurich, N.: A simple arterial occluder, J. Appl. Physiol. 24, 838-839 (1968)

6. Bartels, H. and Harms, H.:Sauerstoffdissoziationskurven des Blutes von Säugetieren, Pflügers Arch. ges. Physiol. 268, 334-365 (1959)

7. Strauss, J., Beran, A.V., Katurich, N., Brown, C.T.: Renal regional O_2-consumption under "normal" and hemorrhagic shock conditions (Abstract) Am. Soc. Nephrol. 1967, p.63

8. Kessler, M.: Oxygen supply to tissue in normoxia and in oxygen deficiency, Microvasc. Res. 8, 282 (1974)

9. Rowe, M.I. and Strauss, J.: The renal response of the newborn to hypoxia (Abstract), Pediat. Res. 7: 41/183 (1973)

CORNEAL OXYGEN SUPPLY CONDITIONS

J. Grote and R. Zander

Institute of Physiology
University of Mainz
65 Mainz

Pronounced cornea hypoxia induces swelling and a loss of transparency. Hypoxia of longer duration causes necrosis, particularly of the corneal endothelium. These findings were observed after ligation of the cilial arteries and the arteria carotis interna, after reduction of oxygen tension on the anterior corneal surface as well as after prolonged wearing of ill-fitted contact lenses (11, 15, 18, 22, 23). Because the normal function of the corneal endothelium plays a central role in maintaining transparency, an insufficient endothelial oxygen supply can directly influence vision (3, 17).

The problem of corneal oxygen supply has been investigated by Fatt et al. (6, 7, 19) and Barr et al. (1, 2). Both groups arrived at partially divergent results. The investigations of Fatt et al. led to the conclusion that the corneal endothelium under conditions of open eyelids as well as closed eyelids is primarily supplied with oxygen by the aqueous humor. On the other hand, Barr et al. maintain that under the conditions of open eyelids the entire cornea receives oxygen from the air, this conclusion being based on measurements of oxygen tension in the anterior chamber and investigations of the corneal oxygen diffusion.

Since the O_2 diffusion constants of the cornea and the O_2 solubility coefficient α of the aqueous humor were to date unknown or not exactly determined, previous investigations had to be based on assumptions which in turn had very significant consequences for the conclusions. We therefore took up the question of oxygen diffusion in the cornea and the problem of oxygen transport in aqueous humor and determined in 2 separate experimental series the exact values for the corneal O_2 diffusion coefficients K and D as well as the O_2 solubility coefficient α of the aqueous humor.

EXPERIMENTAL INVESTIGATIONS

Using an experimental arrangement going back to THEWS (9, 20) we measured the O_2 diffusion coefficients K and D on 26 freshly excised bovine corneae under temperature conditions of 30° C and 37° C. The eyes were obtained immediately after slaughter.

The results of the investigation are summarized in Table 1.

Table 1. Diffusivity of oxygen in bovine cornea. $\bar{x} \pm s_{\bar{x}}$ are given.

t (° C)	n	$K \cdot 10^5$ (ml/cm min atm)	n	$D \cdot 10^5$ (cm^2/sec)
30	26	1.80 ± 0.29	21	1.70 ± 0.24
37	24	1.95 ± 0.25	17	1.95 ± 0.32

The derived values for the O_2 diffusion coefficients K and D are smaller than the comparable constants for other tissues and for the blood (9, 20). They approximate those for tumor tissue (10). The corneal diffusion coefficient K as reported by HEALD and LANGHAM (11) is significantly smaller than that which we measured, and lies far below all to date determined tissue values.

In a second experimental series, we determined the O_2 solubility coefficient α for bovine aqueous humor using a modified VAN SLYKE method for small sample volumes. The values for the O_2 solubility coefficient under the temperature conditions of 30° C and 37° C are contained in Table 2. These values compare well with those of plasma and water (24).

Table 2. O_2 solubility coefficient of bovine aqueous humor

$\bar{x} \pm s_{\bar{x}}$ are given.

t (° C)	n	$\alpha \cdot 10^2$ (ml/ml atm)
30	6	2.46 ± 0.01
37	18	2.26 ± 0.04

THEORETICAL INVESTIGATIONS

The measured data together with the values taken from the literature for the oxygen uptake rate and the thickness of the various layers of the cornea from the basis for determining the oxygen tension profiles in the cornea. Assuming the cornea to be a plane tissue layer of uniform thickness, we calculated the mean oxygen tension decrease through the cornea under the conditions of:

1. Mean oxygen tension of 150 mmHg on the border of the lacrimal fluid and the cornea as to be expected under the conditions of opened eyelids.
2. Mean oxygen tension of 90 mmHg on the border of the lacrimal fluid and the cornea for the conditions of closed eyelids. The assumption was made that the lacrimal fluid oxygen tension corresponds to that of the arterial blood.
3. Mean oxygen tension of 40 mmHg in the aqueous humor of the anterior chamber. This value correspond to the mean value taken from the literatur (reviews. 1, 12). Considering the more recently determined values (approximately 32 mmHg, 1, 12), the results of the investigations are not essentially affected.

We assumed the thickness of the entire cornea to be 550 µm, the thickness of the epithelium to be 75 µm and the thickness of the endothelium to be 10 µm (s. 23). For the oxygen consumption rates of the various layers of the cornea the values summarized in Table 3 were used. These values are mean values derived from the literature (review s. 4, 8). In order to convert the data given in very diverse dimensions into mlO_2/100 g w.wt. min and mlO_2/100 ml min, we assumed the mean corneal water content to be 76 % and the mean corneal density to be 1.1 g/cm^3 (5, 16). To adjust the data from literature to the conditions of 30° C and 37° C Q_{10} = 2 (8) was used.

Table 3. Oxygen consumption rate of various corneal layers at 30° C and 37° C.

	Epithelium	Stroma	Endothelium
30° C (mlO_2/100g w.wt.min)	1.34	0.14	2.45
30° C (mlO_2/100ml min)	1.48	0.15	2.70
37° C (mlO_2/100g w.wt.min)	1.88	0.20	3.43
37° C (mlO_2/100ml min)	2.07	0.22	3.78

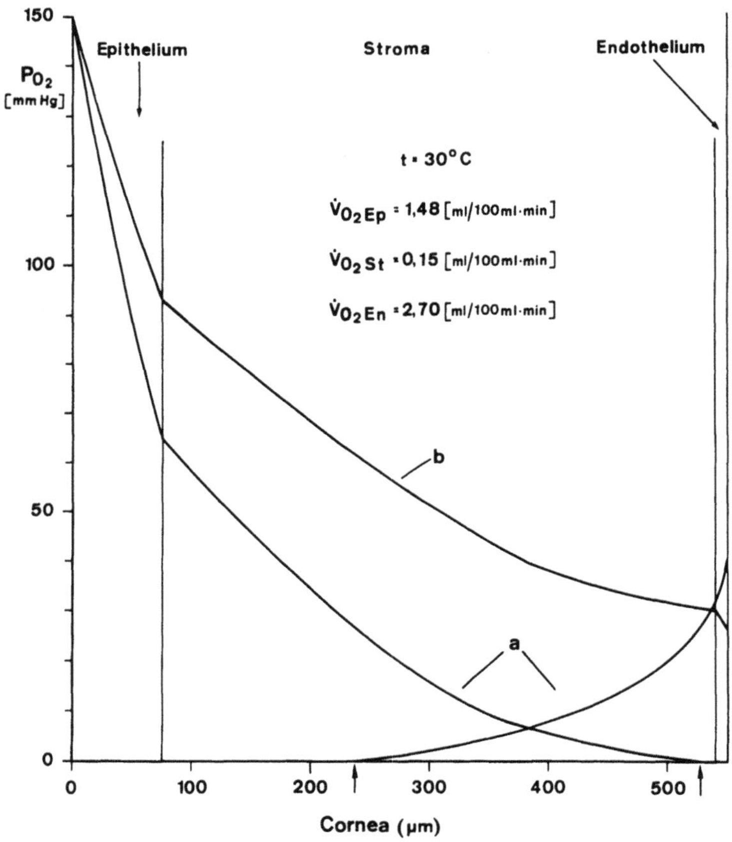

Fig. 1. Oxygen tension profiles through the cornea under the conditions of opened eyelids.
a) Taking into account the corneal O_2 diffusion constants.
b) Taking into account the O_2 diffusion constants of water.
The thickness of the limiting layer of oxygen diffusion is marked with an arrow.

Using the described data we were able to calculate the mean oxygen tension profile within the cornea as well as the thickness of the limiting layer of oxygen diffusion (21). For the conditions of open eyelids and a corneal temperature of 30° C the data in Fig. 1, curve a, were obtained. As can be seen in the figure, it is to be expected that the corneal endothelium with open eyes will primarily be supplied with oxygen from the aqueous humor. Even when assuming the corneal diffusivity to be that of water (curve b) the calculations still lead to the same conclusion. When one employs the O_2 diffusion coefficient K from HEALD and LANGHAM[2] (11) then the oxygen tension profile lies below curve a, Fig. 1, indicating even worse corneal oxygen supply conditions.

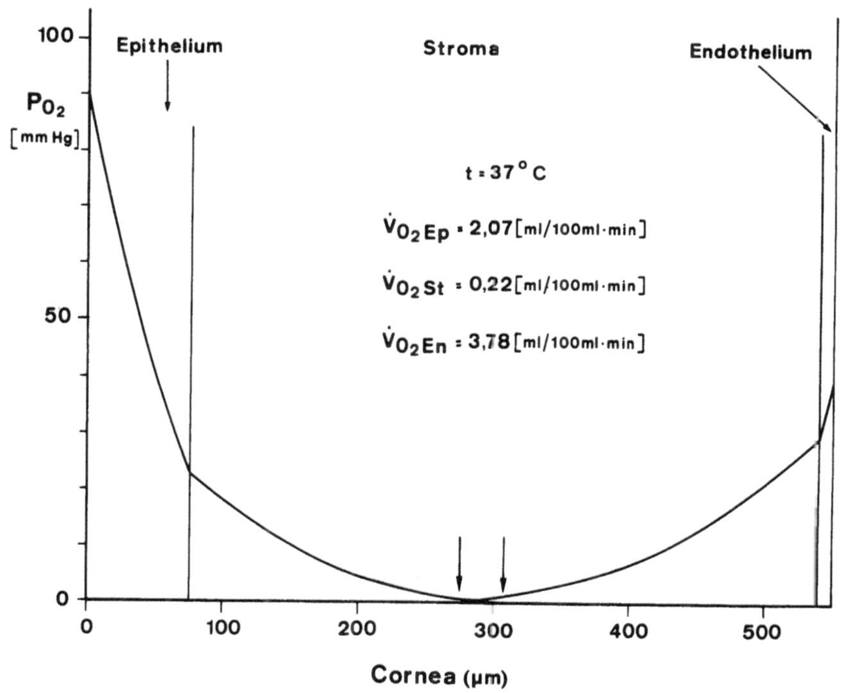

Fig. 2. Oxygen tension profile through the cornea under the conditions of closed eyelids. The thickness of the limiting layer of oxygen diffusion is marked with an arrow.

Under the conditions of closed eyelids, a corneal temperature of 37° C, and the assumption of a mean oxygen tension in the lacrimal fluid which corresponds to that of the arterial blood, the data in Fig. 2 were derived. The calculations lead to the conclusion that under these conditions not only the corneal endothelium but also parts of the corneal stroma have to be supplied with oxygen from the aqueous humor.

The results of the theoretical investigation of the corneal oxygen diffusion support the view of FATT et al. (6, 7, 19), that the corneal endothelium is primarily supplied with oxygen by the aqueous humor of the anterior chamber by both closed as well as open eyes. The oxygen tension profile derived for the condition of open eyelids corresponds in its course to the measured data of KWAN et al. (14).

The question arises as to whether a sufficient amount of oxygen reaches the posterior surface of the cornea by diffusion and convection. Because the net flow of aqueous humor between the capillaries of the ciliar body and the canal of SCHLEMM is only 2.5 μl/min, this was answered negatively by different authors. When one takes into consideration that in addition to the net fluid flow, a fluid exchange in the order of 50 μl/min exists between the ciliar body capillaries and the iris on the one side and the aqueous humor on the other side (13, 23), then a total fluid exchange of about 52,5 μl/min is to be expected. When one further assumes that this exchanged fluid reaches the anterior and posterior chambers with an oxygen tension corresponding to that of arterial blood, then a mean oxygen transport rate of 0.14 μl O_2/min is obtained, taking into account the determined oxygen solubility coefficient of aqueous humor.

Whereas the mean oxygen transport rate into the aqueous humor is about 0.14 μl O_2/min, the oxygen demand of the entire corneal endothelium is only approximately 0.025 μl O_2/min or, using FREEMAN's relatively high endothelial oxygen consumption rate (8), 0.045 μl O_2/min. If these assumptions are correct then the quantity of oxygen transported per minute into the aqueous humor is approx. 3 - 5 times greater than the endothelial oxygen demand per minute. Therefore a sufficient oxygen supply of the corneal endothelium through the aqueous humor is possible, taking into consideration a lenticular oxygen consumption rate of 0.065 μl O_2/min (23).

REFERENCES

1. Barr, R.E., and I.A. Silver: Invest. Ophthal. 12, 140 (1973)
2. Barr, R.E., and E.L. Roetman: Invest. Ophthal. 13, 386 (1974)
3. Dikstein, S., and D.M. Maurice: Israel. J. Med. Sci. 8, 1523 (1972)
4. Duane, T.D.: Arch. Ophthal. 41, 736 (1949)
5. Duane, T.D.: Am. J. Ophthal. 32, 203 (1949)
6. Fatt, I., and M.T. Bieber: Exp. Eye Res. 7, 103 (1968)
7. Fatt, I., R.D. Freeman and D. Lin: Exp. Eye Res. 18, 357 (1974)
8. Freeman, R.D.: J. Physiol. (Lond.) 225, 15 (1972)
9. Grote, J.: Pflügers Arch. ges. Physiol. 295, 245 (1967)
10. Grote, J., R. Süsskind and P. Vaupel: Pflügers Arch. 347, R41 (1974)
11. Heald, K., and M.E. Langham: Brit. J. Ophthal. 40, 705 (1956)
12. Jacobi, K.W.: Albrecht v. Graefes Arch. klin. exp. Ophthal. 169, 350 (1966)
13. Kinsey, V.E., M. Grant and D.G. Cogan: Arch. Ophthal. 27, 242 (1942)
14. Kwan, M., J. Niinikoski and F.K. Hunt: Invest. Ophthal. 11, 108 (1972)
15. Langham, M.E.: J. Physiol. (Lond.) 115, 65P (1951)
16. Langham, M.E., and I.S. Taylor: Brit. J. Ophthal. 40, 321 (1956)
17. Maurice, D.M.: J. Physiol. (Lond.) 221, 43 (1972)
18. Smelser, G.K., and D.K. Chen: Arch. Ophthal. 53, 676 (1955)
19. Takahashi G.H., and I. Fatt: Exp. Eye Res. 4, 4 (1965)
20. Thews, G.: Pflügers Arch. ges. Physiol. 271, 227 (1960)
21. Thews, G.: In: D-Glucose und verwandte Verbindungen in Medizin und Biologie. Hrsg: H. Bartelheimer, W. Heyde und W. Thorn. Stuttgart: Enke 1966
22. Weekers, R.: Ophthalmologica (Basel) 100, 136 (1940)
23. Zander, R.: Albrecht v. Greafes Arch. klin. exp. Ophthal. 195, 215 (1975)
24. Zander, R.: Habil.-Schrift, Mainz 1975

SUMMARY OF DISCUSSION - SESSION VIII:

OXYGEN SUPPLY OF DIFFERENT ORGANS

Chairmen: I. A. Silver, J. Strauss, and Ch. Weiss

The discussion on the papers by Dr. Tsacopoulos and Dr. Barr initiated by Dr. Zander was concerned mainly with diffusion of oxygen through the vitreous body and whether or not there was any diffusion from the ciliary body to the retina or from the retina to the lens but this problem was not resolved. The questions concerning diffusion that were posed to Dr. Barr came mainly from Dr. Grote and referred to his short presentation which followed Dr. Barr's talk. In considering the equation that had to be solved to produce the curves shown by Dr. Grote it was pointed out that for a second order differential equation two specified boundary conditions were needed to derive each curve. One boundary condition was shown on the figure and Dr. Grote indicated that the other boundary condition was zero. Dr. Barr pointed out that in these circumstances each curve must necessarily go to zero at those surfaces. Dr. Grote agreed with this but indicated that his calculations were only preliminary and he now proposed to combine the two curves.

Dr. Goldstick was concerned that during measurement some injury might have been occasioned to the epithelium on the deep surface of the cornea but Dr. Barr reassured him that great care had been taken not to wrinkle or traumatise the cornea during handling and emphasised that during measurements the corneal thickness had remained almost constant and had not swollen. This suggested that the epithelium was intact and functioning normally.

The major questions which were discussed in relation to the paper by Dr. Flower were technical points commented on by Professor Lübbers and Professor Kunze. These participants were concerned with the problems of calibrating a bare pulsed oxygen electrode in the retina when there was neither a recess to the electrode nor a membrane. There was also concern about protein deposition on bare electrodes and whether a particular scheme of "pulsing" was used to polarise the electrode. Dr. Flower answered these questions by referring to his Figure 3 which showed that current flow through the electrode following stepwise application of a polarising potential was initially very high but dropped exponentially as the oxygen in the barrier layer immediately adjacent to the platinum surface was depleted. If the polarising pulse was very long a steady state current flow was finally achieved which was limited by oxygen diffusion through the medium. The amount of oxygen reaching the electrode under these conditions depended not only on the PO_2 but also on the oxygen diffusion coefficient of the media. The purpose of a membrane was to make the steady state current dependent only on the PO_2 of the medium by providing the electrode with a relatively thick barrier layer of known constant oxygen diffusion coefficient. Dr. Flower said that if he covered his electrode with a membrane it would reduce his ability to record LERG activity. In order to overcome the problems associated with bare electrodes he had recorded the current very shortly after application of the polarising potential, i.e. before the current flow became diffusion limited. Theoretically this method was not as sound as the use of a membrane since in practice it was not possible to read the instantaneous current flow at time zero but the closer to time zero that the electrode currents were determined the less dependant should the current be on oxygen diffusion through the media. He also considered it possible that the entire current profile shown in Figure 3 might contain meaningful information about diffusion of oxygen through the different media.

With regard to calibration of bare electrodes his experience had been that the application of very short pulses had given stable readings regardless of the time after application of the potential at which the current determinations were made. Determination of the current at a very precise interval after application of the polarising was possibly because of the high stability of solid state circuitory now available. He had used both long and short duration pulses and found the calibration curves equally stable in both cases although of course the slopes differed depending on the interval between application of the potential and the current reading. His sequence of polarising potentials were applied either as single pulses or chains of pulses. He did not ordinarily pulse continuously because of the greater danger of "poisoning" the electrode surface.

He adopted the old technique of applying a positive potential exactly equal to the value of the negative polarising potential in an attempt to "clean" the electrode surface. He agreed that there was no absolute proof that this technique prevented deposition of protein but it certainly did no harm. Because of the relatively short duration of the pulses the amount of protein deposition should be relatively small.

A number of general comments were made concerning the undesirability of using bare electrodes and questioning the assertion that protein deposition was not important in pulsed electrodes. One contributor thought that protein deposition probably occurred almost immediately the electrode was placed in the tissue and might well act as a kind of natural membrane.

The second part of the session was concerned with oxygenation of the kidney. Professor Weiss asked whether Dr. Strauss had performed any renal function studies in his experiments on isolated perfused kidneys and was told that unfortunately Dr. Strauss' group had not been very successful in their attempts at measuring renal function. In the case of the drug injections the experimental period was too short while with the haemorrhagic shock experiments it was not possible to obtain acurately measured and timed urine output even with an indwelling bladder catheter. However some studies which he had performed with Dr. M. Rowe in piglets during hypoxia showed that both sodium resorbtion decreased and urine volume increased in a marked and significant fashion. It was for this reason that Dr. Strauss had been interested in Professor Weiss' observation that when kidneys were perfused with hydroxyethyl starch, sodium resorbtion and urine output increased simultaneously.

Dr. Versmold commented in relation to the paper by Weiss et al that increased oxygen uptake might well have indicated uncoupling of oxidative phosphorylation rather than improved O_2 supply. He suggested that the infusion of atractyloside, which blocks ADP influx from the cytosole into the mitochondria could serve as a control experiment to determine the coupling state of oxidative phosphorylation in the perfused kidney.

In a comment on the same paper Dr. Beran said that he and his colleagues had performed experiments where they had exchanged blood to 3% Htc with emulsified FC-47 and they observed that while arterial PO_2 remained within normal values oxygen content decreased during perfusion, which suggested either elimination of FC-47 particles or a coating of the particles by protein which decreased the O_2 carrying capacity of the perfusate. If this had happened in the experiments under discussion, it might have explained the constant VO_2.

Dr. Sinagowitz was questioned as to what was meant by the term "tissue saturation" and he was also asked how he measured renal blood flow. In his reply he stated that "tissue oxygen saturation" was perhaps better referred to as the local oxygen saturation in the capillary blood and was a term first coined by Professor Kessler

(Kessler et al., 1973) in order to obtain linear values for an analysis of the regulation of oxygen supply and micro circulation in tissue. PO_2 along a capillary declinedin a non-linear fashion which was caused mainly by the presence of haemoglobin, whereas oxygen saturation showed a linear decrease. Since, at the present time, no direct measurements on local oxygen saturation were available this could only be estimated by using the O_2 dissociation curve of haemoglobin in blood in conjunction with measured local tissue PO_2. Because the PO_2 gradient in tissue was not known exactly the estimated values of local oxygen saturation included a systematic error of approximately 10%. He thought that further development of photometric methods might lead to real measurements of the local oxygen saturation in the capillaries.

With regard to measurements of blood flow in single kidneys he had instruments from Micron and Devices which employed the paramagnetic principle. The different results obtained in rabbits and rats might have been due to species variation or to the degree of hypoxic hypoxia. In dogs 5% oxygen in the inspired gas mixture caused a distinct decrease in renal blood flow (Kessler, M. et al., 1973).

REFERENCES

Kessler, M. et al. (1973) Adv. exp. Med. Biol. 37A, 351-360.

Common Aspects of Oxygen Supply

CELLULAR OXYGEN CONCENTRATION

Rolf Zander

Institute of Physiology
University of Mainz
65 Mainz, F.R.G.

At low oxygen levels the intracellular or intramitochondrial concentration of molecular oxygen together with the amount of reduced cytochrome oxydase determines the rate of oxygen utilization. Below the so-called "critical oxygen concentration", i.e. the value, at which a drop in the rate of oxygen uptake has its first evidence, the kinetic is described by the oxygen affinity (K_m) of the respiratory chain, i.e. the concentration value for half maximal rate of oxygen uptake.
On principle, the concentration value in each case is a function of both oxygen partial pressure and oxygen solubility. In spite of the variation of the latter, which is the reason for JÖBSIS's remark (1964) that oxygen concentration should rather be used for describing critical oxygen supply conditions than oxygen partial pressure, the so-called "critical P_{O_2}" is obviously used more often in physiological literature.
In order to evaluate the possible changes of oxygen solubility at 37°C in different fluids, oxygen solubility coefficients (ml/ml atm) were measured by the classical VAN SLYKE technique in our laboratory previously.
Some values are shown in figure 1.
The total range shown on the left side reaches from about 5×10^{-1} ml/ml atm for fluorocarbon to a value below 2×10^{-4} ml/ml atm for saturated aqueous solutions of different electrolytes.

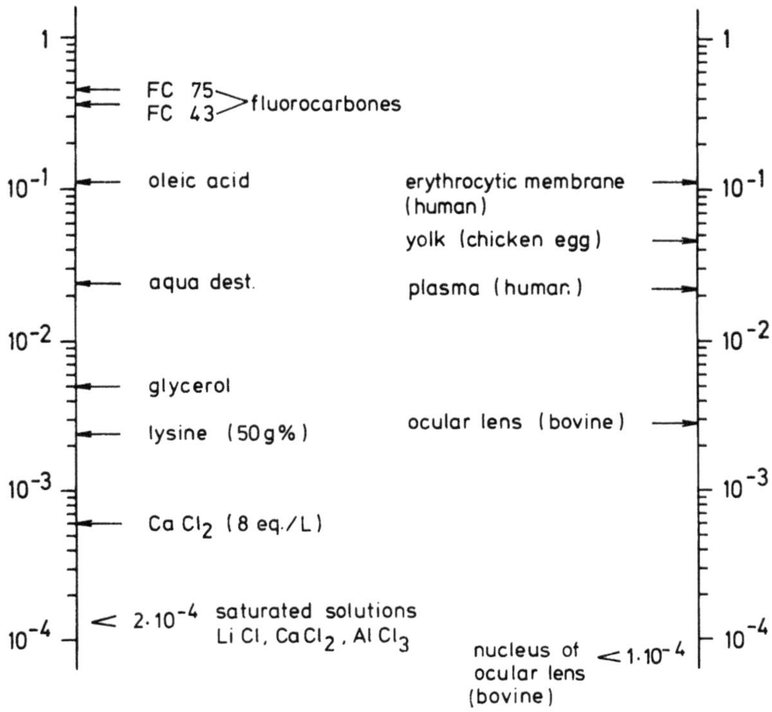

Fig. 1. O_2 solubility coefficients (ml/ml atm) at 37°C of different fluids (left) and biological systems (right)

This is more than 3 decimal power. Some values for the biological range of oxygen solubility are shown on the right side of figure 1.
Here the range reaches from the value for the human red cell ghost (POWER et al., 1970) to the value for the nucleus of the bovine ocular lens.
According to this surprising finding of great variability of oxygen solubility data we were interested in answering the question, which values for oxygen solubility are valid for different human tissues, especially the intracellular space.
For this reason we measured oxygen solubility coefficients by the same VAN SLYKE technique in homogenates of different human tissues. Since undiluted homogenates cannot be equilibrated with pure oxygen the

autopsy material of human subjects was diluted after freeze drying to relative concentrations from zero (i.e. aqua dest.) to 60% with a solution of 0.02 mole/l of $NaNO_2$. This sodium nitrite solution prevents chemical binding of oxygen (Hb, Mb) and its oxygen solubility value is the same as that of pure water. With the measured values of oxygen solubility at relative concentrations up to 60% an exponential or linear function was approximated and used for extrapolation to the undiluted state, if the function was highly significant. Using literature data of the extracellular space of tissues, i.e. the erythrocyte and the plasma volume as well as the volume of the interstitial space, and also measured values for oxygen solubility in these fluids, the oxygen solubility values for intracellular conditions were calculated.

Together with some other values (erythrocyte value of GROTE and THEWS, 1962) the results are shown in figure 2. As can be seen, the intracellular oxygen solubility reaches from 3×10^{-4} ml/ml atm for the liver to 2.8×10^{-2} ml/ml atm for the white matter of the brain.

With the exception of those tissues which contain a greater lipid fraction, a linear correlation is found between the measured percental water content and the oxygen solubility. Consequently an oxygen solubility value of zero must be assumed at a percental water content of 55 - 60%. Is this a realistic value for oxygen solubility in the biological field ? Does such a great fractional water volume exist which can be called nonsolvent water for oxygen, water which is not available for the solution of molecular oxygen ? Indeed, the examples of the saturated electrolyte solutions (shown in fig. 1) with a percental water content of 53 - 63% as well as the shown lysine solution with a percental water content of about 55% show such great water volume, which can be called "bound water" and which, therefore, is not available for the solution of molecular oxygen.

The results and consequences of our findings are as follows:

1. The intracellular oxygen solubility varies much more from cell to cell than it was supposed before. At a uniform oxygen partial pressure of e.g. 1 mmHg the intracellular oxygen concentration at body temperature, therefore, reaches from about 1.8 μmole/l (brain) to 0.018 μmole/l (liver).

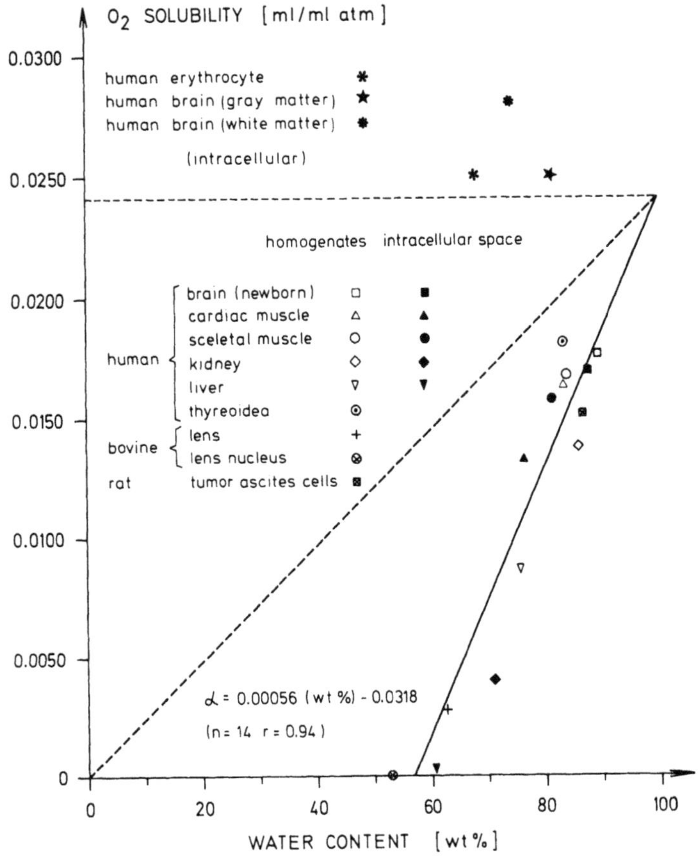

Fig. 2. O_2 solubility coefficients (ml/ml atm) of homogenates and intracellular spaces at 37° C

2. Comparing the critical oxygen supply conditions of different tissues, cells or subcellular particles such as mitochondria, the intracellular or intramitochondrial oxygen concentration should be used rather than the extra- or intracellular oxygen partial pressure.

3. From the knowledge about oxygen solubility in lipids, especially phospholipids, as well as about the protein-lipid-structure of the mitochondrial membrane system, we can assume that the physical properties alone cause very high local oxygen concentration values within mitochondria. If you consider the oxygen solubility value of the red cell membrane of POWER et al. (1970) valid for the mitochondrial cristae, local concentration gradients between the mitochondrion and the nucleus of 50 : 1 may exist. The nucleus contains only 55% water (rat liver cell, LANGENDORF et al., 1961) and, therefore, a low oxygen solubility value according to fig. 2 is expected.

With regard to intracellular oxygen distribution the mitochondrion may act as a "perfect sink" (see CHANCE et al., 1968) in the sense that low oxygen partial pressure is coupled with relatively high oxygen concentration.

References

CHANCE, B., PRING, M.: In: Biochemie des Sauerstoffs Springer, Berlin/Heidelberg/New York 1968

GROTE, J., THEWS, G.: Pflügers Arch. ges. Physiol. 276, 142 (1962)

JÖBSIS, F. F.: In: Handbook of Physiology, Respiration Vol. I Am. Physiol. Soc., Washington 1964

LANGENDORF, H., SIEBERT, G., LORENZ, L., HANNOVER, R., BEYER, R.: Biochem. Z. 335, 273 (1961)

POWER, G. G., STEGALL, H.: J. Appl. Physiol. 29, 145 (1970)

THE ROLE OF CAROTID CHEMORECEPTORS IN THE REGULATION OF ARTERIAL OXYGEN TRANSPORT UNDER HYPOXIA WITH AND WITHOUT HYPERCAPNIA*

Heidrun Kiwull-Schöne, Peter Kiwull,
Klaus Mückenhoff, and Wolfgang Both

Institut für Physiologie, Ruhr-Universität
463 Bochum, Fed. Rep. Germany

In a previous paper (Schöne et al., 1973) we reported that the effectiveness of the carotid chemoreflex drive of ventilation - defined as $\Delta PaO_2/\Delta\dot{V}$ for a given inspiratory pO_2 - decreases with the degree of oxygenation. This is due to the shape of 'ventilatory hyperbolas' counteracting the chemoreflex induced response curve of ventilation. The effectiveness of chemoreflex drive of ventilation on the O_2 transport capacity of hemoglobin can be described as $\Delta SO_2/\Delta\dot{V}$, which in contrast to the $\Delta PaO_2/\Delta\dot{V}$-relation, seems to increase with the degree of hypoxia. Therefore we now investigated the O_2-saturation of hemoglobin in rabbits with intact chemoreflexes, compared to animals with eliminated chemoreflexes, unable to increase pulmonary ventilation under hypoxia. In addition the influence of augmented CO_2 was tested.

Methods

Experiments were carried out in two groups of rabbits, with either intact (n = 10) or cut (n = 12) sinus nerves, anesthetized with pentobarbital sodium. For control, the animals first were breathing pure oxygen and then O_2 with increased CO_2-concentrations. Subsequently hypoxic O_2/N_2 mixtures, yielding constant PaO_2 values of about 45 Torr, controlled by continuous measurement in the arterial blood, again with and without increased CO_2 concentrations, were given.

In order to get steady state conditions, every gas mixture was inspired for about 10 minutes. The following variables were determined: Arterial oxygen pressure, endtidal CO_2-con-

*Supported by the Deutsche Forschungsgemeinschaft, SFB 114 'Bionach'

centration, tidal volume, respiratory rate, arterial blood pressure, heart rate and pH_a. $PaCO_2$, actual and standard bicarbonate were determined numerically by a computer program analogous to usual nomograms. pH_a was corrected for hypoxia as proposed by von Mengden et al. (1969), using numerical iteration. Hb concentration was measured photometrically and O_2 saturation of hemoglobin was calculated from the oxygen content, determined by an oxygen sensor (Lexington Instruments), and corrected for the physically dissolved amount.

For the purpose of statistical evaluation, data were interpolated linearily between two adjacent measured values at always the same $\Delta PaCO_2$, averaged for each animal under hyperoxia (means of two courses of experiments, before and after hypoxia), and compared with the respective values during hypoxia. These data were averaged for the whole population and the significance of difference calculated by a t-test.

Results

1. Respiratory and circulatory parameters (means ± S.E.) are shown in fig. 1. Under hyperoxia the basic ventilation ($\dot{V}_o$) and arterial CO_2 pressure ($PaCO_2$) of the animals with intact sinus nerves were 306 ± 18.8 [$ml \cdot min^{-1} \cdot kg^{-1}$], and 34.8 ± 1.5 [Torr] respectively. The same parameters in the animals with cut sinus nerves were 275 ± 16.1 [$ml \cdot min^{-1} \cdot kg^{-1}$] and 36.1 ± 2.0 [Torr]. Mean arterial pressure (MAP) and heart rate (HR) of the intact group were 83 ± 2.3 [Torr] and 247 ± 8.4 [min^{-1}] respectively, in the group with cut sinus nerves, both values were higher, 99 ± 3.7 [Torr] and 275 ± 4.6 [min^{-1}].

Under hypoxia, in the animals with intact sinus nerves (PaO_2 44.0 ± 0.2 [Torr]), ventilatory minute volume was augmented (+ 66.5 %) by peripheral chemoreflex drive. Concomitantly $PaCO_2$ was lowered by 11.0 ± 1.3 [Torr]. The animals with eliminated chemoreflexes(PaO_2 = 44.7 ± 0.9 [Torr]) changed ventilatory minute volume only insignificantly (+ 9.0 %) with no significant lowering of $PaCO_2$ (- 0.9 ± 0.9 [Torr]). With regard to the circulatory effects no significant changes in MAP and HR could be observed in the chemoreflex intact animals. In the denervated animals, however, both MAP and HR were depressed significantly by 12.0 ± 3.5 [Torr], and 11.1 ± 5.0 [min^{-1}] respectively.

Augmenting $PaCO_2$ under hyperoxia as well as under hypoxia, in both groups led to a distinct increase of ventilation. The slopes of the CO_2-response curves under either level of oxygenation, over a wide range of $\Delta PaCO_2$, were practically equal. In the animals with intact sinus nerves - according to the hypoxic chemoreflex drive - an additional parallel shift to the left could be seen.

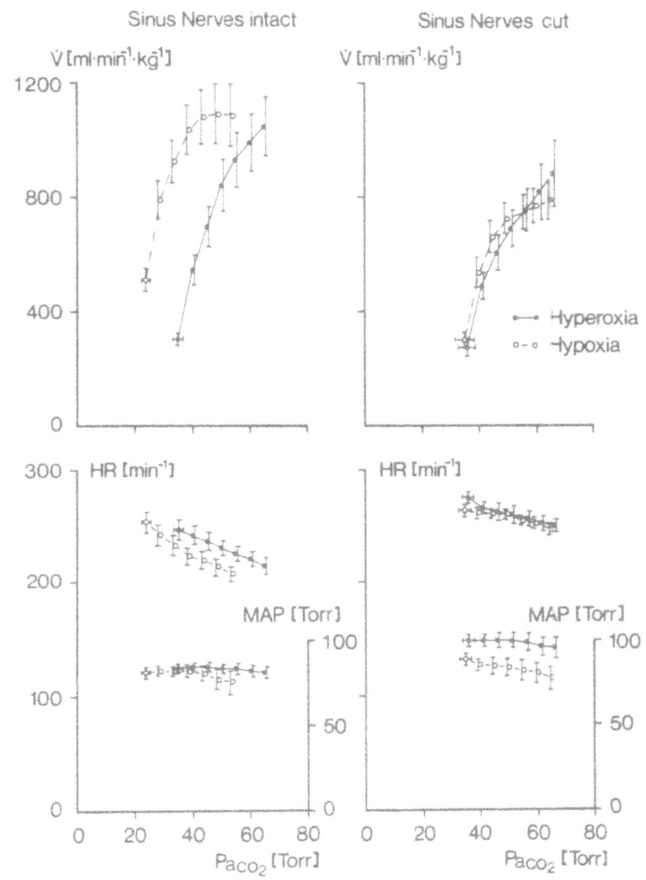

Fig. 1

CO_2-response of ventilation ($\dot{V}$), mean arterial blood pressure (MAP) and heart rate (HR) under hyperoxia and hypoxia (left diagrams: Pa O_2 = 44.0 ± 0.2 [Torr] ; right diagrams: Pa O_2 = 44.7 ± 0.9 [Torr]). Mean values ± S.E. of 10 rabbits with intact sinus nerves and 12 rabbits with both sinus nerves cut.

MAP in the chemoreflex intact animals remained unchanged under raised $PaCO_2$, whereas HR was significantly depressed, the depression being more pronounced under hypoxia than under hyperoxia. In animals with cut sinus nerves, hypercapnia did not significantly alter MAP, whereas HR was significantly lowered, less pronounced under hypoxia, than under hyperoxia. In this group, the depression was generally less than under comparable conditions in the intact group.

2. Arterial acid-base values are shown in fig. 2. In the animals with intact sinus nerves under hyperoxia, mean concentrations of actual bicarbonate $[HCO_3^-]_a$, standard bicarbonate $[HCO_3^-]_{st}$ and hydrogen ions $[H^+]_a$ were 22.3 ± 1.0 [mmol/l], 23.5 ± 0.8 [mmol/l] and 3.758 ± 0.149·10^{-8} [mmol/l]. In the group with cut sinus nerves the same parameters were 19.2 ± 1.3 [mmol/l], 19.9 ± 1.0 [mmol/l] and 4.577 ± 0.144·10^{-8} [mmol/l], respectively.

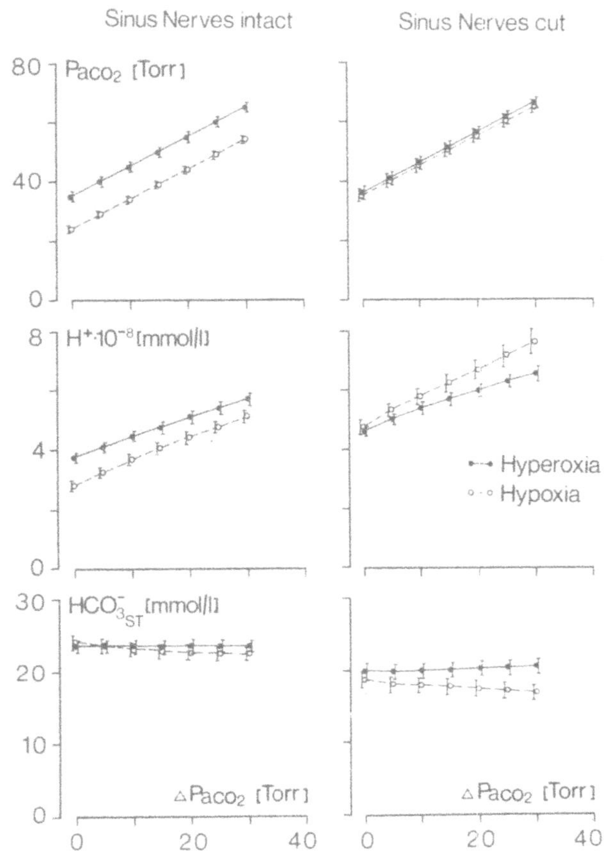

Fig. 2

Absolute arterial CO_2-pressure ($PaCO_2$), H^{+}-ion concentration and standard bicarbonate concentration ($[HCO_3^-]_{st}$) plotted against the change of $PaCO_2$ under hypoxia and hyperoxia. Mean values ± S.E. of the same populations as in fig. 1.

If hypoxia was compared with hyperoxia in the chemoreflex intact group, no metabolic but only respiratory changes could be seen, i.e. no significant change of $[HCO_3^-]_{st}$, but, due to the loss of CO_2 induced by chemoreflex hyperpnea, a distinct decrease of $[H^+]_a$ and $[HCO_3^-]_a$, $-0.932 \pm 0.120 \cdot 10^{-8}$ [mmol/l] and -1.8 ± 0.6 [mmol/l], respectively.

In the animals with cut sinus nerves in contrast, only a small, insignificant respiratory loss of $PaCO_2$ occured, but a significant metabolic decrease of $[HCO_3^-]_{st}$ (-1.2 ± 0.5[mmol/l]). Consequently, there was also a significant decrease of $[HCO_3^-]_a$ (-1.3 ± 0.5 [mmol/l]), but no change of $[H^+]_a$.

Raised $PaCO_2$ under hyperoxia in both groups of rabbits, did not lead to a significant change of $[HCO_3^-]_{st}$. In combination with hypoxia, the animals with intact sinus nerves showed a small but significant loss of $[HCO_3^-]_{st}$ by maximally -1.0 ± 0.4 [mmol/l], only in the higher range of $PaCO_2$ ($\Delta PaCO_2$

15 to 30 Torr). With the same increase of CO_2, the changes in $[H^+]_a$ were more distinct under hypoxia than under hyperoxia, averaging $0.081\cdot10^{-8}$ [mmol/l/Torr] and $0.067\cdot10^{-8}$ [mmol/l/Torr] respectively. In the group with cut sinus nerves, under hypoxia combined with increased $PaCO_2$ ($\Delta PaCO_2$ 5 to 30[Torr]), $[HCO_3^-]_{st}$ was lowered by maximally 3.7 ± 0.5 [mmol/l] . This led to a stronger increase of $[H^+]_a$ (average $0.0104\cdot10^{-8}$ [mmol/l/Torr]), as compared with hyperoxia ($0.072\cdot10^{-8}$ [mmol/l/Torr]), and also as compared with the animals with intact sinus nerves under hypoxia (see above).

3. The O_2-Hb-saturation (SO_2) in both groups of rabbits at the same level of hypoxic PaO_2 (fig. 3) was distinctly different. In the animals with intact sinus nerves, which developed respiratory alkalosis ($[H^+]_a = 2.826 \pm 0.148\cdot10^{-8}$ [mmol/l]), SO_2 was $78.4 \pm 1.2\%$. In the animals with cut sinus nerves, subjected to metabolic acidosis ($[H^+]_a = 4.680 \pm 0.199\cdot10^{-8}$ [mmol/l]). SO_2 was $68.9 \pm 2.1\%$.

With an additional raise of $PaCO_2$, yielding a corresponding raise of $[H^+]_a$, SO_2 was diminished. This decrease, in relation to $[H^+]_a$ was more pronounced in the chemoreflex intact group (average $-7.5\%/10^{-8}$ [mmol/l]) than in the chemodenervated group (average $-2.2\%/10^{-8}$ [mmol/l]).

In the range of $PaCO_2$ between 36.3 and 51.3 [Torr] (absolute values), SO_2 in animals with intact sinus nerves was between 68.7 and 61.5%, in animals with cut sinus nerves between 68.9 and 65.5%. The $[H^+]_a$ values, corresponding to this CO_2-range were distinctly more acid in the denervated group.

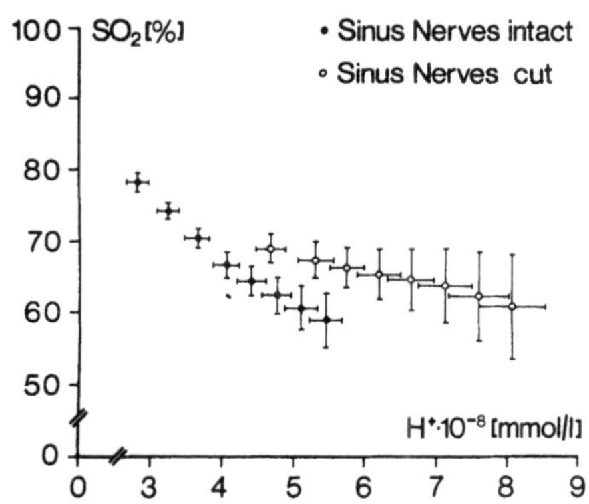

Fig. 3

O_2-Hb saturation at PaO_2 44.0 ± 0.2 [Torr] (sinus nerves intact) and 44.7 ± 0.9 [Torr] (sinus nerves cut) as a function of plasma H^+-ion concentration. Same populations as in fig. 1 and 2.

Discussion

In order to interprete the different SO_2 values - indicating a different O_2 transport capacity - in rabbits with either intact or eliminated chemoreflexes at the same level of arterial hypoxia, first of all, the role of these reflexes on ventilation and circulation must be discussed.

Ventilatory minute volume in the intact group under hypoxia was augmented by chemoreflex drive, followed by a passive decrease of $PaCO_2$. Consequently, in the animals with intact sinus nerves, respiratory alkalosis existed at all levels of hypoxic hypercapnia, but not in the animals with cut sinus nerves. In the denervated group no change of $PaCO_2$ occured, since ventilation remained constant. Under all other experimental conditions, in spite of changed ventilation, no spontaneous changes of blood gas tensions appeared, since PaO_2 and $PaCO_2$ were experimentally controlled (functional open-loop system).

As regards circulation, the marked decrease of MAP in the chemodenervated animals under hypoxic conditions was prevented by chemoreflex drive in the intact animals. It is well known that in rabbits peripheral chemoreflexes stimulated by hypoxia and hypercapnia, are important in maintaining arterial blood pressure (Korner, 1965; Wiemer a.o., 1973). Strong inhibitory chemoreflex effects on heart rate in our experiments must have been partly masked by vagal afferents, which were activated by hyperventilation (Crocker a.o., 1968). Higher heart rate values in the denervated animals, may be due to the elimination of chemo- and baroreflexes, mediated by sinus nerve afferents (Korner, 1965).

With regard to acid-base conditions, the most important difference between both groups under hypoxia concerns respiratory alkalosis in the intact and metabolic acidosis in the denervated group. Respiratory alkalosis could be clearly explained by an effective ventilatory chemoreflex (see above). Metabolic acidosis, however, since ventilatory changes must be excluded, might be caused by circulatory events. The absolute amount of decrease in MAP, together with even higher HR, is not suitable to explain possible insufficient blood supply of organs. It must be assumed that elimination of chemoreflexes alters distribution of blood flow to vital regions (Chalmers a.o., 1967) and probably even particularly to the brain vessels (Ponte and Purves, 1974).

The question arises, in which manner the different acid-base conditions in both groups, determine the O_2-Hb affinity with and without experimentally added CO_2. The interpretation is very complicated, because of the complexity of oxygen transport mechanisms. In order to analyse our findings, we compared the measured O_2-Hb saturation with theoretically calculated data. A suitable numerical approach seemed to be that of Mückenhoff (1973). For description of the O_2-transport system it includes a great number of equations, defining Donnan-equilibrium of all diffusible ions between erythrocytes and plasma, active transport of Na^+- and K^+-ions, interaction between CO_2 and O_2 equilibrium curves, carbamate formation, O_2 saturation as a function of PaO_2 and intracellular pH, and finally titra-

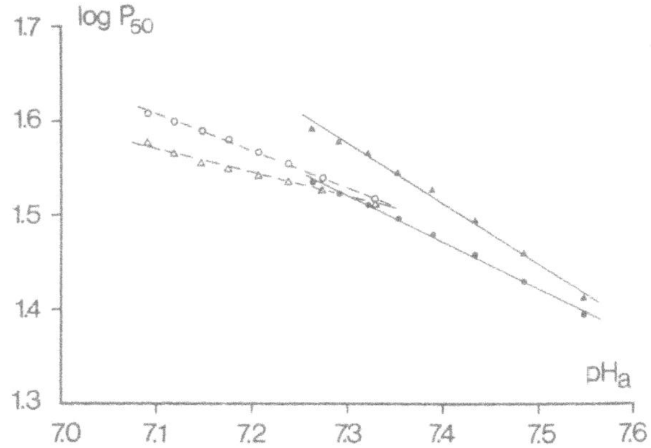

Fig. 4

Relation between log P_{50} and arterial pH in rabbits with intact (filled symbols) and eliminated (open symbols) chemoreflexes. Comparison of measured values (triangles) and theoretically derived data (cycles). Same populations as fig. 1, 2, 3.

tion functions of hemoglobin in relation to O_2-saturation. Using this model the theoretical O_2-equilibrium curves were calculated on the basis of the experimentally given blood gas and acid-base values. Bohr-coefficients ($\Delta logP_{50}/\Delta pHa$) based on these calculated curves were higher in intact, lower in denervated rabbits, being -0.50 and -0.39 respectively (slopes of regression lines as shown in fig. 4). This is in agreement with the findings of Wranne a.o. (1972), indicating that Bohr-coefficients are lower, if the same pH changes are induced by fixed acids and not by CO_2. In comparison with the theoretically derived data, Bohr-coefficients based on our measured values of O_2-Hb saturation, however, yielded a greater difference between both groups, higher values in the chemoreflex intact, lower values in the denervated animals (regression lines, see fig. 4). This may be due to certain factors of the in vivo experiments - not taken into account for the theoretical model - probably changes in 2,3-diphosphoglycerate (DPG) concentration. As shown by Duhm (1973), augmented DPG quantitatively increases Bohr-coefficients (and intracellular H^+), and consequently decreases O_2-Hb affinity. Since in man at high altitude (Lenfant a.o., 1971) higher DPG concentrations are induced by respiratory alkalosis, and can be experimentally lowered in subjects made metabolically acidotic, we suggest - although we did not measure DPG directly - that a similar mechanism may be involved in the oxygen transport system of rabbit blood.

We conclude that the influence of carotid chemoreceptor afferents on pulmonary ventilation and blood-pressure prevents metabolic acidosis due to hypoxia and improves the O_2-saturation of hemoglobin. Without peripheral chemoreflexes, however, the oxygen transport system of the blood seems to be able to compensate partly for an insufficient oxygen supply of the organism under hypoxia and hypercapnia.

Acknowledgements

We are indebted to Miss K. Axt, Mr. W. Balster, Mrs. E. Balster-De Beer and Miss A. Funk for their expert technical assistance.

References

CHALMERS, J.P., P.I. KORNER, S.W. WHITE: Local and reflex factors affecting the distribution of the peripheral blood flow during arterial hypoxia in the rabbit. J. Physiol. 192, 537-548 (1967)

CROCKER, E.F., R.O. JOHNSON, P.I. KORNER, J.B. UTHER, S.W. WHITE: Effects of hyperventilation on the circulatory response of the rabbit to arterial hypoxia. J. Physiol. 199, 267-282 (1968)

DUHM, J.: 2,3-DPG-induced displacements of the oxyhemoglobin dissociation curve of blood: Mechanisms and consequences. In: 'Oxygen Transport to Tissue' (Bicher, H.I., Bruley, D.F. eds.) Advanc. Exp. Med. Biol. 37 A, 179-186 (1973)

KORNER, P.I.: The role of the arterial chemoreceptors and baroreceptors in the circulatory response to hypoxia of the rabbit. J. Physiol. 180, 279-303 (1965)

LENFANT, C., J. TORRANCE, C. REYNAFARJE: Shift of the O_2-Hb dissociation curve at altitude; mechanism and effect. J. appl. Physiol. 30, 625-631 (1971)

v. MENGDEN, H.-J., D. SCHULTEHINRICHS and G. THEWS: Dependence of plasma pH on oxygen saturation. Respir. Physiol. 6, 151-159 (1969)

MÜCKENHOFF, K.: Die Berechnung des Säure-Basen-Status des menschlichen Vollblutes mit Hilfe eines numerischen Verfahrens. Thesis, Bochum (1973)

PONTE, J., M.J. PURVES: The role of the carotid body chemoreceptors and carotid sinus baroreceptors in the control of cerebral blood vessels. J. Physiol. 237, 315-340 (1974)

SCHÖNE, H., W. WIEMER, P. KIWULL: Role of the carotid chemoreflexes in the regulation of arterial oxygen pressure. In: 'Oxygen Transport to Tissue' (Bicher, H.I., Bruley, D.F. eds.) Advanc. Exp. Med. Biol. 37 A, 603-608 (1973)

WIEMER, W., H. SCHÖNE, P. KIWULL: Role of the carotid chemoreceptors in the adjustment of arterial blood pressure to hypoxia. In: 'Oxygen Transport to Tissue' (Bicher, H.I., Bruley, D.F. eds.) Advanc. Exp. Med. Biol. 37 A, 617-622 (1973)

WRANNE, B., R.D. WOODSON, J.C. DETTER: Bohr effect: interaction between H^+, CO_2 and 2,3-DPG in fresh and stored blood. J. appl. Physiol. 32, 749-754 (1972)

Pulmonary Tissue Oxygen Requirement

P.R.B. Caldwell and J.S. Schwartz
College of Physicians and Surgeons
Columbia University, N.Y., N.Y. 10032

T.S. Cottrell
New York Medical College, Vahalla, N.Y. 10591

and

B.A. Wittenberg
Albert Einstein College of Medicine

Earlier studies in an animal model of granulomatous lung disease demonstrated that at normal alveolar oxygen pressure the diseased lung apparently consumed oxygen but did not produce lactate, whereas under hypoxia oxygen consumption diminished and lactate production developed (1-3). Although oxygen uptake decreased when the alveolar oxygen pressure fell below 100 mm Hg, no conclusion was possible regarding the exact tissue oxygen pressure at which this response to hypoxia was manifest. The present studies in lung slices were designed to determine more precisely the oxygen requirement for pulmonary tissue respiration.

The lung disease was produced in albino rabbits by intravenous injection of complete Freund's adjuvant (0.2 ml/kg) on two successive days (2,4,5). Three to four weeks later the animal was sacrificed, the pulmonary vascular bed was perfused with normal saline and tissue slices (400μ) were cut with a McIlwain-Buddle chopper (Brinkman Instruments Westbury, N.Y.) for metabolic and pathologic study. The lung weight to body weight ratio was, on the average, 3.6 times greater in the diseased than the control groups. The surface of the diseased lungs was purplish in color and filled with small nodules 2 mm in diameter. Microscopic examination revealed epithelioid granulomata occasionally surrounded by lymphocytes, plasma cells, polymorphonuclear leukocytes and eosinophils. There were no areas of absess formation. Morphometric measurement showed that, on the average, 90% of the diseased lungs were involved with the proliferative granulomatous process.

Oxygen consumption of the lung slices was measured in a Yellow Springs Model 53 Monitor System (Yellow Springs Instrument Co. Yellow Springs, Ohio). Since the fluid reservoir containing modified Krebs-Ringer phosphate solution and oxygen is not replenished, the measurement is made during an unsteady state in which oxygen pressure falls continously and non-linearly. To standardize the conditions of measurement we first equilibrated the tissue in solution by bubbling with a known oxygen mixture, using previously analyzed tank sources. After 10 minutes of bubbling the gas supply was stopped, the chamber was sealed and the recording of the fall in oxygen pressure with time was begun. Only the first 10 seconds of the recorded trace was used to extrapolate a straight line slope from which the rate of oxygen uptake was calculated. The value of the initial oxygen pressure imposed by the choice of gas mixture was taken as the oxygen pressure for the run. The tissue aliquot was then homogenized in 1% sodium lauryl sulfate,using a hand glass grinding apparatus, filtered and the soluble protein was measured by the Lowry method (6). Four separate cuvettes were used for each lung with duplicate determinations on each cuvette. All tissues were studied within one hour of sacrifice.

The oxygen consumption at 150 mm Hg of diseased lung was 9.4 ± 1.6 ml O_2/mg protein/hr and the value for normal lung was 6.3 ± 0.6 (DF = 18, t = 6, $p < .001$) as shown in Figure 1.

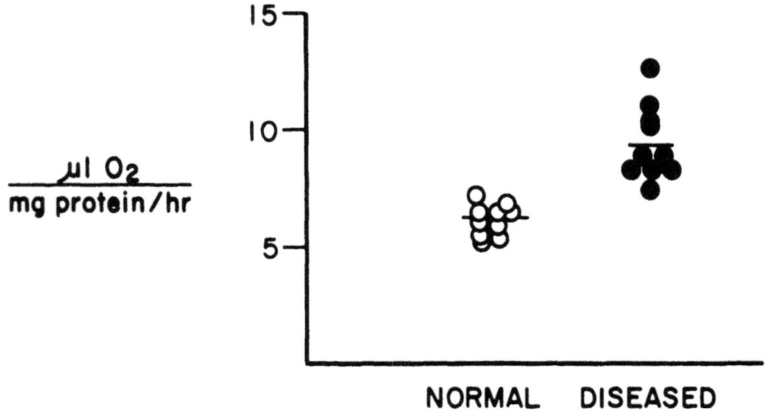

Figure 1

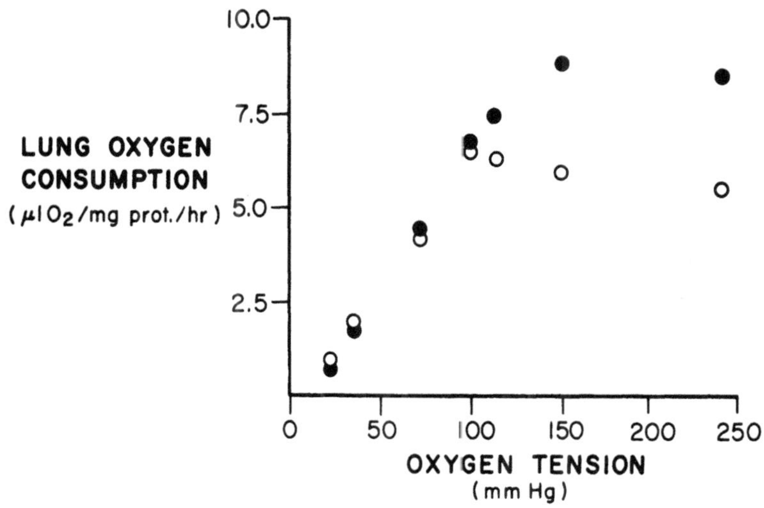

Figure 2

There were no differences in the ratios of protein:wet weight or wet weight÷dry weight between the diseased and normal lung tissue. The relationship of oxygen uptake to oxygen pressure is shown for both diseased and normal tissue in Figure 2. (• diseased, o normal). Here each point represents a mean value for four or more animals. The decrease in oxygen consumption below an initial oxygen pressure of about 100 mm Hg is demonstrated in both diseased and normal pulmonary tissues.

Since Warburg (7) has emphasized the importance of tissue slice thickness in the measurement of tissue respiration we investigated the effect of slice thickness on these measurements. The settings on the McIlwain-Buddle chopper were changed to cut varying thickness. The average thickness was determined by counting the number of slices made at any one setting from a measured length of tissue (1 cm). Since tissue slice thickness might be expected to play a more critical role under conditions of limiting oxygen pressure, measurements of oxygen uptake were made at an oxygen pressure of 36 mm Hg (•) as well as at 150 mm Hg (o). The results for normal lung tissue are shown in Figure 3 and those for diseased lung are shown in Figure 4.

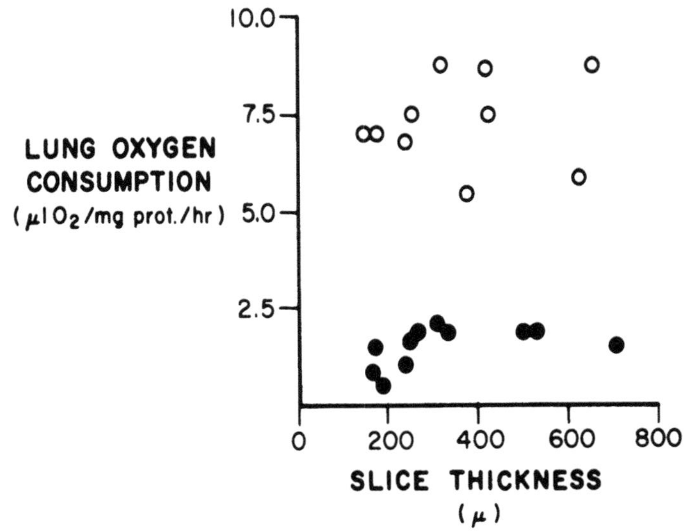

Figure 3

In these figures each point represents a single aliquot of tissue at a given thickness. The thinner slices below 300μ are difficult to prepare intact from the lung and the reduction in oxygen consumption of these thin slices may reflect their fragmentation. Between 300-800μ, however, no discernible effect of tissue slice thickness is seen, even when low oxygen is limiting respiration.

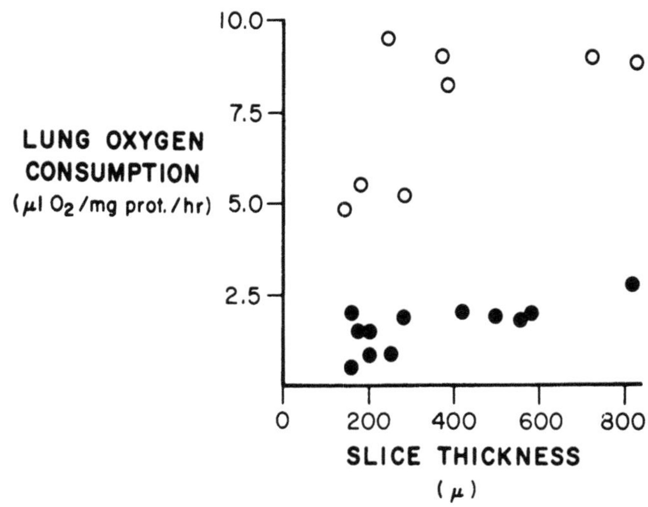

Figure 4

These results are similar to those of Levey and Harvey who found no effect of slice thickness over a similar range on rat lung metabolism studied in the Warburg apparatus (8).

Since oxygen consumption of both diseased and normal pulmonary tissues decreased at oxygen pressures less than 100 mm Hg in these in vitro studies we questioned whether pulmonary tissues might have a unique requirement for oxygen. To investigate this question we designed a special apparatus for measurement of tissue slice respiration under steady state conditions of oxygen pressure (9). This was achieved by having a perfusate which replenishes the oxygen supply in the tissue chamber. The perfusate oxygen pressure is regulated by tonometry with a pre-selected tank oxygen mixture. When the inflow of oxygenated perfusate balances the tissue consumption of oxygen, a steady state of oxygen pressure is achieved. The rate of oxygen uptake can be calculated from the difference between in-flow and out-flow of oxygen through the tissue chamber. Studies of rat tissues, including brain cortex, heart muscle, diaphragm, liver, kidney cortex and lung, demonstrate that the oxygen uptake of each of these tissues decreases monotonically with oxygen pressure below a value of about 100 mm Hg (10). Further, when these data are normalized to the maximal oxygen consumption, a single curve fits the data for each tissue. We conclude, therefore, that there is no evidence that any of the tissues studied has a unique oxygen requirement for respiration. Rather, each organ tissue shows the same relation of oxygen uptake to oxygen pressure in the hypoxic range, where oxygen is limiting.

The results in diseased lung tissue slices support the earlier observations, already cited, on the metabolic behavior in vivo of experimentally produced granulomatous disease in dogs (1-3). The relevance of these studies to human disease is that they afford a model for the interpretation of investigations by Fritts and co-workers (11-13), Rochester and co-workers (14) and Strauss (15). Their investigations showed an increase in intrapulmonary metabolism in patients with diffuse proliferative pulmonary disease. In addition, the presence of appreciable pulmonary oxygen uptake, as much as 12% of the resting total body oxygen consumption (3,13), introduces an error in those tests of cardiorespiratory function which are based on the assumption that the oxygen utilized by diseased lung is negligible. Finally, the independence of tissue oxygen consumption from tissue slice thickness demonstrated here and previously described by others indicates that intracellular oxygen transport requires a fuller description than one based on current models.

Acknowledgement: These investigations were supported by Grants HL-2001, Pulmonary SCOR HL-15088 and HL-5443 from the National Heart and Lung Institute, and by Grant GB 36571 X from the National Science Foundation and a grant from the Muscular Dystrophy Association of America (B.A.W.).

References

1. Caldwell, P.R.B., U. Echeverri and H.W. Fritts, Jr. Trans. Assoc. Am. Phys. 80:97, 1967.

2. Strauss, B., P.R.B. Caldwell and H.W. Fritts, Jr. J. Clin. Invest. 49:1305, 1970.

3. Caldwell, P.R.B., U. Echeverri, M.M. Kilcoyne and H.W. Fritts, Jr. J. Clin. Invest. 49:1311, 1970.

4. Laufer, A., C. Tal and A.J. Behar. Brit. J. Exptl. Path. 40:1, 1959.

5. Rupp, J.C., R.D. Moore and M.D. Schoenberg. Arch. Path. 70:57, 1960.

6. Lowry, O.H., N.J. Rosebrough, A.L. Farr and R.J. Randall. J. Biol. Chem. 193:265, 1951.

7. Warburg, O. Biochem, Ztschr. 142:317, 1923.

8. Levey, S.E. and E. Harvey. J. Appl. Physiol. 37:239, 1974.

9. Wittenberg, B.A., J.W. Wittenberg and P.R.B. Caldwell. In preparation, 1975.

10. Caldwell, P.R.B. and B.A. Wittenberg. Am. J. Med. 57:447, 1974.

11. Fritts, H.W., Jr., P. Harris, C.A. Chidsey, R.H. Clauss and A. Cournand. Circulation 23:390, 1961.

12. Fritts, H.W., Jr., D.W. Richards and A. Cournand. Science 133:1070, 1961.

13. Fritts, H.W., Jr., B. Strauss, W. Wichern, Jr. and A. Cournand. Trans. Ass. Am. Phys. 76:302, 1963.

14. Rochester, D.F., W.A. Wichern, Jr., H.W. Fritts, Jr., P.R.B. Caldwell, M.L. Lewis, C. Giuntini and J.W. Garfield. Am. Rev. Resp. Dis. 107:442, 1973.

15. Strauss, B. J. App. Physiol. 19:503, 1964.

OXYGEN DELIVERY AND UTILIZATION IN HYPOXIC DOGS MADE ACIDEMIC AND ALKALEMIC [1]

Stephen M. Cain

University of Alabama Medical Center

Birmingham, Alabama, USA

A long-standing point of discussion in studies of oxygen transport and delivery during hypoxia has been the relative importance of the driving pressure or PO_2 and the quantity available at the tissue or volume of oxygen delivered per unit time. Because the position of the oxyhemoglobin dissociation curve governs to some extent the ease with which oxygen is loaded at the lung and its driving pressure when unloaded at the tissue, acidemia and alkalemia imposed during hypoxia should affect the quality and quantity of oxygen delivery by their effect upon the position of the dissociation curve, the Bohr effect. To judge whether either condition offers an advantage at a similar level of hypoxia, hypoxic survival time and oxygen uptake were compared to usual parameters of oxygen availability and transport in anesthetized and paralyzed dogs ventilated on an oxygen mixture too low to support the control level of oxygen uptake.

A typical experiment is shown in fig. 1. After the animal was anesthetized with pentobarbital, paralyzed with succinylcholine, and ventilation adjusted to keep end-tidal PCO_2 between 35 and 40 mmHg, a control collection of data for 30 min was begun once stable levels of gas exchange and blood gas tensions were achieved. At the end of the 30 min control period, the intake port of the respirator was abruptly turned to the hypoxic gas mixture, in this case 9.3% O_2 with 7.1% CO_2 in N_2. This was maintained until the animal went into a circulatory crisis of rapidly falling mean arterial pressure (MAP on the figure) when room air

1 Supported by Research Grant HL14693, National Heart and Lung Institute.

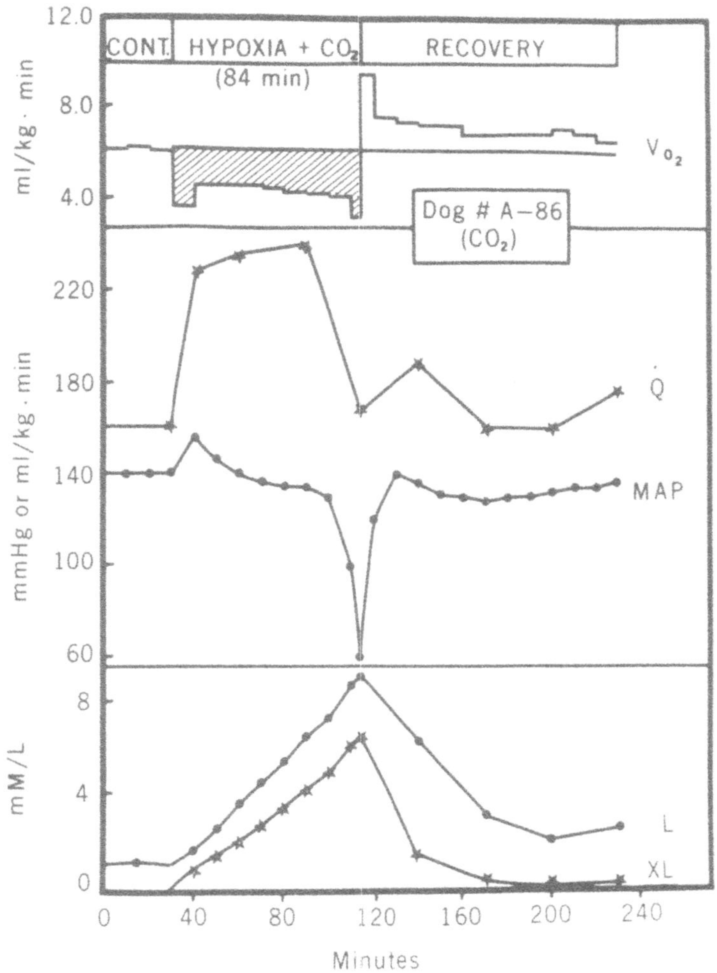

Fig. 1. The course of a typical experiment during control (CONT), experimental, and recovery periods in a dog ventilated with 9.3% O_2 and cardiac output ($\dot{Q}$), mean systemic arterial pressure (MAP), arterial lactate (L) and excess lactate (XL) levels are shown.

was restored as pressure fell below 70 mmHg. That was the time noted as survival time, 84 min in this experiment. Recovery was then followed for 2 hrs.

Gas exchange was measured from expired gas collected in Douglas bags and analyzed every 10 min. Oxygen uptake, after an initial dip in hypoxia that represented O_2 stores utilization, remained near a new steady state level below that of control until the final moments as the animal failed. Cardiac output ($\dot{Q}$) as measured by direct Fick was elevated in this experiment, falling only toward the end of the hypoxic period. Both lactate and excess lactate (XL) rose linearly as the oxygen deficit also increased linearly with time in hypoxia.

In all, three groups of animals were run. The acidemic group, (CO_2 group) which was just described had 10 in number and had an average pH of 6.99 during hypoxia. Alkalemic hypoxia was achieved in a second group of 10 by hyperventilation on 5.2% O_2 at 2.7 times the control ventilation with 7.5% sodium bicarbonate infused so that pH was kept at 7.54 during hypoxia (HV + HCO_3 + β-BL). A third group of 9 was kept at control ventilation on 9.1% O_2 (NO HV+ β-BL) and had an average pH of 7.21 during hypoxia. The latter two groups were given the beta-adrenergic blocking agent propranolol (1 mg/kg per hr) to prevent the calorigenic action of sympathoadrenal stimulation which was largely prevented by acidemia alone in the CO_2 group (2).

In table 1, the ratio of alveolar to total ventilation was calculated from arterial and mixed expired CO_2 fractions measured during the hypoxic steady state. Increasing ventilation by increasing the respiration rate at constant tidal volume resulted in a significantly lower ratio of effective to total ventilation in the HV + HCO_3 + β-BL group. As an estimate of the total flow of oxygen available for gas exchange, the product of F_{IO2} and the inspired alveolar ventilation was compared between groups. This was necessary because of differences in inspired O_2 fractions and ventilations during hypoxia. The CO_2 group in this comparison had a significantly greater oxygen availability than either of the other groups. There was also a significantly greater cardiac output during hypoxia, based on time-weighted averages, in the CO_2 group and this was probably attributable to the use of propranolol in the other two groups. When total oxygen delivery, the product of cardiac output and arterial oxygen content, was compared, however, there were no significant differences between groups. This undoubtedly resulted from the decreased loading of oxygen in the acidemic CO_2 group which thus lost its advantage in oxygen availability.

As total oxygen delivery is a measure of the quantity of oxygen presented to the tissue per unit time, the PO2 might be considered a measure of the quality of oxygen transport. In table 2,

Table 1: Average values (±S.D.) during hypoxia for ratio of effective to total ventilation ($\dot{V}_A/\dot{V}E$), total O_2 availability ($\dot{V}_{AI} \cdot F_{IO2}$), cardiac output, and total O_2 delivery ($\dot{Q} \cdot CaO_2$)

GROUP	$\dot{V}_A/\dot{V}_E$	$\dot{V}_{A_I}$ F_{IO_2} (ML/KG · MIN)	$\dot{Q}$ (ML/KG · MIN)	$\dot{Q} \cdot Ca_{O_2}$ (ML/KG · MIN)
HV + HCO_3 + β − BL	0.43 ± 0.05	8.0 ± 1.2	141 ± 37	6.1 ± 1.8
CO_2	0.74 * ± 0.11	10.9 * ± 2.0	183 * ± 25	6.2 ± 1.1
NO HV + β − BL	0.62 * ± 0.05	7.2 ± 1.1	140 ± 69	5.6 ± 1.7

* Significantly different from HV + HCO_3 + β−BL ($P < 0.05$)

both the CO_2 and NO HV + β-BL groups had higher quality O_2 transport in that arterial PO_2 was significantly greater than in the HV + HCO_3 + β-BL group. From the averages during the hypoxic steady state, PO_2 was 8 mmHg higher in the CO_2 and 5 mmHg higher in the NO HV + β-BL groups. Although mixed venous PO_2 was greater in both those groups also, statistical significance was achieved only by the CO_2 group in comparison to the HV + HCO_3 + β-BL group. As one of the experimental variables, group averages of H^+ concentration all differed significantly from one another. Although the CO_2 group had significantly more O_2 availability and higher arterial and mixed venous values of PO_2, survival time in hypoxia was almost exactly the same as that of HV + HCO_3 + β-BL group. In fact, no group differed from the others significantly in survival time just as all groups had the same average total O_2 delivery.

In that the deficit in O_2 uptake can be related to the hypoxic survival time when additional energy demanding actions such as catecholamine calorigenesis are prevented during hypoxia (3), the relationship of the percent decrease in oxygen uptake and the rate of total O_2 delivery (cardiac output times arterial O_2 content) was

Table 2: Average values (±S.D.) of arterial and mixed venous PO_2, arterial H^+ concentration, and survival time in hypoxia.

GROUP	Pa_{O_2} (mm/Hg)	$P\bar{v}_{O_2}$ (mm/Hg)	$[H^+]_a$ (nM/L)	SURVIVAL TIME (min)
HV + HCO_3+ β–BL	14.5 ± 1.4	7.7 ± 1.4	29.1 ± 5.7	78 ± 28
CO_2	22.6 * ± 1.9	9.6 * ± 1.8	102.6 ± 16.9	77 ± 39
NO HV + β–BL	19.7 * ± 3.4	9.4 ± 2.5	61.2 ± 7.4	111 ± 51

* Significantly different from HV + HCO_3+β–BL ($P<0.05$)

examined in figure 2. The values plotted here are the average for each animal obtained while O_2 uptake was relatively constant in hypoxia. A linear relationship with correlation coefficient of 0.89 was found with all groups equally distributed around the regression line obtained by the method of least squares. In other words, below a critical value of oxygen delivery, oxygen uptake was directly dependent on the volume of oxygen presented to the tissues per unit time. This was true irrespective of the PO_2 at which oxygen was delivered within the values measured in these experiments, a range of 12.4 to 25.1 mmHg PO_2 because the percent of oxygen uptake was not significantly correlated with arterial PO_2. For that matter, neither did percent of oxygen uptake correlate with mixed venous PO_2, cardiac output, nor the alveolar oxygen availability. The critical value of total oxygen delivery was obtained by extrapolating the line of best fit to 100% of oxygen uptake and it was 10.8 ml/kg·min. In some earlier published work, a similar critical value of total oxygen delivery of 12.0 ml/kg·min was found for experiments in which dogs were subjected to anemic hypoxia by reducing circulating hemoglobin and hypoxic hypoxia by reducing inspired O_2 fraction (1). In those experiments, there were much wider ranges of arterial and

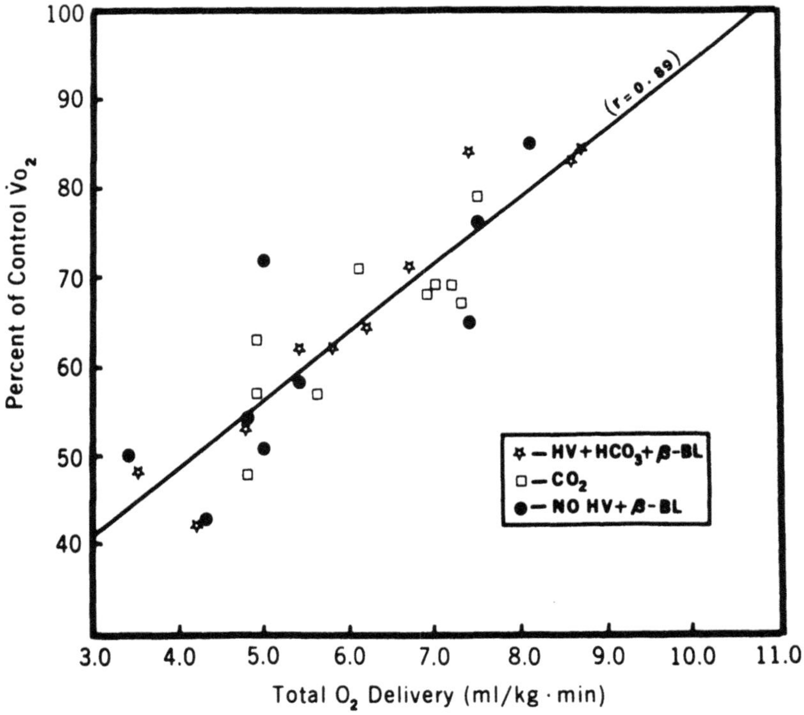

Fig. 2: The percent of control level O_2 uptake during hypoxia in relation to the rate of total O_2 delivery ($\dot{Q} \cdot Ca_{O2}$).

mixed venous PO_2 at which an energy deficit was incurred. More recently, sublethal doses of cobalt chloride in anesthetized and paralyzed dogs kept at constant ventilation on room air produced a transient stagnant hypoxia by reduction of cardiac output and this caused oxygen uptake to decrease below control only as total oxygen delivery fell below 12.0 ml/kg·min (4).

In summary, as tissue hypoxia produced by any means becomes severe enough to limit aerobic metabolism, oxygen uptake becomes wholly dependent upon volume delivery. As oxygen uptake falls, the Krogh-Erlang equation (5) indicates a lessening dependence upon the partial pressure gradient for oxygen. Further, with severe hypoxia and the consequent depression of centrally mediated reflexes, local tissue responses would dominate so that diffusion distances would lessen as capillary beds were maximally utilized (6). These responses would also lessen the importance of the oxygen driving pressure as a supply factor until, finally, it is only the volume delivery of oxygen which sets its rate of uptake.

REFERENCES

1. Cain, S.M. Appearance of excess lactate in anesthetized dogs during anemic and hypoxic hypoxia. Am. J. Physiol. 209:604-610, 1965.

2. Cain, S.M. Diminution of lactate rise during hypoxia by PCO_2 and β-adrenergic blockade. Am. J. Physiol. 271:110-116, 1969.

3. Cain, S.M. Survival time of hypoxic dogs given epinephrine or propranolol. Am. J. Physiol. 225:1405-1410, 1973.

4. Cain, S.M. Oxygen delivery and utilization in dogs with a sublethal dose of cobalt chloride. J. Appl. Physiol. 38: 20-25, 1975.

5. Krogh, A. The number and distributions of capillaries in muscles with calculations of the oxygen pressure head necessary for supplying the tissue. J. Physiol. (Lond.) 52:405-415, 1919.

6. Shepherd, A.P., H.J. Granger, E.E. Smith, and A.C. Guyton. Local control of tissue oxygen delivery and its contribution to the regulation of cardiac output. Am. J. Physiol. 225: 747-755, 1973.

EVIDENCE AGAINST LOCAL CONTROL OF INTESTINAL TISSUE OXYGENATION BY MYOGENIC MECHANISMS

A. P. Shepherd and W. W. Pawlik

Department of Physiology, The University of Texas Health Science Center, San Antonio, Texas and Institute of Physiology, Medical Academy, Krakow, Poland

The proposed basis for the myogenic theory of local blood flow control is that vascular smooth muscle will actively contract if stretched by increased transmural pressure. Critical experiments to test the myogenic hypothesis have employed elevated venous pressure to raise transmural pressures in the microvasculature. In isolated loops of small bowel, elevated venous pressure has been reported to cause an increase in total resistance to blood flow (1). Subsequent studies of capillary filtration showed that the increase in resistance occurred on the precapillary side. Such resistance changes in response to elevated venous pressure are thought to result from a myogenic constriction of resistance vessels (2). In addition to resistance vessels, precapillary sphincters are thought to respond to elevated venous pressure. By measuring the rate of fluid filtration at various venous pressures, and by determining the isogravimetric capillary pressure with a stop-flow technique, Johnson (3) was able to calculate capillary filtration coefficients for small intestine. His study showed that, although the filtration rate increased with increased venous pressure as expected, the calcualted capillary filtration coefficients fell with increased venous pressure. The proposed mechanism to explain the reduction in capillary filtration coefficients was a myogenic constriction of precapillary sphincters in response to the increased venous pressure. Thus, the myogenic closure of precapillary sphincters would reduce the number of perfused capillaries and therefore reduce the capillary filtration coefficient which depends upon the capillary permeability and capillary surface area.

In previous studies, both with mathematical models and in animal experiments, we have shown that the density of the perfused capillary bed can be reduced with vasoconstrictor agents (4,5,6).

Since the oxygen flux from capillary to cell depends on the capillary surface area and the capillary-to-cell diffusion distance, vasoconstrictor-induced reductions in the density of the perfused capillary bed depress oxygen extraction even in isolated gut loops perfused at a constant blood flow rate. Thus, the purpose of this work was to determine if the so-called myogenic response at the capillary level has any effect on the oxygenation of intestinal tissue.

METHODS

Fasted mongrel dogs were anesthetized with sodium pentobarbital (30 mg/kg, i.v.). The femoral arteries were catheterized to obtain blood for perfusing the isolated loops of small bowel, and the femoral veins were cannulated for returning blood to the animal. A segment of jejenum or ileum was exteriorized, placed on saline-soaked gauze, and covered with a plastic film. The artery and vein of the gut loop were cannulated after heparin administration (10 mg/kg, i.v.). Collateral vessels in the gut wall were eliminated by ligating the ends of the gut loop.

The isolated gut segments were perfused with a peristaltic pump (Cole-Parmer, No. 7545) at a constant rate of blood flow. Arterial and venous pressures were measured with transducers connected by T-tubes to the perfusion circuit. The arteriovenous oxygen difference was monitored continuously with a photoelectric device. The level of the venous outflow was initially set to produce a venous pressure of 5 mmHg. Blood flow rates were determined by collecting the venous effluent. To determine ^{86}Rb extraction, a coil of the venous tubing was placed in a well-counter so that venous radioactivity could be monitored continuously. The output of the well-counter fed into a ratemeter and the ratemeter's output was recorded on a Beckman RM recorder along with venous pressure, arterial pressure, and arteriovenous oxygen difference.

Perfusion pressure and arteriovenous oxygen difference were allowed to stabilize for 15 to 30 minutes. Venous pressure was then elevated to approximately 25 mmHg by raising the level of the venous outflow. The elevated venous pressure was maintained for approximately 10 minutes and then restored to the control level. The monitored parameters usually reached new steady-state levels during the period of elevated pressure and they generally returned to the control level when venous pressure was restored to control.

To determine rubidium extraction, a bolus of radioactive ^{86}RbCl in saline was injected into the arterial circuit. The radioactivity appearing in the venous blood was recorded as a time-concentration curve. The arteriovenous ^{86}Rb extraction ratio was determined by planimeter measurements of the area under the washout curve. From the arteriovenous ^{86}Rb extraction ratio (E), Renkin's (7) capillary transport coefficient (PS = permeability x surface area) was calculated as PS = -Q ln (1 - E) where Q is blood flow (ml/min/100g). After each experiment, the perfused gut segment was weighed and its blood flow expressed in ml/min/100g of tissue weight.

RESULTS

Control data from these experiments, expressed as mean ± standard error of mean, were as follows: arteriovenous oxygen difference, 6.6 ± 0.5 ml O_2/100 ml blood; blood flow, 18.5 ± 2.1 ml/min/100g; arteriovenous ^{86}Rb extraction ratio, 0.78 ± 0.03; and oxygen consumption rate 1.20 ± 0.1 ml O_2/min/100g.

Figure 1 shows the record of an experiment in which venous pressure was elevated. In the control period, venous pressure was held at 5 mmHg, and the arterial perfusion pressure was approximately 70 mmHg. The arteriovenous oxygen difference was approximately 6 ml O_2/100 ml during the control period. (It should be noted that changes in arteriovenous oxygen difference at a constant rate of blood flow are equivalent to changes in the oxygen consumption rate.) When the volus of ^{86}Rb was injected, a washout curve was produced and as the figure indicates, the ^{86}Rb arteriovenous extraction ratio calculated for the control period was approximately 69%. When venous pressure was elevated from 5 to 25 mmHg, arterial pressure rose by essentially the same amount. The arteriovenous oxygen difference reached a new steady-state approximately 3 ml O_2/100 ml above the control level. When the bolus of ^{86}RbCl was injected, a washout curve during the period of elevated venous pressure produced an arteriovenous ^{86}Rb extraction ratio of 80%. Thus, elevating the venous pressure from 5 to 25 mmHg produced essentially no change in resistance, but it increased the extraction of oxygen and the extraction of ribidium by the perfused gut loop.

Figure 2 shows the mean values from five experiments with gut loops perfused at a constant rate of blood flow. As Figure 2 indicates, elevating the venous pressure from 5 to 25 mmHg caused the arteriovenous oxygen difference and hence the oxygen consumption rate to increase 28 ± 4.2%. Similarly, the increase in venous pressure was associated with a 19 ± 5% increase in the capillary transport coefficient (PS).

DISCUSSION

In previous studies, we have shown that a number of vasoconstrictors not only increase vascular resistance, but also depress oxygen and rubidium extraction in isolated gut loops perfused at a constant rate of blood flow (5,8). These findings are consistent with the view that vasoconstrictors close precapillary sphincters

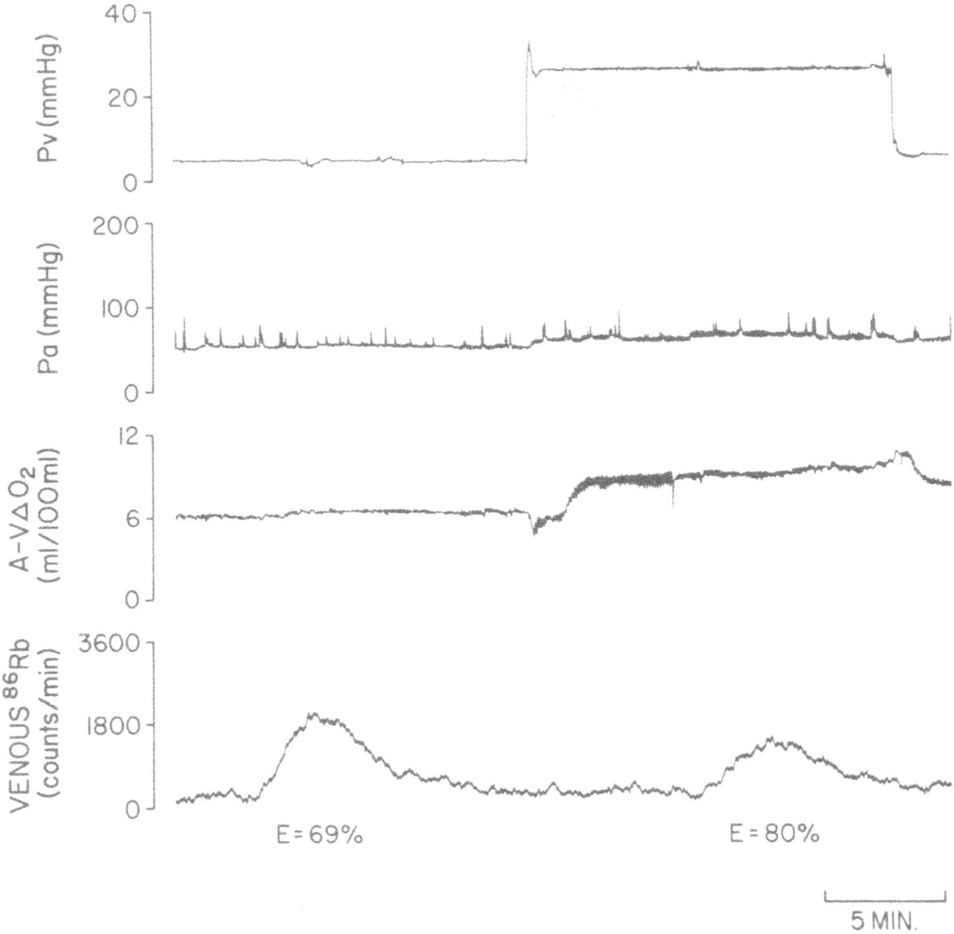

Figure 1. Record of an experiment in which venous pressure was elevated during constant-flow perfusion of an isolated gut loop. Raising venous pressure (Pv) from 5 to 25 mmHg caused arterial pressure (Pa) to increase by approximately the same amount. With the step-increase in venous pressure, the arteriovenous oxygen difference (A-V ΔO_2) increased from 6 ml O_2/100 ml blood to 9 ml O_2/100 ml, and the rubidium extraction ratio (E) increased from 69 to 80%.

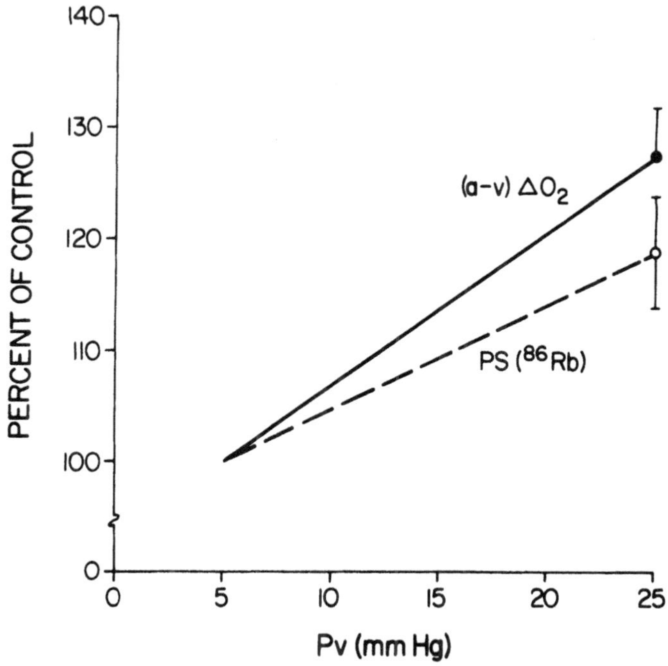

Figure 2. Effect of venous pressure elevation on oxygen and rubidium extraction. When venous pressure was raised from 5 to 25 mmHg, the arteriovenous oxygen difference [(a-v) ΔO_2] increased to 128% of control and the capillary transport coefficient (PS) increased to 119% of control. (Mean values ± standard errors from five experiments are shown.)

and reduce the number of perfused capillaries. Furthermore, our calculations confirm that if the density of the perfused capillary bed falls below a critical level, the diffusion parameters (capillary surface area and capillary-to-cell diffusion distance) will limit oxygen extraction (4,6).

Because increased venous pressure has been reported to cause marked reductions in the density of the perfused intestinal capillary bed (3,9), as indicated by changes in the capillary filtration coefficient (K_f), one would expect elevated venous pressure to depress oxygen extraction in gut loops perfused at constant flow. The present results, however, show that raising venous pressure from 5 to 25 mmHg consistently <u>increased</u> oxygen extraction (Figure 1). Furthermore, the increases in oxygen extraction were consistently associated with increased rubidium extraction (Figure 2). Since the capillary transport coefficient (PS) for rubidium has been shown to reflect changes in the density of the perfused capillary bed (7), the present results indicate that increased venous pressure opened unperfused capillaries and thus allowed greater extraction of both oxygen and rubidium.

Although previous studies used constant arterial pressure perfusion while constant flow was employed in the present study, it is not apparent why the two indices of capillary density (PS and K_f) should undergo dissimilar changes in the two types of studies. Nevertheless, our preparations maintained resistance despite increased transmural pressure, an indication of a mild myogenic response, and they were responsive to vasoactive agents. In view of the responsiveness of the preparation and the failure of elevated venous pressure to reduce oxygen and rubidium extraction, we feel it is doubtful that "myogenic mechanisms" play a role in the local control of oxygen delivery to intestinal tissues.

REFERENCES

1. Johnson, P. C. Myogenic nature of increase in intestinal vascular resistance with venous pressure elevation. Circ. Res. 7: 992-999, 1959.
2. Johnson, P. C. Effect of venous pressure on mean capillary pressure and vascular resistance in the intestine. Circ. Res. 16: 294-300, 1965.
3. Johnson, P. C. and K. M. Hanson. Capillary filtration in the small intestine of the dog. Circ. Res. 19:766-773, 1966.
4. Shepherd, A. P. and H. J. Granger. Autoregulatory escape in the gut: A systems analysis. Gastroenterology 65:77-91, 1973.
5. Shepherd, A. P., D. Mailman, T. F. Burks and H. J. Granger. Effects of norepinephrine and sympathetic stimulation on extraction of oxygen and ^{86}Rb in perfused canine small bowel. Circ. Res. 33:166-174, 1973.
6. Shepherd, A. P., D. Mailman, T. F. Burks and H. J. Granger. Sympathetic nervous control of intestinal O_2 extraction. In: Oxygen Transport to Tissue, H. I. Bicher and D. F. Bruley, Eds., Plenum Press, New York, 1973, pp. 423-428.
7. Renkin, E. M. and S. Rosell. Influence of sympathetic adrenergic vasoconstrictor nerves on transport of diffusible solutes from blood to tissues in skeletal muscle. Acta Physiol. Scand. 54: 223-240, 1962.
8. Pawlik, W., D. Mailman, A. P. Shepherd, T. Burks and E. D. Jacobson. Effects of vasoconstrictors on mesenteric hemodynamics and oxygen consumption. Fed. Proc. 33:338, 1974 (abstract).
9. Mortillaro, N. A. and A. E. Taylor. Interactions of the vascular, interstitial, and lymphatic systems in the cat intestine. The Physiologist 16:401, 1973 (abstract).

EFFECT OF IONIZING RADIATION ON LIVER MICROCIRCULATION AND OXYGENATION

Bicher, H.I.*+, Dalrymple, G.V.+, Ashbrook, D.+, Smith, R*, and Harris, D.+
*Department of Pharmacology, +Department of Radiology
University or Arkansas Medical Center, Little Rock, Arkansas, USA

Ionizing radiation causes destruction of mammalian tissue by two mechanisms (11): 1) inhibition of the proliferative capacity of rapidly dividing cells, and 2) irreversible damage to elements of the microcirculatory system. Organs such as liver, kidney, and brain, not characterized by rapidly proliferating cells, exhibit a relatively pronounced radiosensitivity in spite of a very slow rate of cellular turnover. The radiosensitivity of the microcirculation could provide the reason for the radiosensitivity of the entire organ or tissue.

In previous publications (1,2,4,5) we have described microcirculatory damage to parenchymatous organs induced by intravascular platelet and red cell aggregation, as these processes tend to interfere with tissue oxygenation. The objective of this investigation was to elucidate the effects of Co^{60} ionizing radiation on liver microcirculation, function and oxygenation.

METHODS AND MATERIALS

Oxygen Determinations

The oxygen electrodes used in this series of experiments consist of a teflon coated Pt/Ir wire (120 μ diam, 2 cm long) that is advanced into the liver tissue through the lumen of a 26 G needle after the needle has penetrated the liver capsule. The electrode is allowed to "float" with the normal respiratory excursions of the liver and is attached to the instrumentation by a 40 μ gold wire which will not hamper this movement. The electrodes are coated with Rhoplex AC 35 (a water carrying, highly adhesive, oxygen pervious material, obtained from Rohm & Haas, Philadelphia, Pa.) which is used to delay the "poisoning" of the electrode surface by protein electrophoresis.

The reference electrode is composed of a pure silver wire coated with AgCl and encased in an agar-KCl bridge. This reference electrode is placed inside the abdominal cavity or subcutaneously.

The electrode is calibrated in vitro prior to insertion into the liver using the technique developed by Silver (12).

Reoxygenation times (RT, period of time required for TpO_2 to return to its original level after a 60 second period of anoxic anoxia) was determined as previously described (6). This measurement has been found to be a good indicative parameter of the ability of the microcirculation to deliver oxygen to tissue. In each experiment 5 determinations were made at 4 different locations in the liver.

Determination of Platelet Adhesiveness and Aggregation

Photoelectric Method Platelet Aggregation. The photoelectric method to determine platelet aggregation in platelet-rich plasma (PRP) has been described by Born (8). Continuously stirred PRP is placed in a transilluminated test tube, and the amount of light transmitted is measured with a photocell. Platelet aggregation is induced by ADP. The aggregates change the amount of light received by the photocell, and can thereby be recorded.

To determine platelet reactivity to ADP in animals pre or post irradiation, a dose response curve is carried out for a sample from each animal, using increasing ADP concentrations from 0.1 μg per milliliter to 10 μg per milliliter. The concentration is determined that gives a response midway between a minimum response and a maximal response. The ADP concentration giving a "mean" response is thus determined.

Rolling tube platelet adhesiveness test. In this method, previously described (2), a volume of 1.0 ml/tube of anti-coatulated blood is placed in a series of 10 ml, 1.2 cm diameter non-siliconized test tubes containing no drug (control), and varying concentrations of ADP and ATP. These concentrations are less than, equal to, and more than the amount of ADP required for aggregation as determined by the photoelectric method. After rotation, adhesive platelets adhere to the wall of the test tube, and those remaining in the blood are counted. The differences between the platelet counts of the control and the tubes containing ADP indicates percentages of of platelet adhesiveness caused by the drug. The effective dose of ADP to induce an increase in platelet adhesiveness is thus determined. A change in the required amount of ADP to induce this effect in an individual post irradiation animal as compared to that animal's pre irradiation requirement indicates the increase in platelet adhesiveness.

Histology, Liver Function Tests and Blood Chemistries

Tissue samples were obtained, fixed and stained using standard histological techniques for microscopy studies. Liver function tests and blood chemistries performed include LDH, SGOT, Bilirubin, Total Colloid, Serum Albumin, Total Serum Protein, A/G Ratio, Prothrombin Time, Alkaline Phosphatase, HCT, WBC, RBC, BUN, Na+ and K+. Standard methodology was used in all tests. Blood samples were drawn before and after radiation treatments for testing.

General Experimental Plan

The experiments were performed on female beagle dogs, 1 year old when treatment was started. All determinations were performed prior to radiation, and then again two weeks after radiation treatments ended.

Whole liver radiation was performed through parallel lateral opposing ports after radiological confirmation of field localization. The animals were treated to 4600 rads delivered in 23 treatments, total treatment time being 35 days. A Co^{60} Teletherapy HVL 11 pb unit at a SSD of 50 cm was used. Isodose curves were determined for each animal.

When determining TpO_2 the animals were under barbituate anesthesia with tracheal intubation and cannulation of the femoral artery and vein. Blood samples for <u>in vitro</u> studies were obtained from the cannulated femoral vein. All surgical procedures were done under sterile conditions.

RESULTS AND DISCUSSION

At the present time, pre and post irradiation studies have been completed in 9 beagles.

Reoxygenation times: It was found that the normal reoxygenation time in the dog's liver is 2.14 minutes. This figure is larger than the RT in the cat's brain (0.68 min.) as previously reported (7). After ionizing radiation the liver RT is significantly prolonged, to an average of 3.26 minutes (See Table 1, Figs. 1 and 2).

TABLE 1

AVERAGE BEAGLE REOXYGENATION TIMES - LIVER

DOG	PRE-IRRAD.	POST-IRRAD.	P VALUES
A-5	1.56 ± 0.42	3.36 ± 1.11	< .001
A-6	2.53 ± 1.35	4.87 ± 1.21	< .001
A-7	1.30 ± 0.20	5.50 ± 1.89	< .001
A-8	2.00 ± 1.13	1.84 ± 0.45	< .7
A-9	1.60 ± 0.49	2.72 ± 0.65	< .001
A-10	2.72 ± 1.54	2.17 ± 0.71	< .3
A-11	2.80 ± 0.84	3.15 ± 0.90	< .001
A-12	3.26 ± 0.88	3.79 ± 0.92	< .001
A-13	1.58 ± 0.21	2.98 ± 0.93	< .001
Avg.	2.14 ± 1.12	3.26 ± 1.54	< .001

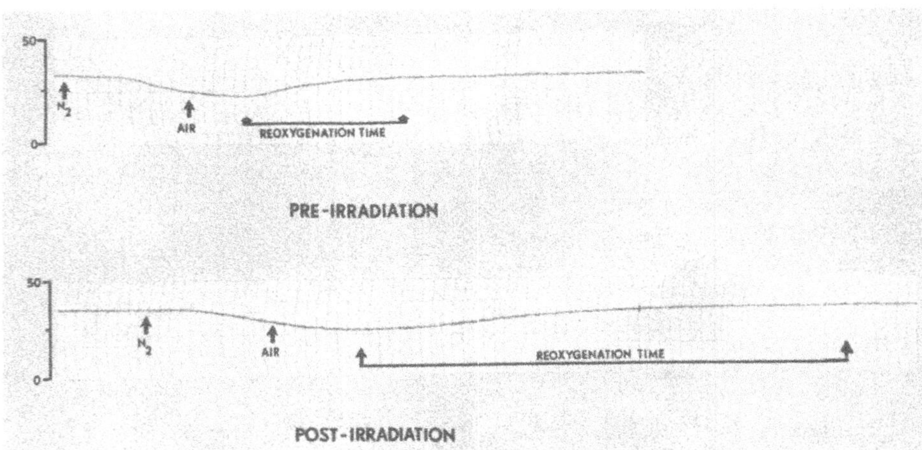

Fig. 1: BEAGLE REOXYGENATION TIMES. Note prolonged RT after irradiation. For explanation see text.

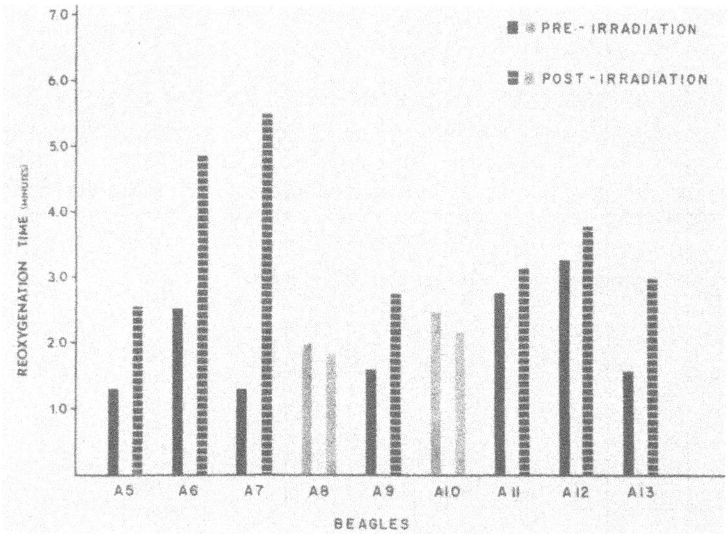

Fig. 2: REOXYGENATION TIMES IN LIVER, PRE & POST IRRADIATION.

Platelet aggregation and adhesiveness: Both platelet aggregation and adhesiveness increased markedly after irradiation. The mean effective dose (MED) of ADP to induce 50% aggregation or adhesiveness decreased from 2.5 μg/ml to 1.3 μg/ml. The adhesiveness induced by the pre-irradiation MED was 46.6% before irradiation and 86.2% after irradiation (See Table 2).

Histology and Blood Chemistry: No significant changes were observed histologically in pre and post irradiation sections. The only significant changes in blood chemistry were: a decrease in albumin from 3.11 mg% to 1.91 mg% in 6 out of 9 dogs; alkaline phosphatase increased from 56 to 300 units in 7 out of 9 dogs. All other parameters were unchanged.

Recently Ingold (9) demonstrated that the liver is not radioresistant to ionizing radiation, but rather one of the more sensitive tissues. Ingold's studies indicated that the sensitivity of the liver is comparable to that of bone marrow, lymphoid tissue, germinal tissue and the kidneys.

Kinzie et al. (10) reported results which indicate that the prevention of intravascular coagulation (by heparinization) greatly reduced the impact of radiation upon the livers of rats. The apparent mechanism is the prevention of ischemic atrophic changes which would follow the post irradiation obliteration of the microcirculation. Although these results would seem to indicate a principle of considerable importance in clinical oncology, additional

TABLE 2

RADIATION INDUCED CHANGES IN PLATELET AGGREGATION
IN VIVO UTILIZATION OF OXYGEN AND GLUCOSE BY NEOPLASTIC TISSUE

DOG	DOSE ADP CAUSING MAXIMUM AGGREGATION		% PLATELETS ADHERING (With Pre-Irrad. Dose for Maximum Aggregation)		% PLATELETS ADHERING (With Post-Irrad. Dose for Maximum Aggregation)
	Pre-Irrad.	Post-Irrad.	Pre-Irrad.	Post-Irrad.	
A-5	2.0 ug	2.0 ug	44.5	93.2	70.6
A-6	2.0 ug	0.25 ug	56.1	91.6	33.7
A-7	1.0 ug	0.5 ug	46.4	85.6	64.9
A-8	1.0 ug	0.5 ug	61.1	86.5	38.9
A-9	5.0 ug	2.5 ug	44.4	95.8	69.1
A-10	3.0 ug	1.5 ug	22.6	84.1	49.9
A-11	2.0 ug	2.0 ug	51.3	66.7	60.1
Avg.	2.3 ug	1.3 ug	46.6	86.2	54.7

information is not available.

The present studies clearly demonstrate that ionizing radiation induces profound deleterious changes in the ability of the microcirculation to oxygenate liver tissue. This is indicated by the marked prolongation in reoxygenation time, a sensitive parameter of this function (3). The microcirculation disturbance could probably be mediated by increased intravascular blood cell aggregation, as indicated by the increase in platelet aggregation and adhesiveness hereby reported.

SUMMARY

Platelet aggregation and adhesiveness, as well as TpO_2 responses to hypoxia were measured as microcirculation parameters in beagle dogs subject to Co^{60} ionizing radiation to a dose of 4600 rads in 5 weeks. Simultaneously, changes in blood chemistry and coagulation were also determined. Marked changes in all studied parameters in the post radiation period lead to the conclusion that radiation liver damage is at least in part mediated through microcirculation disturbances.

REFERENCES

1. Bicher, H.I. Prevention of sludge induced myocardial damage by an anti-adhesive drug. Bibl. anat., 10:202, 1969.

2. Bicher, H.I. Anti-adhesive drugs in thrombosis. Throm. et Diath Haem., Suppl. 42:197, 1970.

3. Bicher, H.I. Brain oxygen autoregulation: A protective reflex to hypoxia. Microvasc. Res., 8:291-313, 1974.

4. Bicher, H.I. and Beemer, A.M. Induction of ischemic myocardial damage by red cell aggregation (sludge) in the rabbit. J. Atherosclerosis Res., 7:409, 1967.

5. Bicher, H.I. and Beemer, A.M. Prevention by an anti-adhesive drug of thrombosis caused by blood cell aggregation. Angiol., 21:413, 1970.

6. Bicher, H.I., Bruely, D.F., Reneau, D.D., and Knisely, M.H. Effect of microcirculation changes on brain tissue oxygenation. J. Physiol., 217:689-707, 1971.

7. Bicher, H.I., Marvin, P., Hunt, D.H., and Bruley, D.F. Autonomic and pharmacologic control of oxygen autoregulation mechanisms in brain tissue. ISOTT Symposium, Mainz, Germany, 1975. (To be published by Plenum Press, N.Y.)

8. Born, G.V. Quantitative investigations into aggregation of blood platelets. J. Physiol., 162:67p, 1962.

9. Ingold, J., Reed, G. and Kaplan, M.D. Am. J. Roentgenology, 93:200, 1965.

10. Kinzie, J., Studer, R.K., Perez, B. and Potcher, E.J. Non-cytokinetic radiation injury; anticoagulants as radio-protective agents in experimental radiation hepatitis. Science, 175:1481, 1972.

11. Rubin, P. The radiographic expression of radiotherapeutic injury. An overview. Seminars in Roentgenology, 1:5, 1974.

12. Silver, I. A simple microelectrode for measuring pO_2 in gas or fluid. Med. Electron. Biol. Eng., 1:547, 1963.

A FACTOR IN LONGITUDINAL TISSUE GRADIENTS: RED CELL CARRIAGE

Carl A. Goresky and Glen G. Bach

McGill University Medical Clinic in the
Montreal General Hospital; and the
Departments of Medicine and Mechanical Engineering
McGill University
Montreal, Quebec Canada

The uptake of oxygen and other substrates from a microcirculatory channel will result in a falling gradient in concentration, from input to output, both within the vascular lumen and within the adjacent tissue. When the materials being extracted are being carried both within the plasma and the red cell, and when the exchange between the red cell and plasma is not instantaneous, a part of the material will be temporarily sequestered within the red cell and will be carried somewhat further along the channel than otherwise would have occurred, before being released to the plasma phase, for removal. The phenomenon of red cell carriage (the trapping and translocation of material within the red cells) will occur, in the case of oxygen, because of both the relatively slow rate of release from oxyhemoglobin and a limiting permeability at the red cell membrane.

Before this important problem can be explored in detail, the constraining effect of red cell carriage upon the distribution of materials into tissue, in a system in which there is no net uptake, must be explored. We have examined this problem, both from an experimental and theoretical point of view, in the liver, and present our findings here. We have examined the exchange of two labeled low molecular weight substances, thiourea and urea. The liver was selected as an organ suitable for this kind of examination because the hepatic parenchymal cells are, in general, much more permeable to low molecular weight substances than are the red cells. The constraining effect of limited red cell permeability then becomes accentuated and more easily liable to quantification.

METHODS AND RESULTS

In these experiments the rapid single injection multiple indicator dilution technique was used (1). Catheters were placed in the portal vein (for injection of materials) and in the common left hepatic vein (for collection of serial blood samples) of an anesthetized dog, and the abdomen was closed. In each experiment we injected simultaneously three substances: ^{51}Cr-labeled red cells, as a vascular indicator, a substance which marks out the transit pattern of labeled red cells; the substance under study, either labeled thiourea or urea, which enters the extravascular space of the liver freely, but is limited in its passage across the red cell membrane; and a second reference substance, labeled water, which freely enters both the liver cells and the red cells. A single injection mixture is made up, with a hematocrit equivalent to that in the animal, and is pre-incubated at 37°C for 10 minutes, a period sufficient to assure complete equilibration of the labeled thiourea or urea across the red cell membrane. This mixture was then injected into the portal vein as rapidly as possible, and serial effluent hepatic venous blood samples were collected over the next 30 to 60 seconds. The samples and standards prepared from the injection mixture were analyzed for their contained activity, in an appropriate fashion.

Dilution patterns corresponding to each of the substances injected were detected in the hepatic venous blood. In order to normalize these patterns, from one to another, the outflowing activity of each indicator will be expressed as a fraction of the injected amount of activity, per milliliter of blood.

The results from two labeled thiourea experiments, in animals with high and low hematocrits, are presented in Figure 1.

In each experiment the outflow fraction per milliliter for labeled red cells rises to the highest and earliest peak and decays rapidly until recirculation occurs. For labeled water the initial outflow delay is larger, and the material emerges in a symmetrically delayed and spread-out fashion. The downslopes of each of these curves are corrected for recirculation, by linear extrapolation on semilogarithmic plots, as suggested by Hamilton, Moore, Kinsman, and Spurling (2). The areas under the resulting primary labeled red cell and water curves are equivalent.

The thiourea curves, in contrast, are bimodal. A first higher peak occurs in relation to the labeled red cell curve; and a second later and lower component reaches its peak at a time substantially later than does the labeled water. The curves exhibit visual evidence of the phenomenon of red cell carriage: the proportion of labeled thiourea in the first peak is much higher when the red

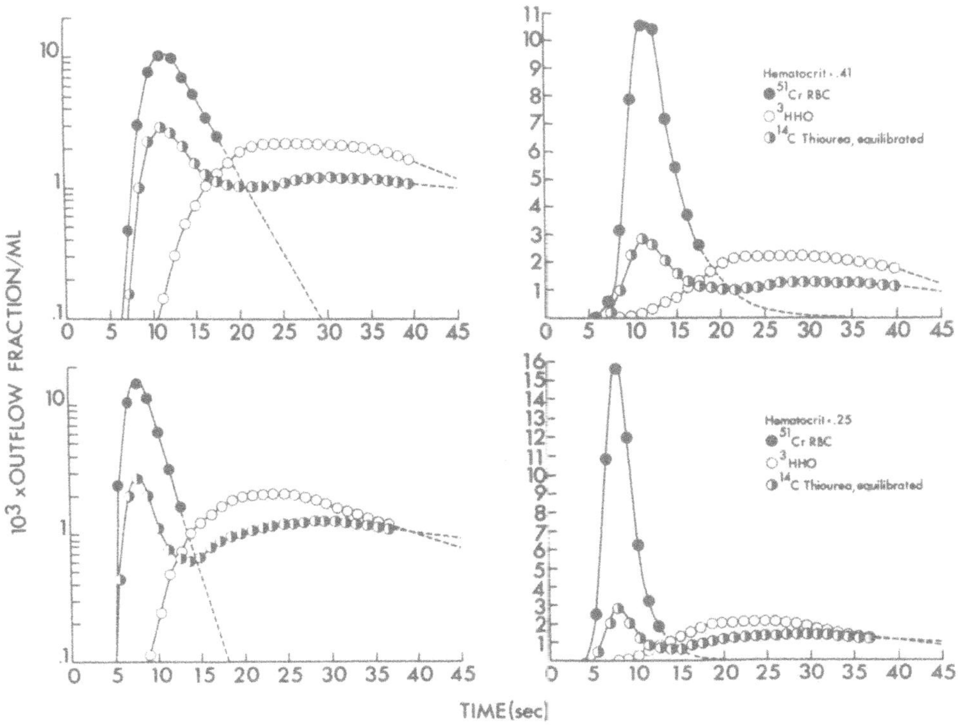

Figure 1. Sets of dilution curves from two typical thiourea experiments. Each experiment is presented, utilizing a logarithmic ordinate scale on the left and a linear scale, on the right. Reproduced from (3) with permission of The American Heart Association, Inc.

cells make up a larger proportion of the blood, when the hematocrit is higher, and the first peak of the thiourea curve greatly resembles the labeled red cell curve, on the semilogarithmic panel.

We have carried out a detailed mathematical model analysis of the phenomenon of red cell carriage (3). This analysis indicates that the outflow mean transit time for the labeled thiourea will be expected to be the same as that for the labeled water; and that, for a material like thiourea, the outflow curves will consist of three parts (one which has been carried through the organ in the red cells; a second fraction, which has not entered the red cells, but which has been delayed by flow-limited distribution from the plasma into the extravascular space; and a third part, which consists of moieties which have exchanged between red cells and plasma, and which emerge in spread-out fashion between the other two parts [3]). We have used this analysis to obtain from the

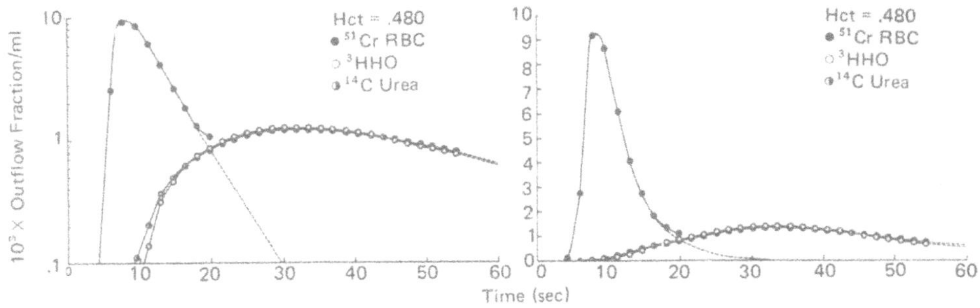

Figure 2. The dilution curves from a typical urea experiment. Reproduced from (3), with permission of The American Heart Association, Inc.

thiourea outflow curves, by a fitting procedure, estimates of the permeability of dog red cells to this substance. We have obtained a mean value fo 2.6×10^{-6} cm sec^{-1}.

Our model analysis indicates that, as the permeability of the red cells to the indicator increases, the initial component, trapped in the red cells and the later component, which has not entered the red cells, will be replaced by an intermediate component which approaches in form that for a label which very rapidly crosses the red cell membrane, labeled water (4). Labeled urea would be expected to equilibrate across the red cell membrane much more rapidly than thiourea (5). The results of an experiment with labeled urea are portrayed in Figure 2. As expected, the labeled urea curve very closely approaches that for labeled water, in form. Only a tiny vestige of the red cell carriage phenomenon remains. The urea curve increases on the upslope slightly more quickly than the labeled water curve, the peak is slightly lower than that for labeled water and the downslope decreases in a slightly slower manner.

The urea data were fitted by means of our model analysis and, from this, an estimate of the permeability of dog red cells to urea was secured. The value obtained was 640 cm sec^{-1}, an estimate 220 times that for thiourea.

DISCUSSION

We have presented an exploration of the effect of limited red cell permeability on the distribution of substances in the liver. We have shown that, when the exchange rate across the red cells is slow, the phenomenon of red cell carriage will limit the entry into liver cells of the material being carried along in the red cell.

For substances not removed and metabolized by the liver, the effect will be of little importance. However, for substances which are consumed by the liver, red cell carriage is potentially of great importance. The material being carried along in the red cells will not be available to the removal process and this lack of availability will modify the steady state distribution of material within the liver lobule.

Previously, we explored the effect of intracellular metabolic sequestration, and showed that this resulted in a concentration gradient within the hepatic lobule, both within the sinusoids and the liver cells (6). If the rate of release of oxygen from oxyhemoglobin and the permeability of the red cell membranes have a constraining effect on the release of oxygen from the red cells to plasma (7), the longitudinal gradient resulting from oxygen consumption will be flattened out. There will be a less marked decrease in concentration from entrance to exit, and the area around the terminal hepatic venules will, correspondingly, receive more oxygen than if this effect did not exist. The phenomenon will tend to keep the oxygen tension in the areas around the terminal hepatic venules from falling to very low levels and will be, in this sense, beneficial. This effect deserves further exploration.

ACKNOWLEDGEMENTS

These studies were supported by grants from the Medical Research Council of Canada and the Quebec Heart Foundation. The authors wish to acknowledge the superb assistance of Mrs. Brita Nadeau and to thank Miss Margaret Mulherin for typing this manuscript.

REFERENCES

1. Goresky, C.A. A linear method for determining liver sinusoidal and extravascular volumes. Am. J. Physiol. 204: 626-640, 1963.

2. Hamilton, W.F., J.W. Moore, J.M. Kinsman, and R.G. Spurling. Simultaneous determination of the pulmonary and systemic circulation times in man and of a figure related to the cardiac output. Am. J. Physiol. 84: 338-344, 1928.

3. Goresky, C.A., G.G. Bach, and B.E. Nadeau. Red cell carriage of label: its limiting effect on the exchange of materials in the liver. Circ. Res. 36: 328-351, 1975.

4. Paganelli, C.V., and A.K. Solomon. The rate of exchange of tritiated water across the human red cell membrane. J. Gen. Physiol. 41: 259-277, 1957.

5. Jacobs, M.H., H.N. Glassman, and A.K. Parpart. Hemolysis and zoological relationship. Comparative studies with four penetrating non-electrolytes. J. Expt. Zool. 113: 277-300, 1950.

6. Goresky, C.A., G.G. Bach, and B.E. Nadeau. On the uptake of materials by the intact liver: the transport and net removal of galactose. J. Clin. Invest. 52: 991-1008, 1973.

7. Roughton, F.J.W. Diffusion and simultaneous reaction velocity in hemoglobin solutions and red cell suspensions. In Progress in Biophysics. Volume 9, pp 55-104, 1959.

EFFECTS OF DOPAMINE AND EPINEPHRINE ON INTESTINAL BLOOD FLOW AND OXYGEN UPTAKE

W. W. Pawlik, A. P. Shepherd, D. Mailman,
L. L. Shanbour and E. D. Jacobson
Institute of Physiology, Medical Academy, Krakow, Poland, and Departments of Physiology, The University of Texas Health Science Centers, Houston & San Antonio, Texas

The cardiovascular effects of dopamine (3,4-dihydroxyphenylethylamine) have been studied by numerous investigators and because of its effects on splanchnic hemodynamics, dopamine has been suggested as a therapeutic agent in cardiovascular shock (1). In normal, anesthetized dogs and in shocked dogs, dopamine is a potent vasoconstrictor in the intestinal circulation (2,3), but the effects of dopamine on the delivery of oxygen to the gut are unknown.

We have previously shown that many vasoconstrictors suppress intestinal oxygen uptake even in isolated gut loops perfused at a constant rate of blood flow. A direct inhibition of tissue oxygen demand by vasoconstrictors and true anatomical arteriovenous shunting of blood flow have been ruled out as possible explanations for this finding (4). Thus, since the vasoconstrictors studied also depressed both capillary filtration coefficients and rubidium extraction by perfused gut loops, the most likely explanation for their effects on oxygen extraction is that they close precapillary sphincters. If sufficient precapillary sphincters constrict in response to the vasoconstrictor, the density of the perfused capillary bed will be so diminished that the blood-to-tissue flux of oxygen will be limited by the diffusion parameters, e.g., capillary surface area and capillary-to-cell diffusion distance (5).

The purpose of the present study was to determine if dopamine, like other vasoconstrictors, can reduce the delivery of oxygen to intestinal tissues and to compare its effects in the intestinal circulation with those of epinephrine.

METHODS

The subjects of our experiments were 27 mongrel dogs of both sexes weighing 15 to 23 kg. All animals were fasted for 24 hours before the experiments and all were anesthetized with sodium pentobarbital (30 mg/kg). A terminal trunk of the superior mesenteric artery supplying a segment of distal ileum (weight: 81±28 g) was exposed through a midline laparotomy. The ends of the gut segment supplied by the artery were ligated to block intramural collateral vessels. A noncannulating electromagnetic blood flow probe (Micron Instruments) was installed on the artery. A lateral branch of the artery was cannulated proximal to the probe for intra-arterial infusion of the agents. Zero flow was obtained by occluding the artery distal to the flow probe at the beginning and end of each experiment. A vein draining the intestinal segment was cannulated along with a femoral artery. Following heparin administration (100 units/kg + supplements), blood was withdrawn from both of these vessels at a constant rate and passed through the cuvettes of a photometric arteriovenous oxygen difference analyzer (Oxford Instrument Co.). The effluent from this instrument was returned to the animal via a femoral vein. This preparation has been described in more detail elsewhere (6). After the surgical preparation, mesenteric arterial blood flow, arterial pressure and arteriovenous oxygen difference were allowed to stabilize for 20 to 30 minutes. Then the intra-arterial infusion of either dopamine or epinephrine was begun. These agents were dissolved in 0.9% saline and the infusions were carried out for 10 minutes. The doses of dopamine used were 1.0, 5.0 and 20.0 μg/kg/min. Epinephrine was infused at a rate of 0.05 μg/kg/min. After control responses to dopamine were recorded, haloperidol (2.0 μg/kg, McNeil) was administered over a 5-minute period directly into the mesenteric artery. Ten minutes later, the same dose of dopamine was again administered. Thirty minutes later, propranolol (0.5 mg) was infused over a five-minute period and the effects of dopamine were again determined. After each experiment, the gut loops were weighed and the blood flow expressed in ml/min/100g of tissue weight. The oxygen consumption rate was calculated as the product of the blood flow rate and the simultaneously measured arteriovenous oxygen difference. The data were expressed in terms of a mean ± standard error.

RESULTS

Initial control values were as follows: mean systemic arterial pressure = 135 ± 15 mmHg; superior mesenteric artery blood flow = 31.5 ± 6.3 ml/min/100g; and intestinal oxygen consumption rate = 2.7 ± 0.6 ml/min/100g. Figure 1 shows the effects of a 10-minute infusion of dopamine (20 μg/kg/min). As the figure indicates, vasoconstriction in the mesenteric vascular bed occurred during the infusion. Since the vasoconstriction occurred quite rapidly and

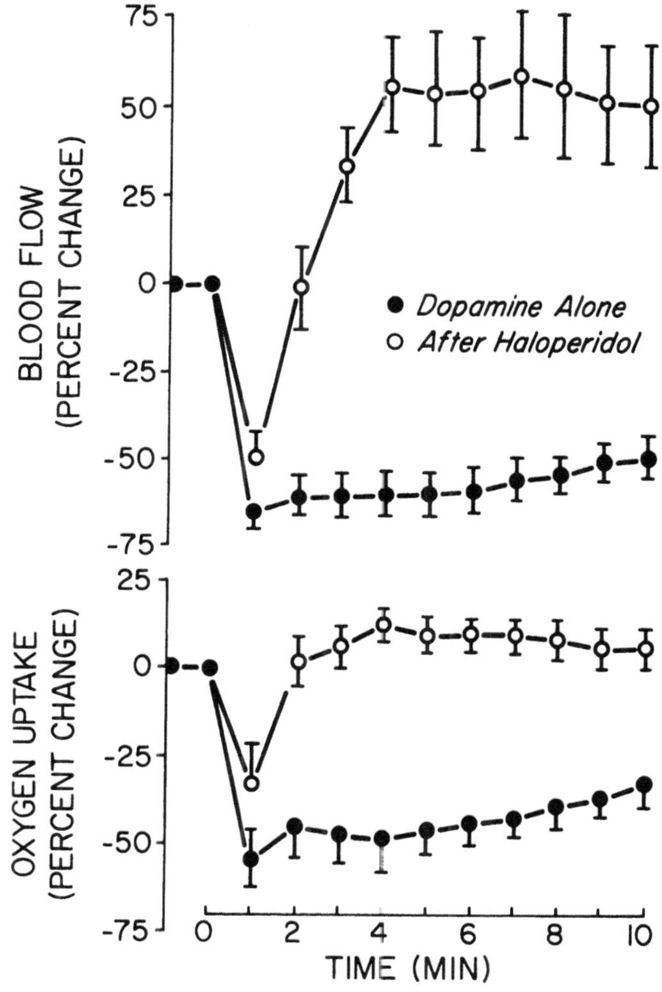

Figure 1. Effects of dopamine (20 μg/kg/min) on intestinal blood flow and oxygen uptake.

because the mean arterial pressure (not shown) was unaltered, dopamine acts directly to constrict intestinal resistance vessels. Dopamine reduced blood flow by approximately 56% at the end of the infusion. Following the initial vasoconstriction there was a degree of "escape" as mesenteric blood flow returned very slightly towards the control level. When dopamine was infused in doses less than 20 μg/kg/min, a post-infusion hyperemia was observed, but blood flow returned slowly to the control value without displaying a post-infusion hyperemia following 20 μg/kg/min dopamine. Figure 1 also shows that dopamine infusion not only reduced blood flow, but also reduced intestinal oxygen uptake. At the end of the 10-minute infusion, oxygen uptake was reduced by approximately 45%. Figure 2 shows a dose-response relationship between dopamine and its effects on intestinal oxygen uptake and mesenteric blood flow. As this figure indicates, dopamine in doses of 1, 5 and 20 μg/kg/min reduced intestinal blood flow by 10, 36 and 56% respectively. These reductions in blood flow were associated with concomitant reductions in intestinal oxygen uptake of 10, 30 and 45%, respectively.

The effects of dopamine-receptor blockade with haloperidol are shown in Figure 1. Following administration of haloperidol, dopamine reduced mesenteric blood flow during the first minute of infusion. Then mesenteric blood flow rapidly increased to a steady-state value 50% above control. Thus, haloperidol reversed the intestinal blood flow response to dopamine, converting it from a vasoconstrictor into a vasodilator. The intense vasodilation produced by dopamine after haloperidol was associated with a small (10%) increase in intestinal oxygen consumption. Beta adrenergic blockade with propranolol did not significantly alter the response to dopamine (not shown).

Intra-arterial epinephrine (0.05 μg/kg/min) reduced intestinal blood flow by 19%, but oxygen consumption was unchanged. After beta adrenergic blockade, the same dose of epinephrine reduced intestinal blood flow by 41% and oxygen consumption by 33%. These results are compared with those for dopamine in Figure 3. As the figure indicates, the 1.0 μg/kg/min infusion of dopamine produced a 10% reduction in blood flow and a 10% reduction in oxygen uptake. All other vasoconstrictors that we have studied produced essentially the same effect as dopamine, e.g., reduced blood flow and suppressed oxygen uptake. The one exception to this rule is epinephrine. Epinephrine significantly reduced blood flow (19%); however, the rate of oxygen consumption was essentially unaltered. Higher doses of epinephrine depressed both intestinal blood flow and oxygen consumption.

DISCUSSION

The predominant effect of dopamine in most vascular beds is

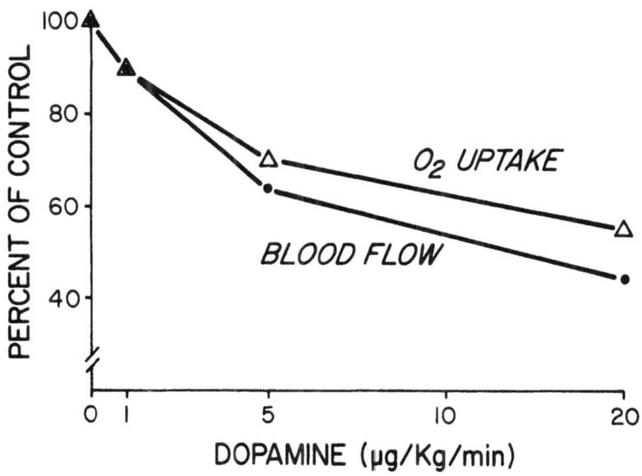

Figure 2. Dopamine produced dose-dependent reductions in both intestinal blood flow and oxygen uptake.

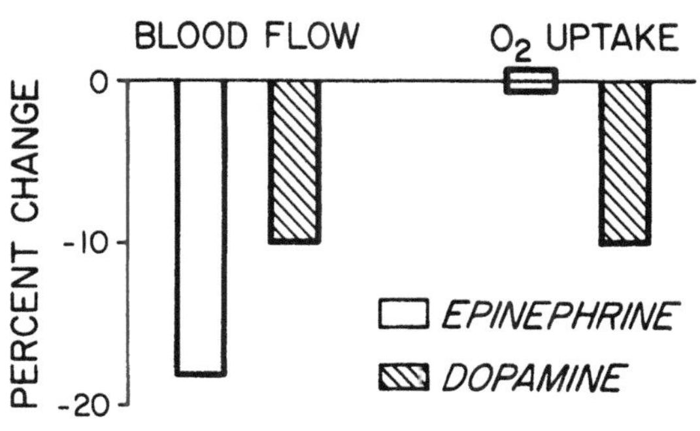

Figure 3. Dopamine (1 µg/kg/min) reduced both blood flow and oxygen delivery, whereas epinephrine (0.05 µg/kg/min) lowered blood flow without depressing oxygen uptake.

vasoconstriction through alpha adrenergic receptors (1). Dose-response studies show that with large enough doses, the vasoconstrictor effect of dopamine predominates over its vasodilating effects (1). Previous investigators have reported that dopamine is a vasodilator in the intestinal circulation; however, their data are not directly comparable to ours because they employed small doses of dopamine injected as a bolus (1,7). In our experiments, small doses of dopamine produced an early increase in blood flow which was followed by a subsequent and well-maintained decrease in blood flow. Thus, our results indicate that dopamine is a potent vasoconstrictor in the intestinal circulation when administered as a continuous infusion. Our results also indicate that the mesenteric vascular response to dopamine is not significiantly reffected by beta adrenergic blockade but that haloperidol reverses the response to dopamine, converting it from a vasoconstrictor into a vasodilator.

Our results also show that in addition to reducing mesenteric blood flow, dopamine also depresses intestinal oxygen uptake. Like most other vasoconstrictors which we have studied, dopamine reduced intestinal oxygen uptake when it was administered in a dose sufficient to produce vasoconstriction. The exceptional vasoconstrictor is epinephrine. Of all the vasoconstrictors studied, epinephrine alone has proved capable of reducing mesenteric blood flow without depressing intestinal oxygen uptake (8). Preliminary studies in our laboratory indicate that vasoconstrictors depress intestinal oxygen and rubidium extraction in gut loops perfused at a constant blood flow (4). These findings are consistent with vasoconstrictor-induced closure of precapillary sphincters and a reduced density of the perfused capillary bed. Thus, in constant pressure perfusion, vasoconstrictors not only reduce blood flow, but also prevent oxygen extraction from increasing sufficiently to maintain oxygen delivery. Since dopamine has been shown to reduce intestinal blood flow and oxygen uptake, it has a potential for deliterious effects on intestinal tissues. Therefore, before dopamine is employed in states of circulatory insufficiencies, its effects on tissue oxygenation should be thoroughly investigated.

REFERENCES

1. Goldberg, L. I. Pharm. Rev. 24:1-30, 1972.
2. Shanbour, L. L. and D. Parker. Canad. J. Physiol. Pharmacol. 50:599-602, 1972.
3. Ulano, H. B., et al. Gastroenterology 62:39-47, 1972.
4. Shepherd, A. P., et al. Circ. Res. 33:166-174, 1973.
5. Shepherd, A. P. and H. J. Granger. Gastroenterology 65:77-91, 1973.
6. Pawlik, W., et al. Gastroenterology 67:100-106, 1974.
7. Higgins, C. B., et al. Amer. J. Physiol. 225:432-437, 1973.
8. Pawlik, W., et al. Fed. Proc. 3:338, 1974 (Abstract).

SUMMARY OF DISCUSSION - SESSION IX:

COMMON ASPECTS OF OXYGEN SUPPLY

Chairmen: Duane F. Bruley and Reinhard Wodick

The session had broad coverage and therefore cannot be discussed with a particular aspect of oxygen transport to tissue as a focus. The topics were of interest and the presentations well done however discussion from the audience was limited because of the late start of the session.

A few selected comments made during the discussion periods will now be summarized.

Dr. Jobsis (Durham) inquired about how the low solubility or rather the bound state of water affects the diffusion of oxygen. Dr. Zander (Mainz) referred to existing knowledge about the exponential decrease of oxygen diffusivity D (cm^2/sec) with decreasing percentage of water content in biological solutions, as well as the linear decrease of oxygen solubility with decreasing water content. He stated that one can expect a very strong decrease of the oxygen conductance K (mlO_2/cm min atm) when the percentage water content at a biological structure decreases.

Dr. Kreuzer (Nijmegen) wondered what effect a shift in the oxygen dissociation curve might have on the interpretation of Dr. Cains' results. Dr. Cain (Birmingham) replied that the shift in dissociation curves was implicit and desired in the experimental design. It was the means to alter the upper end of the Po_2 gradient which drives O_2 to the sites of utilization, at the same time keeping the volume delivery of oxygen in the same range among the three experimental groups. The dependence of the percent reduction in oxygen uptake upon the volume delivery rate of oxygen in spite of differing values of Pao_2, Pvo_2 and thereby $Pcapo_2$ was the somewhat surprising result. Higher P_{O_2} did not necessarily support better oxygen uptake.

Dr. Meldon (Odense) asked if Dr. Goreskys' (Montreal) finding of a good agreement with known RBC membranes permeability for urea proves that there was no intra-erythroytic or intraplasma diffusion resistance. Dr. Goresky said no, only that the major and measurable resistance was at the red cell membrane. From the magnitude of the diffusion coefficient for urea in the plasma and in the red cell the time for equilibration would be expected to be negligibly small. The slight decrease in the diffusion coefficient for urea, inside the red cell, secondary to the high concentration of hemoglobin present there would not be great enough to produce a noticeable effect.

For oxygen, however, the problem might assume another character!

Respiratory Gas Exchange and Metabolism in Tumor Tissue I

IN VIVO UTILIZATION OF OXYGEN AND GLUCOSE BY NEOPLASTIC TISSUE

Pietro M. Gullino

Laboratory of Pathophysiology
National Cancer Institute
National Institutes of Health
Bethesda, Maryland 20014

EXPERIMENTAL APPROACHES

The biological role of oxygen utilization and glucose consumption in the survival and growth of tumors was first emphasized by Warburg (1,2). For many years the experimental approach in this field relied upon manometric techniques, tissue slices, and homogenates. The overriding preoccupation of investigators was the aerobic glycolysis as a lesion pathognomonic of neoplastic transformation. Only in 1961 (3) was a tumor preparation developed which permitted measurements of oxygen and glucose consumption by solid tumors *in vivo* following standard physiological procedures (4-9).

This preparation consists of three steps: (1) surgical isolation of a pedicle containing only one artery and one vein, (2) transplantation of a tumor fragment at the distal end of the pedicle, and (3) wrapping of the transplant with a sheet of paraffin to form a sack in which the tumor does grow, isolated from surrounding tissues and connected to the host by only one artery and one vein. The preparation which we call "tissue isolated tumors" permits several types of experiments. The efferent vein can be cannulated, thus tumor blood flow can be measured directly. Concentration changes of blood constituents can be determined in the arterial and venous compartments for several hours upon recirculation of the tumor efferent blood. Thus consumption *in vivo* can be calculated. Both the artery and vein of the tumor pedicle can be cannulated and the tumor can be transferred into a perfusion system as an organ totally separated from the host (10,11).

To improve our ability of assessing *in vivo* the status of the pericellular fluid and relating it to changes in the vascular and cellular compartments, a method for sampling the tumor interstitial fluid was developed (10). It is based on a property peculiar to all the neoplastic tissues we studied. When a chamber with walls constituted by millipore filters is placed in a pouch of the subcutaneous tissue with 100 to 200 mg of tumor fragments, the neoplastic cells grow against and around the chamber which then becomes incorporated into the growing tumor. The cells adhere to the filter but cannot penetrate into the chamber because of the pore size (0.45 μ average). The fluid surrounding the cells, however, does flow into the chamber and can be sampled. We designate this fluid, tumor interstitial fluid (TIF) and believe it represents the pericellular fluid phase interposed between the vascular walls and the cell outer membrane.

Oxygen Supply and Utilization

Data available permit the following generalizations which are applicable to carcinomas as well as sarcomas. Similar to normal organs, oxygen consumption by tumors depends on supply through the vascular system and local removal capacity by the tissue. Contrary to normal organs, the vascular system of the tumor undergoes continuous changes (9,13-15). As the tumor mass increases, the volume of the vascular network proportionately decreases. The vessels become shorter but larger relative to the unit mass, the exchange surface area of the capillaries decreases, and the intercapillary distance increases. Consequently, as the tumor grows, oxygen supply per unit mass decreases, as does consumption. Thus, absolute values of consumption levels are meaningful only when determined in small tumors or when tumor size is known. On the other hand, tumors grow as parasites of normal tissues which are being destroyed by the invading neoplastic cells. One must be aware that small tumors can, indeed, be a mixture of neoplastic cells and host cells which are not yet destroyed and interfere with the measurements.

The second important parameter which controls consumption concerns local tissue conditions. In tumors, oxygen removal from blood is particularly efficient for the special acid-base equilibrium of TIF (Table 1). The fluid surrounding neoplastic cells *in vivo* has always been found to be more acid than aortic plasma; among the tumors we have studied (16), the difference was 0.25 to 0.45 pH units. Dissolved CO_2 and pCO_2 values in TIF almost doubled that of arterial plasma. Under these conditions one would expect a large yield of oxygen from the oxyhemoglobin passing through the tumor network. In fact, a large utilization of oxygen

Table 1

Acid-base status of interstitial fluid in rat hepatocarcinomas

Treatment of rats[a]	pH		pCO_2 (mm Hg)	
	AP[b]	TIF[c]	AP	TIF
None	7.38 ±0.09[d]	6.95 ±0.17	43 ±3	80 ±10
Air + CO_2	7.08 ±0.02	6.67 ±0.03	103 ±10	226 ±17
$NaHCO_3$	7.35 ±0.02	6.84 ±0.05	55 ±4	123 ±7

[a] 175-240 g rats bearing hepatocarcinomas (9.6-18.8 g) containing the micropore chamber for TIF sampling. Comparison of acid-base balance when animals were breathing normal air (Hb >90% saturated), or Air + CO2 (9:1), or receiving NaHCO3 in drinking water (0.1%) for 10 days prior to sampling.

[b] Aortic plasma

[c] Tumor interstitial fluid

[d] Mean ± S.D.

could be induced in tumors made acidotic by $NaHCO_3$ (Table 2) (16). Thus, the low pH of TIF should be kept in mind when assessing pO_2 measurements in neoplastic tissues.

Experiments with tumors perfused _ex vivo_ revealed that blood dilution with cell culture media (17) or 0.85% NaCl impaired the ability of tumors to remove blood oxygen (Table 3). We have no explanation for this observation which, nevertheless, may be important in assessing _in vivo_ data. For instance, rapid intravenous injection of 3 to 4 ml of a solution into a 200 g rat, which usually has about 10 ml of circulating blood, induces a blood dilution which may momentarily impair oxygen utilization and interfere with whatever determination is being made, including oxygen consumption.

Table 2

Oxygen utilization during acidosis

Rat No. / Tumor weight (g)	Before treatment[a] Oxygen available (mmoles/hr/100 g)	Before treatment[a] Oxygen utilized (mmoles/hr/100 g)	%[b]	After treatment[a] Oxygen available (mmoles/hr/100 g)	After treatment[a] Oxygen utilized (mmoles/hr/100 g)	%[b]
1/6.3	18.4	7.4	40	4.3	3.6	84
2/4.4	10.7	3.1	29	7.6	6.9	91
3/4.0	31.8	10.9	34	12.5	8.3	66
4/5.0	13.2	1.5	11	30.4	4.4	14
5/2.5	24.6	5.7	23	93.1	40.6	43
6/11.6	4.5	1.2	27	4.2	3.6	86

[a] The animal was anesthetized with urethan (1 mg/g). The abdomen was opened, the tumor vein was punctured with a thin needle and sufficient suction was applied with a syringe to remove all blood flowing out of the tumor for a period of several minutes. Thus, blood flow was measured as the venous sample was withdrawn. Simultaneously with venous blood sampling, aortic blood was removed with a catheter introduced through the common carotid artery. The needle was then withdrawn from the tumor vein, hemorrhage was stopped by application of pressure for a few minutes,and the abdomen was closed. Treatment with $NaHCO_3$ followed: 3 doses of 100 mg each given by stomach tubing at 1-hour intervals. One hour after the third dose, blood sampling was repeated. Oxygen available to the tumor was calculated from blood flow and hemoglobin saturation of arterial blood; oxygen utilized was calculated from blood flow and the difference in saturation between arterial and tumor blood. In the same tumor available oxygen changed depending on the time of sampling but the amount of oxygen utilized was always larger in the acidotic stage.

[b] Percent utilized over available oxygen.

Table 3

Effect of blood dilution on oxygen utilization by W256 carcinomas.

Tumor weight range		Oxygen (mmoles/hr/100 g)		
		Available	Utilized	% Utilization
In vivo[a]	8.3 (5.2-12.4)	5.3±1.2[b]	2.38±0.94	45
In vitro[c] perfusates:				
Whole blood	9.8 (4.5 15.4)	4.5±1.0	1.96±0.51	44
Blood + Eagle's medium 2:1	7.7 (4.3 11.8)	3.5±1.6	0.85±0.20	27

[a]Twenty tumors grown as tissue isolated preparations. Blood supply and utilization calculated as in Table 2.

[b]Mean ± S.D.

[c]Six tumors each group, perfused continuously for 4 hours. Utilization was calculated for the 4-hour period.

Blood dilution reduced oxygen utilization to about one-half that expected from the available supply.

Another possible error related to assessing oxygen utilization and metabolic activity in vivo may occur when a tumor is acutely deprived of oxygen (Table 4). CO_2 elimination increases very sharply, much over the oxygen supply, suggesting that oxygen from other sources is being extensively utilized as an emergency hydrogen acceptor. The possible consquences produced by such drastic conditions must be taken into consideration.

The oxygen consumption by tumors in vivo is reported in Table 5. Tumors perfused ex vivo with whole blood consumed oxygen as those in vivo (Table 3). An increasing oxygen supply augmented consumption (5,9). Doubling of blood flow improved oxygen consumption from 15 to 50% in perfused Walker carcinomas (10,12). In vivo reduction of oxygen supply by acute anemia elicited an increase of utilization but no appreciable increment of blood supply in 6 out of 7 experiments (Table 6). Compensation

Table 4

Effect of acute deprivation of oxygen on CO_2 elimination by W256 carcinomas *in vivo*.

Experiment No.	mmoles/hr/100 g			
	Oxygen available		CO_2 eliminated	
	Before[a]	After[a]	Before[a]	After[a]
1	6.7	0.5	4.3	12.3
2	7.1	0.5	2.4	11.0
3	26.2	6.5	5.7	10.0
4	12.6	3.2	4.9	9.9
5	7.2	2.1	0.9	4.3
6	15.0	4.0	2.5	4.6

[a]Acute deprivation of oxygen produced by substitution of 3-5 ml blood with 3-5 ml serum. Second determination done 10 minutes after onset of anemia. Double sampling and determination of blood flow as in Table 2.

Table 5

In vivo oxygen consumption by rat tumors

Tumor	Tumor weight range (g)	Q02 µl O_2/hr/mg dry tumor	Reference
DS carcinosarcoma	3.2-13	2.6-0.36	(9)
Walker 256 carcinoma	2.0-9.8	4.3-2.3	(5)
Hepatocarcinoma 5123	3.8-7.0	7.9-2.7	(5)
Fibrosarcoma 4956	5.0-12.7	0.94-0.12	(5)

Table 6

Oxygen utilization and blood flow during acute anemia[a]

Rat No.	Oxygen available (mmoles/hr/100 g)		Oxygen utilized as % available		Blood flow (ℓ/hr/100 g	
	Before[b]	After[b]	Before[b]	After[b]	Before[b]	After[b]
1	7.2	2.1	42	90	1.6	1.3
2	12.6	3.2	28	44	2.4	1.7
3	6.7	5.0	42	64	1.6	1.9
4	15.0	4.0	31	60	2.3	2.6
5	6.8	2.7	24	74	1.3	0.6
6	7.1	3.0	52	73	1.2	0.8
7	7.1	0.5	37	40	1.4	4.3

[a]W256 carcinomas, 4.4 to 8.6 g weight range.

[b]Before and after substitution of 3 to 5 ml blood with 3 to 5 ml serum in host vascular bed. Sampling procedure as in Table 2.

of anoxia by improved circulation was not commonly observed in tumors. A reduction in saturation of afferent hemoglobin from 95 to 60% induced a decrease of saturation in the efferent hemoglobin from about 60 to 30% when Walker carcinomas were perfused with whole blood at a constant flow rate. Reduction of hemoglobin saturation in vivo was also followed by a sharp reduction in hemoglobin saturation in the efferent tumor blood. Thus, the capacity of tumors to remove oxygen from circulating blood was very efficient during a sudden decrease of supply. A chronic reduction in oxygen supply, which usually occurs in vivo because of host anemia, produced a decrease in consumption per unit weight. Oxygen utilized by tumors in anemic rats decreased proportionately to the hemoglobin content of blood (5).

Glucose Supply and Utilization

Glucose consumption in vivo, as measured in tissue isolated tumors of normoglycemic hosts, varied quite extensively depending on tumor type and size (Table 7). Hypoglycemia or low supply always produced a reduction in glucose consumption; contrary to oxygen uptake, the tumor is unable to increase removal of glucose from blood when the supply is reduced. Acute hyperglycemia or high supply always produced an increase of consumption. Present data (6,8,9) sustain these generalizations. Chronic hyperglycemia can be induced in rats by alloxan (18). With blood glucose at about twice the physiological concentration, consumption in Walker carcinomas and hepatomas 5123 stabilized at about 30% above the normoglycemic level but fibrosarcomas 4956 reduced consumption to about 30% below normoglycemic levels (6).

As an attempt to better understand the regulation of glucose uptake by the solid tumor, glucose concentration in TIF was measured at several levels of glycemia and consumption. In normoglycemic hosts, glucose content was very low and often negligible in the TIF of all tumors studied (19) despite large consumption. During an acute hyperglycemia, produced by a single intravenous injection of glucose, we failed to detect free glucose in TIF. Probably the time needed for diffusion into the sampling chamber was too long for detecting a rapid peak of concentration. Accumulation of free glucose in TIF was observed only after several hours of hyperglycemia at about twice the physiological levels. In animals made diabetic by alloxan treatment, glucose concentration in TIF was only about 10% lower than blood glycemia, or about 300 mg/100 ml (6). When insulin was injected into these animals to produce a normo- or hypoglycemia, the level of free glucose in TIF during the first 12 to 24 hours, was found to be only 10 to 20% lower than in blood. However,

Table 7

Glucose consumption and lactate elimination by tumors growing in normoglycemic rats. (mmoles/hr/100 g)

Tumor	Tumor weight range (g)	Glucose		Lactate eliminated in tumor efferent blood
		Supplied	Consumed	
Walker 256 carcinoma	2.0–11.5	18.9 (21.7–16.1)[a]	5.4 (6.4–4.3)	3.8 (4.3–3.3)
Hepatocarcinoma 5123	3.4–7.0	13.3 (17.8–8.9)	3.1 (4.9–1.8)	2.0 (2.5–1.4)
Fibrosarcoma 4956	5.0–12.7	7.8 (11.7–3.9)	2.5 (3.9–0.9)	1.67 (2.8–0.6)

[a]95% confidence limits for 65, 23, and 19 determinations, respectively.

3683 HEPATOCARCINOMA

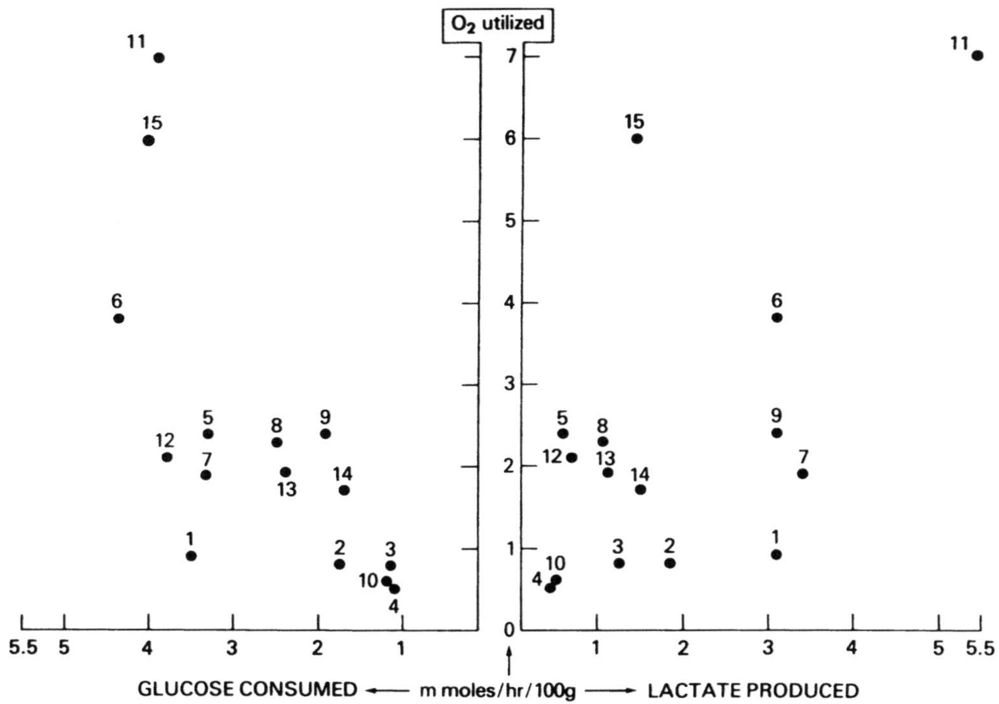

Chart 1. Oxygen utilization compared with glucose consumption and lactate production. Each experiment indicated by the same number.

if normo- or hypoglycemia was maintained for more than 24 hours, TIF of insulin-treated diabetic animals again had negligible amounts of free glucose (6). The simplest interpretation of these data is that neoplastic cells of the solid tumor utilize very rapidly all glucose crossing the vascular wall, thus a sharp gradient between blood and TIF is usually found. When hyperglycemia is induced, more glucose crosses the capillary wall and more is utilized until cell saturation is reached. The glucose accumulates in TIF to concentrations just slightly lower than in plasma. Under these conditions the ability of the vascular wall to maintain a gradient is overcome. When normo- or hypoglycemia is reinstated, about 24 hours are needed for the capillary wall to recuperate the ability to maintain the gradient. We postulated that glucose transfer from blood to neoplastic cells may be "regulated" at the capillary level. In our experience the interstitial fluid is free of glucose only in tumors. The micropore chambers, placed in the subcutaneous tissue, samples a fluid with only 10 to 15% less glucose than in plasma (6,19).

Glycolysis

Large production of lactate as well as high consumption of glucose *in vivo* is usually observed in tumors also utilizing high amounts of oxygen (Chart 1). The fraction of consumed glucose which is elininated in blood as lactate varies considerably from a relatively small amount (Chart 1, Nos. 15,8,13) to a large percentage (Chart 1, Nos. 9,2,3).

The role of glycolysis in the life of cells has traditionally been considered as an energy yielding process coupled with oxygen consumption or lack thereof. The reasons sustaining this interpretation are well known. Inhibition of glycolysis by oxygen (Pasteur effect) or inhibition of oxygen utilization by increased glucose concentration in the media (Crabtree effect) have been repeatedly observed *in vitro* and reproduced *in vivo* (9). However it is also well known (11) that when the energy supply is increased to respiring ascites cells, the energy loss due to reduced oxygen consumption is roughly replaced by the energy produced by glycolysis; but when oxygen supply is increased to glycolyzing ascites cells, oxygen consumption replaces 3- to 6-fold the energy lost because of the inhibited glycolysis. A convincing explanation of this discrepancy is not known. *In vivo*, the fraction of consumed glucose eliminated as blood lactate not only differs greatly among tumors of the same type but varies with time for each tumor. For instance, in perfused tumors where conditions are better controlled, one can observe results as in Table 8. During a 3 hour period, while oxygen utilization remained constant (±10%), glucose consumption decreased by 50% and lactate

Table 8

Walker 256 carcinoma (5.5 g) perfused at 37° C

Hours of perfusion	mmoles/hr/100 g			
	Oxygen utilized	Glucose consumed	Lactate produced	%[a]
1	2.05	5.48	4.60	42
2	2.11	3.20	1.82	28
3	1.87	2.71	2.61	48

[a]Percent of utilized glucose eliminated as lactate in the efferent blood and calculated as: 2M lactate eliminated = 1 M glucose consumed.

Hb saturation, 96 to 98%. Glucose level in perfusate at the end of each hour: 125, 94, and 150 mg/100 ml.

production, during the second hour, differed greatly from the first and the last hours.

A comparison of the data obtained _in vivo_ and in the _ex vivo_ perfusion system (Table 9) suggests that, in general, tumor manipulation and perfusion with media different from physiological blood tend to increase the percentage of glucose transformed into lactate. The amount of lactate production could not be correlated with either oxygen or glucose consumption (Table 10).

Another observation which does not fit with the concept of glycolysis strictly as an energy yielding process concerns lactate production by the same tumor when subjected to profound hypoglycemia followed by hyperglycemia (7). Insulin was injected into tumor-bearing animals to pr oduce a hypoglycemia of 30 to 40 mg % for several hours. During this time the small amount of glucose utilized by the tumor could be entirely accounted for in the lactate eliminated through the efferent blood. Glucose was then injected into the host to produce a 300 to 400 mg % hyperglycemia. In the next 10 to 15 minutes, glucose consumption increased up to 10-fold but

Table 9

Oxygen utilization, glucose consumption, and lactate production by Walker 256 carcinoma.

	mmoles/hr/100 g							
	Oxygen			Glucose			Lactate	
	Available	Utilized	% Utilization	Available	Utilized	% Utilization	Produced	% of Utilized glucose
In vivo	5.3 ±1.2[a]	2.38 ±0.94	45	18.9 ±1.2	5.4 ±0.9	29	3.8 ±0.6	35
Perfusion media:								
Whole Blood	4.5 ±1.0	1.96 ±0.51	44	5.5 ±1.0	2.3 ±0.5	42	2.4 ±0.6	52
Blood + Eagle's medium (2:1)	3.5 ±1.6	0.86 ±0.20	27	3.2 ±1.1	1.4 ±0.3	44	2.2 ±0.2	79
Erythrocyte-free perfusate (Eagle's medium)[b]	0.26 ±0.08	0.08 ±0.02	31	4.1 ±1.2	1.3 ±0.4	32	2.0 ±0.5	77

[a]Mean ± S.D.

[b]Eagle's basal medium (17).

Table 10

In vivo oxygen or glucose consumption and lactate production compared with growth rate.

Tumors	Weight doubling time (hr)[a]	mmoles/hr/100 g		
		Oxygen	Glucose	Lactate
Walker 256 carcinoma	33	2.4	5.4	3.8
Hepatocarcinoma 5123	196	4.2	3.1	2.0
Fibrosarcoma 4956	61	0.8	2.5	1.7

[a]Calculated from the semilog plot of time: dry weight increase over the maximal growth period (subcutaneous transplants).

lactate production became very small and, in some cases, tumor efferent blood had less lactate than aortic blood. Within one hour, lactate production returned to the levels common to the hyperglycemic state. Lactate production, in this case, appeared to be related to glucose starvation.

Induction of high lactate production was obtained in the absence of a tumor when chambers constituted by millipore filters (10) were implanted in a pouch of the rat subcutaneous tissue. During the first week of implant, the fluid collected by the chamber contained glu cose in concentrations which were only about 20% less than in blood. From the second week on, however, glucose concentration decreased while lactate content increased several-fold over the aortic level and became similar to the concentration in tumors (100 to 150 mg/100 ml). When the millipore chambers were left *in situ*, primary fibrosarcomas arose around them in 4 out of 5 animals during a period of 12 to 18 months after chamber implantation. Thus, high lactate concentration was observed for one year before any tumors appeared. Whether a correlation between the two events does exist is not known (20), but a persistent increment of lactate could be obtained in the absence of any demonstrable neoplastic transformation of the connective tissue embedding the chamber.

Since continuous, unrestrained growth is the major symptom of neoplastic disease, it seemed reasonable to inquire if a correlation existed between the growth rate of the tumors studied and oxygen utilization, glucose consumption, or lactate production. We found none (Table 10).

REFERENCES

1. Warburg, O. "The Metabolism of Tumours." R.R. Smith, Inc., New York, 1931.

2. Warburg, O. "Uber die katalytischen Wirkungen der lebendigen Substanz." J. Springer, Berlin, 1928.

3. Gullino, P.M., and Grantham, F.H. Studies on the exchange of fluids between host and tumor. I. A method for growing "tissue-isolated" tumors in laboratory animals. J. Nat. Cancer Inst. 27: 679-693, 1961.

4. Vaupel, P., Günther, H., and Grote, T. Atemgaswechsel und Glucosestoffwechsel von Tumoren (DS-Carcinosarkom) in vivo. I. Experimentelle Untersuchungen der versorgungsbestimmenden Parameter. Z. Gesamte Exp. Med. 156: 283-294, 1971.

5. Gullino, P.M., Grantham, F.H., and Courtney, A.H. Utilization of oxygen by transplanted tumors in vivo. Cancer Res. 27: 1020-1030, 1967.

6. Gullino, P.M., Grantham, F.H., Courtney, A.H. Glucose consumption by transplanted tumors in vivo. Cancer Res. 27: 1031-1040, 1967.

7. Gullino, P.M., Grantham, F.H., Courtney, A.H., and Losonczy, I. Relationship between oxygen and glucose consumption by transplanted tumors in vivo. Cancer Res. 27: 1041-1052, 1967.

8. Vaupel, P., Günther, H., and Grote, J. Einfluss einer Hyperglykämie auf die Sauerstoff- und Glucoseaufnahme von Implantationstumoren (DS-Carcinosarkom) in vivo. Z. Krebsforsch. 77: 17-25, 1972.

9. Vaupel, P. Atemgaswechsel und Glucosestoffwechsel von Implantationstumoren (DS-Carcinosarkom) in vivo. Akademie der Wissenschaften und der Literatur, Mainz, 1974.

10. Gullino, P.M. Techniques for the study of tumor physiopathology. In: H. Busch (ed), "Methods in Cancer Research," vol. 5, pp. 45-91. Academic Press, New York, 1970.

11. Aisenberg, A.C. "The Glycolysis and Respiration of Tumors," pp. 159-179. Academic Press, New York, 1961.

12. Gullino, P.M. In vitro perfusion of tumors. In: J.C. Norman, J. Folkman, W.G. Hardison, et al (eds.), "Organ Perfusion and Preservation," pp. 877-898. Appleton-Century Crofts, New York, 1968.

13. Hilmas, D.E., and Gillette, E.L. Morphometric analyses of the microvasculature of tumors during X-irradiation. Cancer 33: 103-110, 1974.

14. Vogel, A.W. Intratumoral vascular changes with increased size of a mammary adenocarcinoma: New method and results. J. Nat. Cancer Inst. 34: 571-578, 1965.

15. Vogel, A.W., and Haynes, J. Mammary adenocarcinoma (72j) blood flow in mice treated with thioTEPA. J. Nat. Cancer Inst. 37: 293-300, 1966.

16. Gullino, P.M., Grantham, F.H., Smith, S.H., and Haggerty, A.C. Modifications of the acid-base status of the internal milieu of tumors. J. Nat. Cancer Inst. 34: 857-869, 1965.

17. Eagle, H. Amino acid metabolism in mammalian cell cultures. Science 130: 432-437, 1959.

18. Goranson, E.S., and Tilser, G.J. Studies on the relationship of alloxan-diabetes and tumor growth. Cancer Res. 15: 626-631, 1955.

19. Gullino, P.M., Clark, S.H., and Grantham, F.H. The interstitial fluid of solid tumors. Cancer Res. 24: 780-798, 1964.

20. Libenson, L., and Jena, M. Extracellular pH and neoplastic transformations. Cancer Res. 34: 953-957, 1974.

O_2 SUPPLY CONDITIONS IN TUMOR TISSUE IN VIVO

G. Thews and P. Vaupel

Institute of Physiology
University of Mainz
65 Mainz, Federal Republic of Germany

During the last few years O_2 supply of tumor tissue has very carefully been investigated using GULLINO's model of a "tissue isolated" implantation tumor (GULLINO and GRANTHAM, 1961; GÜNTHER et al., 1972; VAUPEL et al., 1971; VAUPEL, 1974). We analysed the O_2 supply for a DS-Carcinosarcoma in the rat kidney by two methods:

1. direct measurement of O_2 pressures in the tissue by means of gold micro-electrodes,
2. P_{O2} calculation according to diffusion laws considerring the experimentally determined parameters in the arterial and venous blood.

There seemed to be a discrepancy between the directly measured and the calculated values for the mean tissue P_{O2} . The following statements are to show that the calculated and measured values approximate, if inhomogeneities of the supply parameters are consistantly taken into account.

1. Experimental results

Local P_{O2} measurements in tumor tissue reveal mainly very low values. The P_{O2} histograms show a typical frequency distribution shifted to the left. Fig. 1 illustrates this pattern of P_{O2} distribution in four tumors of different weight. It is obvious that with increasing tumor weight, i.e. age of tumor growth, the histograms are shifted to lower values. This regularity is particularly evident, if the mean O_2 pressure in the tissue $\bar{P}_{O2}$ is decribed as a function of the tumor weight. Fig. 2 shows that there exists a significant logarithmic interdependence between these two parameters.

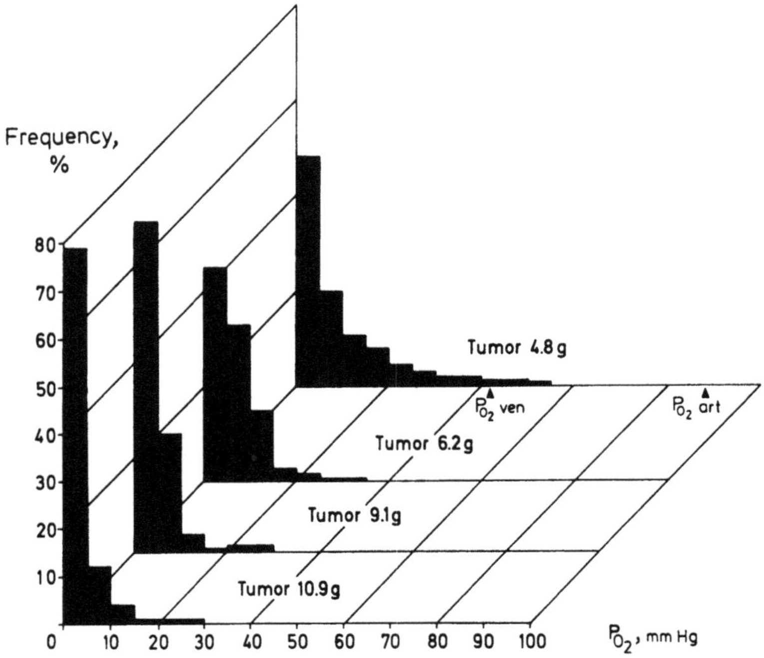

Fig. 1: P_{O2} frequency distribution in implantation tumors of different age of growth (characterized by the corresponding tumor weights).

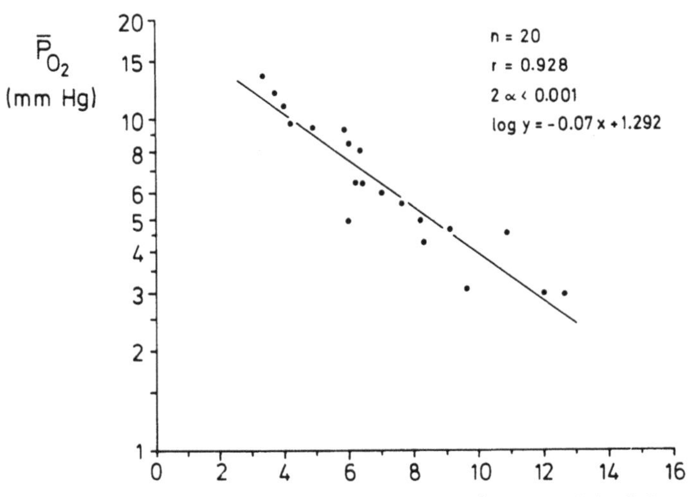

Fig. 2: Dependence of the mean O_2 pressure $\bar{P}_{O2}$ in the tumor tissue on the respective tumor weight.

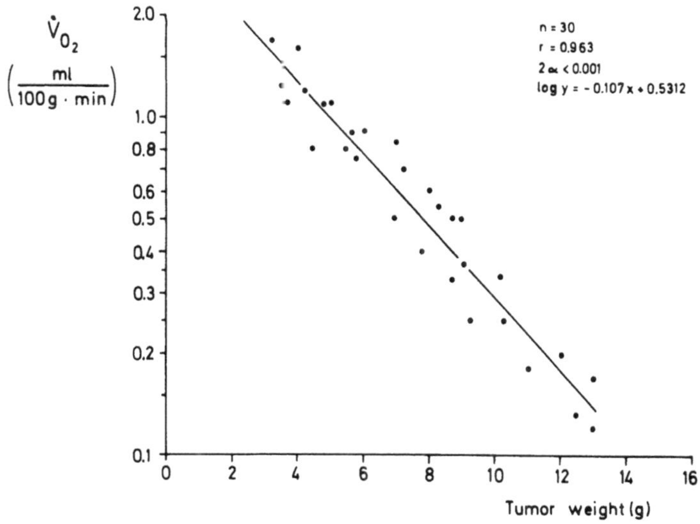

Fig. 3: Dependence of the mean O_2 consumption $\dot{V}_{O2}$ by the tumor tissue on the respective tumor weight.

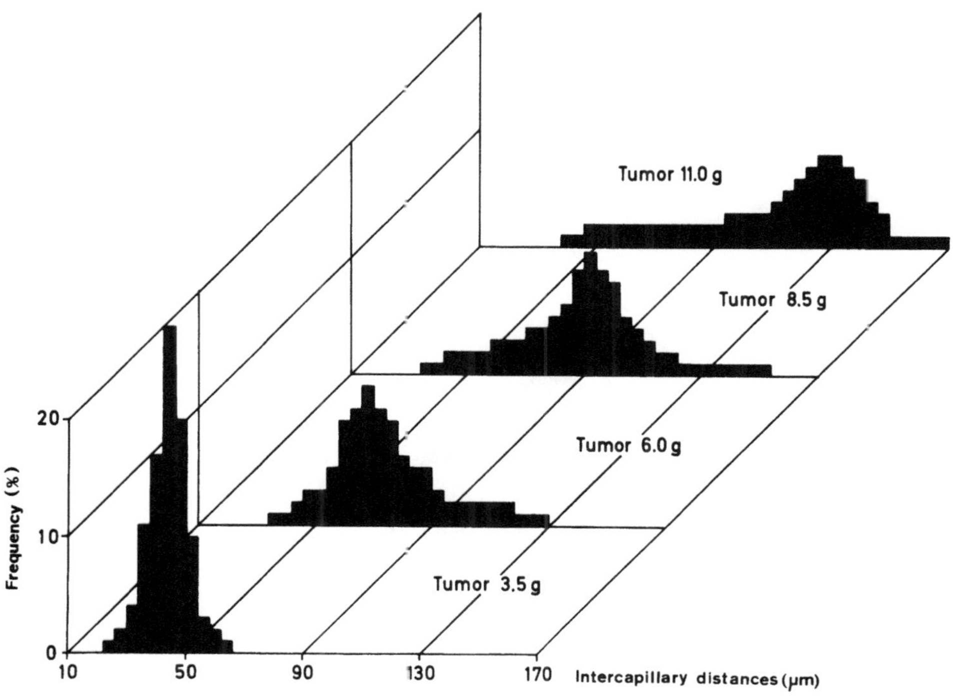

Fig. 4: Frequency distribution of intercapillary distances in implantation tumors of different weight.

Such a logarithmic dependence on the tumor weight is also valid for many parameters, on which depend the values of tissue P_{O2}. As an example Fig. 3 shows the logarithmic decrease of O_2 consumption with increasing tumor weight.

The capillary architecture attracted our special attention. Thus, the intercapillary distances as well as the lengths and radii of the capillaries were examined by morphometric methods. In Fig. 4 frequency distributions of intercapillary distances for tumors of various age are presented. Accordingly mean distances as well as inhomogeneities increase with advancing age. So we must base our consideration on the fact that the supply areas of the single capillaries vary considerably. As can be seen in Fig. 5, the capillary lengths show similar variations.

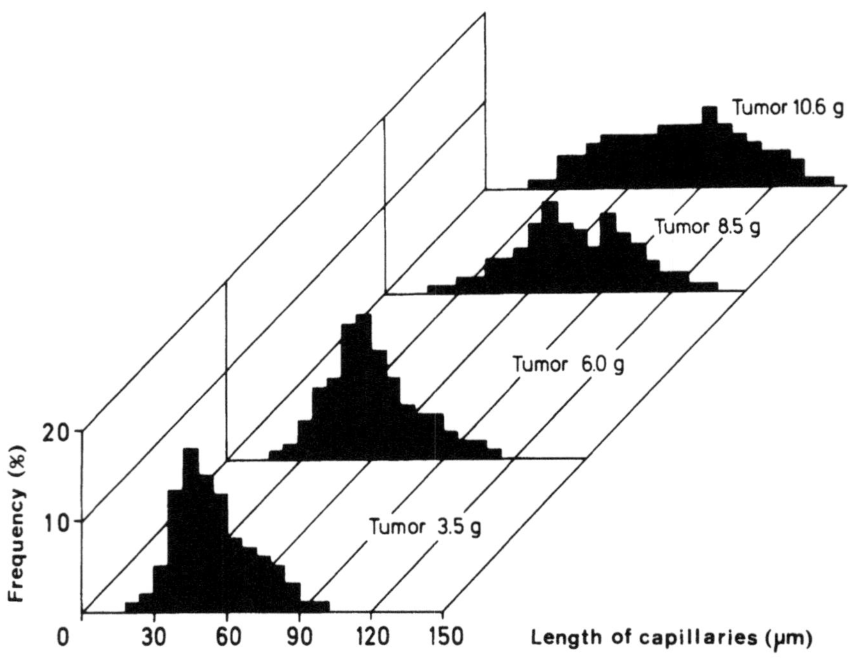

Fig. 5: Frequency distribution of capillary length in implantation tumors of different weight.

2. Results of the calculations

We calculated the local O_2 pressures on the basis of the present data for the relevant parameters of O_2 supply. These calculations were made according to KROGH's cylinder model, since the influence of inhomogeneities can best be made clear by means of this model. As an additional basis for our calculations we took the data of younger tumors, since their areas of deficient O_2 supply are still relatively small unlike those of older tumors. According to the results of our measurements the mean values given in Table 1 are valid for this example. If the mean O_2 pressure of the tissue is calculated on this basis, there results a value of 41 mmHg. But the mean value for younger tumors measured polarographically amounts to 10 - 15 mmHg.

In order to clear up this considerable discrepancy, we took different factors of influence into additional account. First of all a shunt-perfusion in the tumor tissue is to be expected. It may not be neglected, since in respect of the total perfusion its rate is estimated at about 15 % by several authors. With regard to this value the mean tissue P_{O_2} decreases by 3 mmHg.

Table 1: O_2 supply parameters for young tumors (mean values)

arterial O_2 pressure P_{aO_2}	: 88 mmHg
arterial O_2 content C_{aO_2}	: 16,0 vol%
venous O_2 pressure P_{vO_2}	: 41 mmHg
venous O_2 content C_{vO_2}	: 8,1 vol%
O_2 consumption $\dot{V}_{O_2}$	: 1,5 ml/100 g/min
O_2 conductivity (KROGH's diffusion coefficient) K	: $1{,}5 \cdot 10^{-5}$ ml/cm·min·atm
radius in KROGH's cylinder model R	: 47 µm

Inhomogeneities of the intercapillary distances are expected to have a more considerable influence on the tissue P_{O_2}. Fig. 6 gives an impression about variations of the supply radii. The distribution approximately corresponds to the situation in younger tumors. Here it must be taken into consideration that the mean tissue P_{O_2} in large cylinders are shifted to small values for two reasons: 1. Capillary O_2 pressure is lowered by an increased O_2 uptake. 2. There is a considerable P_{O_2} de-

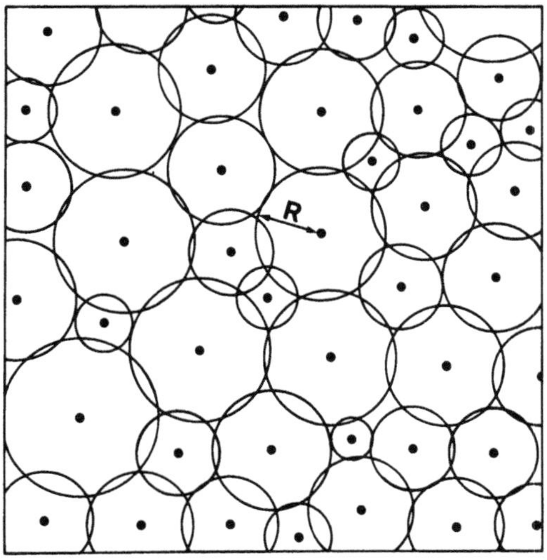

Fig. 6: Variation of supply radii of the single capillaries in tumor tissue. The schematic representation approximately corresponds with the distribution of intercapillary distances in younger tumors.

crease in radial direction of the tissue cylinder. Since we know the variation of the intercapillary distances, both the effects can be calculated. Fig. 7 shows the method. Based on frequency distribution of the intercapillary distances (A), the distribution of the end-capillary O_2 concentration (B) can be calculated first. By taking the O_2 dissociation curve and the BOHR effect into account, the mean intracapillary O_2 pressures (C) are calculated. To get the frequency distribution of the mean local O_2 pressures in the tissue (D), the mean radial P_{O2} decrease must finally be determined within tissue cylinders, which vary in size (THEWS, 1953).

The calculation procedure becomes simplified using an alignment nomogram for the parameters of the respiratory gas transport in rat blood (BORK et al., 1975). This nomogram (Fig. 8) gives the interdependence of P_{CO2}, pH, P_{O2} and S_{O2}. If two of these values are known, the nomogram permits the reading of the remaining parameters from the intersection line with the corresponding scales.

The results of these investigations are as follows: If inhomogeneities of the supply radii are taken into account, the calculated mean tissue P_{O2} is 12 mmHg below the calculated value assuming homogeneous supply conditions. A similar analysis can be conducted to determine the influence of different capillary lengths. Such an analysis shows that, if frequency distribution of the capillary lengths is taken into consideration, the mean tissue P_{O2} is below the value of homogeneous conditions by another 2 mmHg.

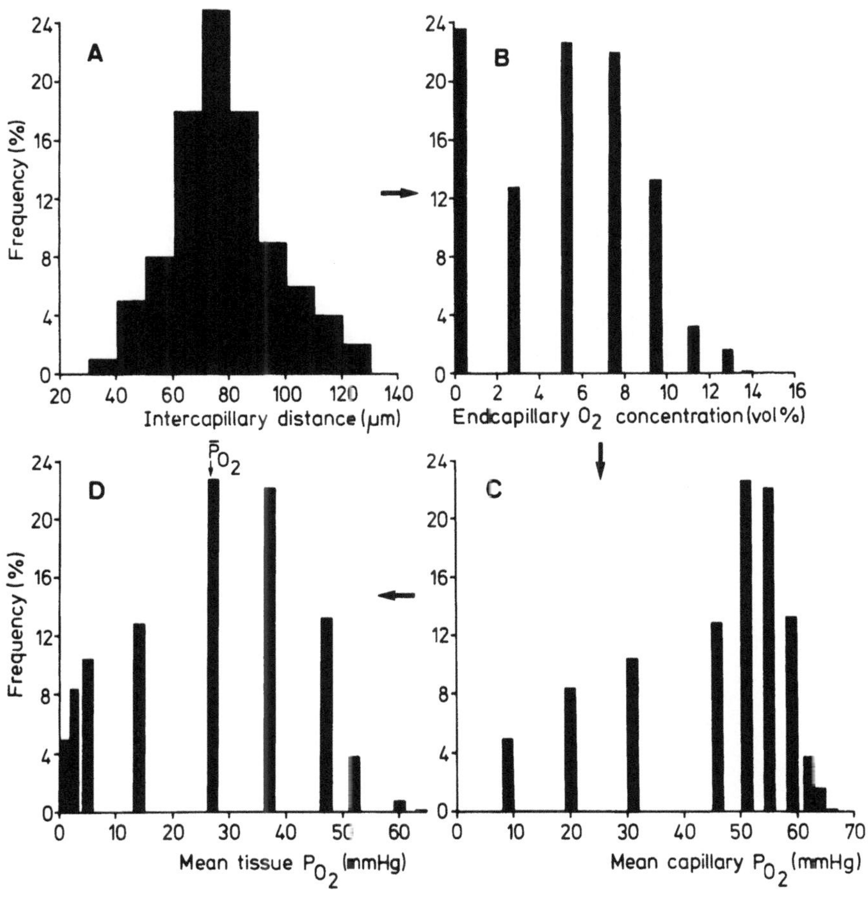

Fig. 7: Calculation of the mean tissue P_{O_2} ($\bar{P}_{O_2}$) taking inhomogeneous distribution of the supply radii into consideration. The values are calculated by determining frequency distributions of intercapillary distances (A), endcapillary O_2 concentrations (B) mean intracapillary O_2 pressures (C), and mean O_2 pressures in the tissue cylinders of different size (D).

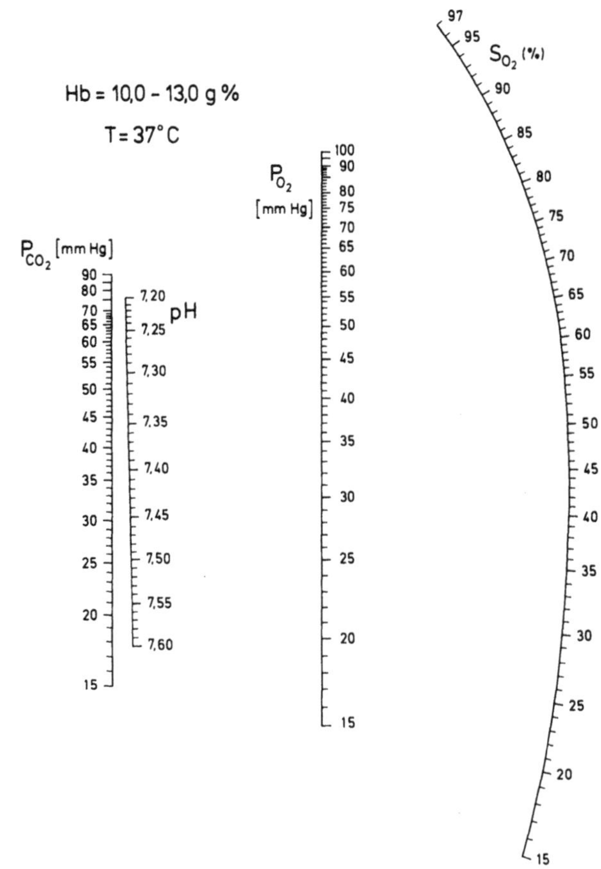

Fig. 8: P_{O_2} - P_{CO_2} - pH nomogram for rat blood at 37°C (Hb concentration : 10 - 13 g%)

All the factors that can cause a P_{O_2} decrease in the tissue, are once again put together in Table 2. In addition to shunt-perfusion as well as inhomogeneities of perfusion oxygen consumption may also influence the tissue P_{O_2}. But experimental data for a quantitative analysis of the factors mentioned last have not yet been determined. Nevertheless, we found reliable criteria indicating that well-supplied tumor cells have higher O_2 consumption in vitro than it is measured in vivo. This hints at inhomogeneities of O_2 consumption by the tumor tissue. Thus we draw the following conclusions:

1. Inhomogeneities of the supply parameters in tumor tissue have considerable influence on O_2 pressures in the tissue .

Table 2: Factors causing P_{O_2} depression in tumor tissue

	P_{O2} depression in young tumors
Shunt Perfusion	- 3 mmHg
Inhomogeneities of	
supply radii	- 12 mmHg
length of capillaries	- 2 mmHg
capillary perfusion	
intracapillary hematocrit	
perfusion of greater areas	
O_2 consumption	

2. Mathematical analysis shows that taking these aspects into account the measured low P_{O2} values are quite plausible.
3. Neglecting those inhomogeneities can falsify P_{O2} calculation just as choosing an inadequate supply model.

References:

BORK, R., VAUPEL, P., THEWS, G.: Atemgas-pH-Nomogramme für das Rattenblut bei 37°C. Anaesthesist 24, 84 -90 (1975)

GÜNTHER, H., VAUPEL, P., METZGER, H., THEWS G.: Steady state distribution of P_{O2} values in tumor tissue (DS- Carcinosarcoma). I. Measurements in vivo using gold microelectrodes. Z. Krebsforsch. 77, 26 - 39 (1972)

GULLINO, P. M., GRANTHAM, F. H.: Studies on the exchange of fluids between host and tumor. I. A method for growing "tissue - isolated" tumors in laboratory animals. J. Nat. Cancer Inst. 27, 679 - 693 (1961)

THEWS, G.: Über die mathematische Behandlung physiologischer Diffusionsprozesse in zylinderförmigen Objekten, Acta biotheor. (Leiden) 10, 105 - 138 (1953)

VAUPEL, P.: Atemgaswechsel und Glucosestoffwechsel von Implantationstumoren (DS- Carcinosarkom) in vivo. Experimentelle Untersuchungen und theoretische Analysen zur Frage der kritischen Sauerstoff- und Glucoseversorgung im Tumorgewebe. In: Funktionsanalyse biologischer Systeme (Vol. 1). Ed.: G. Thews (Steiner, Wiesbaden 1974)

VAUPEL, P., GÜNTHER, H., GROTE, J., AUMÜLLER, G.: Respiratory gas exchange and glucose metabolism of tumors (DS- Carcinosarcoma) in vivo. Z. ges. exp. Med. 156, 283 - 294 (1971)

PATHOPHYSIOLOGICAL ASPECTS OF GLUCOSE UPTAKE BY THE TUMOR TISSUE UNDER VARIOUS CONDITIONS OF OXYGEN AND GLUCOSE SUPPLY

P. Vaupel and G. Thews

Institute of Physiology, University of Mainz

D - 65 Mainz, Saarstrasse 21, Fed.Rep. Germany

Earlier examinations of the glucose uptake in neoplastic tissue by isolated DS- Carcinosarcoma implanted into the rat kidney had the results as follows (VAUPEL, 1974):

1.An increase of the tumor mass from 3 to 13 g wet weight caused an exponential decrease of the glucose consumption by the tumor tissue from 44.4 to 6.7 μmoles per 100 g/min; very young tumors of 3 - 4 g had uptake rates from 27.8 to 44.4 μmoles/100 g/min.

2.Simultaneous measurements of the mean actual glucose concentrations in the tumor tissue showed that in the very young tumors the concentration still ranged from 1.75 to 2.25 μmoles/g wet weight, whereas those in old tumors drop as low as 0 to 0.17 μmoles/g. From the observations on the exponential fall of the mean glucose uptake rate and on the mean glucose concentration we conclude that in the course of tumor growth an increasing rarefaction of the terminal vascular bed which is accompanied by an exponential widening of the intercapillary distances, and a rapid depletion of the glucose supply in the tissue take place. During this period the mean lactate concentrations in the neoplastic tissue rise from 14.4 to 22.2 μmoles/g.

3.The theoretical analysis of the critical supply conditions in DS- Carcinosarcoma showed that O_2 as well as glucose can be regarded as limiting substrates of tumor metabolism, glucose supply of the tissue being even more poor than oxygen supply. Therefore, both the substrates must be held responsible for the declining of the growth rate as well as for the enlarging of tissue areas showing cytolysis and necrosis, the phenomena running in parallel with increasing of tumor weight.

4.Even if the kinetics of O_2 and glucose uptake at the very low levels of O_2 and glucose concentrations were taken into account it becomes obvious that regional deficiency in O_2 and glucose imminently occurs during tumor cell proliferation.

The aim of the present investigations was to elucidate (a) the interconnection of glucose and O_2 supply, and (b) the extend of the maximal glucose uptake under conditions of an excess of substrate supplied. The point of the second series of experiments is the fact that the cancer cells are maintained in a state of "glucose hunger" in vivo (SHAPOT, 1972)

IN VIVO INVESTIGATIONS ON THE PASTEUR EFFECT IN IMPLANTATION TUMORS:

Today the PASTEUR effect is usually defined as the inhibition of glycolysis by oxygen in tissues showing both the aerobic and anaerobic pathway of glucose breakdown. In the presence of O_2, glycolysis is restricted in favour of the oxidative pathway. Since the aerobic pathway is the most economic and effective way to utilize glucose, the glucose consumption by the cell can generally be limited, if there has been no previous absolute or relative glucose deficiency. Our in vivo investigations on the inoculated DS- Carcinosarcoma in the rat kidney also show a typical PASTEUR effect when the conditions were changed from arterial normoxemia (see table; t- test is based on paired observations). Increasing the arterial O_2 partial pressure from 89 to 480 mmHg we observed a drop in glycolytic rate (GR) by about 10%, although the improved O_2 supply benefits only the first quarter of the area surrounding a capillary, i.e. the arterial end of the capillary. The release of lactate ($\dot{V}_{La}$) from the tumor tissue into the blood is reduced as a consequence of the diminished glycolytic rate; the lactate- pyruvate- ratio is dropping correspondingly.

No significant reduction of the glucose uptake ($\dot{V}_{Gl}$) was observed. A decrease in the glucose uptake could not be expected under the above conditions because of a deficient glucose supply to the tumor cell in vivo.

Table: Parameters of glucose metabolism and respiratory gas exchange during normoxia and hyperoxia (n = 11; tumor weight: 4.0 ± 0.7 g)

	normoxia		hyperoxia		t-test
	$\bar{x}$	$\pm s_{\bar{x}}$	$\bar{x}$	$\pm s_{\bar{x}}$	2p <
TBF (ml/100 g/min)	11.9	2.4	11.8	2.0	--
art. pO_2 (mmHg)	89	8	480	12	0.001
$\dot{V}_{O_2}$ (ml/ 100 g/min)	1.25	0.38	1.42	0.47	0.005
$\dot{V}_{gl}$ (μmoles/100 g/min)	26.7	10.6	26.1	10.0	--
$\dot{V}_{la}$ (μmoles/100 g/min)	27.8	10.0	21.1	11.1	0.05
La/Pyr ven.	40.7	10.9	34.5	8.3	0.01
GR (%)	51.4	19.7	42.5	17.3	0.005

Thus, a drop of the glucose consumption together with an improvement of the O_2 supply conditions will remain the privilege of well- supplied cells in vitro, where sufficient glucose supply is guaranteed.

IN VIVO INVESTIGATIONS ON THE CRABTREE EFFECT IN IMPLANTATION TUMORS:

Having investigated tumor metabolism under in vitro conditions CRABTREE (1929) found that the O_2 uptake by neoplasms decreased after the addition of glucose to the incubation medium. These findings were interpreted as an inhibition of endogenous respiration, i.e. inhibition of the oxidation of endogenous substrates, such as fatty acids and/or amino acids by glycolysis (CRABTREE effect).

The initial decrease of O_2 consumption by the tumor cells in vivo (observed in our experiments after the arterial glucose concentration had been raised) largely corresponds to phenomena observed under in vitro conditions. Up to now the CRABTREE effect (or "reversed PASTEUR effect") has not been demonstrated under in vivo conditions. Therefore, it has been held to be characteristic of the in vitro metabolism of cancer cells. Our findings disprove such a view.

In accordance with the in vitro data, the extend of inhibition of the endogenous respiration and duration of this effect depend on the intracellular glucose concentration (COE, 1966; COE et al., 1966), i.e. on the amount of glucose added. The phenomenon turned out to be reversible. Like KIELER (1960) we also found an inhibition of the CRABTREE effect at high CO_2 pressures or acidosis (see fig. 1). But we cannot decide now which

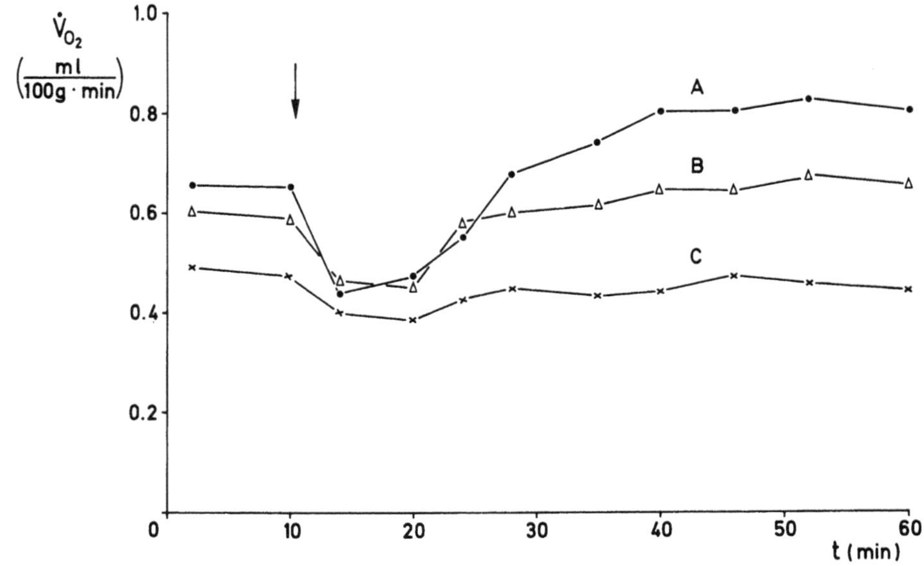

Fig. 1. Effect of gas parameters in the arterial blood on the CRABTREE effect. The time of glucose addition is marked by an arrow.
A: pCO_2 = 39 mmHg, pO_2 = 91 mmHg
B: pCO_2 = 51 mmHg, pO_2 = 81 mmHg
C: pCO_2 = 62 mmHg, pO_2 = 72 mmHg

of the parameters (pCO_2, pH or pO_2) which change during alveolar hypoventilation of the tumor- bearing animals are responsible for the diminishing and eventually disapparence of the CRABTREE effect.

GLUCOSE UPTAKE BY YOUNG TUMORS OF DS- CARCINOSARCOMA ON HYPERGLYCEMIA:

In "tissue- isolated" preparations of implanted tumors, 3 to 4 g of weight, a continuous arterial hyperglycemia maintained for several hours (27.8 to 33.3 μmoles/ml) induces a maximal glucose uptake rate of 0.16 to 0.20 mmoles/100g /min. Below these arterial glucose concentrations glucose uptake decreases continually. Thus, when the solid tumor is supplied with glucose only by the capillary network glucose uptake attains the maximal rate at concentrations which are 4 to 5- fold of that on normoglycemia.

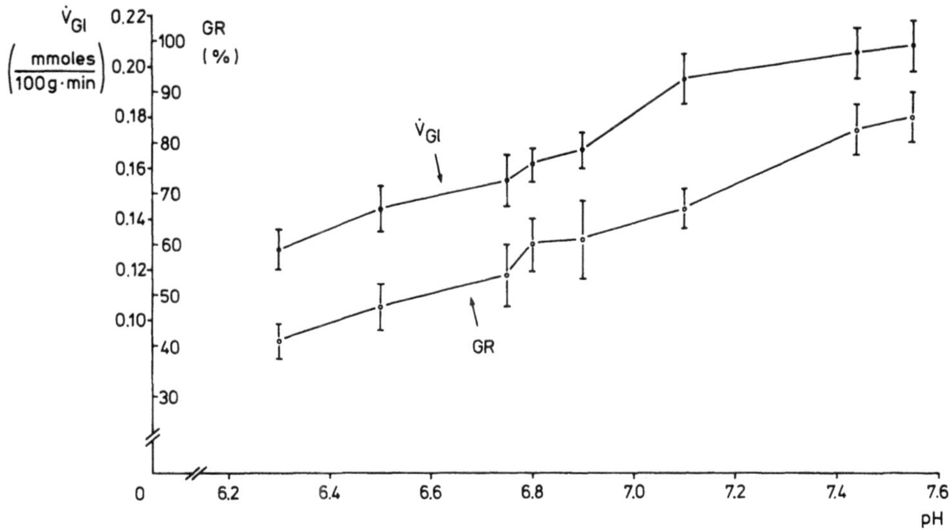

Fig.2. Relationship between pH of the medium and the amounts of glucose utilized ($\dot{V}_{Gl}$) and glycolytic rate (GR) by ascites cells of DS- Carcinosarcoma. Values are means $\pm$ SE, n = 10.

GLUCOSE UPTAKE BY DS- CARCINOSARCOMA ASCITES CELLS:

To avoid the consequences of the limited transport of glucose (and O_2) in solid tumors which affect uptake of the above substances by the neoplasm, ascites form of the same tumor (DS- Carcinosarcoma) was used. They were suspended in Eagle's medium (20 mmoles/l Hepes, 6 to 26 mmoles/l $NaHCO_3$, 20% calf serum) for eight hours. The glucose concentration in the medium was constantly maintained at 7.5 to 7.8 μmoles/ml for the period of the experiment in order to imitate in vivo conditions (normoglycemia). To the medium 20% calf serum was added to provide the ascites cells with insulin and amino acids, since it is well-known that these substances can stimulate glucose utilization and glycolytic rate (BLAKER et al., 1971; TEMIN, 1967; van VENROOIJ et al., 1972). Variation of the pH value in the medium is achieved by adding 6 to 26 mmoles/l $NaHCO_3$. The suspended cells were equilibrated with a water saturated gas mixture containing 21vol% O_2, 6 vol% CO_2 and 73 vol% N_2 at 37°C. The optimum convection in the medium was guaranteed.

The results of this series of experiments are shown in fig.2. A pH- dependent glucose utilization ($\dot{V}_{Gl}$) by the ascites cells can be observed: glucose consumption by the cells decreased in a reverse correlation with acidosis in the medium. This process is to be attributed to the fact that glycolysis is inhibited with H^+ concentration increased. This effect was proved previously by PAUL et al. (1966) and ZWARTOUW and WESTWOOD (1958) for other cells.

In the in vitro experiments with glucose concentrations in the medium corresponding to that in the blood of tumor- bearing rats, observed under usual conditions, ascites cancer cells have been shown to consume glucose at the same rate as do similar cells, belonging to a solid tumor, only when a high hyperglycemia in the host was induced.

Thus, we are left with the conclusion that the factors limiting glucose (and O_2) uptake by the cancer cells is the transport of the above substances to the solid tumor (a low and insufficient blood flow, impaired microcirculation as well as great diffusion distances between blood vessels and cancer cells) rather than an impairment of the metabolism.

References:

BLAKER, G.J., BIRCH, J.R., PIRT, S.J.: The glucose, insulin and glutamin requirements of suspension cultures of HeLa cells in a defined culture medium. J. Cell. Sci. 9, 529 - 537 (1971)

COE, E.L.: Correlation of glycolytic and respiratory events after addition of a small amount of glucose to Ehrlich ascites carcinoma. Cancer Res. 26, 269 - 275 (1966)

COE, E.L., IBSEN, K.H., DIXON, M., McKEE, R.W.: Glycolysis of a small amounts of glucose by Ehrlich ascites carcinoma cells. Cancer Res. 26, 276 - 281 (1966)

CRABTREE, H.G.: Observation on the carbohydrate metabolism of tumors. Biochem. J. 23, 536 - 545 (1929)

KIELER, J.: Influence of CO_2 tension on the respiration of Yoshida ascites tumor cells. J. Nat. Cancer Inst. 25, 161 - 176 (1960)

PAUL, J., BROADFOOT, M.M., WALKER, P.: Increased glycolytic capacity and associated enzyme changes in BHK21 cells transformed with polyoma virus. Int. J. Cancer 1, 207 - 218 (1966)

SHAPOT, V.S.: Some biochemical aspects of the relationship between the tumor and the host. Adv. Cancer Res. 15, 253 - 286 (1972)

TEMIN, H.M.: Studies on carcinogenesis by avian sarcoma virus. VI. Differential multiplication of uninfected and of converted cells in response to insulin. J. Cell. Physiol. 69, 377 - 384 (1967)

VAUPEL, P.: Atemgaswechsel und Glucosestoffwechsel von Implantationstumoren (DS- Carcinosarkom) in vivo. Experimentelle Untersuchungen und theoretische Analysen zur Frage der kritischen Sauerstoff- und Glucoseversorgung im Tumorgewebe. In: Funktionsanalyse biologischer Systeme (Vol. 1). Ed.: G. Thews (Steiner, Wiesbaden 1974)

van VENROOIJ, W.J.W., HENSHAW, E.C., HIRSCH, C.A.: Effects of deprival of glucose or individual amino acids on polyribosome distribution and rate of protein synthesis in cultured mammalian cells. Biochim. Biophys. Acta 259, 127 - 137 (1972)

ZWARTOUW, H.T., WESTWODD, J.C.N.: Factors affecting growth and glycolysis in tissue culture. Brit. J. exp. Path. 39, 529 - 539 (1958)

SOLUTION OF THE DIFFUSION FIELD EQUATION OF SUBSTRATE CONCENTRATION IN THE INTERCAPILLARY REGION CONSIDERING THE DECREASE IN SUBSTRATE CONSUMPTION IN THE UNSATURATED REGION OF CANCER CELL GLYCOLYSIS AND RESPIRATION

A. von Ardenne and M. von Ardenne

Forschungsinstitut Manfred von Ardenne
Dresden

8051 Dresden Zeppelinstr. 7, GDR (Germany)

1. GENERAL

In the few papers written by reason of theoretical statements to the concentration microtopography of glucose and O_2 in the intercapillary region of tumor tissue, especially from THEWS [1] and, somewhat later, VAUPEL [2], it is assumed that substrate consumption remains constant up to the periphery of the considered cylindrical space around the capillary, i. e. within the socalled KROGH's cylinder.

Because of the short capillary distances, normal healthy tissue shows to be in such a good supply situation that constant substrate consumption can be taken for granted. Here we speak of a saturated substrate consumption. In tumor tissue, on the other hand, proliferation will yield distances that must result in critical supply regions.

2. GLYCOLYSIS AND RESPIRATION CHARACTERISTICS

As pointed out in previous papers of M. VON ARDENNE [3] consumption of the offered substrate in tumor tissue reduces proportional to substrate concentration when a particular limit

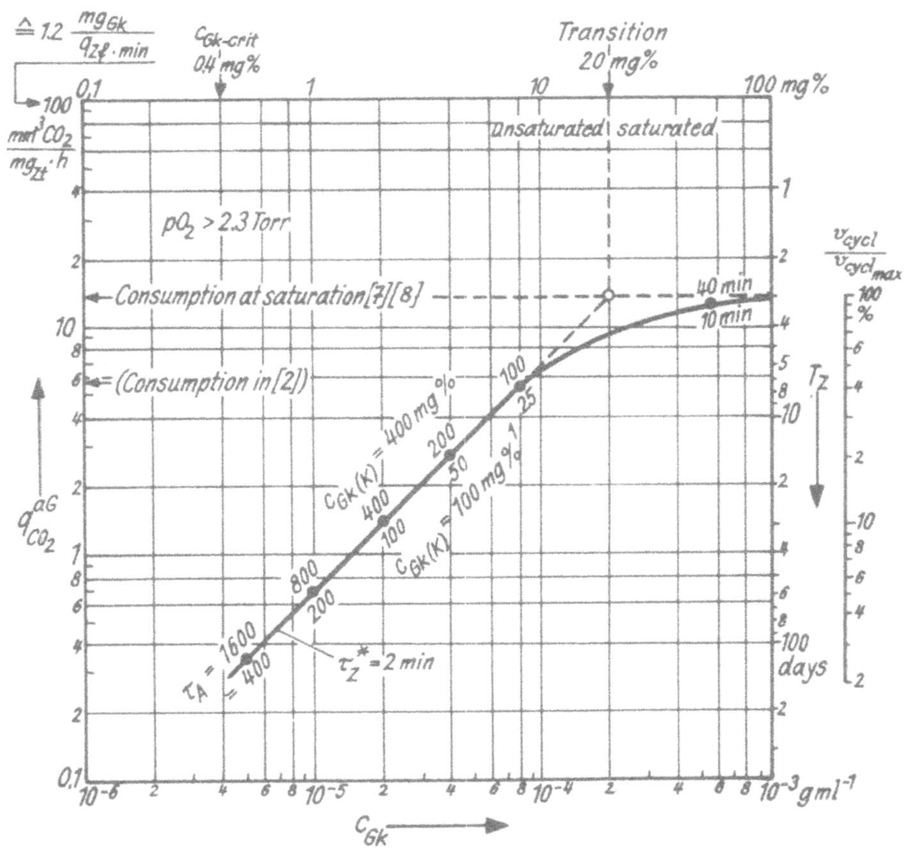

Fig. 1: Characteristic $q^{aG}_{CO_2} = f(c_{Gk})$ of Human Cancer Cells at a Glucose Consumption Time Constant of $\tau^*_Z = 2$ min.
(Averaged Model).
Guide on the relationship between glucose concentration in the intercapillary region c_{Gk}, glucose fermentation $q^{aG}_{CO_2}$ and cell reduplication T_Z or cycling rate ϑ_{cycl}-Working points for various values of time constant τ_A of glucose/lactic acid exchange between circulation and tumor tissue at glucose concentrations in blood of $c_{Gk(K)}$ = 100 and 400 mg%, respectively.

---

1 $\tau_A = \tau^*_Z \dfrac{c_{Gk(K)}}{c_{Gk}}$

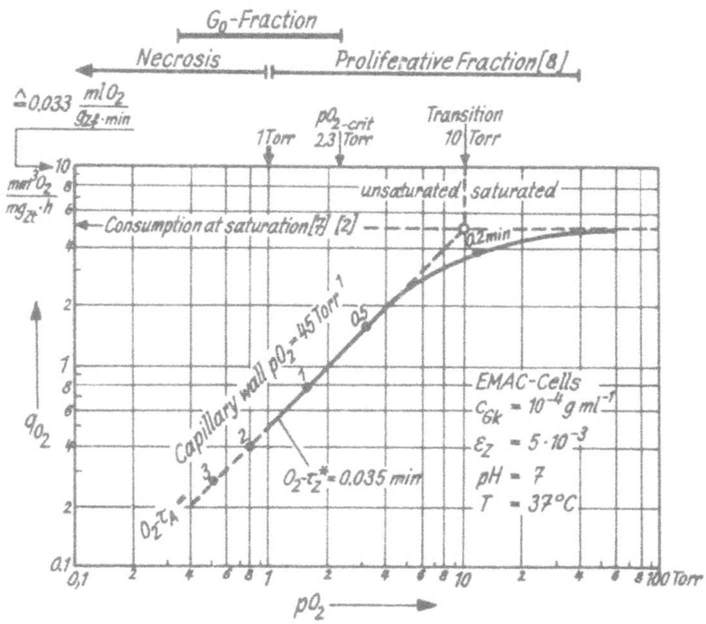

Fig. 2: Characteristic $q_{O_2} = f(pO_2)$ of Cancer Cells. Transition from saturated to unsaturated cancer cell respiration at about $pO_2 = 10$ Torr.

- ∘ Measuring points. Electrochemical measurement [3, p. 228].
- • Working points for equilibrium between offer and consumption.

$O_2\text{-}\tau_Z^*$ = time constant of O_2 consumption in tumor tissue.

$O_2\text{-}\tau_A$ = time constant of O_2 exchange between circulation and tumor tissue.

concentration is underpassed. This holds true for both glucose [4] and oxygen consumption [3, p. 228] and means that, below the said limit concentration, there is an unsaturated substrate consumption.

In the following it shall be shown that diverse ideas on substrate consumption in the critical supply regions have led to various quantitative assessments.

---

1 $$O_2\text{-}\tau_A = \tau_Z^* \cdot \frac{pO_2 \text{ at capillary wall}}{pO_2}$$

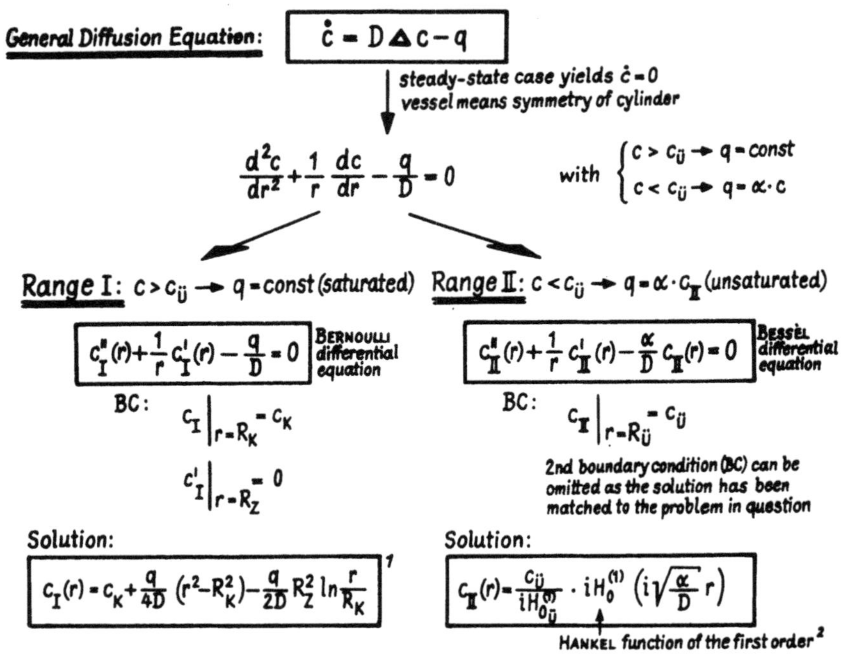

Fig. 3: Solution of the Diffusion Field Equation for Substrate Concentration in the Intercapillary Region Considering the Reduced Substrate Consumption in the Unsaturated Region of Cancer Cell Glycolysis and Respiration

Depicted in Fig. 1 is the "Glycolysis Characteristic" in human cancer cells for tumor species of medium growth rate (cell cycling time in the saturated region approx. 70 hours). Plotted on the ordinate is the glucose consumption and on the abscissa the glucose concentration.

Within the saturation range, i.e. at a glucose concentration higher than $20 \cdot 10^{-5}$ g/ml (= 20 mg%), glucose consumption in tussue remains almost constant. Should the concentration drop below the aforementioned level, glucose consumption also reduces proportional to glucose concentration. In the figure it is shown that the critical glucose concentration of $0.4 \cdot 10^{-5}$ g/ml is far below the transition point of $20 \cdot 10^{-5}$ g/ml.

---

1 See [1][2][9]

2 To determine $H_0^{(1)}$ see [5]

Fig. 2 gives the "Respiration Characteristic" of cancer cells. Plotted on the ordinate is the O_2 consumption and on the abscissa the O_2 pressure. Same as with glucose consumption, O_2 consumption drops proportional to the O_2 pressure after a certain limit pressure - here 10 Torr - has been underpassed. In this case the critical O_2 pressure of 2.3 Torr occurs at about 25 % of the pressure at the transition point.

3. SOLUTION OF THE DIFFUSION FIELD EQUATION CONSIDERING BOTH SATURATED AND UNSATURATED SUBSTRATE CONSUMPTION

Let us consider the diffusion of glucose or O_2 in a cylindrical tissue pattern having a capillary in its centre. For this, the diffusion field equation (given in Fig. 3) is to be solved. As it is only the steady-state case with the applied cylinder symmetry of the examined arrays, this equation can be substantially reduced.

With constant glucose or O_2 consumption one obtains a BERNOULLI differential equation. Its solution is rather simple and gives the diffusion into the supply region of the so called KROGH's cylinder. THEWS and VAUPEL have used this solution as starting point for various considerations on the concentration distribution in tissues interspersed with vessels.

But if the drop in substrate consumption in the unsaturated region of cancer cell glycolysis and respiration is also taken into consideration, BERNOULLI's differential equation is transformed to a BESSEL differential equation. Its non-trivial solution contains the HANKEL function of the first kind as tabulated in JAHNKE-EMDE [5].

Both solutions then allow the quantitative determination of glucose and O_2 concentration in tumor tissue that surrounds a capillary.

Shown in Fig. 4 is the qualitative behaviour of substrate concentration in tumor tissue. On the boundary of the capillary (R_K) the substrate concentration reaches the value c_K. Starting from R_K, the substrate then diffuses into the tumor tissue.

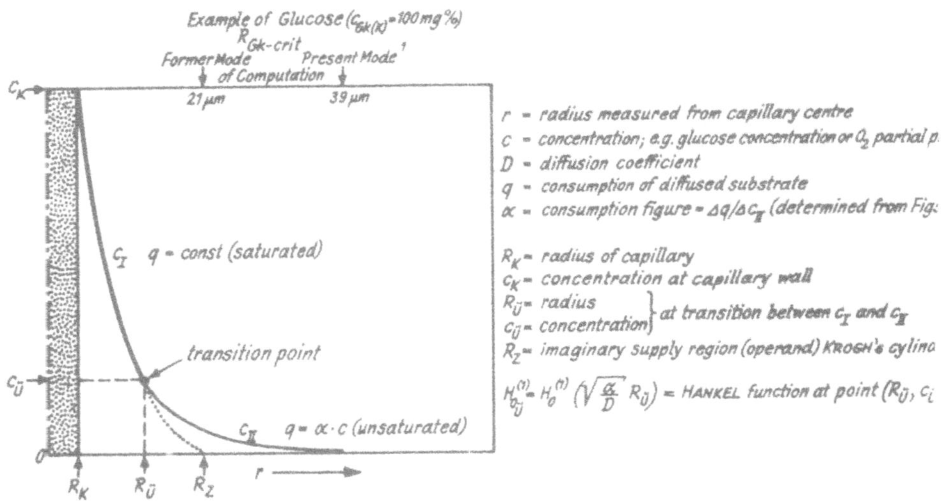

Fig. 4: Symbols used in the General Solution of the Diffusion Field Equation

Constant substrate consumption in the saturated region then causes the concentration to drop to the limit concentration $c_Ü$. From there on, substrate consumption in the unsaturated region will reduce with the concentration according to knowledge gained from Fig. 1 and Fig. 2.

If the range of constant substrate consumption is expanded to a concentration c= 0 we obtain the hitherto supposed concentration behaviour which reaches the periphery of KROGH's cylinder at R_Z.

The example of glucose diffusion given on top of the diagram clearly reveals that it is very important to consider the nonconstant glucose consumption in the unsaturated region.

Because according to VAUPEL [6] a capillary distance of 180 µm has been determined in tumors having a weight of more than 8 g whereas our computation only result in critical concentrations around a value of 40 µm, it is possible to disregard a superposition of the diffusion cylinders.

---

1 Ratio: radii 1.9 : 1 and volumina 3.6 : 1! Parameters as in Para 2.5

Tumor tissue		Glucose					O_2				
		c_{Gk-K}	$c_{Gk-Ü}$	D_{Gk}	$q_{Gk(satur)}$	$c_{Gk-crit}$	pO_2	$pO_{2-Ü}$	D_{O_2}	$q_{O_2(satur)}$	pO_{2-crit}
		$10^{-5} g ml^{-1}$ (mg %)	$10^{-5} g ml^{-1}$ (mg %)	$cm^2 s^{-1}$	$\frac{mg}{100g \cdot min}$	$10^{-3} g ml^{-1}$ (mg %)	Torr	Torr	$cm^2 s^{-1}$	$\frac{ml}{100g \cdot min}$	Torr
intact		100 400 (CMT)	20	$9 \cdot 10^{-9}$ (v. Ardenne-Vaupel)	16	0.4	45 62 (CMT)	10	$3 \cdot 10^{-6}$ ($0.6 \cdot 10^{-6}$ Vaupel) ($0.8 \cdot 10^{-6}$ Rieger)	1.6	2.3 to 1.0
after therapy	without mesenchym incorp.	100	20	$2 \cdot 10^{-8}$	8 (L = 50%)	0.4	45	10	$6 \cdot 10^{-6}$	0.8 (L = 50%)	2.3 to 1.0
	with mesenchym incorp.	100	20	$9 \cdot 10^{-9}$ to $2 \cdot 10^{-8}$	8 (L = 50 to 95%)	0.4	45	10	—	—	2.3 to 1.0

Fig. 5: Numerical values of the equation-parameters

4. PARAMETERS OF THE DIFFUSION FIELD EQUATION AND THEIR SELECTION

Diffusion coefficients, concentrations and consumption constants as given in the table of Fig. 5 have been used for computing the substrate concentration in the intercapillary region. The symbols denote:

c_{GK-K}: Glucose concentration on the boundary of the capillary.
Concentration parameters were chosen with due consideration of the fact that - from the arterial to the venous end of the capillary - there is a substantial depletion of glucose and O_2 in blood (see also [2]). So the most unsuitable supply situation will be found at the venous end and all concentration values have been selected accordingly.

$c_{GK-Ü}$: Glucose concentration at the transition point between constant and nonconstant substrate consumption as per Fig. 1.

D_{GK}: Diffusion coefficient for glucose.

$q_{GK(satur)}$: Glucose consumption in the region of constant substrate consumption.

$q_{GK-crit}$: Limit concentration of glucose below which cancer cell proliferation almost ceases.

Similar explanations apply to the symbols used for the O_2 parameters.

Apart from the diffusion in still intact tumor tissue, two other cases were treated theoretically after application of our CMT Concept, viz:

1. Immediately after therapeutic treatment with high cancer cell killing rate prior to mesenchyme incorporation and

2. after therapeutic treatment and subsequent mesenchyme incorporation which obstructs the diffusion process.

Numerical values given for therapeutically treated tissue have been derived by extrapolation from the values of still intact tumor tissue.

The solution of the diffusion field equation obtained from the values given in Fig. 5 has been briefly discussed in [10].

References

[1] G. Thews, Acta biotheor.(Leiden) 10, 105, 1953.

[2] P.Vaupel, Habil.-Schrift,Universität Mainz, 1973.

[3] M. von Ardenne, 2nd Edition. VEB Verlag Volk und Gesundheit, Berlin, 1970/71.

[4] M. von Ardenne - F.Rieger, Z.Naturforschg. 21b, 472, 1966.

[5] E.Jahnke - F.Emde, Teubner, Leipzig, 1952.

[6] P.Vaupel et al, 7th Europ.Conf.Microcirculation, Aberdeen 1972, Part II.Bibl.anat. 12, 527, 1973.

[7] F.Rieger, Archiv Geschwulstforschg. 43, 52, 1974.

[8] P.Vaupel et al, Z.Krebsforschg. 77, 17, 1972.

[9] G.Thews, Enke-Verlag, Stuttgart, 1966, p. 250.

[10] M.von Ardenne - A.von Ardenne, Computation of glucose and O_2 concentration distribution in the intercapillary region of intact tumor tissue ... Vortrag auf d.2nd Intern.Conf.on Oxygen Transp. to Tissue, Mainz, 12.- 14.3.1975.

COMPUTATION OF GLUCOSE AND O_2 CONCENTRATION DISTRIBUTION IN THE INTERCAPILLARY REGION OF INTACT TUMOR TISSUE CONSIDERING THE DECREASE IN SUBSTRATE CONSUMPTION IN THE UNSATURATED REGION OF CANCER CELL GLYCOLYSIS AND RESPIRATION

M. von Ardenne and A. von Ardenne

Forschungsinstitut Manfred von Ardenne
Dresden

8051 Dresden Zeppelinstr. 7, GDR (Germany)

1. MICROTOPOGRAPHY COMPUTATION OF THE SUBSTRATE CONCENTRATION

With the aid of the diffusion field equations and the numerical values of the equation parameters given in the preceding paper [1] we have calculated the microtopography of glucose and O_2 concentration in the intercapillary region of intact tumor tissue, taking into account that substrate consumption decreases in the unsaturated region of cancer cell glycolysis and respiration. The result is shown in Fig. 1 B. The critical supply radii $R_{Gk} = 0.4$ mg% and $R_{O_2} = 2.3$ / 1 Torr for maintained proliferation - compared to former computations [2] - increase by a factor of almost 1.8. Fig. 1 A shows the variation in distance R between capillary centre and cancer cells obtained with tumors in their various stages (model DS-Carcinosarcoma) and with healthy tissue as measured in [2].

Computing the decrease in substrate concentration also in the unsaturated region permits to give the scales of time constants for substrate exchange between circulation and tumor tissue based on [1][3] as a function of the capillary distance R. These scales for the glucose and O_2 tissue constants Gk-τ_A and

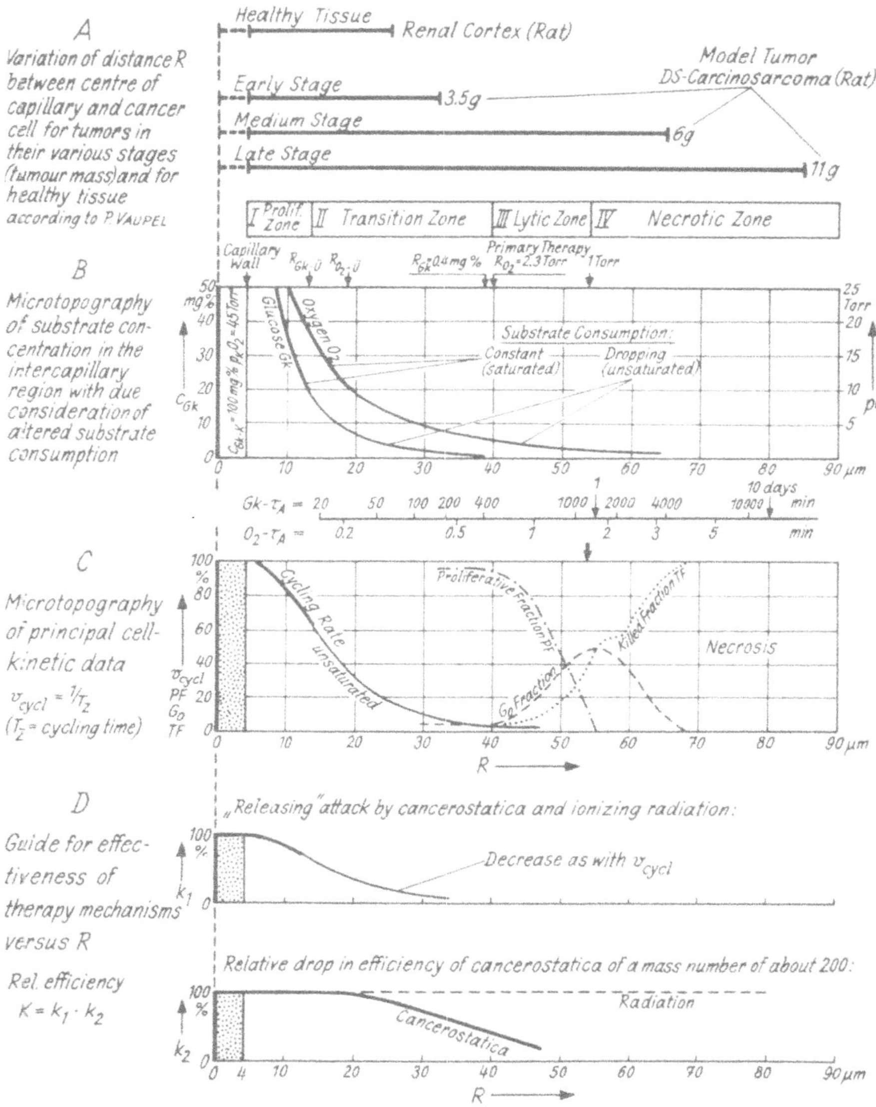

Fig. 1: Regularities of Substrate Concentration (B), Cancer Cell Kinetics (C) and Efficiency of Cancerostatica or Ionizing Radiation (D) in the Intercapillary Region of Tumor Tissue Considering the Altered Substrate Consumption in the Unsaturated Region of Cancer Cell Glycolysis and Respiration.
For comparison, (A) contains the variation of the distance to the capillary centre for tumors in their various stages. Guede values.

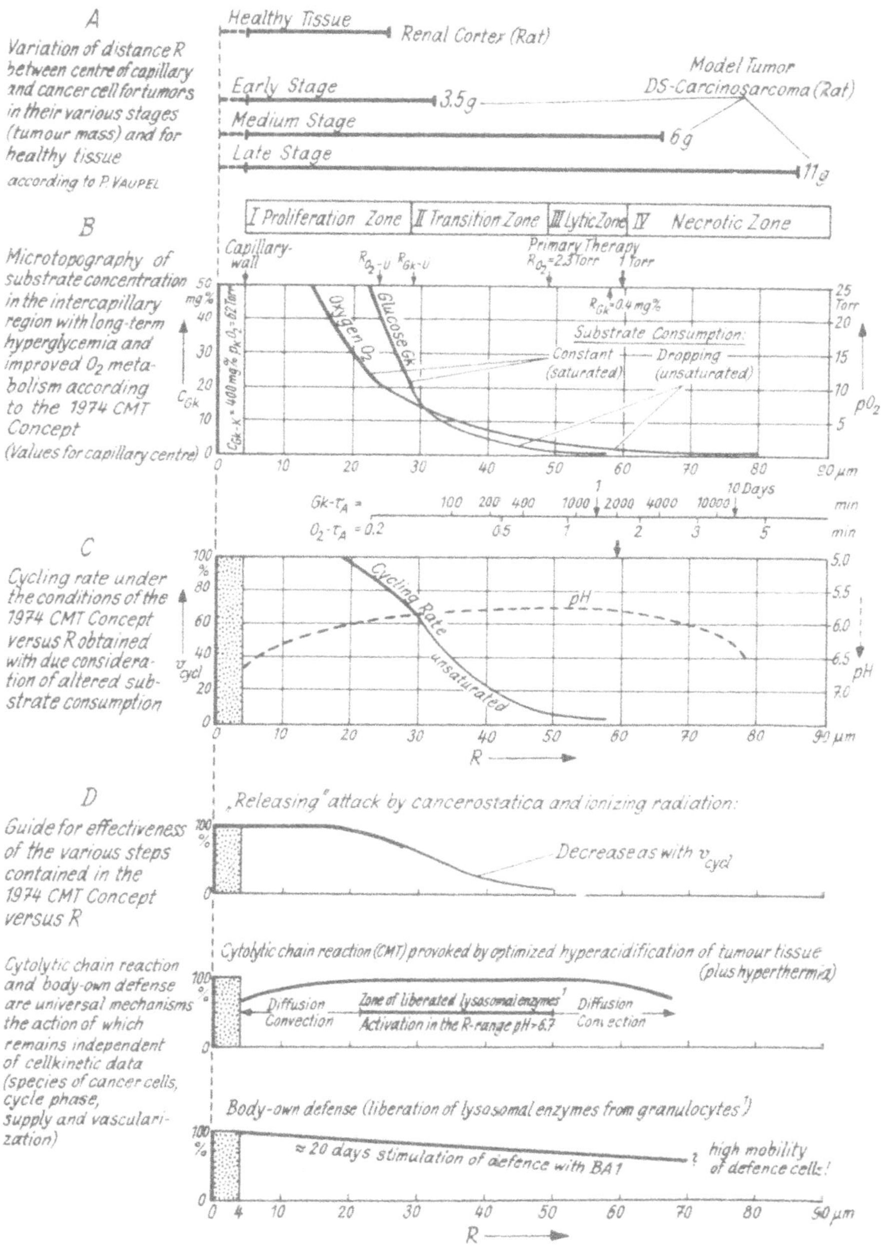

Fig. 2: Regularities of Substrate Concentration (B) and Therapy Parameters of Effects (C and D) in the Intercapillary Region of Tumor Tissue under the Conditions of the 1974 CMT Concept Considering the Altered Substrate Consumption in the Unsaturated Region of Cancer Cell Glycolysis and Respiration. Guide values.

O_2-τ_A are plotted at the bottom of Fig. 1 B. With a distance of R ≈ 39 μm and more it can be estimated that the time constant τ_A of glucose/lactic acid exchange approaches a level of Gk-τ_A>400 min.

This is why stimulation of glycolysis through hyperglycemia becomes fully effective also in tumor tissue located farther from the capillaries only in cases where hyperglycemia duration is greater than the abovementioned value of the time constant.

The computed microtopography of glucose and O_2 concentration in the intercapillary region of tumor tissue with long-term hyperglycemia and improved O_2 metabolism according to the 1974 Concept [5] of our Cancer Multi-step Therapy (CMT) is shown in Fig. 2 B. In our example we find critical R-values for normal conditions of R_{Gk} = 0.4 mg% = 38 μm and of R_{O_2} = 2.3/1 Torr = 40/54 μm and for CMT conditions of R_{Gk} = 0.4 mg% = 57 μm and R_{O_2}=2.3/1 Torr = 48/59 μm, respectively.

According to these values the critical R for glucose is lower than the critical R for O_2. This statement holds almost true even under CMT conditions where the blood glucose concentration has been raised to 4 times its normal level. So it is not the O_2 supply but the glucose supply which - as we have assumed since 1966 [3][4][6] - determines the proliferation rate of cells in cancer tissue. With the 4-capillary model this statement receives a still better foundation due to summation [7]. Our result shows that, under CMT conditions, it is possible to temporarily increase cancer cell glycolysis (hyperacidification, proliferation rate) in tissue ranges with larger R-values. With 27-h hyperglycemia [5], where the time constant Gk-τ_A is very high, the steady state of glucose concentration and of the cell kinetics is nearly reaches also for R-values near the necrotic regions.

2. GLUCOSE DIFFUSION FIELD, CELL KINETICS AND CANCER THERAPY

Based on the assumption that cancer cell proliferation is almost proportional to the cell glycolysis level [1][4][6] the decrease of the cell cycling rate may be extrapolated as a function of the capillary

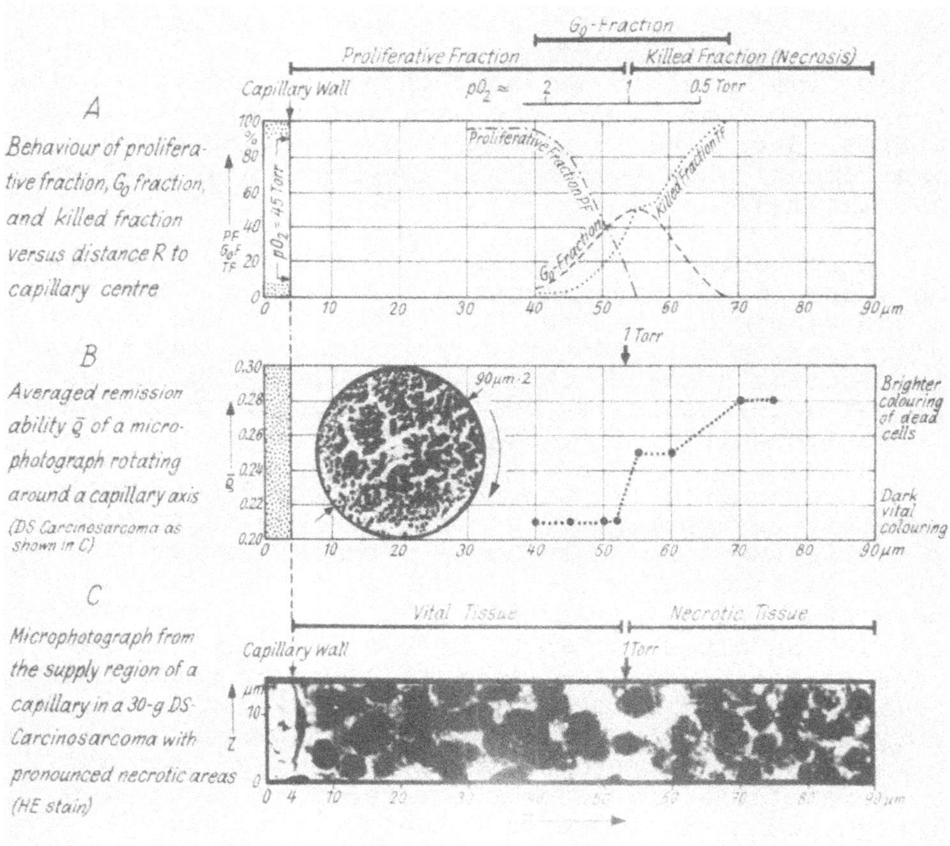

Fig. 3: Variation of Vital Cancer Cell Fractions (PF, G_0) in a DS Carcinosarcoma during its Late Stage versus Distance R to Capillary Centre according to this Paper (A) and in Compliance with Microphotographs of Stained 6-µm Sections (B and C).

distance R. This is done in Fig. 1 C and Fig. 2 C. From this combination results the active part of a cancer growing balance theory. To check our theory and the numerical values of the equation parameters we have prepared microphotographs of HE stained sections from a tumor in its late stage (large intercapillary distance) to evaluate them according to Figs. 3 B and C. According to Figs. 1 B and C, transition from vital to necrotic tissue should take place at R-values near 50 µm. The same value has been found in Figs. 3 B, C as an average from 50 micrometric measurements made in the said preparation and analogous material.

A comparison between Fig. 1 C and Fig. 2 C shows that, due to CMT Hyperglycemia, the cell cycling rate in tissue regions between R ≈ 15 to 50 µm has been multiplied. Hence, sensitivity to ionizing radiation and cancerostatica is enhanced especially in tissue regions being decisive for the therapeutic resistance of the tumor (Fig. 1 D, Fig. 2 D).

According to [7] the cancer cell portions with extremely low proliferation rate and the major part of the G_0-fraction, both being responsible for cancer recurrence, will be found at a capillary distance of $R_{O_2} = 2.3$ Torr and $R_{O_2} = 1$ Torr, respectively; i.e. on sites marked by arrows in Fig. 1 B. Because of their very low sensitivity to cancerostatica and ionizing radiation, these fractions can hardly be damaged by a single conventional therapeutic shock. So it is only an improved supply situation that has to be maintained for one or several days (long-time hyperglycemia and improved O_2 metabolism, also in connection with a cell cycle synchronization method [8] against cells of the G_0-fraction) and the utilization of therapeutic mechanisms being independent of cell kinetic data (lysosomal cytolytic chain reaction [4][9], body-own defence) that offer a way out of this dilemma. Such an expedient has been used in the CMT Concept [5] and, from the viewpoint of our theory, partially outlined in Fig. 2 D.

If it is assumed that, for reaching steady-state glucose concentration and cell kinetics, therapeutic action on the cancer cells ceases, for instance, when cycling rate or efficiency have dropped to 20 % of their maximum, our computation gives the following results: - As compared to standard conditions, the volume of tumor tissue directly attacked by cancerostatica or ionizing radiation (reduced dose) in compliance with the CMT Concept increases by a factor of 2.9.

Superposed on the reduction in effectiveness of cancerostatica versus R (lowered cell cycling rate) is the decrease in efficiency due to pharmaco-kinetic reasons. The decline in effective dose of cancerostatica with high diffusion coefficient and low consumption in the tumor tissue has been assessed and plotted in Fig. 1 D based on one of our previous contributions [10]. This decline is likely to underpass 20 % in the R-interval containing the critical cancer cell portions of the G_0-fraction. When using ionizing radiation, however, this decline in effective dose does not occur. For this reason it seems feasible, either alone or in combination, to use ionizing radiation during primary therapy directed against tumor tissue with high substrate exchange time constants (τ_A discernible by measurements according to [11]; e.g. against tumors in their medium or late stages (tumor dose of, say, 1000 r).

The chance to kill the high resistive cells near the necrosis region (G_0-fraction, cells with low proliferation rate) by repeated therapeutic treatment is reduced by resistance development phenomena. According to [12] the mesenchyme incorporation close to the capillaries [13], reducing the substrate diffusion coefficients, contributes to the developing resistance in tumor tissue when therapy processes are repeated. Therefore therapeutically untouched tumor tissue should be attacked by a single, superstrong blow [5]!

A highly efficient additional step to kill the critical resistive cells near the necrosis region seems to be the stimulation of immune-defence with the 1974 discovered BA 1 substance [14][15] over a posttherapeutic interval of nearly 20 days (long migration time for the defence cells, long R-way). Better than by diffusion processes these critical cells will be reached by defence cells owing to their self-mobility.

R e f e r e n c e s

[1] A. von Ardenne - M.von Ardenne, Vortrag auf der 2nd Intern.Conf.on Oxygen Transp. to Tissue. Mainz, 12.-14.3.1975.

[2] P.Vaupel, Habilitationsschrift der medizinischen Fachbereiche. Universität Mainz, 1973.

[3] M. von Ardenne - F.Rieger, Z.Naturforschg. 21b, 472, 1966.

[4] M. von Ardenne, 2nd Edition, VEB Verlag Volk und Gesundheit, Berlin, 1970/71.

[5] M. von Ardenne, Radiobiol.Radiother. 16, ,1975.

[6] M. von Ardenne, Z.Naturforschg. 27b, 1547, 1972.

[7] M. von Ardenne, Wiener Klin.Wochenschr. 86, , 1974.

[8] M. von Ardenne, Naturwiss. 60, 483, 1973.

[9] M. von Ardenne - P.G.Reitnauer, Z.Naturforschg. 29c, 425, 1974.

[10] M. von Ardenne - A. von Ardenne, Arzneimittelforschg. 24, , 1974.

[11] M. von Ardenne, Z.ärztl.Fortbildg. 68, , 1974.

[12] M. von Ardenne - A. von Ardenne, Archiv Geschwulstforschg. 43, , 1974.

[13] S.Peel - D.M.Cowen, Brit.J.Cancer 27, 72, 1973.

[14] M. von Ardenne - P.G.Reitnauer, Arzneimittelforschg. 25, , 1975.

[15] M. von Ardenne - W. Krüger, Archiv Geschwulstforschg. 45, , 1975.

MESENCHYME THEORY ON THE INCREASE IN RESISTANCE EXPERIENCED DURING REPETITION OF CANCER THERAPY PROCESSES

M. von Ardenne and A. von Ardenne

Forschungsinstitut Manfred von Ardenne
Dresden

8051 Dresden Zeppelinstr. 7, GDR (Germany)

Experimental observations of pronounced mesenchyme incorporation near the capillaries of cancer tissue occurring three days after therapeutic treatment with a tumor cell killing rate of 50 % (Fig. 1, 2) have led to the conclusion that mesenchyme reaction is one of the most likely causes of the known increase in resistance found with repeated cancer therapy processes.

Mesenchyme incorporation especially diminishes the glucose diffusion coefficient and therefore weakens the glucose diffusion field around the capillaries so that proliferation and sensitivity of tumor cells to cancerostatica and radiation will decrease to a very high degree.

The in [1] given solution of the diffusion field equation permits for glucose a quantitative presentation of regularities and therapeutic results about mesenchyme incorporation, which surrounds a capillary till a distance from the capillary axis of $R \approx 30$ µm (Fig. 3). So it has been calculated that, in steady-state, a transition to the conditions obtained with Cancer Multi-step Therapy (CMT) will increase the volume of tumor tissue being accessible to a therapeutic process by a factor of more than 2.5.

Viewed from theoretical aspects, the CMT Concept therefore seems to be one of the most promising

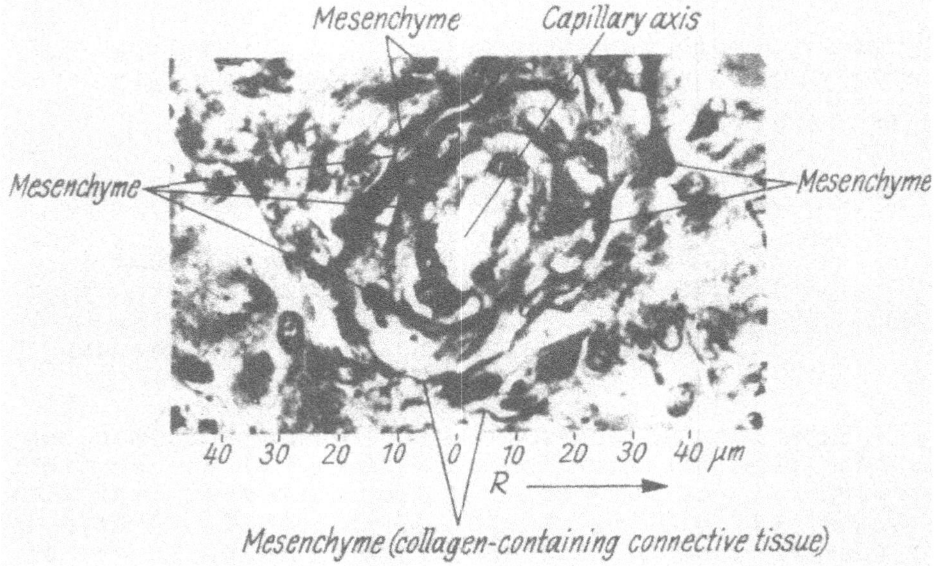

Fig. 1: Tissue of DS carcinosarcoma with capillary showing axially symmetric mesenchyme incorporations near the capillary (to about R = 30 µm) three days after therapeutic treatment with 150 mg/kg Ifosfamid.

Photograph : P. G. Reitnauer
Capillary-radius: $R_K \approx 4$ µm
Indicator : Azan stain

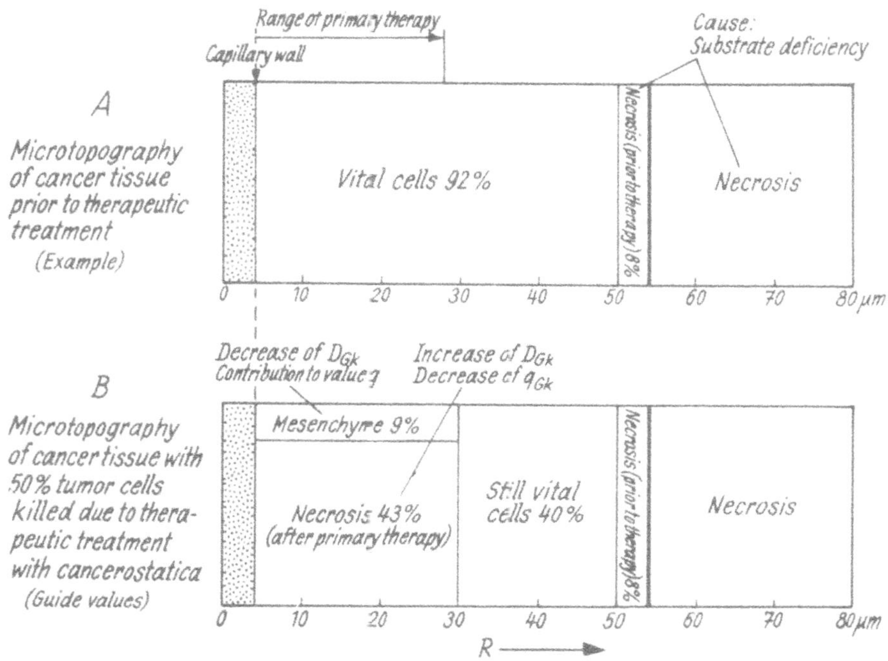

Fig. 2: Ideas on the microtopography of cancer tissue prior therapy (A) and 3 days after 50 % of tumor cells have been killed by therapeutic treatment (B).
Numerical values acc. to S. Peel and D.M. Cowen, Brit.J.Cancer 27, 72, 1973. (Fibrosarcoma RIB_5 in rats, single dosage of 100 mg/kg Cyclophosphamide. Δt = 3 days).

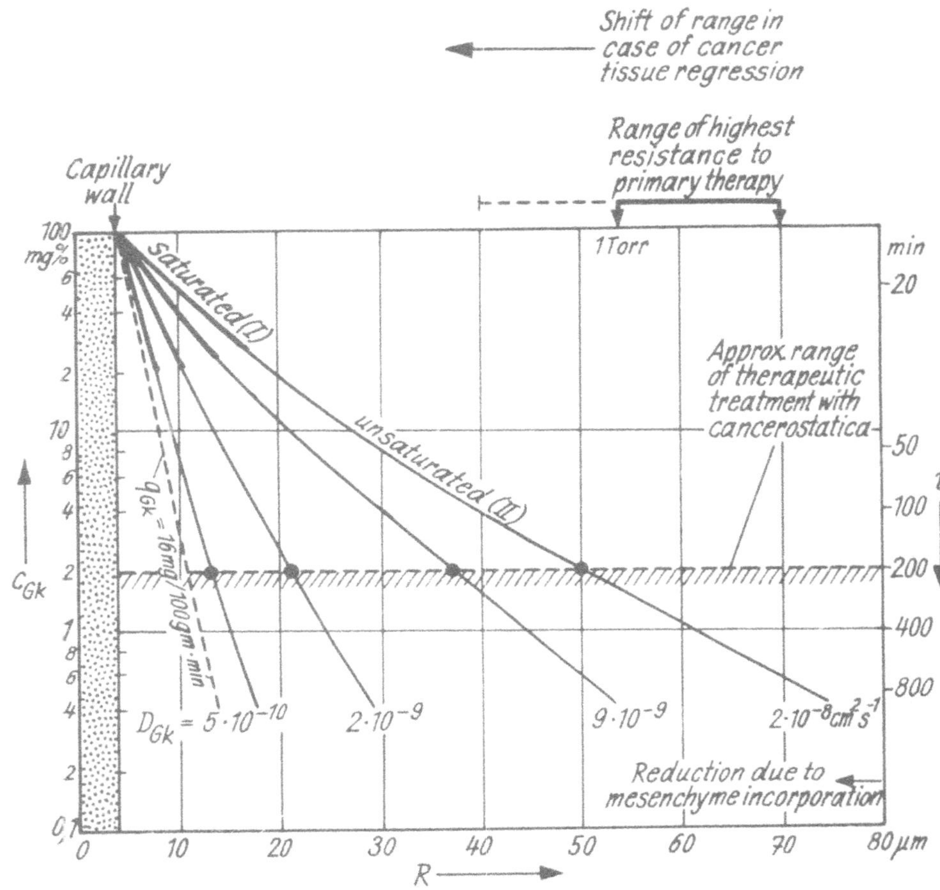

Fig. 3 Glucose concentration c_{Gk} and guide values of Gk-τ_A versus distance R to the capillary wall after 50 % of tumor cells have been killed by therapeutic treatment (Gk consumption q_{Gk} = 8 mg/100 gm min) determined for various diffusion coefficients D_{Gk}.

possibilities to overcome the (mesenchyme) resistance of tumor tissues. This is the more so as this give a real chance to demage therapeutically untreated cancer tissue by a single shock to such a degree that the (stimulated) body-own defence is able to overcome the surviving cancer cells.

References

[1] A. von Ardenne - M. von Ardenne, Lösung der Diffusionsfeldgleichung der Substratkonzentration im Interkapillarraum unter Berücksichtigung der Abnahme des Substratverbrauches im ungesättigten Bereich von Glykolyse und Atmung der Krebszellen.
Vortrag auf der 2nd Intern. Conf. on Oxygen Transport to Tissue, Mainz, 12. - 14.3.1975

SUMMARY OF DISCUSSION - SESSION X:

RESPIRATORY GAS EXCHANGE AND METABOLISM IN TUMOR TISSUE I

Chairmen: P. M. Gullino and M. Von Ardenne

Lübbers: Changes in oxygen and glucose consumption by perfused tumors could be due to a local disturbance of the microcirculation and necrosis may exert such an influence.

Gullino: This is certainly possible. However, glucose utilization or lactate production may change while oxygen consumption remains constant or vice versa. Alterations in microcirculation would probably modify all three parameters. We have no data on the effects of necrotic material on tumor microcirculation.

Siesjö: Under conditions of hypoglycemia, neoplastic cells could use other substrates or stored glycogen. What are the data available?

Gullino: The rat mammary and hepatocarcinomas we studied have very little stored glycogen. The respiratory quotient of Walker 256 carcinoma is 1.25; of hepatocarcinoma 5123, 1.00; of fibrosarcoma 4956, 0.76.

Tannock: In determining the mean pO_2 of neoplastic tissues, the electrode may be placed in necrotic areas where pO_2 may be zero. Was this taken into consideration?

Thews: In small tumors there is very little necrosis; in large tumors necrosis is more common. In our measurements we could not see a clear difference between the two conditions.

Erdmann: We have become very critical of the methodology of absolute pO_2 measurements in tissues since we could not obtain consistent pO_2 values in equally equilibrated solutions of glycerin or bovine serum at different concentrations. The recessed electrode that we have now developed, appears to correct for errors due to differences in diffusion coefficients.

Versmold: The importance of knowing pO_2 values of neoplastic tissues in vivo, as measured by Dr. Thews, is emphasized by the observation of Brauser and coworkers indicating that $K_{\frac{1}{2}}$ (O_2) of cytochrome aa_3 is the same in rat liver mitochrondria, either isolated or left in intact cells.

Gosalvez: Inhibition of respiration caused by administration of high doses of glucose was transient. Is this due to rapid utilization of glucose? How much glucose is necessary to obtain the Crabtree effect in vivo?

Vaupel: We inject 100 mg glucose in 1 ml solution into a rat with about 10 ml of circulating blood. I believe the transient effect on respiration is due to rapid glucose utilization by the tumor.

Siesjö: When the glycolytic rate decreases after a fall in pH, what happens to oxygen consumption?

Vaupel: We have no data to answer this question.

Gullino: Tumor pH may be reduced by increasing the glucose supply. In this case, Walker carcinomas augmented oxygen utilization. If the glucose supply was increased to a tumor previously starved of glucose, glycolysis was sharply reduced while glucose consumption as well as oxygen utilization were increased.

Moll: How does the supply of oxygen and glucose affect the growth rate of tumors?

Vaupel: We have not yet investigated the growth rates of DS-carcinosarcomas after supply conditions were improved. However, I believe that oxygen as well as glucose are limiting substrates and a deficient supply should limit growth.

Gullino: In several types of rat tumors we have been unable to see a direct correlation in vivo between growth rate and either oxygen utilization, glucose consumption or lactate production.

Tannock: We observed reduction of tumor growth in hypoxic animals. However, these animals were in poor health. Cell death in tumors is probably due to a combination of factors and the emphasis placed on diffusion distances for oxygen or glucose within the neoplastic tissues, as a way of explaining cell death and reduction of growth rate, is probably excessive. This impression is derived from the long survival of neoplastic cells despite hypoxic conditions.

Respiratory Gas Exchange and Metabolism in Tumor Tissue II

STUDIES ON THE ABILITY OF THE TUMOR RESPIRATION IN VIVO TO FULFILL ITS PHYSIOLOGICAL FUNCTIONS

V.S. Shapot

Department of Biochemistry
Institute of Experimental and Clinical Oncology
Moscow II5478, USSR

There is no doubt that the tumor growing in the host finds itself under conditions of severe hypoxia (Vaupel, 1974) due to scarce O_2 supply. It is likely that hypoxia would prevent the respiration of cancer cells from fulfilling in vivo its normal physiological functions.

We tried first to answer the question whether extra O_2 supply will increase protein synthesis in ascites cancer cells. Both O_2 and ^{14}C-lysine were administred intraperitoneally. Then the incorporation of the radioactive amino acid into proteins of the host's liver and ascites rat and mouse cancer cells (ovaria and Ehrlich carcinomas) was measured.

Extra O_2 supply exerted an insignificant effect on ^{14}C-lysine incorporation into host's liver proteins but stimulated markedly (by about 50%) protein synthesis in both kinds of cancer cells within 60 min of observation. Thus, an improvement of O_2 regime seems to elevate tumor respiration to the extent which permits to utilize extra energy for protein synthesis.

The second question to be answered was whether the in vivo glycolysis of cancer cells is restricted by the Pasteur effect. Glucose content of the ascitic fluid of Ehrlich carcinoma is known to be negligible although sufficient to ensure a continuous lactic acid production. The unmeasurably low concentration of glucose in this ascitic fluid was found to be a dynamic one, a result of an extensive consumption of glucose by cancer cells and a relatively slow glucose

Fig. I. IN VIVO DEMONSTRATION OF PASTEUR EFFECT IN CANCER CELLS BY EXTRA O_2 SUPPLY

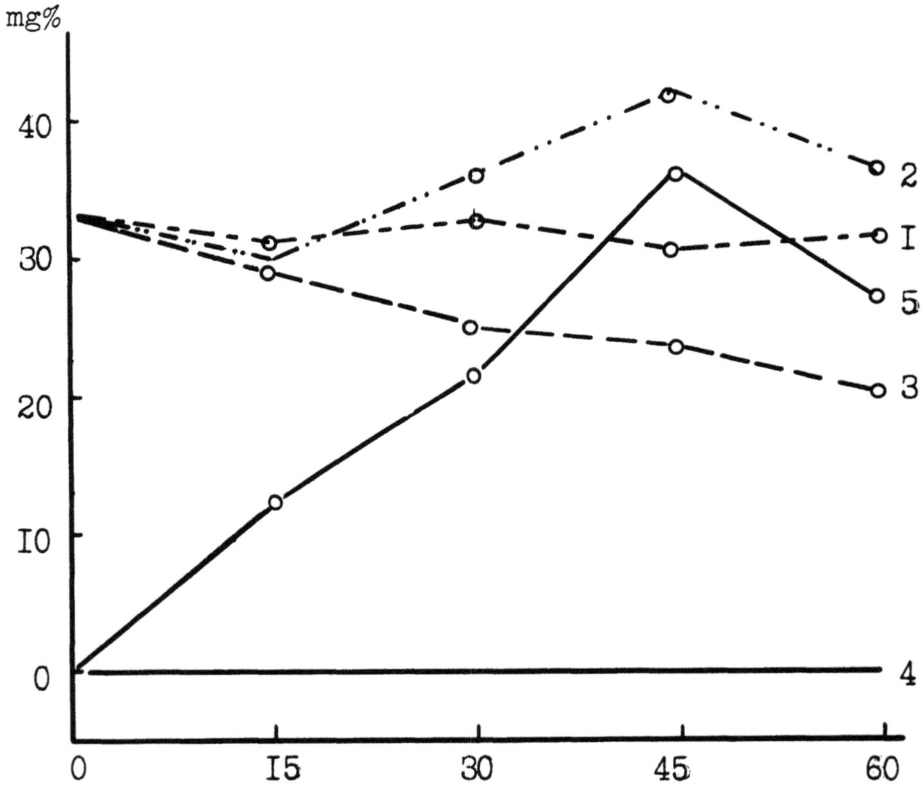

Ascites fluid of ovaria rat carcinoma
Abscissa - time in min; Ordinate - mg%;
I - lactate (usual conditions); 2 - lactate (extra glucose supply - 2 mg/g); 3 - lactate (extra glucose and O_2 supply); 4 - glucose (usual conditions); 5 - glucose (extra glucose and O_2 supply).

influx (Shapot, I972).

When O_2 was introduced intraperitoneally into the mouse with Ehrlich carcinoma the formation of lactic acid was found to slow down whereas glucose appeared in the ascitic fluid accumulating up to 60 mg% within 40 min. It is clear from the above observations that respiration of cancer cells in vivo is not able to affect glycolysis and spare glucose. Only extra O_2 supply induced the Pasteur effect.

Using rat ovaria ascites carcinoma we tried to find out whether the Pasteur effect can be demonstrated in a similar way when substantial amounts of glucose (2 mg/g) were injected into the tumor-bearing animals subcutaneously along with oxygen which was introduced intraperitoneally. Administration of glucose alone resulted in an increase in lactic acid content of the ascitic fluid from the 30-th minute on but no glucose in the fluid could be detected. However, oxygen introduced simultaneously with glucose changed the whole picture. Lactic acid levels gradually decreased and glucose appeared attaining by the 45-th minute the concentration as high as about 40 mg% (fig. I).

The above results indicate that respiration of cancer cells in vivo when supplied with sufficient oxygen is able to suppress their glycolysis elevated by the administration of glucose into the host.

The inability of cancer cell in vivo respiration to arrest glycolysis under usual conditions suggests that extensive anaerobic glycolysis not restricted by the Pasteur effect is the basic source of energy for these cells. A continuous glucose deficiency of cancer cells in vivo endowes them with the capacity to act in the host as a trap for glucose, as a powerful hypoglycemic factor (Shapot, I972).

Here we report on the experiments which clearly show that even in animals with normal blood sugar levels a hypoglycemic pressure on the host exerted by the tumor can be revealed.

Inbred male mice F_I CBA x $C_{57}BL$, 20 to 22 g, were implanted with the Ca-755 tumor syngenic to one of the parent lines, C57BL. By day 20 after implantation liver glycogen reserves in nonstarved mice turned out to be exhausted falling as low as I.87 mg/g liver, i.e. I0-fold.

When glucose (I0 mg/g) was introduced daily liver glycogen increased both in intact and tumor-bearing animals, in the latter-I4-fold. After the administration of glucose was ceased liver glycogen in control

Fig. 2. LIVER GLYCOGEN OF INTACT (I,3) AND TUMOR-BEARING (2,4) MICE

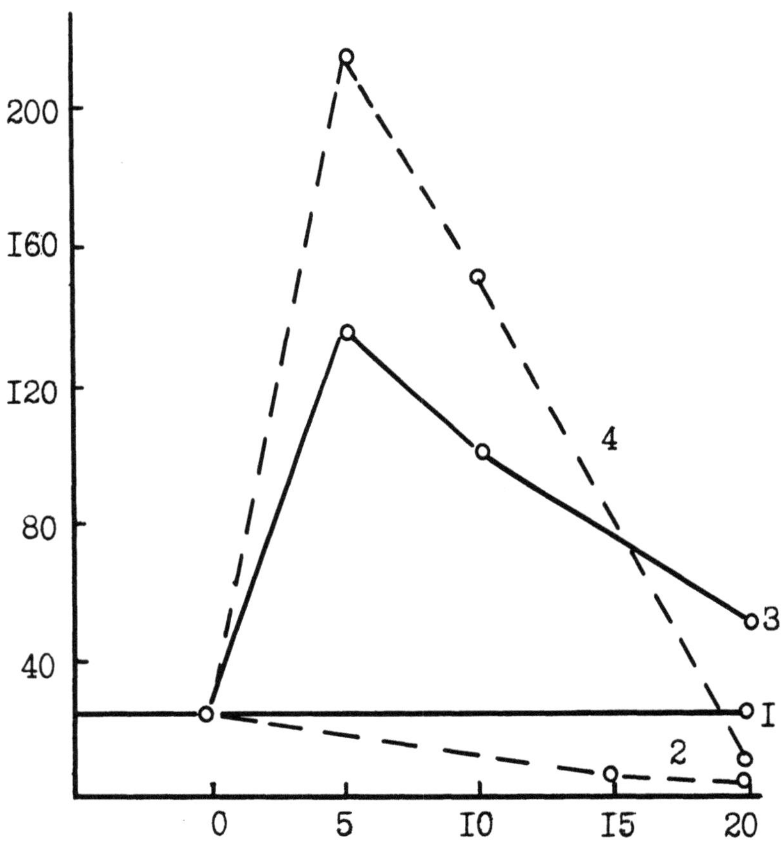

I,3 - intact, 2,4 - tumor bearing mice.
I,2 - usual conditions; 3,4 - glucose administred daily for the first 10 days.
Abscissa - days after transplantation;
Ordinate - glycogen content (mg/g liver).

Fig. 3. FORMATION OF LIVER ^{14}C-GLYCOGEN FROM ^{14}C-TYROSINE IN INTACT AND TUMOR-BEARING MICE (FOR THE METHOD - SEE SHAPOT AND BLINOV, 1974)

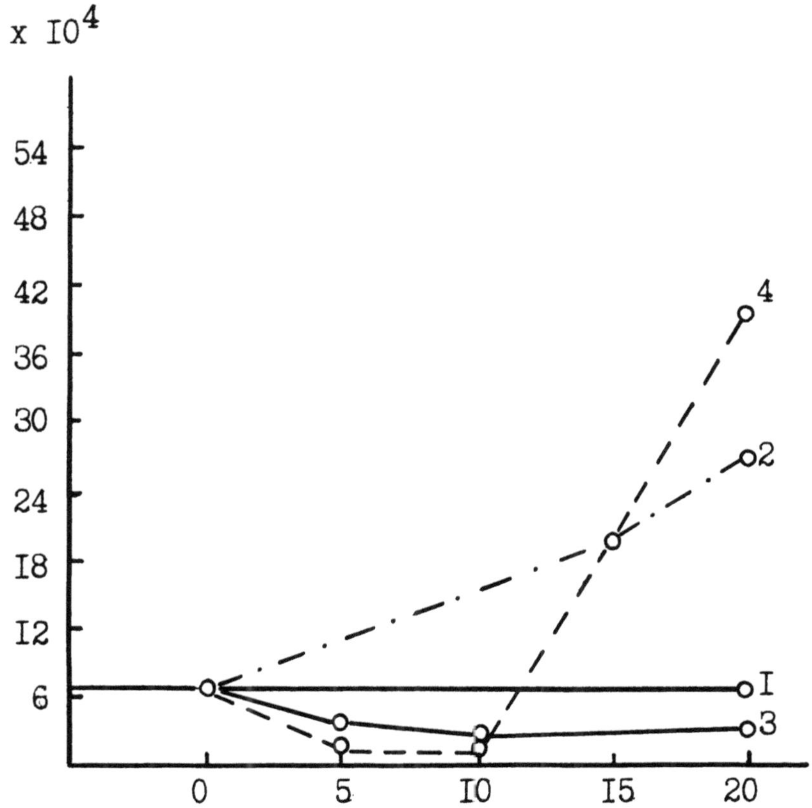

Designations - as in fig.2.
Abscissa - days after transplantation;
Ordinate - specific activity of the newly formed glycogen (cpm/g glycogen).

mice kept at the elevated level for IO days whereas in mice carrying Ca-755 liver glycogen content decreased drastically (fig. 2), obviously as a result of extensive compensatory mobilization of glycogen to counterbalance the tendency to hypoglycemia.

But stimulation of gluconeagenesis from non-carbohydrate sources is to be recognized the basic compensatory mechanism in tumor-bearing animals (Shapot and Blinov, I974). In mice with Ca-755 the content of the radioactive liver glycogen derived from ^{14}C-tyrosine was found by day 20 after implantation to be 4 times higher than that in intact mice.

Intraperitoneal administration of glucose inhibited gluconeogenesis both in tumor-bearing and intact mice. After glucose injections were interrupted the rate of ^{14}C-glycogen formation in the liver of intact animals remained low for IO days while in tumor-bearing ones this rate increased manyfold (fig.3).

Our presentation demonstrates a close connection between oxygen and glucose deficiency characteristic of cancer cells growing in vivo as well as grave consequences of this situation for the host.

References

Shapot V.S. Adv.Cancer Res. I5, 253-286, I972.
Shapot V.S., Blinov V.A. Cancer Res. 34, I827-I832, I974.
Vaupel P. Atemgaswechsel und Glucosestoffwechsel von Implantationstumoren (DS-Carcinosarcom) in vivo, I974.

CONTROL MECHANISMS OF OXYGEN AND GLUCOSE UTILIZATION IN TUMOURS

Mario Gosalvez and Sidney Weinhouse

Bioquimica Experimental, Clinica Puerta de Hierro, Facultad de Medicine, Universidad Autonoma de Madrid, and the Fels Research Institute and Department of Biochemistry, Temple University School of Medicine, Philadelphia

Most living cells depend on oxygen and glucose utilization to obtain the chemical energy necessary to maintain their functions and growth. Tumour cells are no exception to this rule though they may differ from other cell types in their mechanisms of control of oxygen and glucose utilization.

Two major levels for the control of glucose and oxygen utilization can be considered. First are those factors that control the supply of glucose and oxygen to the tumour tissue, and second are the factors that control the degree of utilization of oxygen and glucose by tumour defects (1), which limit diffusion of oxygen, thus creating radioresistent hypoxic areas (2) and limitations of critical respiratory gas exchange are well-known as important control factors, some of which are being analyzed in detail in this symposium. We will circumscribe our presentation to the second level - to the factors which control the degree of utilization of glucose and oxygen by tumour metabolism.

Fifty years ago the great German biochemist, Otto Warburg (3), discovered that tumours are capable of metabolizing glucose to lactic acid in the presence of oxygen. With only a few exceptions (4,5,6), normal cells metabolize glucose to CO_2 and H_2O in the presence of oxygen, and can form lactic acid in the absence of oxygen. The high aerobic glycolysis of cancer cells led Warburg to propose a theory of respiratory impairment in cancer (7) which has had enormous impact and still is guiding efforts at chemotherapy (8,9). Although this theory still remains unproven, nevertheless, the high

1. Aided by U.S. Public Health Service Grant CA-10916 and CA-12227 from the National Cancer Institute, by Grant BC-74 from the American Cancer Society, and by Grants 12-079-73 and 12-914-74 from the Spanish Instituto Nacional de prevision.

aerobic glycolysis of tumours has served as a focus for intensive efforts toward an understanding of the interrelationships between respiration and glycolysis.

Respiration and glycolysis, the conversion of glucose to CO_2 plus H_2O or to lactic acid, are closely interrelated in both normal and neoplastic cells. In the absence of oxygen, tumour cells utilize glucose at maximal rates and convert it virtually quantitatively to lactic acid. The availability of oxygen depresses the glycolytic rate, usually, to one half or one third of the anaerobic rate. This effect of oxygen was termed by Warburg the Pasteur effect (10). The Pasteur effect is much more intense on a percentage basis in normal cells, as glycolysis is nearly totally suppressed by respiration. Alternatively, when tumour cells respire in the presence of sufficient glucose to maintain maximal glycolytic rates, the respiration decreases to about one half. This effect has been termed the Crabtree effect in the name of its discoveror (11). As respiration yields much more chemical energy than glycolysis, the Crabtree effect may represent an energetic disadvantage for the tumour cell. On the other hand, the low Pasteur effect or high aerobic glycolysis of tumour cells characterizes the cancer cell as highly glucose-utilizing.

Although the Pasteur and Crabtree Effects are still not well understood (12), they represent focal points for the deciphering of the relationships between glycolysis and respiration. In 1941, Lynen (13) and Johnson (14) independently suggested that inorganic phosphate and ADP may be the keys to the control of glycolysis as well as to the Pasteur Effect. Since these substances are used both by glycolysis and respiratory oxidative phosphorylation, these processes would compete favorably and thereby decrease the rate of lactic acid production, resulting in the Pasteur Effect. Alternately, a low respiration, coupled with high glycolytic capability, would give rise to a high rate of glycolysis; and favorable competition by the glycolytic system for the available ADP would result in a Crabtree Effect. However, this hypothesis is unable to explain how a decrease in the ADP utilizing transphosphorylation steps would decrease glucose utilization.

In the early sixties, a number of authors (15,16,17,18) discovered that the enzyme phosphofructokinase is allosterically inhibited by ATP, and Passoneau and Lowry (19) proposed that the Pasteur effect was due to the inhibition of phosphofructokinase by the ATP formed by respiration. The inhibition of phosphofructokinase results not only in a blockade of glycolysis, but by causing an accumulation of fructose-6-phosphate, which is in equilibrium with glucose-6-phosphate, would inhibit glucose utilization by hexokinase.

The phosphofructokinase inhibition, in principle, admirably accounts for the Pasteur effect in muscle and brain without invoking competition for ADP and Pi between glycolysis and respiration. However, phosphofructokinase inhibition was unable to explain the high aerobic glycolysis and the Crabtree effect in tumours.

In the meantime, other evidence pointed to pyruvate kinase as a control site in tumours and revived the Lynen and Johnson theory. Studies on a series of rat hepatomas with a wide range of differentiation (20,21,22,23) demonstrated that there is a switch to embryonic isoenzyme forms in the glycolytic enzymes of undifferentiated tumours. Within these changes, the alterations in pyruvate kinase were the most dramatic. Pyruvate kinase is one of the transphosphorylating enzymes of glycolysis, requires ADP as a substrate, and exists in various isoenzyme forms. Pyruvate kinase isoenzyme type III is the main form existing in embryonic tissue and is not allosterically controlled by ATP. Pyruvate kinase isoenzyme type I is the main form existing in adult liver and is subject to allosteric inhibition by ATP. In the poorly differentiated tumours, the activity of pyruvate kinase is extremely high and is isoenzyme type III. The strategic position of pyruvate kinase in the glycolytic chain and its high content in tumours in a form non-inhibitable by ATP, suggested that its level in cells may be a determinant in the regulation of glycolysis through competition with respiration for ADP. Compelling evidence was obtained in an experimental system composed of glycolytic and respiratory fractions which competed for the available ADP in the presence of oxygen, fructose diphosphate and an ADP-regenerating system consisting of 2-deoxyglucose and hexokinase (24). This hypothesis was then tested in a more definitive model system composed of coupled rat liver mitochondria and purified muscle pyruvate kinase (25). Figure 1 shows a summary of the results obtained. Graph A of figure 1 shows the decrease in mitochondrial respiration and graph B shows the increase of pyruvate formation which occurs with increasing activity of pyruvate kinase, when the mitochondrial concentration was fixed. Graph C shows the increase in mitochondrial respiration and graph D shows the decrease in pyruvate kinase activity which occurs with increasing additions of mitochondria to a fixed concentration of pyruvate kinase. These experiments in the model system obviously mimic the Crabtree and Pasteur effects. It was also observed that the decrease of mitochondrial respiration with the increased pyruvate kinase activity was accompanied by a decrease of the ATP/ADP ratio; and this was interpreted to result from a competition for ADP favorable to mitochondria (25,26).

To corroborate whether such competition occurs in living cells, it was necessary to modify _in vivo_ the activity of pyruvate kinase or the activity of mitochondria. This was achieved by using inhibitors of both pyruvate kinase and mitochondria in Ehrlich ascites cells. Figure 2 shows that the pyruvate kinase obtained from these cells is inhibited by the amino acids alanine, cysteine and phenylalanine. As these tumour cells are permeable to these amino acids, it was possible to study the cells _in vivo_ under conditions in which the activity of pyruvate kinase was made to vary in a wide range through the addition of the amino acids.

Figure 3 shows the effect of the amino acids on the respiration of these tumour cells as measured by the oxygen electrode. As the

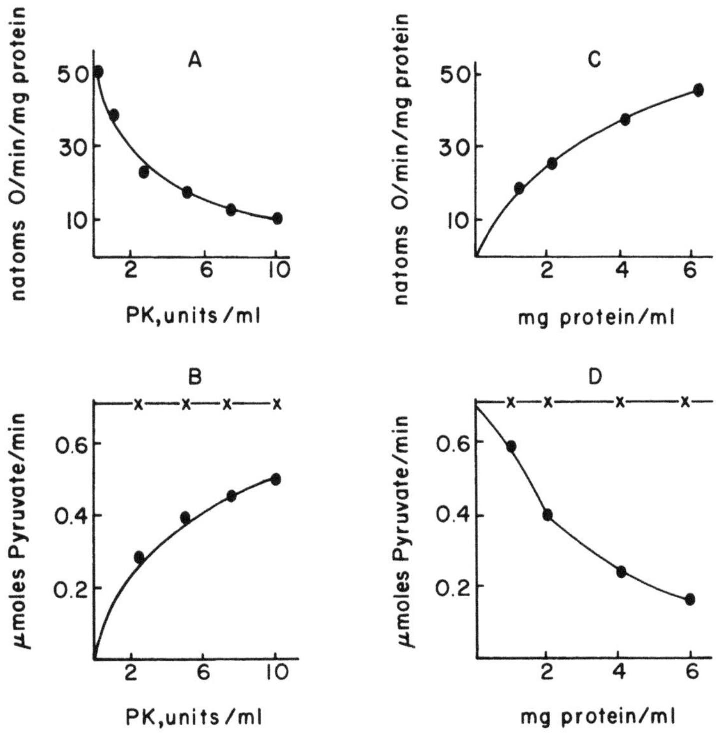

Figure 1. Interaction of mitochondrial respiration and pyruvate kinase activity in a model system. A&B, mitochondria held constant and pyruvate kinase varied; C&D, the same conditions as in A&B but pyruvate kinase constant at 5 units/ml and mitochondrial protein varied as indicated.

trace shows, there is a moderate endogenous respiration; then on addition of glucose, after a momentary increase in respiration, the respiration is inhibited in accordance with the well-known Crabtree effect. The addition of the amino acids, either alanine or phenylalanine, releases the respiratory inhibition caused by glucose, abolishing the Crabtree effect. As shown in the third trace, the addition of cysteine also releases the respiratory inhibition. The stimulation of respiration caused by the amino acid cysteine is reversed by oligomycin and released by dinitrophenol, thus indicating that the effect of this amino acid is to release coupled respiration inhibited by glucose addition. As shown in figure 4, the increase of respiration caused by cysteine is accompanied by an inhibition of the glycolytic rate. In this experiment, the glycolytic rate was measured by H^+ released by lactic acid formation, using a recording pH electrode (27). It can be observed through this kinetic method, that glycolysis starts immediately following the addition of glucose,

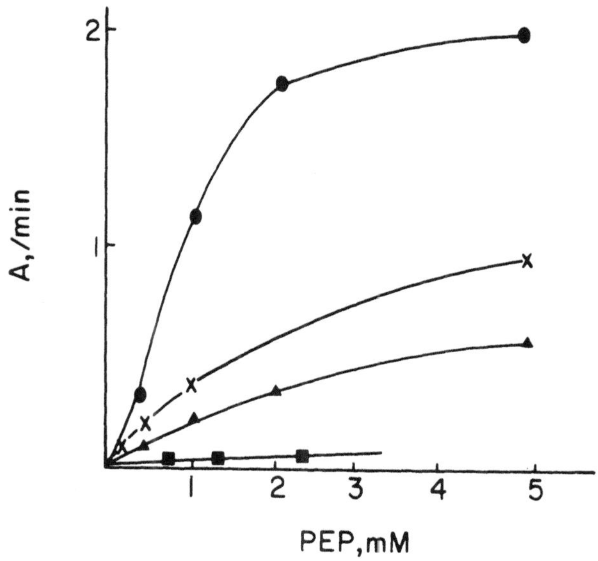

Figure 2. Activity of partially purified Ehrlich ascites cell pyruvate kinase in the presence of 2 mM concentrations of the amino acids cysteine (crosses), alanine (triangles) and phenylalanine (squares). The kinetics of the enzyme in the absence of amino acids (circles) is sigmoid.

first at a very high rate which is transient and almost parallels the transient increase in respiration caused by glucose. This high initial rate of glycolysis decreases to a steady moderate rate, possibly due to partial inhibition of phosphofructokinase by glycolytic ATP. Immediately upon adding cysteine, there is a sharp increase of respiration accompanied by a marked decrease of glycolysis.

The explanation for the reversal of the Crabtree effect by the amino acids can be deduced from the data shown in figure 5. There it can be seen that with increasing concentrations of cysteine, there is a progressive decrease in the glycolytic rate and an increase in the respiratory rate. Figure 6 A and B shows that with increased cysteine concentration there is also progressive inversion of the ratios of pyruvate/PEP and of ATP/ADP. These changes are in complete agreement with an inhibition of pyruvate kinase by cysteine, thus making increased ADP available to mitochondria with consequent increased respiration.

The reversal of the Crabtree effect by decreasing the activity of pyruvate kinase represents direct evidence for the existence of

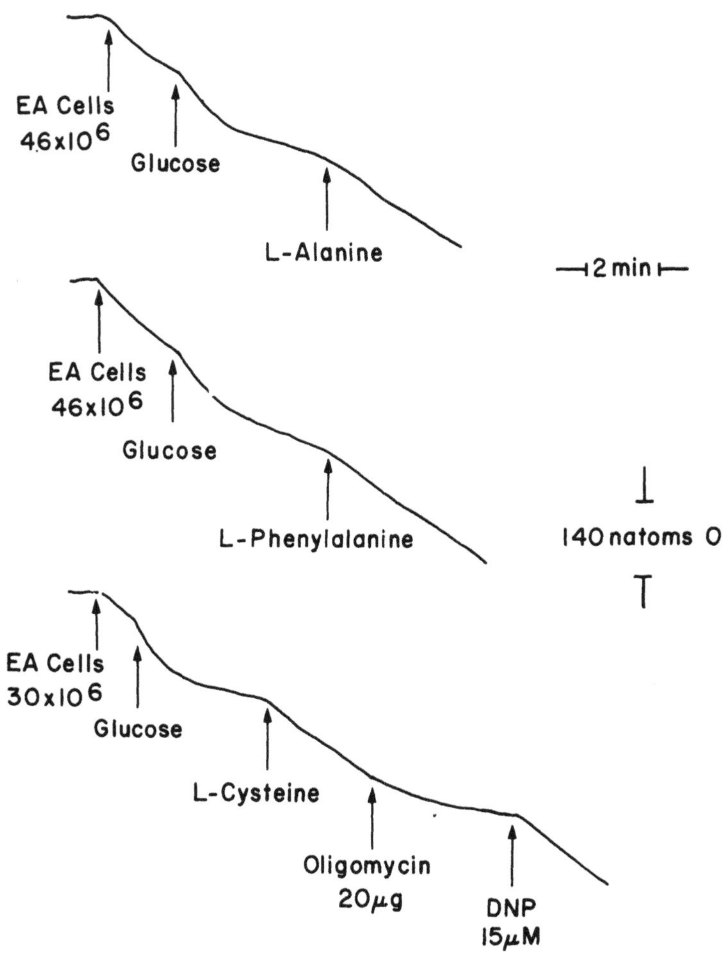

Figure 3. Reversal of the Crabtree effect induced by glucose in Ehrlich ascites cells by the addition of the amino acids alanine, phenylalanine or cysteine.

a competition for ADP between mitochondria and pyruvate kinase. Given the high activity of pyruvate kinase in tumour cells (21,28) and the low respiration of poorly differentiated tumours (4,29,30), it is clear that this competition would be favorable to pyruvate kinase and thus be not only responsible for the Crabtree effect, but also for the high aerobic glycolysis.

The high content of pyruvate kinase in an isozymic form non-inhibitible by ATP, could also play a role in the Pasteur effect as well as being responsible for the high aerobic glycolysis of tumours. It is altogether likely that control of glycolysis is exerted at multiple sites and it is conceivable that it may be affected by the inhibition of both phosphofructokinase and pyruvate

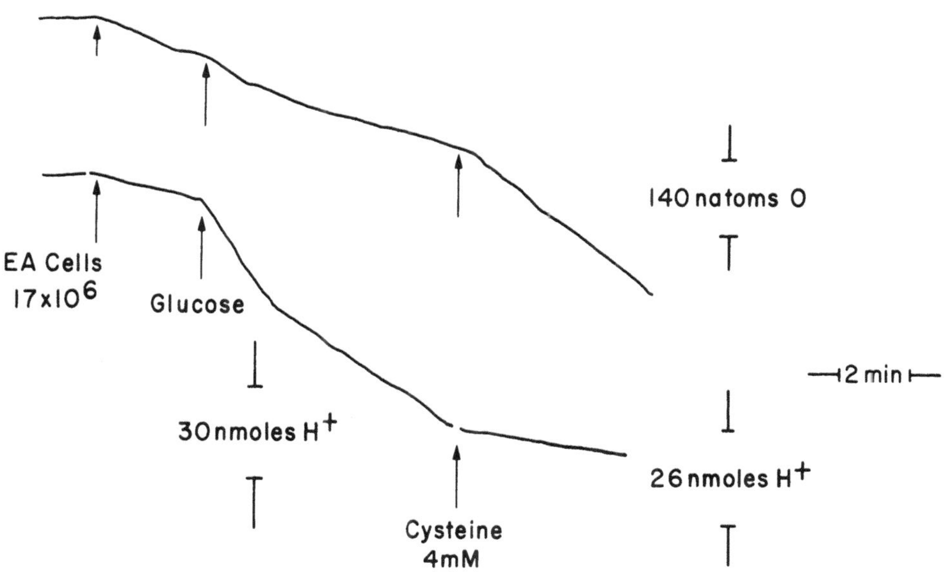

Figure 4. Simultaneous recording of oxygen uptake and acidification by lactic acid production in a suspension of Ehrlich ascites cells.

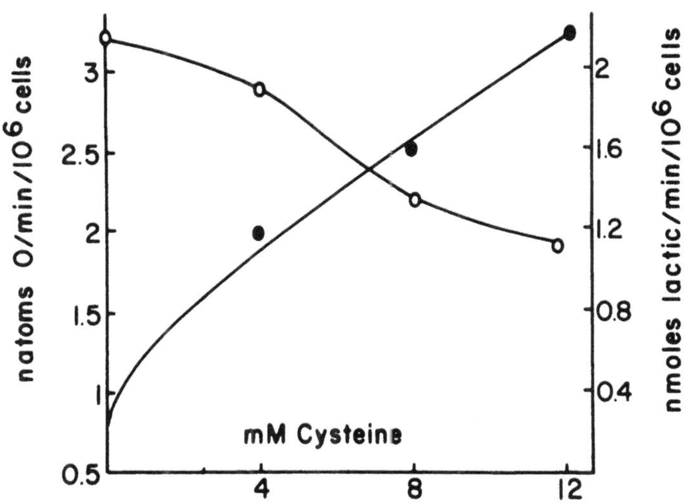

Figure 5. Dependence of respiratory enhancement and glycolytic inhibition on concentration of cysteine in Ehrlich ascites cells.

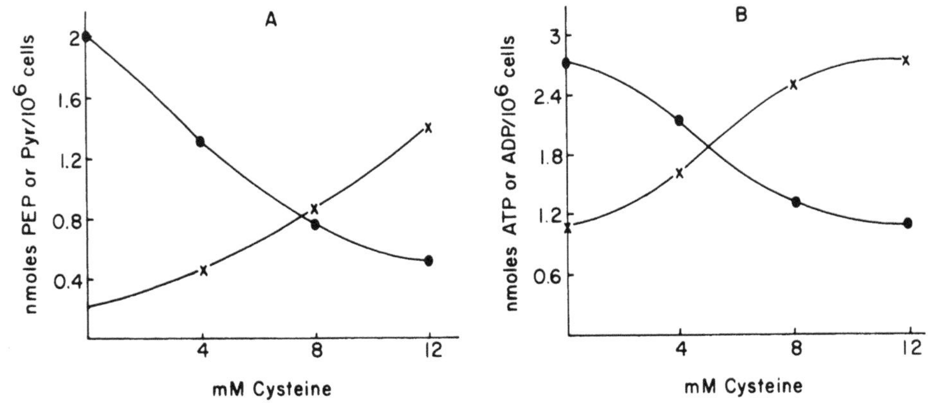

Figure 6. Effect of cysteine concentration on metabolite concentrations after incubation with glucose.

A) Phosphoenol-pyruvate is designated by crosses and pyruvate by circles.

B) ATP is designated by circles and ADP by crosses.

kinase by ATP can be separately de-inhibited by specific allosteric effectors (31).

BIBLIOGRAPHY

1. H. Reinhold. Improved microcirculation in irradiated tumours. Europ. J. Cancer, 8, 267, 1972.
2. M. Gosalvez, R.G. Thurman, B. Chance and H. Reinhold. Regional variation in the oxygenation of mouse mammary tumours in vivo demonstrated by fluorescence of pyridine nucleotide. Brit. J. Radiol., 45, 510, 1972.
3. O. Warburg. The metabolism of tumours. London, Arnold Constable, 1936.
4. F. Dickens and H. Weil Malherbe. Metabolism of intestinal mucous membrane. Biochem. J. 35, 7, 1941.
5. F. Dickens and H. Weil Malherbe. A note on the metabolism of kidney. Biochem. J. 30, 659, 1936.
6. C.N. Graymore. General aspects of the metabolism of the retina. in The Eye (Dawson H. ed.) vol. I, p. 601, Academic Press, New York.
7. O. Warburg. On respiratory impairment in cancer cells. Science, 124, 269, 1956.
8. M.J. Figueras and M. Gosalvez. Inhibition of the growth of Ehrlich ascites tumours with the respiratory inhibitor rotenone. Europ. J. Cancer, 9, 529, 1973.
9. M. Gosalvez, M. Blanco, J. Hunter, M. Miko and B. Chance. Effects of anticancer agents on the respiration of isolated mitochondria and tumour cells. Europ. J. Cancer, vol. 10, 567, 1974.

10. L. Pasteur. Experiences et vues nouvelles sur la nature des fermentation. C.R. Acad. Sci. 52, 1260, 1861.
11. H.C. Crabtree. Observations on the carbohydrate metabolism of tumours. Biochemical J. 23, 536, 1929.
12. H.A. Krebs. The Pasteur effect and the relations between respiration and fermentation. Essays in biochemistry. Vol. 8, 1-34, Academic Press, London, 1972.
13. F. Lynen. Uber den aeroben phosphat bedarf den Hefe. Ein zur kenntnis der pasteur's chen reaction. Justus liebigs Ann. Chem., 546, 120, 1941.
14. M. Johnson. The role of aerobic phosphorylation in the Pasteur effect. Science, 94, 2000, 1941.
15. F. Lynen, G. Hartmann, K.F. Netter and A. Schnegraf. Phosphate turnover and Pasteur effect. In Ciba Foundation Symposium on regulation of cell metabolism (Wolstenholme, G.E.W. and O'Connor, C.M. eds.) pp. 256-273, J.H. Churchill, London.
16. K.K. Lonberg-Holm. A direct study of intracellular glycolysis in Ehrlich ascites tumours. Biochem. Biophys. Acta, 35, 464, 1959.
17. T.H. Bucher. Zellulare Kondination Energie Transformierender Stoffwechselketten. Ang. Chem., 71, 744, 1959.
18. T.E. Mansour and J.M. Mansour.Effects of serotonin (5-hydroxytryptamine) and adenosine 3,5-phosphate on phosphofructokinase from the liver fluke, Fasciola hepatica. J. Biol. Chem., 237, 629, 1962.
19. J.V. Passonneau and O.H. Lowry. Phosphofructokinase and the Pasteur effect. Biochem. Biophys. Res. Commun. 7, 10-15, 1962.
20. S. Weinhouse, J.B. Shatton, W.E. Criss and H.P. Morris. Molecular forms of enzymes in cancer. Biochimie, 54, 685, 1972.
21. F.A. Farina, R.C. Adelman, Chai Ho Lo, H.P. Morris and S. Weinhouse. Metabolic regulation and enzyme alterations in the Morris hepatomas. Cancer Research, 28, 1897, 1968.
22. S. Weinhouse. Glycolysis, respiration, and anomalous gene expression in experimental hepatomas: G.H.A. Clowes memorial lecture. Cancer Research 32, 2007, 1972.
23. J.B. Shatton, H.P. Morris and S. Weinhouse. Kinetic, Electrophoretic, and Chromatographic studies on glucose-ATP phosphotransferases in rat liver and hepatomas. Cancer Research 29, 1161, 1969.
24. C.H. Lo, V.J. Cristofalo, H.P. Morris and S. Weinhouse. Studies on respiration and glycolysis in transplanted hepatic tumors of the rat. Cancer Research 28, 1-10, 1968.
25. M. Gosalvez, J. Perez-Garcia and S. Weinhouse. Competition for ADP between pyruvate kinase and mitochondrial oxidative phosphorylation as a control mechanism in glycolysis. Eur. J. Biochem. 46, 133, 1974.
26. M. Gosalvez, L. Lopez-Alarcon, S. Garcia-Suarez, A. Montalvo and S. Weinhouse. Stimulation of respiration of Ehrlich

27. L. Lopez-Alarcon and M. Gosalvez. A method to measure glycolysis in cell suspensions by means of a sensitive recording pHmeter. Rev. Esp. Fisiol., in press, 1975.
28. J.E. Feliu, J.J. Diaz-Gil, R. Garcia-Canero and M. Gosalvez. Interconvertible forms of Class A pyruvate kinase from Ehrlich ascites tumour cells. Accepted FEBS Letters, January, 1975.
29. P.L. Pedersen. Enzymology, ultrastructure, and energetics of mitochondria from three Morris hepatomas of widely different growth rate. GANN Monograph on Cancer Research, 13, 251, 1972.
30. A.C. Aisenberg. Studies on normal and neoplastic mitochondria I. Respiration. Cancer Research 21, 295, 1961.
31. M. Gosalvez, L. Lopez-Alarcon and S. García-Suarez. In preparation.

OXYGEN DISTRIBUTION IN TUMOURS: INFLUENCE ON CELL PROLIFERATION AND IMPLICATIONS FOR TUMOUR THERAPY

Ian Tannock

Toronto General Hospital

Toronto, Ontario, Canada

Tumour cell proliferation, and the response of individual tumour cells to various types of therapy, are dependent on the local concentration of oxygen and other metabolites. The existence of severely hypoxic but viable cells in solid tumours has been well established in experiments assaying tumour response to radiation: thus the pO2 in viable regions of tumours varies from close to zero to its value in blood. In most tumours the relationship between capillaries, tumour cells and necrotic tissue is complex. However, in some human and animal tumours, cylindrial cords of tumour cells with a central capillary and peripheral necrosis have been observed (Fig. 1); cords with peripheral stroma and central necrosis may co-exist in the same tumour (1-4). Tumours with this rather simple morphology may be used to study relationships between cellular kinetics and the concentration of metabolites or drugs that diffuse from blood vessels.

CELL PROLIFERATION AND METABOLITE DIFFUSION

Experiments were performed on two mouse mammary tumours which contained regions where there were cylindrial cords of tissue surrounded by necrosis. One of these tumours has been studied extensively in experiments with radiation and has been shown to contain severely-hypoxic viable cells (5). Since oxygen diffuses from blood vessels these hypoxic cells are

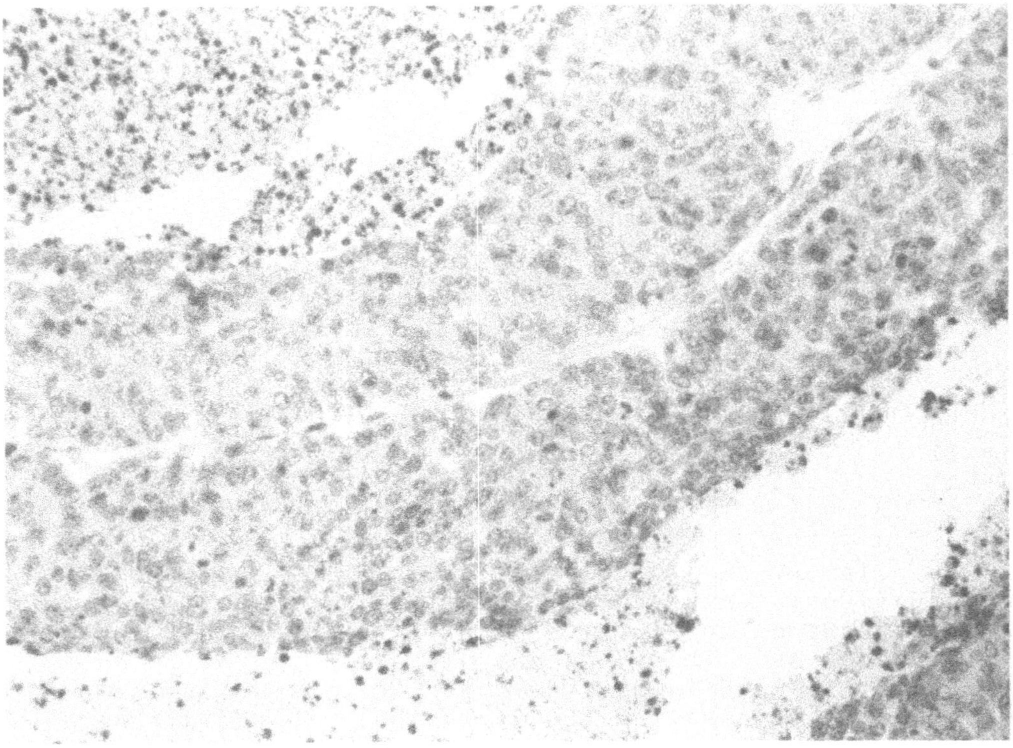

Fig. 1: Tumour Cord With Central Capillary and Peripheral Necrosis.

presumably situated at the periphery of tumour cords, adjacent to necrotic tissue. The mean radius of cords in the two tumours was 85 - 100μ . Estimates of oxygen diffusion radius (defined as the radial distance at which pO_2 falls to zero) are inexact because of dependence on a number of factors that are not known precisely: diffusion coefficient, rate of oxygen consumption, capillary radius and pO_2. However, using published values of these parameters, a range of estimates of oxygen diffusion radius for mouse tumour has been calculated previously (6). This range is 50 - 90μ . The agreement between estimated oxygen diffusion radius and mean cord radius is consistent with hypoxia at the periphery of tumour cords and suggests that hypoxia or anoxia may be one factor involved in tumour cell death and necrosis. However, other essential metabolites (e.g. glucose) diffuse from the blood; low concentrations of these metabolites or toxic concentrations of catabolites, probably also contribute to cell death at the cord periphery(7).

Within tumour cords, the concentration of oxygen and other blood-borne metabolites decreases with increasing radial distance from the axial capillary. Mitotic and thymidine labelling indices in central, intermediate and peripheral regions of tumour cords have been estimated from auto-radiographs and are listed in Table 1. In both tumours the rate of cell proliferation decreases rapidly with distance from the axial vessel, in parallel with the decrease in metabolite concentration. Also the proportion of labelled cells in peripheral regions of tumour cords increases rapidly with time after a single injection of tritiated thymidine (2). This result, analagous to observations that can be made in upper layers of epidermis, suggests rapid migration of tumour cells from well-nourished rapidly-proliferating regions close to a blood vessel to poorly nourished tumour regions where the proliferative rate is low and thence to cell death and necrosis. (Fig. 2).

	BICR/SA1 Tumour		C3H Mammary Tumour	
	L.I.(%)	M.I.(%)	L.I. (%)	M.I. (%)
Region near blood vessel	62	3.1	50	4.3
Intermediate region	42	2.2	30	2.5
Region near necrosis	30	1.2	10	0.6

Table 1: Mean thymidine labelling and mitotic indices in different regions of tumour cords within two mouse mammary tumours.

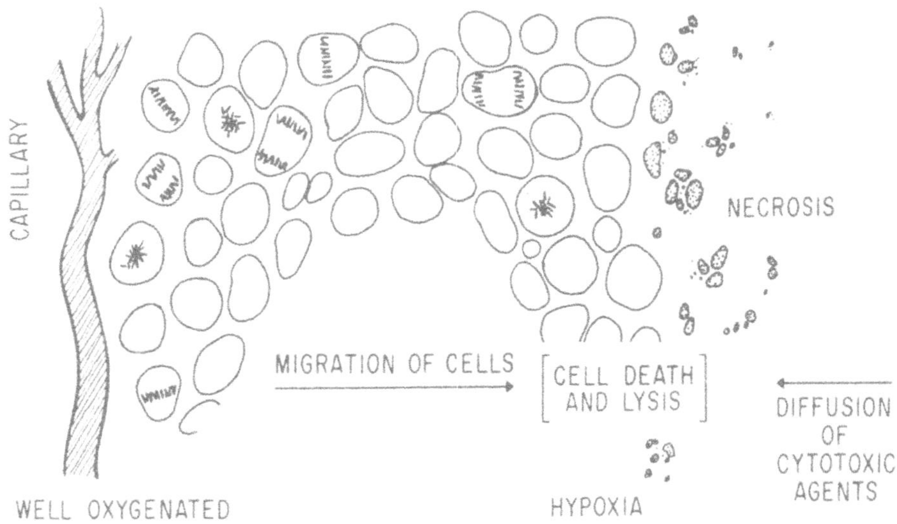

Fig. 2: A model of Cell Proliferation and Cell Death in Solid Tumours

VASCULAR PROLIFERATION AND BLOOD FLOW

The above experiments imply that the rate of tumour cell proliferation, (and hence the rate of tumour growth), is sharply dependent on a supply of nutrients from tumour blood vessels. Delivery of these nutrients depends in turn, on the rate of enlargement of the vascular bed and on the rate of blood flow through it.

Using special staining methods to facilitate recognition of capillaries, the thymidine labelling index of capillary endothelial cells has been measured for the above C3H mouse mammary tumour. The mean value was 11% compared with 50% for neighbouring well-nourished tumour cells (4). These results provide an explanation for the observed slowing of growth rate with increasing tumour size. Initially a focus of tumour cells is probably well supplied with oxygen and other metabolites, and will have a short doubling time equal to the cycle time of the tumour cells. However, proliferation of supporting vasculature is slower so that separation between vessels increases, tumour cell proliferation decreases in intervening regions, and cell death begins to occur. Ultimately tumour doubling time may tend to the rather slower turnover time of vascular endothelial cells.

Vascular stasis may also limit the supply of nutrients to tumour cells. The same histological staining techniques were used to study a rat mammary tumour (BICR/M1) in which there was no simple relationship between capillaries and necrosis. In this tumour, blood vessels were demonstrated within regions of necrotic tissue (8). This paradox was resolved by developing a method whereby Cr 51-labelled red cells could be recognized by autoradiography in sections of tumour tissue: it was found that peripherally-injected radioactive red cells penetrated readily to blood vessels in viable tumour regions, but not to vessels within necrotic tissue. Thus an alternative cause of tumour necrosis may be stasis of blood within the vessels.

STUDIES IN ANIMALS BREATHING 10% OXYGEN

The importance of oxygen concentration on tumour cell proliferation and cell death was studied by constructing a chamber that allowed host animals to breathe 10% oxygen in nitrogen for a week or more (9). There was little effect of hypoxia on growth rate of the rat mammary tumour where necrosis seemed to be related largely to vascular stasis (9). However, the mouse tumour with necrosis surrounding tumour cords grew more slowly in 10% oxygen than in air (Fig. 3). Mean cord radius, and mitotic and thymidine labelling indices were also reduced (Table 2). Animals lost weight in an environment of 10% oxygen and compensated with an increase in hemoglobin, so that some of these results might be non-specific; however, reduction in food intake sufficient to cause a similar loss in body weight did not change significantly the rate of tumour growth (9). Thus, there is a strong suggestion that local tumour pO2 has some direct influence on the rate of cell proliferation and that hypoxia is involved in processes leading to cell death.

	Air	10% Oxygen
Tumour weight at death	2.5 g	0.6 g
Body weight at implantation	26.7 g	25.1 g
at death	27.9 g	18.2 g
Blood hemoglobin at death	10.4 g%	14.2 g%
Tumour cord radius	85.1 μ	75.5 μ
Labelling index of tumour cords:		
Region near blood vessel	65%	50%
Intermediate region	48%	37%
Region near necrosis	30%	23%

Table 2: Mean values of experimentally determined parameters estimated for BICR/SA1 tumours in mice breathing air or 10% oxygen.

IMPLICATIONS FOR THERAPY

Tumour cells situated near regions of necrosis may be therapeutically elusive. Paradoxically, such cells would probably soon die in the untreated tumour (Fig. 2), but there is evidence that they may be the cells from which tumours recur after treatment. These cells are resistant to radiotherapy because they are hypoxic. They are slowly proliferating and are therefore resistant to many cycle-dependent anti-cancer drugs. Also, since these cells are situated far from a blood vessel it may be difficult to achieve adequate concentrations of drugs in their environment. Estimates of mean grain count per labelled cell have shown that tritiated thymidine is concentrated much less by cells in DNA synthesis in peripheral regions of tumour cords than by well nourished cells near blood vessels (2,4). Similar low concentrations of purine and pyrimidine antimetabolites can be expected. The efficacy of these and other drugs may be limited by poor diffusion or poor uptake by cells. Thus therapeutic effectiveness against solid tumours may require development of drugs that are specifically designed to attack hypoxic tumour cells.

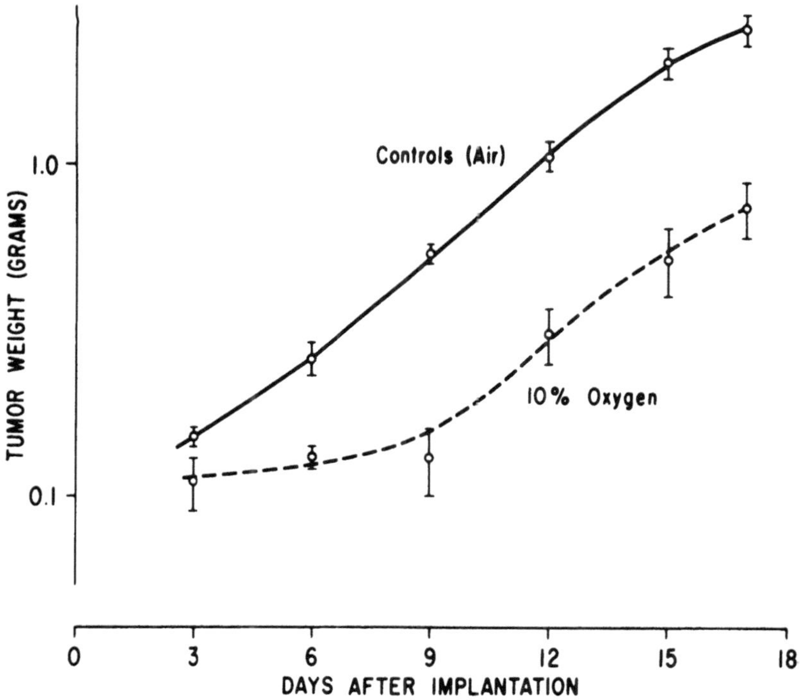

Fig. 3: Growth Curves for the Mouse Mammary Tumour BICR/SA1 in Air and 10% Oxygen. Means and their Standard Errors are Indicated.

REFERENCES

1. Thomlinson, R.H. and Gray L.H., Brit. J. Cancer 9 539, 1955
2. Tannock, I.F., Brit. J. Cancer, 22, 258, 1968
3. Hug, O. and Von Szczepanski, L., In "Radiation - Induced Cancer", P. 85, 1969 (IAEA Symposium)
4. Tannock, I.F. Cancer Res. 30, 2470, 1970
5. Suit, H.D. and Maeda, M., J. Nat. Cancer Inst. 39, 639, 1967
6. Tannock, I.F., Brit. J. Radiol, 45, 515, 1972
7. Vaupel, P. Funktionsanalyse Biologischer Systeme 1, 1974
8. Tannock, I.F. and Steel, G.G., J. Nat. Cancer Inst. 42, 771, 1969
9. Tannock, I.F. and Steel, G.G., J. Nat. Cancer Inst. 45, 123, 1970

PRELIMINARY OBSERVATIONS OF OXYGEN LEVELS IN MICROCIRCULATION OF TUMORS IN C3H MICE

H. W. Puffer, N. E. Warner, L. D. Schaeffer,
R. W. Wetts, and M. Bradbury
Department of Pathology, School of Medicine
Department of Physiology, School of Dentistry
University of Southern California
Los Angeles, California 90033, U.S.A.

Fundamental understanding of the oxygen level in microvasculature and tissues of developing tumors may be of great import in elucidation of observed radioresistance and decreased radiation sensitivity of certain tumors in humans. Frequently radiation therapy which at certain doses causes death of cells in vitro fails to kill the cells in vivo, even though the doses are comparable. L. H. Gray, et al, 1953, demonstrated reduced radiation sensitivity of cells which are oxygen deficient. Therefore, this study was undertaken to demonstrate whether changes in microvasculature and microcirculation play a significant role in the oxygen deficiency of various portions of a tumor in vivo.

Material and Methods

Female C3H/Crgl mice were used throughout this study. This strain of mice spontaneously develops a congenic type of RNA virus induced mammary tumor with an incidence of approximately 90 to 95%. Palpable tumors developed in retired breeders at 7-10 mo and the animals were separated into 3 groups according to tumor size: small, 0.5 cm dia or less; medium, 0.5-1.0 cm dia; and large tumors, 1.0-4.5 cm dia.

Prior to microvascular observations each mouse was anesthetized with pentobarbital, 100 mg/kg, injected intraperitoneally. The hair was removed from overlying skin and an incision made at the base of the tumor. Exposed tissues were bathed with Locke-Ringer's solution at 37°C.

The microcirculation was examined by epi-illumination using an American Optical fiber optic illuminator model 11-80. The microvasculature was observed through a Leitz stereomicroscope equipped with 2, 4, 8 and 12 x objectives and 12.5 x eyepieces and a Leitz monoobjective, trinocular microscope equipped with a 3.8 x objective and 12.5 x eyepieces. The length and diameter of observed vessels was measured using the Leitz monoobjective, trinocular microscope equipped with a 3.8 x objective and a Leitz calibrated 12.5 x filar eyepiece. The trinocular microscope was also equipped with a Leica M-1 camera and an ITP model 148A closed circuit television system for recording observations.

Rate of blood flow in observed vessels was estimated and graded on a scale of 1 to 5 similar to the method of McCusky, et al, (1965) and defined as 1= no flow, no movement of blood cells; 2= very slow to no flow, blood oscillates with individual cells seen; 3= slow flow, steady forward progression of blood cells with individual cells seen; 4= moderate flow, blood cells are blurred; 5= rapid flow blood cells not detected as individual entities.

Volume of blood flow in the field of observation was calculated using the formula $V= \pi r^2 h$ when V= volume, r= radius of vessels and h= length of vessels in the field.

Blood pO_2 in arterioles, venules and adjacent tissue was measured using gold plated, Rhoplex (Rohm and Haas Incorporated) coated, platinum microelectrodes as described by Bicher (personal communication). The electrodes had a tip diameter of approximately 2μm. The gold plated electrode was the cathode in the polarographic system. A separage Ag/AgCl anode was used as the reference electrode.

The electrodes were used in conjunction with microelectrode carriers, model 1108, chemical microsensor model 1201 and calibration cell, model 1251 supplied by Transidyne General Corporation. Values for oxygen levels were continuously recorded on a strip chart recorder, model 7402A supplied by Hewlett Packard Corporation. Oxygen levels were expressed in mm Hg.

Results

Recorded oxygen levels in tumors ranged from 14-42 mm Hg and varied greatly from animal to animal. However, oxygen levels in arterioles tended to be greater in smaller tumors whereas oxygen levels in tissues adjacent to microvasculature did not appear to vary greatly with size of tumor. Oxygen reading obtained with the microelectrode placed deep within the tissue of the tumor, that is near the center of the tumor, often approached zero. The rate of blood flow tended to be slower in larger tumors and the volume of blood tended to be greater in larger tumors. Oxygen levels in tissues surrounding the microcirculation appeared to decrease as the distance from vessels increased.

Discussion

Growth and morphology of the vasculature in spontaneous mammary tumors in C3H mice differs markedly from that in normal mammary tissue. The vessels in tumors are markedly tortuous and the arterioles and venules fail to develop as smooth tapering cylinders. An extreme abundance of capillaries is often found, particularly in early stages of development of the tumors. Sacculations and microaneurysms are sometimes present and increase in number as the tumors develop; rate of flow in these deformed vessels is often reduced. Morphologically the vasculature in advanced tumors is only one or two cell layers thick.

Such abnormal changes in the microcirculation and morphology should be reflected in the metabolism and perhaps in the oxygen levels of these tumorous tissues, an important consideration pertinent to the use of radiotherapy of tumors (Cater, et al., 1962).

In our study the measurement of oxygen levels has been limited primarily to arterioles, venules and adjacent tissues on the surface of developing tumors. The oxygen levels in these arterioles varies greatly from 14-42 mm Hg in each of the 3 groups of small, medium and large tumors. However, oxygen levels tend to be lower as the size of the tumor increases whereas the apparent oxygen level remains more constant in the tissues adjacent to the microvasculature.

In an attempt to explain this we have developed a simple formula which employs the apparent reduced rate of flow and apparent increased volume of blood in larger tumors: that is ODI = (RF)x(VB)x(pO_2) where ODI is oxygen delivery index, RF is rate of blood flow as defined above, VB is volume of blood calculated from measurements of the vessels under observation, and pO_2 is the oxygen level in the most prominent arteriole in mm Hg as measured with microelectrodes. Use of this formula indicates that oxygen levels in the arterioles of small, medium and large tumors appears not to vary significantly (Table 1).

Obviously a number of problems exist. Our measurement of oxygen levels is not always reproducible, possibly as a result of difficulties encountered in the preparation of electrodes. It is also possible that oxygen levels in exposed tissues is being measured too close to the surface of the tissues and oxygen levels may be influenced by the solution bathing them.

We have also ignored a number of important factors relative to tissue oxygenation and the diffusion of oxygen through the vasculature which have been presented in the sophisticated work of others (for example, Grunewald, 1973 and Fletcher, 1973).

TABLE I

Typical Application of Oxygen Delivery Formula

Tumor Size	ODI*	=	RF**	x	VB+	x	pO_2++
Large (greater than 1.5 cm dia)	6848		2		214		16
Medium (0.5 - 1.5 cm dia)	7056		3		98		24
Small (less than 0.5 cm dia)	6580		5		47		28

*ODI: is oxygen delivery index

**RF: rate of blood flow on scale of 1 to 5, 5 is most rapid

+VB: volume of blood calculated from measurement of vessels in field

++pO_2: oxygen level in mm of Hg in most prominent arteriole

Nevertheless we have attempted to explain what appears to be a rather constant oxygen level in the proliferating tumor tissue by relating this to the manner in which the blood flow patterns develop. Our preliminary results appear to indicate such a relationship may exist.

Conclusions

1. Oxygen levels varied greatly from 14-42 mm Hg, however, the variation was constant between the 3 groups according to tumor size.

2. Oxygen levels in tissues surrounding the microcirculation appeared to decrease as the distance from vessels increased. Readings deep within the tumor, that is near the center, often approached zero.

3. As the size of the tumor increased, observations of the microcirculation on the surface indicated that the rate of blood flow decreased and the volume of blood appeared to increase.

4. A simple formula is proposed to explain the relationship of blood flow and oxygen delivery in developing tumors.

Acknowledgements

Supported in part by Special Grant Number 626 from the California Division, Inc. of the American Cancer Society; by Grant DRG 1252 from the Damon Runyon Fund for Cancer Research, Inc.; and by Grant CA 14089 from the National Cancer Institute to the Los Angeles County-University of Southern California Cancer Center.

References

Cater, D.B., Grigson, C.M.B., and Watkinson, D.A. Changes of oxygen tension in tumors induced by vasoconstrictor and vasodilator drugs. Acta Radiologica 58: 401-434 (1962).

Fletcher, J.E. A mathematical model of the unsteady transport of oxygen to tissues in the microcirculation in: Oxygen Transport To Tissue: Pharmacology, Mathematical Studies, and Neonatology, Eds. Bruley and Bicher, Adv. in Exp. Med. Biol. 37B: 819-825 (1973).

Gray, L.H., Conger, A.D., Ebert, M., Hornsey, S. and Scott, O.C.A. Concentration of oxygen dissolved in tissues at the time of irradiation as a factor in radiotherapy. Brit. J. Radiol. 26: 638-648 (1953).

Grunewald, W. Computer calculation for tissue oxygenation and the meaningful presentation of the results in: Oxygen Transport To Tissues: Pharmacology, Mathematical Studies and Neonatology, Eds. Bruley and Bicher, Adv. in Exp. Med. Biol. 37B: 783-792 (1973).

McCusky, R.S., Meineke, H.D., and Townsend, S.F. Studies of the hemopoietic microenvironment. 1. Changes in the microvasculature system and stroma during erythropoietic regeneration and suppression in the spleens of CFI mice. Blood 39: 697-712 (1965).

THE DISTRIBUTION OF OXYGEN CONSUMPTION RATES IN SOME TISSUES BEFORE AND AFTER X-IRRADIATION

T.B. Constable and N.T.S. Evans

Medical Research Council, Cyclotron Unit

Hammersmith Hospital, London

The oxygen consumption rate per unit volume of tissue is one of the factors which determines tissue oxygen tension, the other factors being arterial tension, blood perfusion and the oxygen diffusion constant and solubility. Since the microscopic structure of tumours has an important role in the response to radiation there is a need for developing techniques for measuring the local distributions of these parameters.

The apparatus and basic experimental procedure for the measurement of oxygen consumption rate distributions have been described in a previous presentation to this symposium (1). A sharp blade is used to cut through a sample of freshly excised tissue and the plane cut surface is placed in contact with the polythene membrane of the cuvette. A multicathode electrode measures the oxygen uptake rate in the surface layer of the specimen at an hexagonal array of 91 positions spaced 0.5mm apart.

THE EFFECT OF HAEMOGLOBIN

The non-linear relationship between oxygen tension and the oxygen content of haemoglobin will distort a tissue time response curve. The theory of the method assumes simple oxygen diffusion properties for the sample. There are two ways of circumventing the effect of haemoglobin or myoglobin. The tissue can be initially equilibrated with 100% oxygen and the time course measured during a period when nearly all of the haemoglobin remains saturated, or alternatively the tissue can be exposed to carbon monoxide for a few minutes before equilibration with air. Carbon monoxide binds

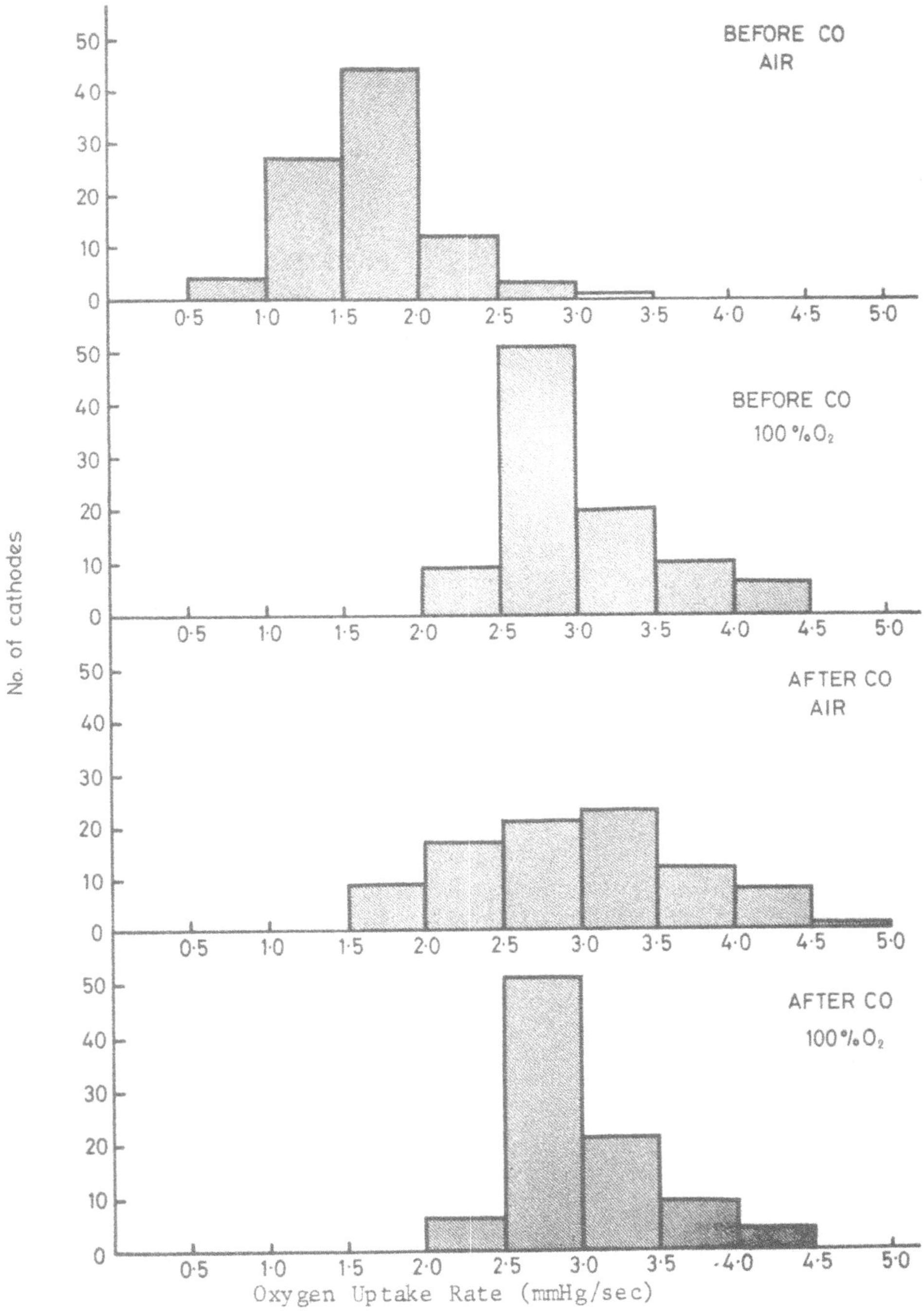

Fig. 1. Distribution of oxygen uptake rates in tumour SSB1a before and after exposure to carbon monoxide. Equilibration with air or 100% O_2.

strongly to haemoglobin but is readily displaced by oxygen from combination with the respiratory enzymes (2). The equilibration of tissues with 100% oxygen results in some loss of spatial resolution of the measurements, since the initial penetration distance is increased by just over a factor of two.

Figure 1 shows a series of histograms of oxygen uptake rates on a sample of the rat fibrosarcoma SSB1a and represents the distribution of the 91 values from all cathodes. The mean values for measurements following 100% oxygen equilibration either before or after exposure to carbon monoxide or following air equilibration after exposure to carbon monoxide are all identical. The values for air equilibration without exposure to carbon monoxide are reduced due to desaturation of oxyhaemoglobin during the time course. The narrower distribution of the values for 100% oxygen equilibration is due to reduced spatial resolution.

OXYGEN UPTAKE DURING TUMOUR GROWTH

The change in the oxygen uptake distribution with tumour growth has been studied in the SSB1a fibrosarcoma. This is a fast growing tumour with a doubling time of about 1½ days and appreciable collagen content. For each measurement the tumour was sliced in half and for tumours up to 10mm diameter one half could be fitted into one of the standard cuvettes. For larger tumours a cylinder of 10mm diameter was bored out from the cut half using a strip razor blade attached to a metal cylinder. For tumours greater than 20mm diameter it was possible to bore out two cylinders, one at the centre and one as close as possible to the edge of the tumour. The electrode measures over an hexagonal area of width 5mm in the centre of each sample placed in the cuvette. Figure 2 shows a plot of oxygen uptake against tumour diameter where W indicates the use of a whole tumour section and E and C the use of cylinders bored from the edge and centre of the tumour respectively. The error bars on figure 2 indicate the standard deviation of the distribution of 91 values thus giving a measure of the spread in oxygen uptake rates within the sampled area.

The mean oxygen uptake rate decreased gradually with increasing tumour diameter and the spread in values increased. For large tumours the oxygen uptake rate was higher towards the edge than in the centre. The decrease towards the centre was due to the existence of areas of low respiration but these were interspersed with areas of the more normal respiration of the tumour edges. The right hand portion of figure 2 shows a series of measurements on tumours which had been irradiated (2500 rads γ-rays) at 10mm diameter and allowed to grow to 25-30mm. The oxygen uptake rate at the edge of these tumours was comparable to that of the unirradiated

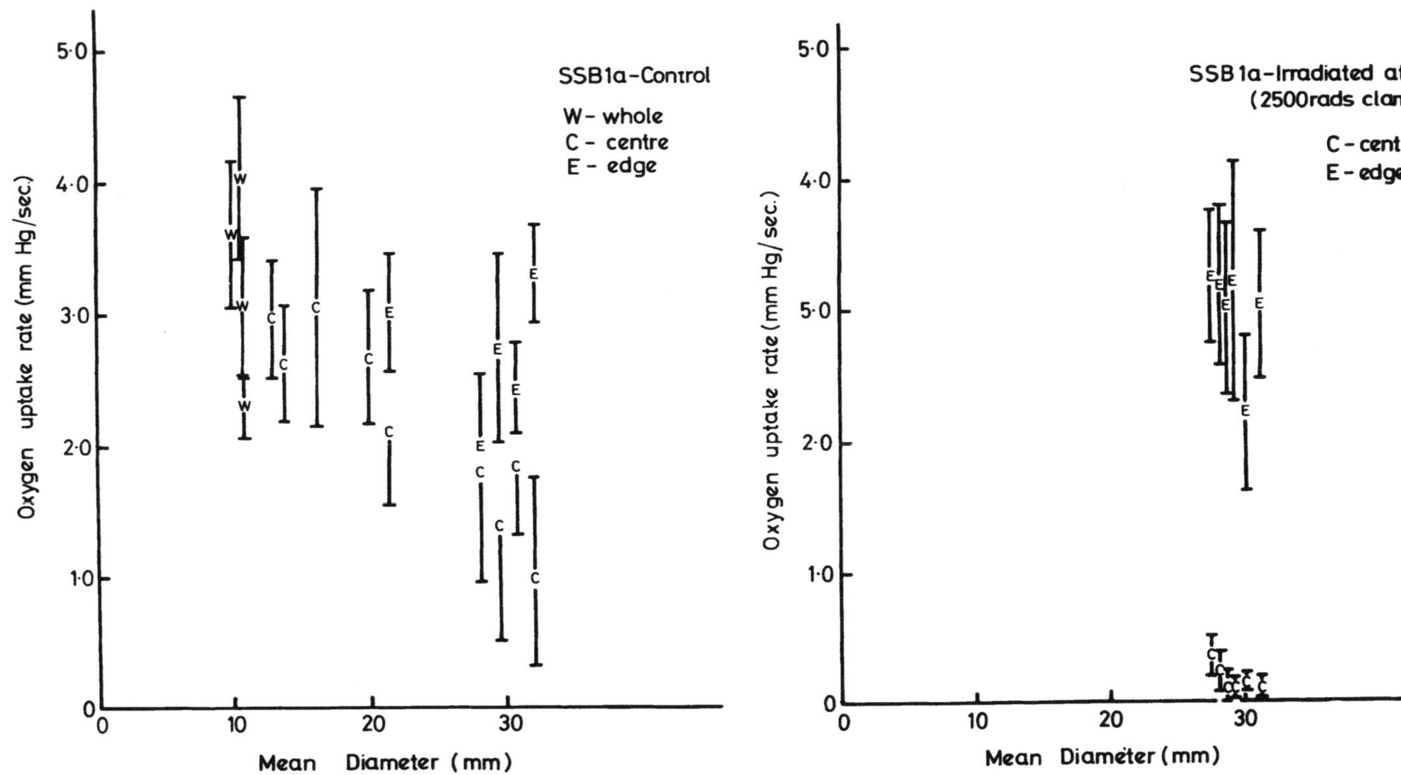

Fig. 2. Variation of oxygen uptake rate of SSB1a with tumour diameter. Comparison with tumours irradiated at 10mm and allowed to regrow to 25 - 30mm.

controls but the respiration throughout the central region was uniformly low without any regions of more normal respiration. This region of low respiration was considerably larger than the size of the tumour at the time of irradiation and indicates radiation damage to some process which occurs during tumour growth. Further investigations will examine the timing of the change in oxygen uptake by looking at irradiated tumours of intermediate sizes.

PATTERNS OF OXYGEN UPTAKE RATE

Oxygen uptake distributions have been measured in samples of liver and several transplanted rat and mouse tumours. The liver samples had high and fairly homogeneous metabolism rates. However, much variation between different tumours has been noted some having uniform and rapid respiration and others having pockets of low oxygen uptake. Figures 3 & 4 show examples of the 'structure' of oxygen uptake distributions for two mouse tumours. The maps are produced by a computer program which interpolates between the measured values at the positions of the hexagonal array. Increasing density of the symbols indicates increasing oxygen uptake. The first generation transplant of a spontaneous mammary tumour in C3H mice (fig. 3) showed mainly high respiration with a region of somewhat lower respiration towards the centre. The mean oxygen uptake of a fat cell sarcoma in CBA mice (fig. 4) was lower than that of the C3H tumour and the regions of highest respiration tended to occur towards the centre. Both tumours were about 8mm in diameter and the oxygen uptake rate was measured at 25°C.

It is necessary to develop techniques for comparing oxygen uptake distributions such as those shown in figures 3 & 4 with the structures of the tissues. It will be necessary to make histological preparations of the surface layer with minimum distortion of the dimensions of the sample and to identify the regions corresponding to each cathode with an accuracy rather better than the 0.5mm cathode spacing. It will then be possible to compare the oxygen uptake distribution with the vascular structure and with regions of necrosis or cellular differentiation.

EFFECT OF RADIATION ON OXYGEN UPTAKE

A change in the oxygen uptake rate per unit volume is one factor which could result in reoxygenation of a tissue during a fractionated irradiation schedule. Alteration in the oxygen consumption rate will depend on a dynamic balance between the rate at which cells cease to respire, the rate at which dying cells are removed or lysed and the extent to which the tissue shrinks as dead cells are removed. The sequence of these events is likely to be different in different types of tumours.

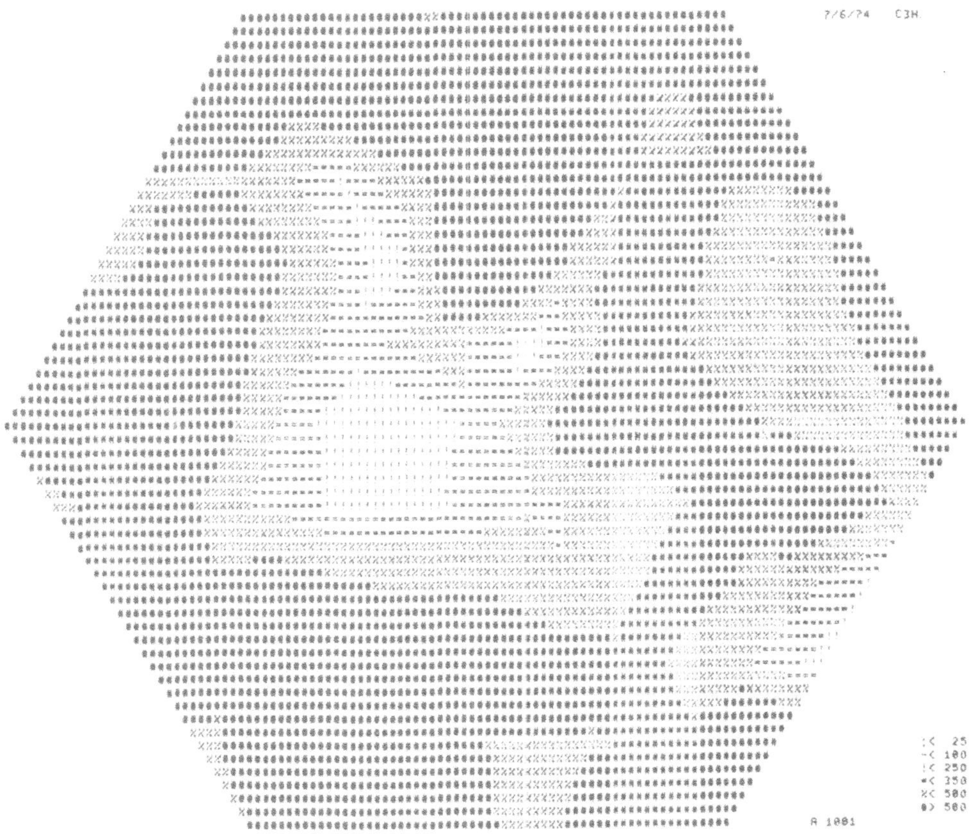

Fig. 3. Map of oxygen uptake in C_3H tumour.
Symbol key refers to oxygen uptake in mmHg/sec x 100.

The oxygen uptake rate of the first generation transplant of the C_3H tumour has been found to show no significant change up to 7 days after a dose of 2000 rads. The volume of the tumour approximately halved during this time and the high cell loss rate of the tumour is likely to be associated with an efficient mechanism for the removal of damaged cells. The rat fibrosarcoma SSB1a maintains its pre-irradiation size for about 10 days after this dose of radiation before regrowing. The mean oxygen uptake rate did not decrease during the first 24 hours but was reduced to 80% of the control value at two days and 70% at five days after irradiation. Further experiments are in progress to examine the timing of these changes in more detail. Changes of this order in the oxygen uptake rate could be sufficient to produce a significant reduction in the number of hypoxic tumour cells.

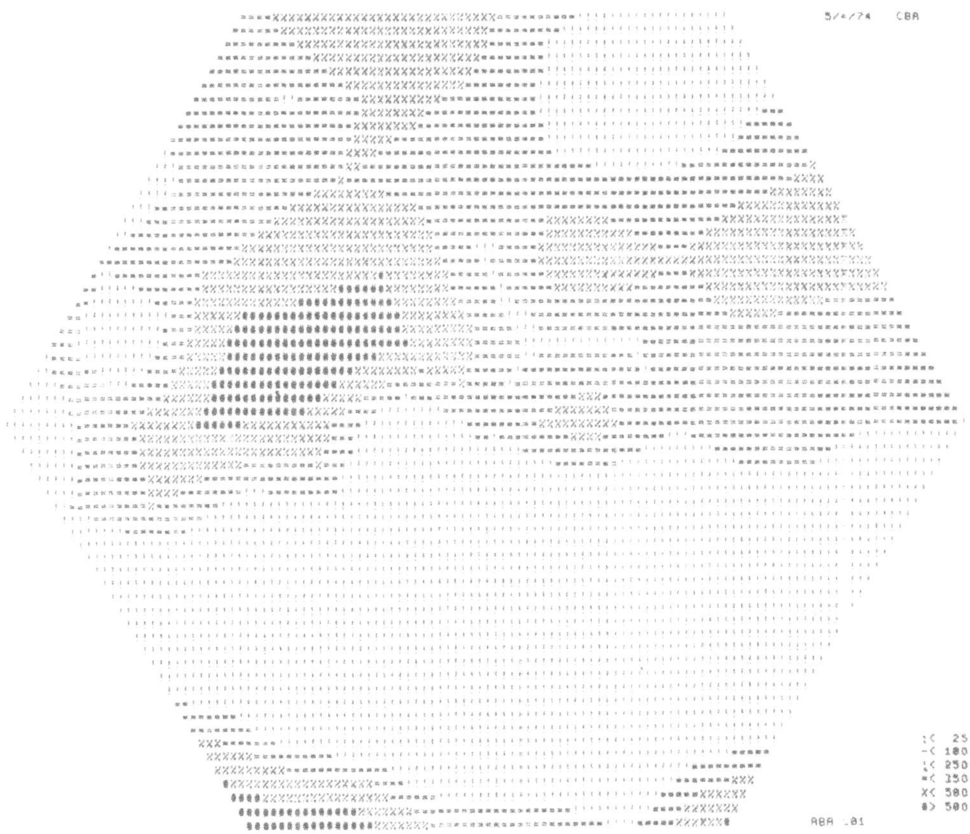

Fig. 4. Map of oxygen uptake in CBA fat cell sarcoma. Symbol key refers to oxygen uptake in mmHg/sec x 100.

REFERENCES

1. N.T.S. Evans and T.B. Constable. A method for measuring oxygen uptake rate distributions over the surface zone of excised tissue using a 91-cathode electrode. This symposium.

2. E.G. Ball, C.F. Strittmatter and O. Cooper. The reaction of cytochrome oxidase with carbon monoxide. J. Biol. Chem., 193, 635-647 (1951).

SUMMARY OF DISCUSSION - SESSION XI:

RESPIRATORY GAS EXCHANGE AND METABOLISM IN TUMOR TISSUE II

Chairmen: V. S. Shapot and P. Vaupel

Additional lines of evidence were provided (I. TANNOCK) as to the dependence of tumor growth in vivo on the supply with nutrients. The proliferation of cancer cells decreased in parallel with the distance of the tumor cells from the axial vessel owing to a poor vascularity and stasis of the blood within the vessels.

The observation that poor oxygen supply affects tumor cell proliferation in vivo is of great interest. NEGELEIN has shown some years ago in the in vitro experiments that O_2 content in the gas phase as low as 3 vol% was sufficient to maintain Ehrlich ascites cell proliferation in the proper medium while the absence of O_2 arrested cell division completely. Severe hypoxia prevents respiration of tumors in vivo to serve as a source of energy but tumor respiration proceeding even at a very low level is presumably needed to enable 3-C- fragments of glucose, formed in the course of glycolysis, to enter Krebs cycle and be transformed into amino acids, precursors of proteins. Indeed, it was shown in the in vitro experiments in my laboratory (ELTZINA) that in case glycolysis coexists with respiration the efficiency of the utilization of the carbon skeleton of 14C- glucose in protein synthesis rised manyfold. Similar observations have been made (SHAPOT, 1972) in the experiments performed in vivo. Thus, in these instances oxidation of glucose or its intermediates serves as a source of plastic materials for the growing tumor mass.

Data have been presented (V. SHAPOT) demonstrating the inability of ascites cancer cells to maintain in vivo their respiration at the level which permits to support protein synthesis and the Pasteur effect because of severe local hypoxia. Only extra O_2 supply to the host enabled the respiration of the cancer cell to fulfill its physiological functions. The point to be emphasized is that there is no aerobic glycolysis in tumors under in vivo conditions - only anaerobic glycolysis can proceed. Thus, there is no reason to ascribe to aerobic glycolysis of cancer cells observed in vitro any biological meaning as did WARBURG and his followers in the past - since severe hypoxia in vivo prevents this phenomenon to manifest itself.

Extensive glucose consumption by the cancer cell in vivo and relatively slow influx of glucose from the host endows the tumor with the capacity to act as a powerful hypoglycemic factor - and this phenomenon could be demonstrated even in the tumor - bearing animals with normal blood glucose levels.

Quite novel findings (GONSALVEZ and WEINHOUSE) on the critical role playing by pyruvate kinase in the regulation of glycolysis by respiration (Pasteur effect) and vice versa (Crabtree effect) were reported. An extremely high activity of the latter, which is not very much sensitive to pH variations, seems to be partially responsible for a mighty glycolysis occurring in many poorly differentiated hepatomas.

The inhibition of pyruvate kinase activity by cysteine or alanine diminished glycolysis and enhanced respiration rate of the cancer cell eliminating Crabtree effect. Sound proves were presented as to the competition of mitochondria respiration with glycolysis (at the stage of the reaction catalyzed by pyruvate kinase) for ADP. This phenomenon was regarded as one of the reasons for the Pasteur effect to occur, in addition to the already known involvement of hexokinase in this effect.

In cancer cells the above competition is favourable to pyruvate kinase owing to its high content and activity and nonsensitivity to the inhibitory action of ATP.

Oxygen Supply of Muscle Tissue

MECHANISMS OF CIRCULATION METABOLISM COUPLING IN SKELETAL MUSCLE

C. R. Honig

University of Rochester
Department of Physiology
School of Medicine and Dentistry
Rochester, New York 14642 USA

Post-contraction vasodilation is unaffected by extrinsic denervation (3). It is therefore believed that local metabolites fully account for the phenomenon. Recently, however, neuronal cell bodies have been identified in the walls of arteries and arterioles (8). The experiments to be described indicate that these intrinsic nerves initiate post-contraction vasodilation. A unifying hypothesis is proposed which assigns specific functions to extrinsic sympathetic nerves, intrinsic nerves and metabolites in control of circulation during muscle contraction.

METHODS

Thirty-four dog gracilis muscles were isolated and perfused at constant flow (5,8). In 8 experiments the venous effluent from 1 gracilis was used to perfuse the other (bioassay mode). No reservoir existed between the 2 muscles. Transit time was 24 sec. In 4 isolated but autoperfused muscles arterial pressure and gracilis flow were measured, and resistance computed "on line."

In some experiments PvO_2 was sampled intermittently; correction for dead space was made in correlating O_2 and resistance data. Acutely denervated muscles were stimulated with supramaximal monophasic square wave pulses to the obturator nerve. Pulse duration was 0.2 msec or less. Such pulses do not excite extrinsic autonomic nerves (5). Chronically denervated muscles were stimulated with an array of needle electrodes. Local anesthetics were infused at 0.5 ml/min. All control data in such experiments were made while saline was infused at the same rate.

RESULTS

To evaluate the role of intrinsic nerves we observed the effect of local anesthetics. In Fig. 1A, 20 twitches at 2/sec produced vasodilation in the donor. If metabolites were released they were below threshold for the resting recipient, whose resistance remained constant. A population of control responses like the one in panel A was obtained as resistance varied spontaneously. We previously showed (7) that for stimuli of constant intensity the fall in resistance (ΔR) is a precise linear function of the initial resistance (Ri). The regression of ΔR on Ri, and its 95% confidence belt, defines the limits of normal response from any Ri. Lidocaine, 2.5 mM in donor perfusate, lowered Ri and virtually abolished post-contraction vasodilation; see panel B. This response is shown as the open triangle on the Ri vs ΔR plot. Note that substantial vasodilation could have occurred despite the effect of lidocaine on Ri. Recovery was 70% complete in 10 min. Lower doses of lidocaine and procaine produced reversible partial block in the same muscle. In this and each of 9 similar experiments, autoregulation of blood flow and post-occlusion vasodilation, both of which appear to be myogenic in nature (4), were completely unaffected when post-contraction vasodilation was blocked. This indicates that the ability of vascular smooth muscle to relax was not impaired by the local anesthetics. The drugs must therefore block

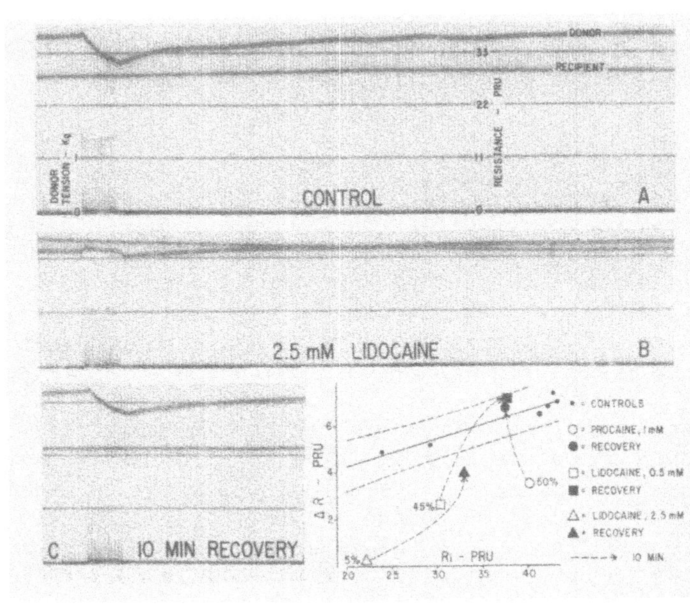

Fig. 1. Block of post-contraction vasodilation by local anesthetics.

intrinsic or extrinsic nerves, or the release of metabolites by skeletal muscle cells.

Extrinsic nerves can be ruled out because the degree of block by procaine was the same in 8 innervated and 5 chronically denervated gracilis muscles. Histologic examination of the denervated muscles revealed that all post-ganglionic fibers from the sympathetic chain had degenerated, and that the remaining fibers originated from neuronal cell bodies in the arteriolar walls (8). The following experiments demonstrate that skeletal muscle cells do indeed release vasodilator metabolites, but the fall in resistance so produced is delayed, and about 10 times slower than that observed when contraction begins. Local anesthetics have no effect whatever on the late, slow metabolic component of vasodilation. By exclusion we conclude that local anesthetics act on intrinsic nerves, and that these structures are responsible for the brisk vasodilation when contraction begins.

Fig. 2 contrasts the time course of vasodilation in a contracting donor with that induced by metabolites in a resting recipient. Note that vasodilation begins less than 1 sec after one twitch. It is hardly possible that metabolites could be produced in sufficient quantity, cross the muscle-cell membrane, diffuse to arterioles and cause vasodilation in so short a time. K^+ is the first dilator metabolite released during contraction (6,10). The calculated (6) increase in K^+ concentration in the interstitial fluid due to one twitch is at least 10 times less than the minimum concentration required to produce vasodilation (10). During phasic contraction the rate at which resistance falls is about 10 times greater in the donor. The arrow indicates when donor blood cleared the dead space. Vasodilation in recipient did not begin until 16 sec later, and its time course paralleled PvO_2. Similar slow, delayed vasodilation can be produced by abruptly lowering PO_2 in the perfusate of a resting muscle. Lidocaine blocked vasodilation in the donor, but had no effect on vasodilation in the

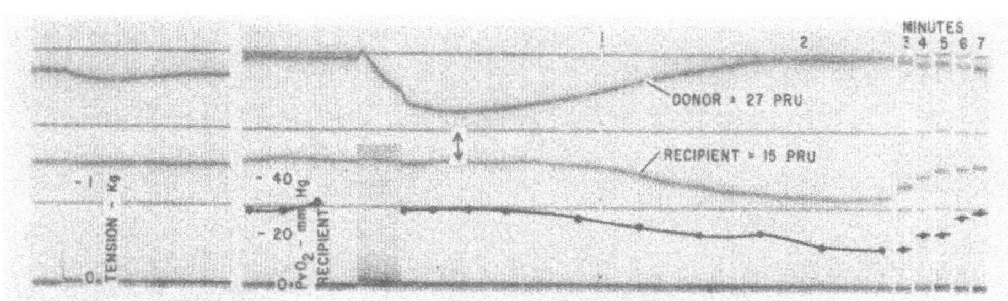

Fig. 2. Time courses of response of contracting donor and resting recipient to a single twitch and to 20 twitches at 2/sec.

recipient, even if infused into recipient perfusate. This result constitutes direct evidence that local anesthetics do not inhibit release of metabolites or the ability of vascular smooth muscle to respond to metabolites. Recovery in the donor was complete in 2 min whereas recovery of the recipient required 6 min.

The effect of flow rate provides further evidence that two distinct mechanisms contribute to post-contraction vasodilation. Fig. 3 shows responses of the same muscle to 120 twitches at 2/sec when autoperfused and during constant flow at 3.9 ml/min. The constant flow rate was chosen to match the measured flow rate at rest during autoperfusion. During contraction peak flow was 350% greater when autoperfused. Nevertheless, resistance followed about the same biphasic time course and reached about the same minimum value in both cases. This minimum resistance was maintained until contraction stopped. Since the additional flow during autoperfusion not only transported more O_2 but also washed out metabolites at a greater rate, it is unlikely that metabolites contributed significantly to the initial fall in resistance. During autoperfusion resistance returned to control in 1.5 min. This is consistent with decay of activity in intrinsic nerves (8). During constant flow, however, recovery was delayed for 3 min and required 8 min for completion.

A more severe stress demonstrates that slow recovery depends on the presence of metabolites. Fig. 4 illustrates the effect of 5 min of contraction at 2/sec during constant flow at 4 ml/min. Minimum resistance was attained in 50 sec. It remained at that level until contraction stopped, even though PvO_2 fell from 14 to 5 mm Hg between 50 sec and 2 min. The decrease in tension after 3 min indicates that $\dot{V}O_2$ was inadequate for the work. Despite the

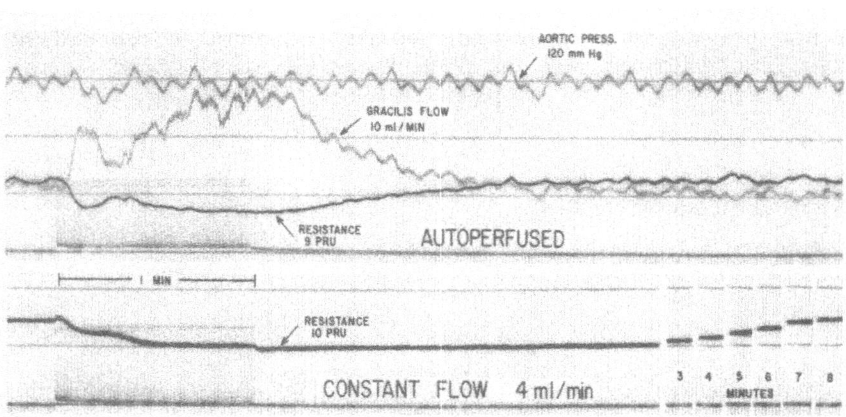

Fig. 3. Time courses of vasodilation and recovery in the same muscle during constant and variable blood flow.

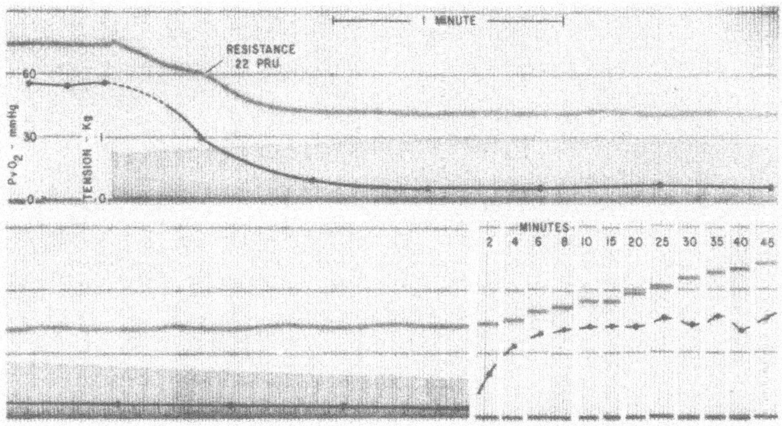

Fig. 4. Correlation of resistance and PvO_2 during and after sustained phasic contraction.

large amount of metabolites released under these conditions (9), resistance remained the same as it was at 50 sec. It appears that the neural mechanism responsible for the rapid initial vasodilation drives resistance to a minimum value before metabolic vasodilation is fully developed. Obviously, metabolites would have played an even less important role during contraction had flow been free to vary, as in the normal animal.

When contraction stopped, PvO_2 began to rise almost immediately. At 2 min it was 4 times its minimum value but resistance remained unchanged. Eight minutes later PvO_2 plateaued, but resistance continued to rise. Evidently resistance is controlled by a metabolite other than O_2 per se. (The metabolite could, of course, be O_2-linked.) PvO_2 remained low, and O_2 extraction therefore remained high, even after resistance returned to normal. This suggests that pre-capillary sphincters rather than arterioles are responsible for repaying the final installments on the O_2 debt.

Fig. 5 suggests that adenosine is at least partly responsible for slow recovery after sustained phasic contraction. Dipyridamol was infused at a rate which enhanced and greatly prolonged vasodilation produced by injected adenosine. Dipyridamol lowered Ri, sometimes quite markedly, but had no effect on the maximum rate at which resistance fell when contraction began. The extent of vasodilation was also unchanged, as judged by Ri vs ΔR plots. Lack of effect on the initial phase of vasodilation is expected, provided the intrinsic nerves do not release a purinergic mediator.

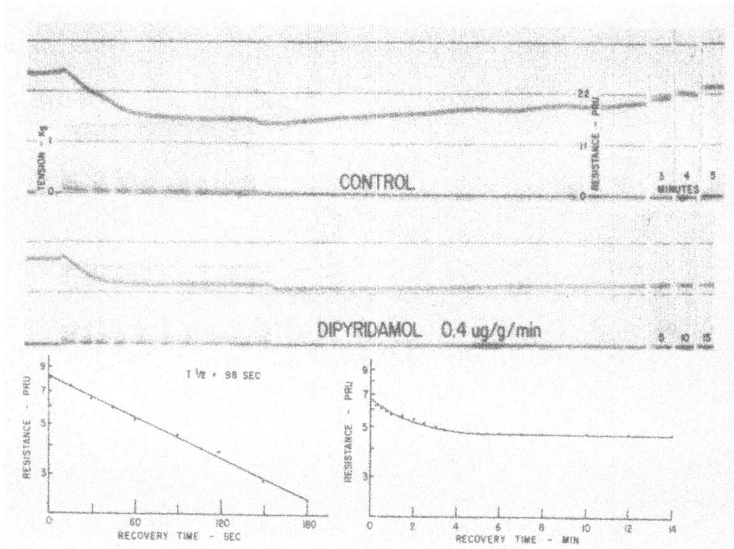

Fig. 5. A constant infusion of dipyridamol lowers Ri and prolongs recovery from contraction during constant flow.

In each of 18 experiments dipyridamol greatly slowed recovery of resistance when contraction stopped. Indeed, in some muscles, like the one in Fig. 5, resistance remained close to its minimum value as long as the dipyridamol infusion was continued. These results are consistent with chemical (2) and bioassay (9) evidence that adenosine contributes to post-contraction vasodilation.

SUMMARY AND UNIFYING HYPOTHESIS

Fig. 6 illustrates the separate time courses of vasodilation evoked in skeletal muscle by extrinsic sympathetic nerves, intrinsic nerves, and metabolites in support of muscle contraction. In our experiments at least 45 sec elapsed before minimum resistance (maximum flow) was attained. During this time the muscles could have acquired a significant O_2 debt. This need not occur in the intact animal, however, for active sympathetic vasodilation can increase flow in <u>anticipation</u> of muscle contraction (1). This extrinsic neural response lasts only 30-45 sec (1,8). A longer response is not necessary, however, for intrinsic nerves are activated once contraction begins; compare solid and dashed curves in Fig. 6. This idea is particularly attractive because recent evidence indicates that post-ganglionic sympathetic vasodilator

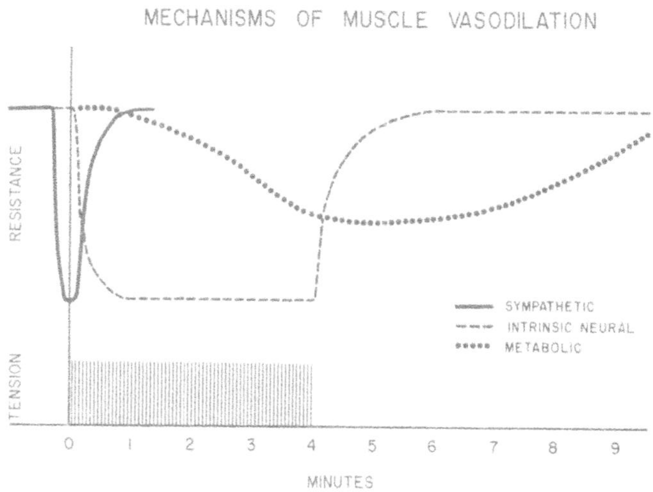

Fig. 6. Schematic representation of circulation-metabolism coupling in skeletal muscle.

(but not constrictor) nerves terminate on the intrinsic neurones rather than on vascular smooth muscle cells (8). Consequently, in the transition between sympathetic and post-contraction vasodilation, only the mode of stimulation of the intrinsic nerves would change.

The dotted line in Fig. 6 indicates the magnitude and duration of metabolic vasodilation, as judged from bioassay experiments and from the vasodilation which persists in the presence of lidocaine. Note that nerves drive resistance to a minimum value before metabolic vasodilation begins. When contraction stops neurogenic vasodilation decays rapidly. Metabolic vasodilation, however, persists for many minutes, and permits repayment of O_2 and substrate debts.

In summary, circulation-metabolism coupling in skeletal muscle requires extrinsic nerves to initiate vasodilation before contraction, intrinsic nerves to maintain maximum vasodilation during contraction, and metabolites to continue vasodilation for an appropriate time during recovery.

REFERENCES

1. Bolme, P. and J. Novotny. Conditional reflex activation of the sympathetic cholinergic vasodilator nerves in the dog. Acta Physiol. Scand. 77: 58, 1969.

2. Dobson, J. G., Jr., R. Rubio, and R. M. Berne. Role of adenine nucleotides, adenosine and inorganic phosphate in the regulation of skeletal muscle blood flow. Circ. Res. 29: 375, 1971.

3. Hilton, S. M. Experiments on the post-contraction hyperemia of skeletal muscle. J. Physiol. (Lond.) 120: 230, 1953.

4. Honig, C. R., J. L. Frierson, and R. F. Rakowski. Mechanism of post-occlusion hyperemia. Fed. Proc. 33: 393abs, 1974.

5. Honig, C. R. and J. L. Frierson. Evidence that neurones intrinsic to arterioles initiate post-contraction hyperemia. Am. J. Physiol. Submitted.

6. Mohrman, D. E. and H. V. Sparks. Role of potassium ions in the vascular response to a brief tetanus. Circ. Research 35: 384, 1974.

7. Myers, H. A. and C. Honig. Influence of initial resistance in magnitude of response to vasomotor stimuli. Am. J. Physiol. 216: 1429, 1969.

8. Myers, H. A., E. A. Schenk, and C. R. Honig. Ganglion cells in arterioles of skeletal muscle: role in sympathetic vasodilation. Am. J. Physiol. Accepted.

9. Scott, J. B., R. M. Daughterty, Jr., J. M. Dabney, and F. J. Haddy. Role of chemical factors in regulation of flow through kidney, hindlimb and heart. Am. J. Physiol. 208: 813, 1965.

10. Skinner, N. S. and W. J. Powell, Jr. Action of oxygen and potassium on vascular resistance of dog skeletal muscle. Am. J. Physiol. 213: 533, 1967.

ACKNOWLEDGMENTS

This research was performed with the help of Mr. J. L. Frierson and Mr. W. Reaves. It was supported by grant H.L.-03290 from the United States Public Health Service.

Spontaneous Oscillations of PO_2 in Muscle Tissue

KLAUS KUNZE

Department of Clinical Neurophysiology
Centre of Neurology, Justus Liebig-University
63 Giessen, Am Steg 14, Fed.Rep.Germany

Oxygen pressure in muscle tissue shows a distribution related to capillaries, metabolic requirements and the technique of measurement as it has been shown by KUNZE (1966, 1969), WHALEN (1967, 1970), VAN LIEW (1973). From these measurements a mean PO_2 can be calculated and mean values of about 38mmHg have been found in the resting human tib.ant.muscle by different techniques. Spontaneous fluctuations are to be seen in most of the intramuscular PO_2-tracings but in most cases these fluctuations seem to be inconstant and there is the question whether they could be artefacts perhaps caused by contractions of muscle fibres. So it is the question whether they are a physiological phenomenon and if this is right it should be taken into account for the concept of a mean oxygen pressure of muscle tissue.

During earlier PO_2-measurements perpendicular to muscle fibres sometimes we have not been convinced about the physiological nature of these fluctuations and measurements with great PO_2-fluctuations have been ruled out. Now by modification in our needle-electrode arrangement we found these fluctuations constantly and we could distinguish between several types of PO_2-oscillations.

METHODS:

Measurements have been performed in the human forearm extensor muscles. The patients lay relaxed in the supine position on the bed. For the measurements they got no drugs. The right arm was fixed that way that gross distortions were impossible but careful isometrical contractions and reflex motor activations of the forearm muscle groups were permitted. The needle-electrodes with a free tip of about 1-2 μ were inserted very flat through the guiding cannula at an angle of about 5-10° so that the PO_2-needle was nearly parallel with the muscle fibres. This could be done by hand or by micromanipulator and for measurements even during slight muscle contractions the connection of the needle with the holding device was flexible. In all cases the guiding cannula served as the reference electrode. Only those measurements in each case corrected to intramuscular temperature of electrodes have been evaluated which showed an unchanged calibration curve after the intramuscular measurements. In each case electrical activity (motor activity) of the muscle and in some cases respiration activity was monitored simultaneously. In the relaxed state there were no muscle contractions respectively discharges of motor units. (fig. 1)

A sensitive needle position in the muscle is found by a good ischemia reaction. During ischemia achieved by a cuff with a pressure up to 250-300mmHg proximal to the needle position PO_2 goes down to values between zero and about 5mmHg and it can be repeated easily. During hyperventilation PO_2 goes up and this PO_2 increase is a little bit dependent on the needle position in muscle tissue and it depends much more on whether the patient really performs a hyperventilation. Besides that there are a rise in muscle-PO_2 caused by sympathetic reflexes or following sensory or electrical stimuli to the skin or the supplying nerve. These stimuli may lead to a discharge of motor units combined with visible muscle contraction or not. During muscle contractions PO_2 rises initially and then falls durings sustained contraction.

RESULTS:

The analysis of PO_2-tracings in resting human skeletal muscle permits to differentiate at least between <u>three types of spontaneous PO_2-oscillations.</u>

FIRST of all there are spontaneous changes in PO_2 which are not related to any visible event in the muscle itself because a continuous simultaneous EMG-monitoring is made. Apparently without any cause intramuscular PO_2 goes up or down. In a part of those cases one can find by exact observation that just at the time of spontaneous PO_2 changes the contralateral arm

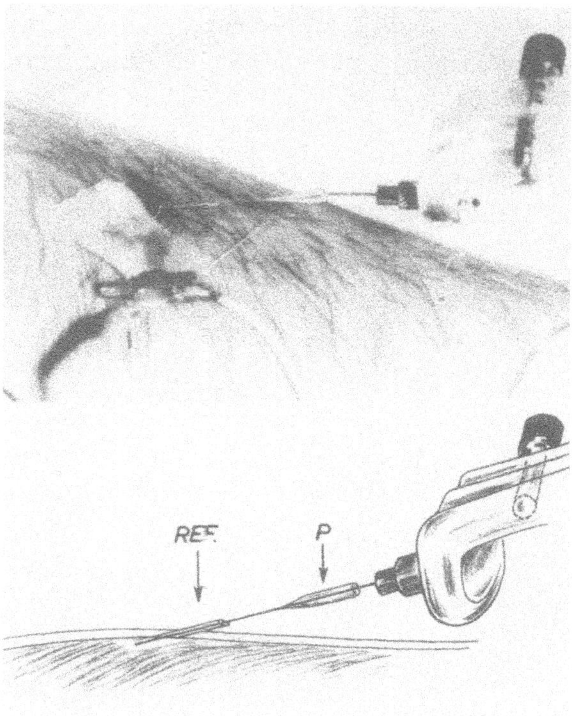

Fig.1: PO_2-needle position in the human forearm extensor muscles with a diagram in the lower part.

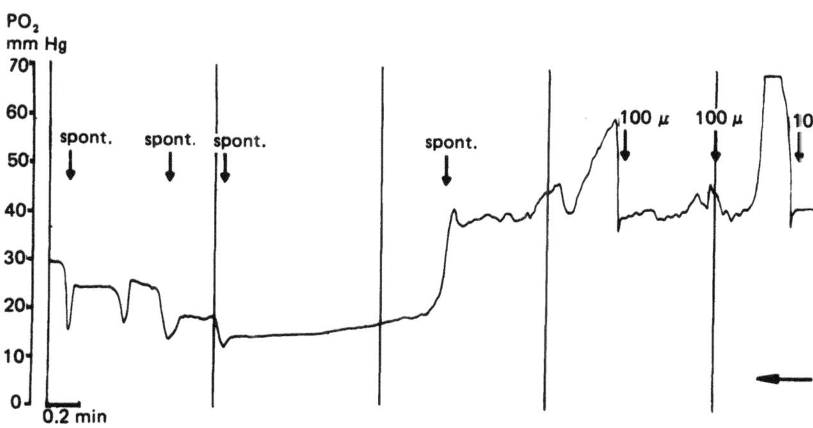

Fig.2: Spontaneous PO_2-fluctuation indicated at the arrow during electrical silence (no motor unit discharge monitcred by simultaneous EMG recordings).

or hand or one of the legs has been moved. Self-evidently these PO_2-changes are not rhythmic. (fig.2)

SECONDLY there are spontaneous rhythmic PO_2-oscillations with a frequency of 0,5-2/min. which show the same frequency range as rhythms of local muscle blood flow measured by local heat clearance which have been described detailed by GOLENHOFEN (1971). In this connexion it should be mentioned that the PO_2-electrodes used in these measurements were not flow-dependent. PO_2-oscillation of this frequency range have been described by WHALEN and NAIR (1970) too. (fig.3)

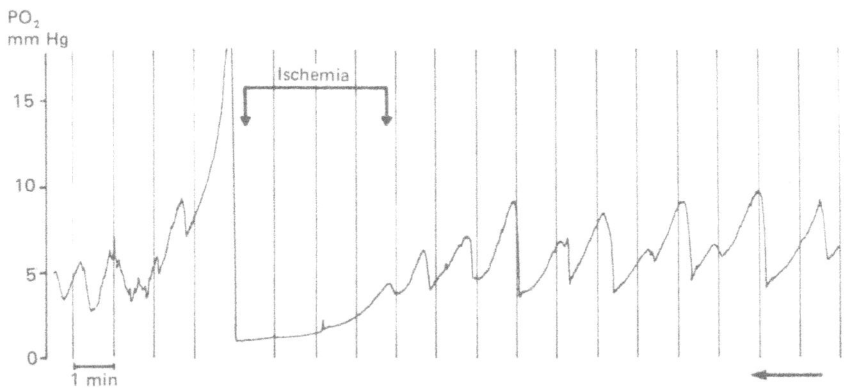

Fig.3: Spontaneous type II PO_2-oscillations and ischemia reaction.

The absolute PO_2-difference in these oscillations is varying with a maximum in our cases up to now to 6mmHg. It seems to be that at low mean PO_2-values these PO_2-differences are smaller. A difference is found during waking and sleeping that way that during the latter state PO_2-changes and frequency of oscillations are smaller. (fig.4)

THIRDLY there are PO_2-oscillations which show a correlation to the respiration cycle. The PO_2-changes of this type increase during a deep breath and decrease during higher respiration frequency resp. hyperventilation and they are extinguished during apnoea. (fig.5) This type of oscillations is found most often in the intramuscular PO_2-monitoring and it is frequency-

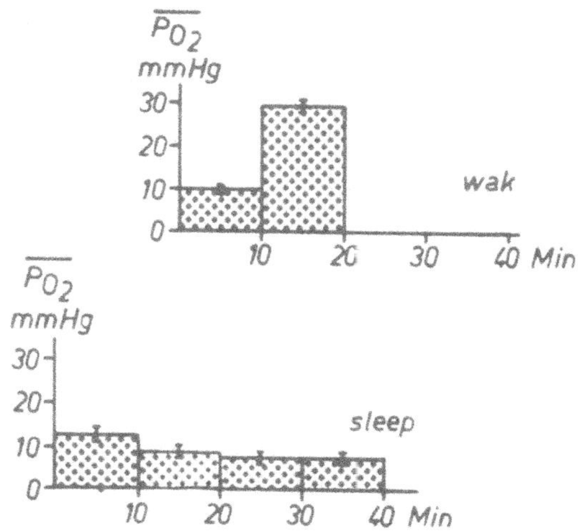

Fig.4: Mean PO_2 during sleeping (oscillat.frequency 1,3-1,7/min) and after this during awaking (oscillat.frequency 2,1-2,8/min.)

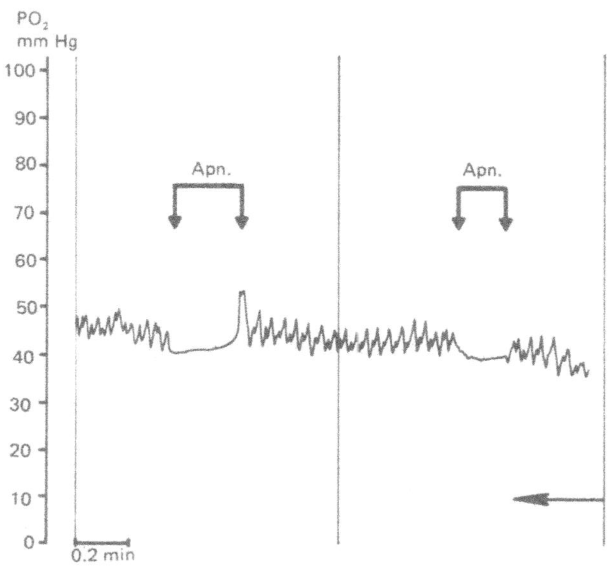

Fig.5: Spontaneous respiratory coupled PO_2-oscillations (type III) with the apncea-test.

modulated by the type II oscillations. (fig.6)

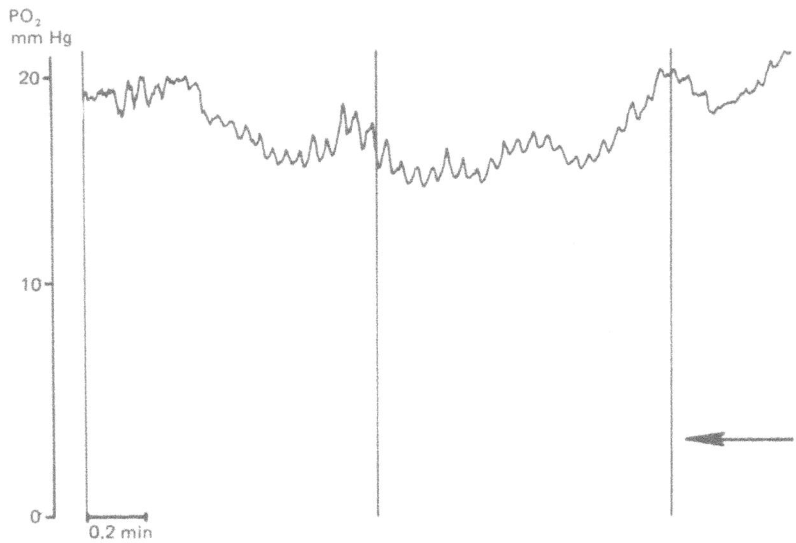

Fig.6: Type II slow PO_2-oscillations modulating fast type III PO_2-oscillations.

Besides that these oscillations are found in different needle positions in the same muscle and during different reactions e.g. sympathetic reflexes and breathing different oxygen mixtures. After ischemia reactions these oscillations are mostly more pronounced. In trying to make a hypothesis about the origin of these oscillations I would like to suppose that they are related to vasomotor nerve activity and they are possibly reflected to tissue via smaller vessels to the capillaries. This may be right in so far as we have seen that after blocking of the supplying muscle nerve these oscillations go off or diminish. This would be in agreement with DELIUS et al (1972) who found in muscle nerves a respiratory coupled activity of vasoconstrictor nerves.

CONCLUSION:

It should be pointed to three types of spontaneous PO_2-oscillations whereas it is possible to test a sensitive intramuscular PO_2-needle position very simply by measuring respiratory coupled PO_2-oscillations and their disappearance during the apnoea-test.

REFERENCES :

DELIUS, W., K.E. HAGBARTH, A. HONGELL and B.G. WALLIN

Manoeuvres Affecting Sympathetic Outflow in Human Muscle Nerves.

Acta Physiol. Scand., 84: 82 (1972)

GOHLENHOFEN, K.

Der Muskelkreislauf.

in: Physiologie des Kreislaufs, 424: 385
Springerverlag, Berlin, Heidelberg, New York 1971
ed.: Bauereisen, E.

KUNZE, K.

Die lokale kontinuierliche Sauerstoffdruckmessung in der menschlichen Muskulatur.

Pflügers Arch. ges. Physiol. 292: 151 (1966)

KUNZE, K.

Das Sauerstoffdruckfeld im normalen und pathologisch veränderten Muskel.

Neurologie, Neurology Series Bd. 3
Springer-Verlag Berlin, Heidelberg, New York 1969

VAN LIEW, H.D.

Regional heterogeneity of PCO_2 and PO_2 in skeletal muscle.

in: Oxygen Transport to Tissue.
ed.: H.J. Bicher and D.F. Bruley
Advances in Exp. Med. and Biol. Vol. 37A
Plenum Press, New York - London 1973

WHALEN, W.J., J. RILEY and P. NAIR

A microeletrode for measuring intracellular PO_2.

J. Appl. Physiol. 23: 798 (1967)

WHALEN, W. and P. NAIR

Skeletal muscle PO_2: effect of inhaled and topically applied O_2 and CO_2.

Am. J. Physiol. 218: 973 (1970)

TISSUE PO_2, VO_2, VENOUS PO_2 AND PERFUSION PRESSURE IN RESTING DOG GRACILIS MUSCLE PERFUSED AT CONSTANT FLOW [1]

W.J. Whalen, D. Buerk, C. Thuning, *B.E. Kanoy, Jr., and *W.N. Duran

St. Vincent Charity Hospital, 2351 East 22nd St., Cleveland, Ohio 44115, and *Dept. of Physiology and Pharmacology, Duke University Medical Center, Durham, North Carolina, 27710

Verzar (14), who studied resting cat skeletal muscle *in vivo*, was the first to report that oxygen consumption ($\dot{V}o_2$) depended on blood flow. A dependent relationship has since been found in blood perfused skeletal muscle preparations of the cat (15,18), and rat (4). However, Nakamura (7) could find no dependency in cat skeletal muscle except at very low flow rates. In dog skeletal muscle Rein and Schneider (9) and Pappenheimer (8) found that $\dot{V}o_2$ was dependent on blood flow in the normal range (4-10 ml/100g tissue/min.). On the other hand Stainsby and Otis (12) reported an independent $\dot{V}o_2$-flow relationship when perfusion pressure was varied in dog skeletal muscle except at very low flow rates (1-2 ml/100g/min.). In a recent study by Duran and Renkin (2) 25 of 35 dog gracilis muscle preparations showed an independent relationship, and one converted spontaneously from a dependent to an independent relationship.

The mechanism of the $\dot{V}o_2$-flow dependency remains obscure. *A priori*, limitation of $\dot{V}o_2$ by O_2 availability would seem to be a plausible mechanism. However, in a previous study in our laboratory (15) we found that $\dot{V}o_2$ in resting cat soleus and gracilis muscles varied directly with blood flow (more than five-fold in some pre-

---

1. Supported in part by grant no HL 12703 and no HL 12749 from the USPHS.

parations - see Figure 1) and yet measurements of tissue Po_2 (TPo_2) revealed few values below 5 mmHg even at the lowest flow rates. Thus, hypoxia in the classical sense (5) was ruled out as a possible mechanism. It could be, however, that the critical Po_2 in vivo is much higher than the 4-5 mmHg determined from studies on isolated mitochondria (5). We hoped that the present study might help to answer this question.

To explain the ephemeral nature of the $\dot{V}o_2$-flow relationship we (16) have suggested that in preparations which show good autoregulation, like those of Stainsby and Otis (12), TPo_2 might be held almost constant. This suggestion is far less tenable as an explanation for the results of Duran and Renkin (2) where constant-flow perfusion was used. It would have to be assumed that when there was no dependency large increments of blood flowed through non-nutritional shunts, thus keeping TPo_2 relatively constant. In those experiments in which $\dot{V}o_2$ was flow dependent, nutritional flow (and, to some extent, TPo_2) would be expected to vary directly with total flow. That this explanation may not be the correct one was suggested in the experiments of Duran and Renkin (2) when vasodilator drugs, which abolished autoregulation, failed to convert independent-type preparations to dependent ones. Nevertheless, we have tried to test this possibility by measuring TPo_2 with our micro O_2 electrode at three levels of constant flow.

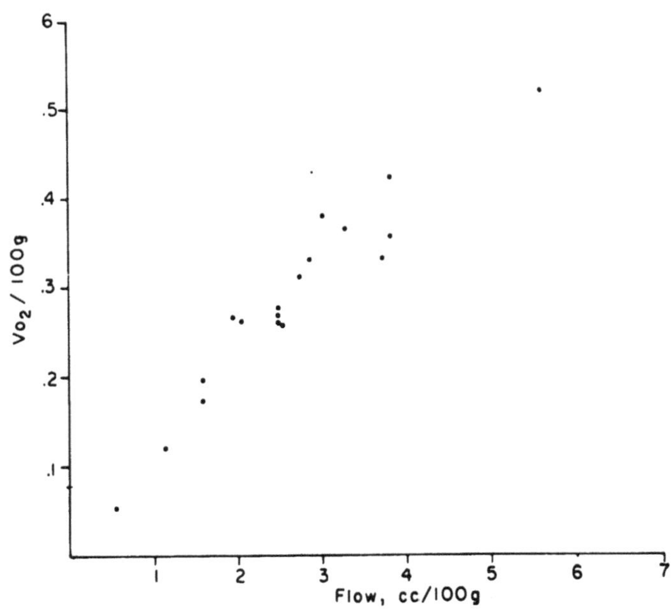

Figure 1: Steady state $\dot{V}o_2$ vs. blood flow in an isolated gracilis muscle of the cat (15).

We chose to use the dog gracilis (rather than the cat) partly to see whether in our hands there was a species difference, and partly because the likelyhood of finding an independent $\dot{V}o_2$-flow relationship was somewhat greater in the dog than in smaller animals (4,15). We hoped that comparison of the TPo_2 values in autoregulating ($\dot{V}o_2$-flow independent?) and non-regulating ($\dot{V}o_2$-flow dependent?) would provide a clue to the possible mechanism. We chose to use constant flow rather than constant pressure so that we could compare the results with those of Duran and Renkin (2), and so that we could enhance the opportunity to force exposure of the muscles to higher Po_2 levels.

In addition to steady-state measurements of TPo_2 we have measured the transient changes in one location during step changes in flow to see whether the pattern would vary with either the $\dot{V}o_2$ or the autoregulatory response. Some measurements of venous Po_2 and the Po_2 at the muscle surface were also made in the hope that the inter-relationships among the several parameters might be revealing.

METHODS.

Dogs were anesthetized with pentobarbital (40 mg/Kg) given intravenously, intubated and artificially ventilated. A heating pad under the animal maintained near normal body temperatures. Cannulas were inserted into the carotid artery and jugular vein. After an initial dose of 1500 U/Kg heparin was given intravenously, supplements of pentobarbital (5 mg/Kg-hr) and heparin (500 U/Kg-hr) were supplied usually by a constant infusion pump. A saline intravenous drip countered fluid losses.

The gracilis muscle was denervated, isolated and removed after cannulating the arterial supply and venous outflow following procedures described in the previous study of cat gracilis muscle (15). Saran tubing (.045" ID) was used for cannulation to minimize gas exchange between blood and environment. The animal was transferred to the experimental table after muscle isolation, and connected to the infusion pump, pressure and temperature transducers. The muscle was placed on a heated stage and connected to the perfusion system shown in Figure 2, where the perfusion rate of the pump was adjusted during the first 10-20 minutes to maintain a perfusion pressure within 80-100 mmHg. Flow was determined from the pump setting and checked with an interrupted beam photocell drop counter.[2] Blood was collected in a siliconized beaker and returned at the same flow rate to the animal via the jugular vein.

The arterial inflow line was jacketed with a heat exchanger,

2. Gilson Medical Electronics, Co., P.O. Box 27, 3000 West Beltline, Middleton, Wisconsin 53562

with venous outflow through a polarographic Po_2 macroelectrode built into the heated stage. The muscle was gently stretched to in situ length and positioned over a multi-cathode macroelectrode also built into the heated stage to monitor Po_2 over a 1" diameter area on the lower surface of the muscle. Under experimental conditions, surface and venous Po_2 equilibrium after a flow change was essentially reached within two to three minutes. Macroelectrodes were checked for linearity and calibrated preceding and following each experiment. Drift was occasionally encountered (often in the surface electrode) and was assumed to be linear during the course of the experiment when determining Po_2 values. Therefore, we do not consider the currents obtained with these macroelectrodes to be absolute measurements of Po_2, but rather, of value mainly in the relative sense. In a few cases venous Po_2 was estimated from the O_2 content and hematocrit.

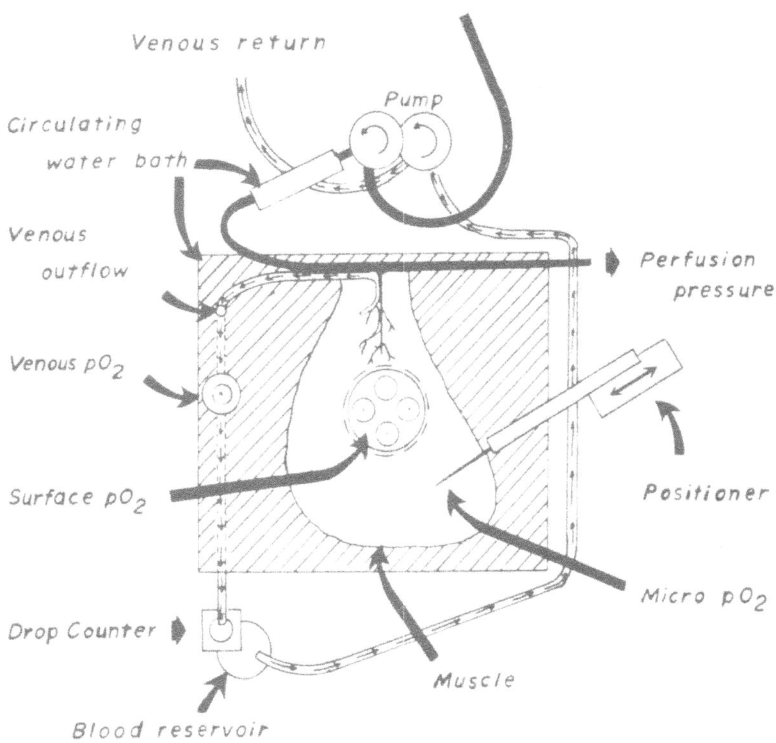

Figure 2: Diagram of constant temperature stage for isolated muscle with built-in venous and surface Po_2 sensors. The surface Po_2 electrode assembly is underneath the surface. The constant perfusion pump supplies blood to the muscle through a short segment of cannula enclosed in a heat exchanger.

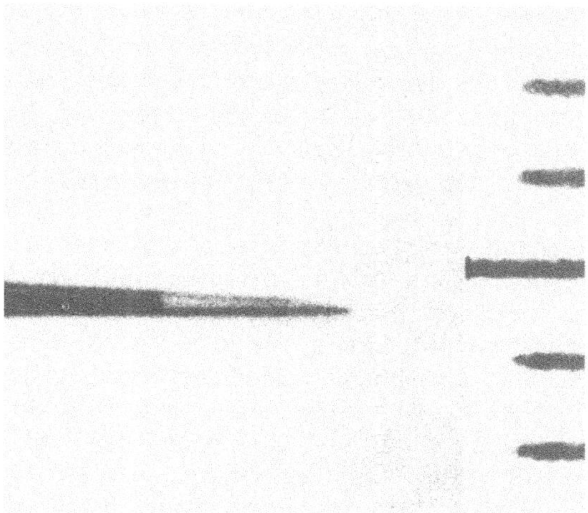

Figure 3: Photograph of the tip of the O_2 microelectrode (17) used. Scale in 10μ divisions, at right.

The muscle was covered with saran wrap to minimize surface evaporation and gas exchange between muscle and environment. A calibration well of Pluronics F127[3] was formed (over a tiny hole in the saran) and filled with saline equilibrated with room air at 37° C during microelectrode calibrations preceding and following each experimental run. A variation of 15% or less was considered acceptable. Microelectrode zeroes were obtained in yeast-agar prior to use and checked in each muscle by stopping the pump.

The construction, testing and use of micro O_2 electrode used to measure TPo_2 has been pre iously described (17). A photograph of the electrode tip is shown in Figure 3. Briefly, the electrode consists of a glass micro-pipette filled with a Woods metal-gold alloy to within about 30μ of the bevelled tip. About 15μ of gold is plated on the alloy. Rhoplex[4] in the recess serves as a filter for large molecules. The O_2 use is very small; the current being about 6×10^{-14} Amps/mmHg. The response time of the electrode is a second or two (slightly damped) and it is stir insensitive.

An experimental run consisted of a control period, followed by one or two step changes in flow, and return to control flow. Flow changes were usually ± 50% of control, allowing 10-12 minutes for each change, so that experimental runs varied from 30-45 min-

3. BASEF Wyandotte, Corporation, Wyandotte, Michigan.
4. Rohm and Haas Co., Independence Mall West, Philadelphia, Pa.

utes. Arterial and venous O_2 contents were determined from 20 ul samples using a total O_2 content analyzer[5]. Arterial pH and hematocrits were determined from samples drawn from the carotid artery before each experimental run at fairly regular intervals. Steady state venous samples were obtained directly from the muscle outflow line 8 to 10 minutes following each change in flow. A-V oxygen content differences obtained in this manner provided the basis for $\dot{V}o_2$ calculations using Fick's principle.

The microelectrode was inserted into the muscle through the small hole in the saran, and the tissue region 1 mm to 4 mm under the tissue surface sampled, avoiding visible blood vessels. The maximum depth of penetration varied from site to site, depending on the degree of tissue compression encountered. The tissue region was sampled by withdrawing the microelectrode from its deepest penetration in 50-60 μ steps every 10-15 seconds, to no closer than 1 mm from the surface, then returning in a similar manner to the deep location. Two to four minutes were required to obtain Po_2 values (the time average at each position) representing 20 to 40 locations per site with an equal number of up and down values. The microelectrode was left at the deep location to observe the time course of tissue Po_2 for at least one minute preceding and 5 minutes following a flow change. The steady state Po_2 distribution was again sampled in the same region, a venous content sample taken and the transient followed for each change and return to post-control.

Four constant flow experiments were conducted at Duke University.[6] In this series, the muscles were left _in situ_, and only measurements of TPo_2, $\dot{V}o_2$, perfusion pressure and flow were made. Unavoidably, the data are less complete in these experiments but are included where appropriate.

RESULTS.

Metabolic information was obtained from 15 dogs, including the four experiments at Duke University. Complete data from six muscles at three flow ranges are summarized in Table 1, Group A. Additional data from 8 muscles, including the Duke series, are included in Group B. Venous and surface Po_2's were not measured in the Duke experiments, and technical problems encountered in four experiments in Cleveland did not allow a full set of Po_2 information. Data from one animal (2/8/74) are not included since shock conditions were encountered. The muscle from the latter dog appeared to be maximally dilated, showing little or no autoregulation. Tissue Po_2's were noticeably higher probably because higher

5. Lexington Instruments Corporation, Waltham, Mass.
6. We wish to thank Dr. Eugene Renkin, then at Duke, for the use of some of his facilities and for his generous help in these experiments.

O_2 delivery rates were possible. The metabolism was not flow dependent, and was one of the two lowest rates encountered.

	Range	n	Flow	Perf. Pr.	O_2 Del.	$\dot{V}o_2$	Ven. Po_2	Surf. Po_2	TPo_2
A	Low	16	3.5±.7	57±18	.6	.24±.04	42	24	16
(N=6)	Cont.	37	7.1±2	91±19	1.2	.23±.06	53	27	21
	High	14	9.4±2	113±21	1.8	.27±.07	56	33	27
B	Low	29	3.4±.9	58±17		.22±.05			
(N=14)	Cont.	57	6.7±2	91±20		.23±.06			
	High	24	9.4±2	116±30		.25±.07			

Table 1: Mean (± S.D.) of steady state values for three ranges of blood flow. Flow, O_2 delivery and $\dot{V}o_2$ are expressed as ml/100g/min; balance of values in mmHg. In the interests of space S.D. omitted from Po_2 values. These ranged from 7.2 to 11.6. Arterial O_2 content for Group A dogs ranged from 11.9 to 21 ($\bar{x}$ = 17.2); pH ranged from 7.32 to 7.48 ($\bar{x}$ = 7.41); hematocrit ranged from 36 to 51 ($\bar{x}$ = 43).

All of the remaining fourteen animals exhibited good transient pressure responses to step changes in flow. Examples of recordings of tissue Po_2 and pressure transients are shown in Figure 4 for decreased and Figure 5 for increased flow. The Po_2 responses to flow changes for 3/4/74 and 2/13/74 show excellent control of tissue Po_2, with different time resporses. The record from 3/4/74 was the fastest response observed. Secondary changes in tissue Po_2 as seen for the flow increase for 1/14/74 were often encoutered, and oscillations, but were seen occasionally less dramatic than the response illustrated by the flow cecrease for 1/14/74. TPo_2 changes were often delayed varying in duration with location but usually less than 12 seconds. A minimum or maximum value in tissue Po_2 (depending on direction of flow change) was observed during the first 3 minutes, with a tendency to stabilize after three minutes. Figure 6 summarizes the Po_2 transients in flow, pressure, and tissue Po_2. It is apparent that there was little tendency for tissue Po_2 to return to the control level, especially with an increase in flow. There appeared to be some tendency for low tissue Po_2 values to exhibit a greater return to control than high

Po_2 values. Undoubtably slow, random time changes in tissue Po_2 distribution are occurring locally, which are difficult to characterize. Overall, the change in tissue Po_2 bore no consistent relationship to the autoregulatory response, as is also apparent from the examples in Figures 4 and 5.

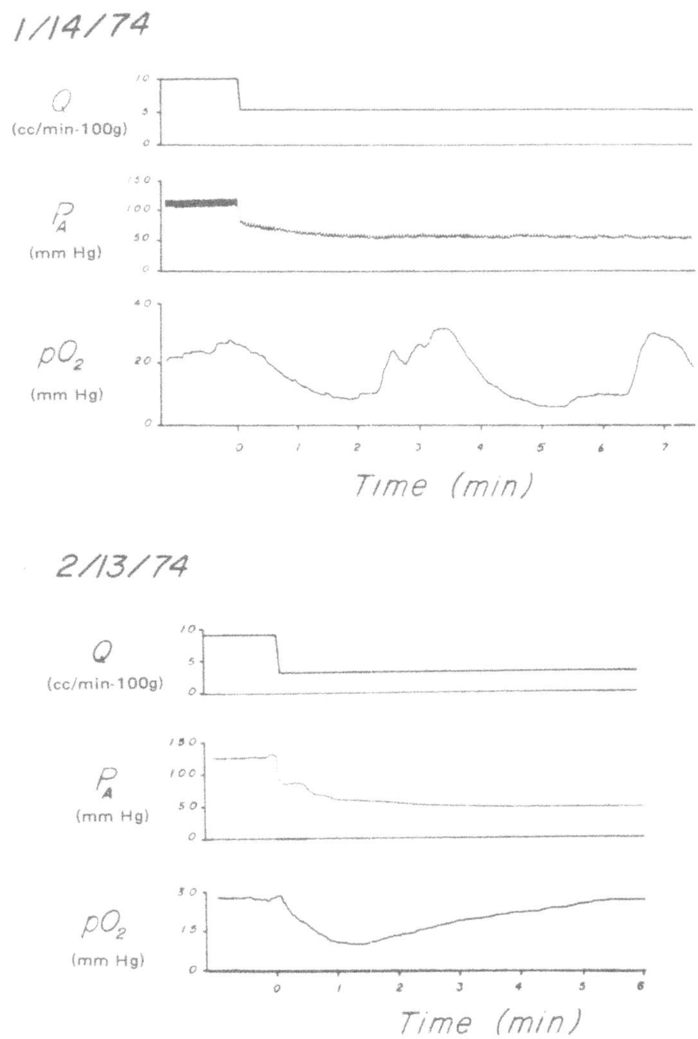

Figure 4: Examples of individual pressure and tissue Po_2 transient responses to following a step decrease in blood flow at $t = 0$; Q = blood flow in cc blood/min/100g tissue; P_A = arterial pressure, mmHg; Po_2 = partial pressure of oxygen in tissue, mmHg. (These symbols used throughout this report.)

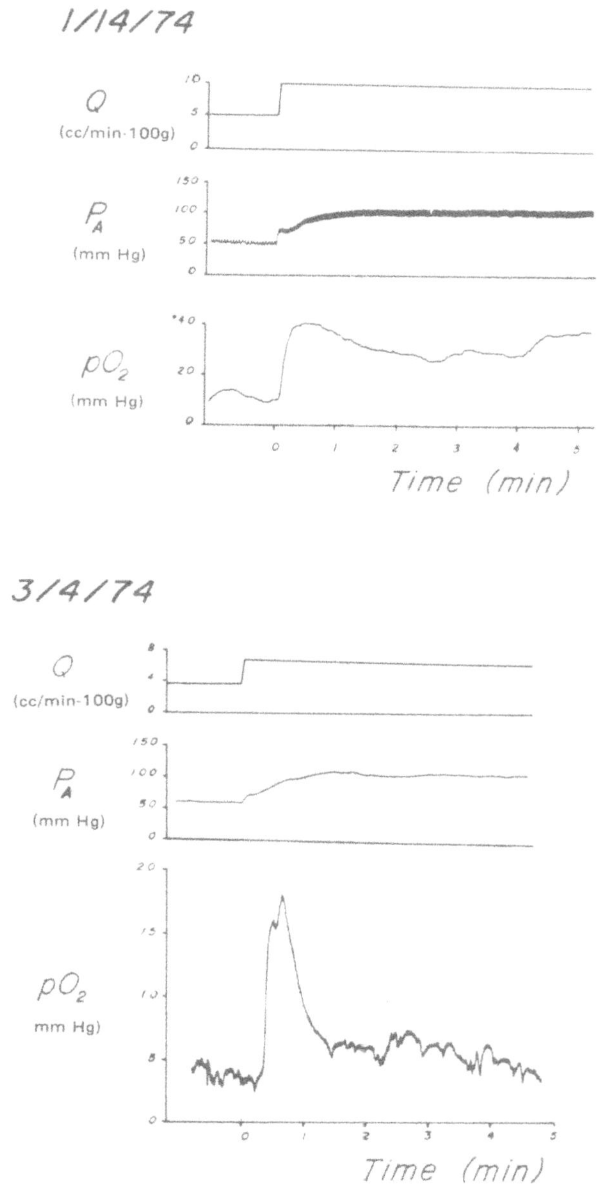

Figure 5: Same as Figure 4, but for a step increase in blood flow.

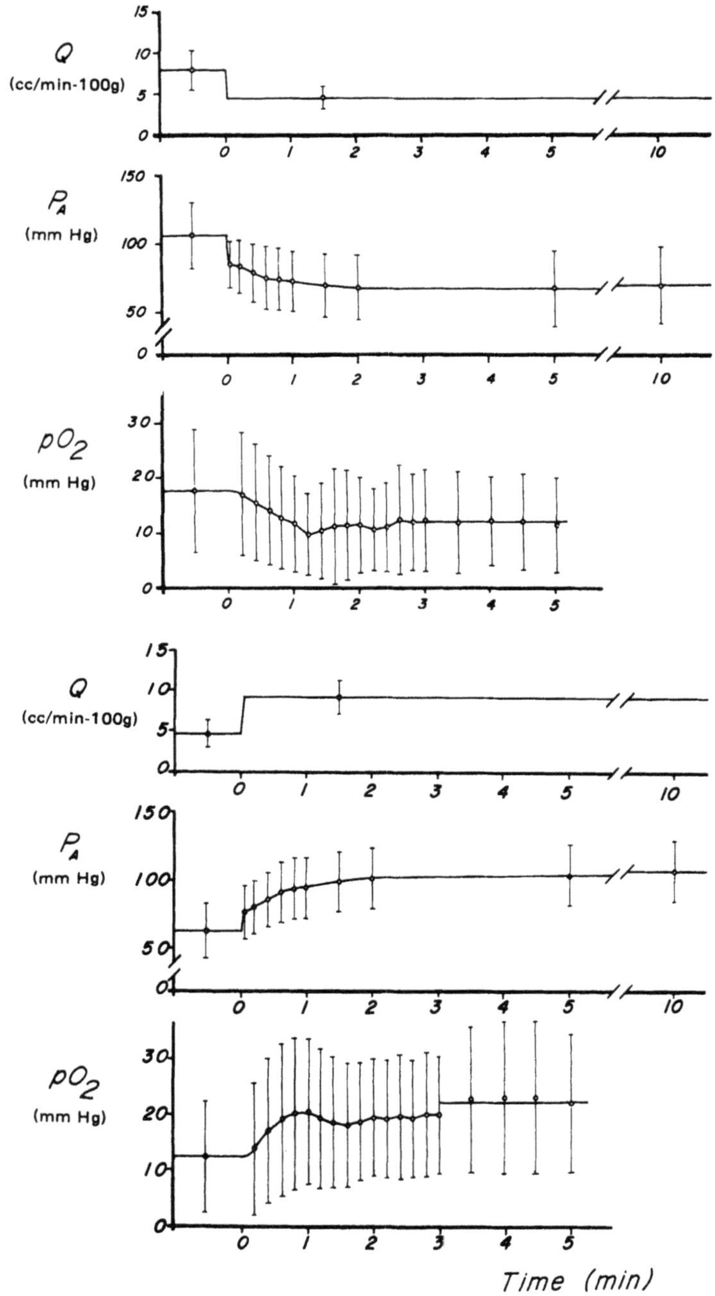

Figure 6: Mean (± S.D.) pressure and TPo_2 transient responses to decreased blood flow (n = 25) or increased blood flow (n = 23). Time in minutes below.

Venous Po_2 changes in 45 of 48 changes were in the direction of flow changes, as expected, with identical results for surface Po_2. A linear correlation of surface Po_2 % changes with venous Po_2 % changes was significant ($r = .78$). Per cent changes in mean steady state TPo_2 had little correlation with venous Po_2 % changes ($r = .30$) or surface Po_2 % changes ($r = .17$). The results of an analysis of variance (one way classification) performed for $\dot{V}o_2$, arterial pressure, surface, venous and mean tissue Po_2 values at three blood flow levels (control, high and low) are presented in Table 2. No significant differences were found between means of $\dot{V}o_2$ and surface Po_2's at the different levels. Significant differences were found between means of pressure, venous Po_2 and TPo_2 at the different levels.

Variable	Group	F-Ratio	P
$\dot{V}o_2$	A (N = 6)	2.87	>.25
	Total (N = 14)	1.53	>.25
P_A	A (N = 6)	33.62	.025<P<.05
	Total (N = 14)	45.16	.005<P<.025
VPo_2	A (N = 6)	12.24	.05<P<.10
SPo_2	A (N = 6)	2.64	>.25
TPo_2	A (N = 6)	6.33	.10<P<.25

Table 2: An analysis of variance (one way classification). (see text)

The steady state $\dot{V}o_2$ values for the three flow ranges summarized in Table 1 (N = 14) are shown in Figure 7 (at left). Time trends were observed for metabolism in individual experiments. Some changes with time were not best characterized as a linear trend over the entire experiment, showing a slight increase before declining. Time trends were determined using linear regression and control $\dot{V}o_2$ along the time trend. Normalization and comparison in this manner more clearly demonstrates the independent nature of metabolism over the flow range investigated, as shown in Figure 7 (at right).

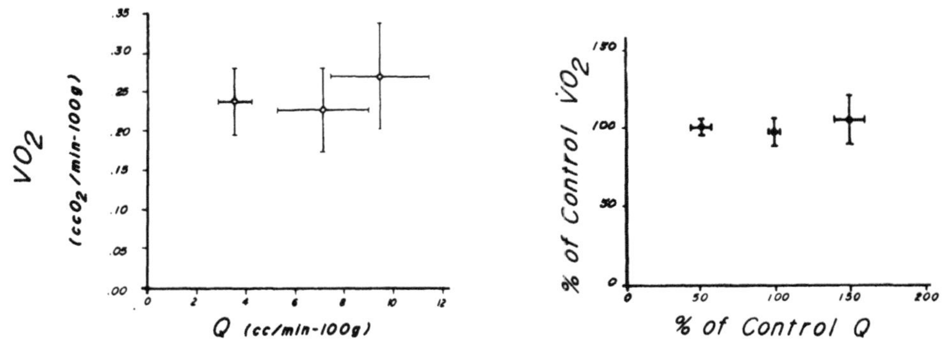

Figure 7: Steady state $\dot{V}o_2$-Q relationships. At left, mean and standard deviation for absolute values of $\dot{V}o_2$ and Q (Group A, 6 animals) low flow (n = 16), control flow (n = 37) and high flow (n = 14). At right, normalized $\dot{V}o_2$-Q relationship, after time trend removal.

Normalized steady-state TPo_2 histograms in 5 mmHg intervals for the three blood flow groups (from group A dogs) are shown in Figure 8. The first interval of each group includes values of 5 mmHg or less, with values of 2 mmHg or less shown as solid bars. It is apparent that there was a shift to the left as blood flow declined. However, the percent of hypoxic locations (2 mmHg or less) did not increase from control.

DISCUSSION.

To the extent that there are data to compare the present results are almost identical to those from the Group I muscle preparations of Duran and Renkin (2), i.e., the muscles which showed an independent relationship between $\dot{V}o_2$ and blood flow. Unfortunately, we found no muscles which gave results comparable to their $\dot{V}o_2$-flow dependent, Group II, preparations. In their group II preparations mean $\dot{V}o_2$ almost doubled as blood flow was increased from about 5 to about 9 ml/100g/min. In the present experiments there was a slight tendency for the $\dot{V}o_2$ to be higher at the higher flow rates, but the change was small and not significant. In none of the 14 muscles we studied did we find the $\dot{V}o_2$ was flow-dependent, and all showed changes in vascular resistance characteristic of autoregulating preparations (2). Thus, our hope to compare the TPo_2, and other parameters, in muscles responding differently was not realized.

However, since TPo_2 increased significantly with increases in flow while $\dot{V}o_2$ remained constant, we can say that O_2 availability

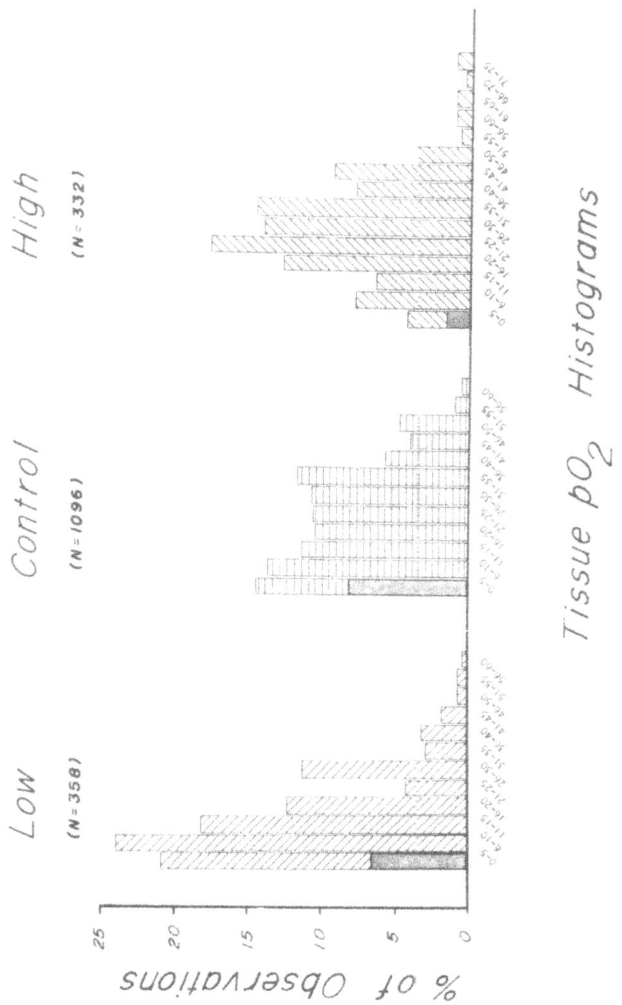
Low
(N=358)
Control
(N=1096)
High
(N=332)
% of Observations
25
20
15
10
5
0
Tissue pO2 Histograms

Figure 8

(above some minimal level) is not, by itself, the rate limiting factor for O_2 uptake in resting dog gracilis muscle.

The values for TPo_2 that we found even at higher levels of arterial pressure ($\bar{x}$ = 113 mmHg) appear to be somewhat lower than those reported by Sinagowitz _et al_ (11) for dog skeletal muscle, and those by Kunze (6) for human skeletal muscle. In both of the latter studies a needle, polarographic electrode was used. Coburn (1) who used a CO-myoglobin technique found very low values for calculated TPo_2 in dog skeletal muscle, _in situ_. Possibly the fact that the muscles in his study were inervated (see 16) and/or untouched, played a role in his experiments. Van Liew (13) who used a gas-pocket technique reported mainly high values in rat leg muscles.

In cat skeletal muscle we have found lower mean values for TPo_2 (16) and values comparable to those in the present study (15). In the cat, however, the great inter-individual variation makes comparison of mean data less than fruitful. There was much less inter-individual variation in the present study. The control average TPo_2 for each animal ranged from about 17 to 28 mmHg.

The lack of a significant relationship between steady state TPo_2 and venous and surface Po_2 deserves comment. It may indicate that there is some shunting of blood in this preparation, either of blood, or O_2 in counter current fashion.

Values for TPo_2 should be helpful in unraveling the mechanism underlying autoregulatory phenomena. Some investigators have suggested that O_2, per se, plays a primary role in the regulation of blood flow (3,10) by providing a metabolic signal for increased blood flow when cellular Po_2 reaches a "critical" level; the critical level being that level of Po_2 at which $\dot{V}o_2$ begins to decline. Jobsis (5) places this level at around 5 mmHg. Granger _et al_ (3) suggest 1 mmHg. In the present study, when flow was decreased, 11 of the 25 locations transiently fell below 5 mmHg; 7 fell to 1 mmHg or less; and 5 locations remained below 5 mmHg. These results can be interpreted as favoring the O_2 hypothesis at low blood flows, i.e., nearing impairment between O_2 supply and $\dot{V}o_2$. It could be argued that these areas of low Po_2 are key locations which provide a continuing signal for vasodilatation. If they were few in number our random penetrations might not have found them in all muscles. On the other hand, when flow was increased, the 6 locations in which the control Po_2 was 5 mmHg or less, all showed a transient increase to at least 5 mmHg in the first minute and remained high, yet vascular resistance continued to increase for several minutes thereafter. If these locations are representative it would seem that either the critical Po_2 for the metabolic signal for blood flow autoregulation must be normally relatively high, or that TPo_2

is not the main signal at normal blood flows.

Our results do provide further evidence that in dogs $\dot{V}o_2$ is most often independent of blood flow at least down to very low flow rates (2,13). The reason for the occasional finding of a dependent relationship (8,9) is not clear. It may be related to the state of acclimatization of the dogs (see 15 for refs.), their size (or species) or some subtle difference in the techniques used. However, Duran and Renkin (2), who found both types, were unable to correlate the type of relationship with any of the above possibilities to the extent that this was possible.

In studies of cat (14,15,18-but see 7) and rat (4) skeletal muscle marked dependency of $\dot{V}o_2$ on blood flow is the rule. The mechanism of this dependency is also unknown. However, it has been reported that for the cat, at least, classical tissue hypoxia ($Po_2 < 5$ mmHg) plays no role. It could be a blood-borne substance (other than O_2 presumably, unless the critical Po_2 is high) which stimulates the $\dot{V}o_2$, and/or that the tissues have a markedly different metabolic pattern.

Whatever, the basis of the dependent $\dot{V}o_2$-flow relationship is, it seems reasonable to conclude that the mechanism(s) of blood flow regulation must be, at least quantitatively, different in the cat (and small animals?) vs. the dog.

1. Coburn, R.F. and L.B. Mayers. Myoglobin O_2 tension determined from measurements of carboxymyoglobin in skeletal muscle. Am. J. Physiol. 220: 66-74, 1971.
2. Duran, W.N. and E.M. Renkin. Oxygen consumption and blood flow in resting mammalian skeletal muscle. Am. J. Physiol. 226: 173-177, 1974.
3. Granger, H.J., A.H. Goodman and D.N. Granger. Intrinsic metabolism regulation of blood flow, O_2 extraction and tissue O_2 delivery in dog skeletal muscle. In: Oxygen Transport to Tissue, ed. by H.I. Bicher and D.F. Bruley, 37A: 451-456, 1973.
4. Honig, C.R., J.L. Frierson and C.N. Nelson. O_2 transport and $\dot{V}o_2$ in resting muscle: sig'ificance for tissue-capillary exchange. Am. J. Physiol. 220: 357-363, 1971.
5. Jobsis, F.F. Basic processes in cellular respiration. In: Handbook of Physiology. Respiration. Washington, D.C.: Am. Physiol. Soc., 1964, sect. 3, vol. 1, chapt. 2, p. 63-124.
6. Kunze, K. Significance of oxygen pressure field measurements in human muscle, with special remarks on Po_2 micro-needle electrodes. Progr. Resp. Res. 3: 153-157.
7. Nakamura, H. The oxygen use of muscle and the effect of sympathetic nerves on it. J. Physiol., London 55: 100-110, 1921.
8. Pappenheimer, J.R. Blood flow, arterial oxygen saturation and oxygen consumption in the isolated perfused hind limb of the dog. J. Physiol. london 99: 283-303, 1941.
9. Rein, H. and M. Schneider. Die Auswirkung Kunstlicher Mangeldurchblutung auf den lokalen Stoffwechsel. Arch. Ges. Physiol. 239: 451-463, 1938.
10. Ross, J.M., H.M. Fairchild, J.J. Weldy and A.C. Guyton. Autoregulation of blood flow by oxygen lack. Am. J. Physiol. 202: 21-24, 1962.
11. Sinagowitz, E., H. Rahmer, R. Rink, L.Gornandt, M.Kessler. Local oxygen supply in intra-abdominal organs and in skeletal muscle during hemorrhagic shock. Advances in Exptl. Med. and Bio., 37A, ed. by H.I. Bicher and D.F. Bruley, 505-511, O.T.T. 1973.
12. Stainsby, W.N. and A.B. Otis. Blood flow, blood oxygen tension, oxygen uptake and oxygen transport in skeletal muscle. Am. J. Physiol. 206: 858-866, 1964.
13. Van Liew, H.D. Regional heterogeneity of PCo_2 and Po_2 in skeletal muscle. Advances in Exptl. Med. and Biol., 37A, ed. by HI.I. Bicher and D.F. Bruley, 457-465. O.T.T 1973.
14. Verzar, F. The gaseous metabolism of striated muscle in warm-blooded animals. J. Physiol., London 44: 243-258, 1912.
15. Whalen, W.J., D. Buerk and C.A. Thuning. Blood flow-limited oxygen consumption in resting cat skeletal muscle. Am. J. Physiol. 224: 763-768, 1973.
16. Whalen, W.J. and P. Nair. Skeletal muscle Po_2: effect of inhaled and topically applied O_2 and CO_2. Am. J. Physiol. 218:

973-980, 1970.

17. Whalen, W.J., J. Riley, and P. Nair. A microelectrode for measuring intracellular Po_2. J. Appl. Physiol. 23: 798-801, 1967.
18. Wright, D.L. and R.R. Sonnenschein. Relations among activity, blood flow, and vascular state in skeletal muscle. Am. J. Physiol. 208: 782-789, 1965.

EFFECT OF A SHIFT OF THE OXYGEN DISSOCIATION CURVE ON MYOCARDIAL OXYGENATION AT HYPOXIA

Z. Turek and F. Kreuzer

Department of Physiology, Faculty of Medicine
University of Nijmegen
Nijmegen, The Netherlands

Krogh's cylindrical model of the tissue (1922) has been widely used for the estimation of tissue oxygen tension (P_{O_2}). The model is based on several assumptions but it probably depicts the major trends in the changes of oxygen tension, even though the absolute values may deviate from reality.

In our following analysis of P_{O_2} in cardiac muscle we are going to use the original Krogh model with the only modification that for the radius of the tissue cylinder the circumferential radius of Thews' hexagon (Thews, 1960) is used rather than half the mean distance between capillaries (diffusion distance). The determinants of tissue oxygen tension are: myocardial oxygen consumption, myocardial blood flow, radius of the tissue cylinder, capillary radius, partial pressure of oxygen in arterial blood, blood oxygen capacity, oxygen diffusion coefficient of the tissue, and also the shape and position of the oxygen dissociation curve necessary for the interconversion of oxygen partial pressure and concentration in capillary blood. Whereas the importance of the other oxygen tension determinants has been analyzed in detail (Kety, 1957; Rakušan, 1971), the significance of the oxygen dissociation curve (DC) for tissue P_{O_2} has been rather neglected. Recently Duvelleroy et al. (1973) have analyzed the behavior of coronary flow due to a change in blood oxygen affinity by using an analog model.

The purpose of the present study is to show the effect of a shift of the DC on tissue P_{O_2} in the heart muscle and to compare it in man (with relatively high oxygen affinity of the blood) and in the rat (an animal with lower blood oxygen affinity). DC's were described according to Adair (1925); the constants of the human DC were taken from a paper by Roughton and Severinghaus (1973), and those of the rat DC from our results (Turek et al., 1973). P_{50}, i.e. the P_{O_2} corresponding to 50% saturation on the standard DC, is 26.6 mm Hg in human and 37 mm Hg in rat blood. In order to make the results comparable we assumed the tissue radius and capillary radius to be the same in both species, the former equal to 14 μm and the latter equal to 4 μm. These values are similar to those given in the literature for man (Rakušan, 1971) and also to values found in the rat in our previous studies. Tissue oxygen consumption was assumed to vary from 0.1 to 0.3 ml/min.g, coronary blood flow from 0.5 to 2.5 ml/min.g, blood oxygen capacity between 15 and 25 ml O_2/100 ml blood, and arterial P_{O_2} between 30 and 90 mm Hg. Arterio-venous pH difference was (unless stated otherwise) 0.04 and concentration of H^+ ions was assumed to increase linearly over the length of the cylinder. With all other parameters unchanged a shift of the DC to the right leads to an increase of tissue P_{O_2} at normoxia and mild hypoxia (favorable effect) but to a decrease of tissue P_{O_2} at severe hypoxia (unfavorable effect), as expected from previous analysis of the effect of a shift of the DC on mixed-venous P_{O_2} (Turek et al., 1973). A shift to the left in general has an opposite effect. In the following only a shift to the right will be considered.

The ambiguous effect of a right shift of the DC on tissue P_{O_2} at the periphery of Krogh's cylinder and its dependence on arterial P_{O_2} is shown in Fig. 1. The DC was shifted by 3 mm Hg to the right and the tissue P_{O_2} before and after the shift was calculated at an arterial P_{O_2} of 70 mm Hg (on the top), 50 mm Hg (in the middle), and 30 mm Hg (on the bottom). On the left part of the graph the situation in man, on the right side that of the rat is shown. It is obvious that at an arterial P_{O_2} of 70 mm Hg the P_{O_2} at the periphery of the tissue cylinder is higher after the shift in both species, i.e. the effect of the DC shift might be considered to be favorable. At an arterial P_{O_2} of 50 mm Hg the shift of the DC remains advantageous in man but, at least at the end of the tissue cylinder, has an unfavorable effect in the rat. The situation in the rat further demonstrates that the effect of a shift of the DC does not necessarily imply the same trend in the entire cylinder. In the proximal part of the tissue cylinder of the rat the shift leads to an increase of tissue P_{O_2}, whereas in the distal part of the cylinder the opposite occurs. At a very low arterial P_{O_2} (30 mm Hg) the shift of the DC is unfavorable in both species, the situation being more severe in the rat.

The most important criterion as to whether a shift of the DC has a favorable or an unfavorable effect is the change of the mean steepness of the physiological DC before and after the shift. The mean steepness of the physiological DC is the slope of a straight line connecting the arterial and venous points in case we are

interested in tissue P_{O_2} at the end of the tissue cylinder, or that of a straight line connecting the arterial point with a capillary point at any particular distance from the beginning of the cylinder. The arterial point is defined by the arterial P_{O_2} and the position of the DC, resulting in the arterial O_2 concentration. The capillary (or venous) point is defined by the oxygen concentration of the blood at a given distance arising from oxygen consumption and coronary blood flow and resulting in the capillary (or venous) P_{O_2}.
A favorable effect of a shift to the right is associated with a steeper slope and an unfavorable effect with a less steep slope of the physiological DC after the shift (Turek et al., 1973). Obviously between the situation where the mean slope increases (mild hypoxia) and that where it decreases (severe hypoxia) due to a shift, a value of the arterial P_{O_2} must exist at which no change of the mean slope after the same shift occurs. We call this the point of inversion. Factors leading to a decrease of this critical P_{O_2} extend the beneficial effect to more severe hypoxia. The opposite is true for factors increasing the P_{O_2} at the point of inversion.

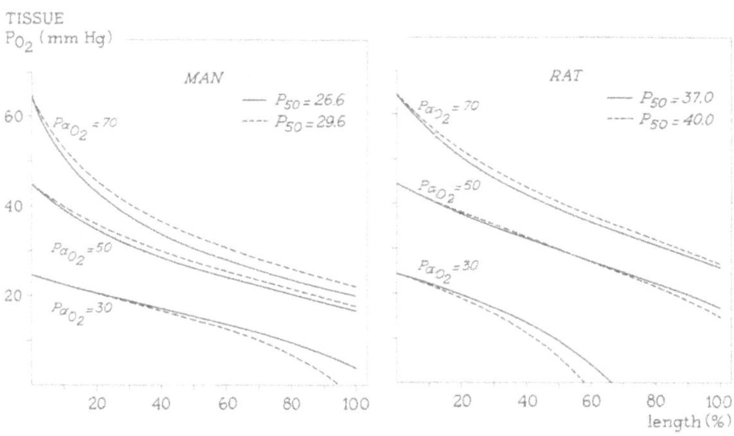

Fig.1. Myocardial tissue oxygen tension (P_{O_2}) at the periphery of Krogh's cylinder in man (on left side) and in the rat (on right side) before (solid line) and after a shift of the dissociation curve to the right by 3 mm Hg (broken line) for three values of the arterial P_{O_2} (Pa_{O_2}). Blood O_2 capacity = 20 ml O_2/100 ml blood, myocardial O_2 consumption = 0.15 ml/min.g, coronary blood flow = 1.5 ml/min.g, arterio-venous O_2 difference = 10 ml O_2/100 ml blood, arterio-venous pH difference = 0.04.

It is interesting to know what determines the P_{O_2} at the point of inversion. Fig. 2 illustrates that the effect of an identical shift to the right depends on the original position of the DC. When the DC is primarily shifted to the right, then a further shift becomes unfavorable even at milder hypoxia. This also explains the divergent results of the same shift in man and rat. The influence of blood oxygen capacity is shown in Fig. 3. During anemia the point of inversion is shifted up and polycythemia helps to extend the beneficial effect of the shift to more severe hypoxia. The rat has a point of inversion at higher P_{O_2} as explained previously. Both an increase of myocardial tissue consumption and a decrease of coronary blood flow elevate the point of inversion due to their effect on the arterio-venous O_2 difference. This is demonstrated in Fig. 4. In heart muscle arterio-venous O_2 difference is physiologically high (Rushmer, 1961) and therefore the unfavorable effect of a shift of the DC to the right is expected to occur at milder hypoxia than in other organs with low arterio-venous O_2 difference, at least at the end of the tissue cylinder. The line for the rat lies higher as expected. An interesting point is that at a very high arterio-venous O_2 difference the P_{O_2} at the point of inversion increases to normoxic values even in man. A disproportion between oxygen need and oxygen supply by the coronary circulation apparently is the most important factor in the pathogenesis of myocardial ischemia and myocardial infarction. It may be shown in man at normoxia that at decreased coronary blood flow a situation might occur where a shift of the DC to the right increases tissue P_{O_2} in a major part of the tissue cylinder but leads to severe hypoxia

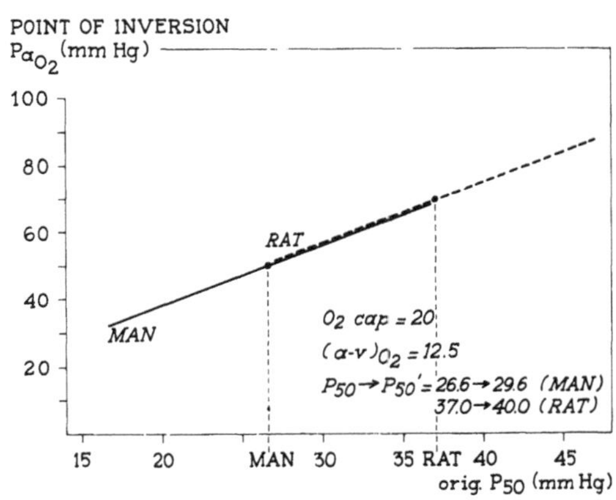

Fig.2. Effect of the original P_{50} (original position of the dissociation curve) on the P_{O_2} at the point of inversion in man and rat. Blood O_2 capacity = 20 ml O_2/100 ml blood, arterio-venous O_2 difference = 12.5 ml O_2/100 ml blood, curves are shifted to the right by 3 mm Hg, arterio-venous pH difference = 0.04.

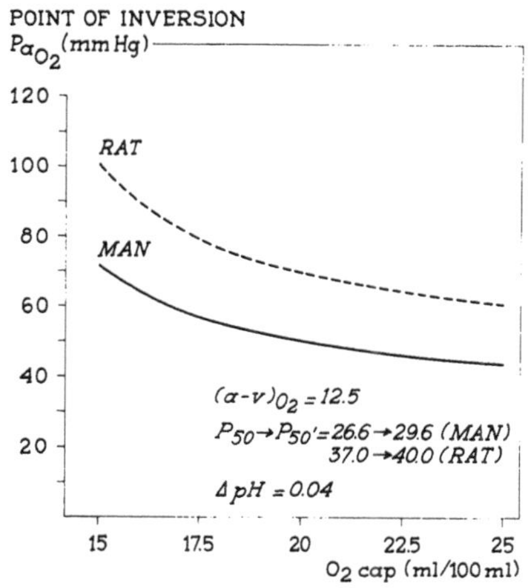

Fig.3. Effect of blood O_2 capacity on the P_{O_2} at the point of inversion in man and rat. Original P_{50} = 26.6 and 37.0 mm Hg in man and rat, resp., curves are shifted to the right by 3 mm Hg, other parameters the same as in Fig.2.

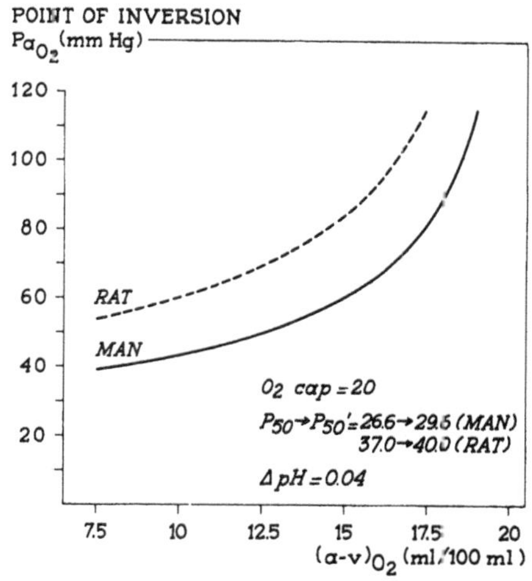

Fig.4. Effect of the arterio-venous O_2 difference on the P_{O_2} at the point of inversion in man and rat. Blood O_2 capacity = 20 ml O_2/100 ml blood, the other parameters the same as in Fig.3.

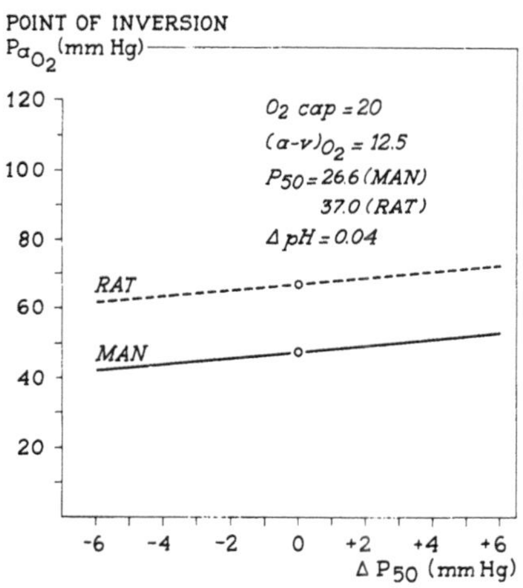

Fig.5. Effect of the extent of a shift to the right on the P_{O_2} at the point of inversion. Arterio-venous O_2 difference = 12.5 ml O_2/100 ml blood, the other parameters the same as in Fig.4.

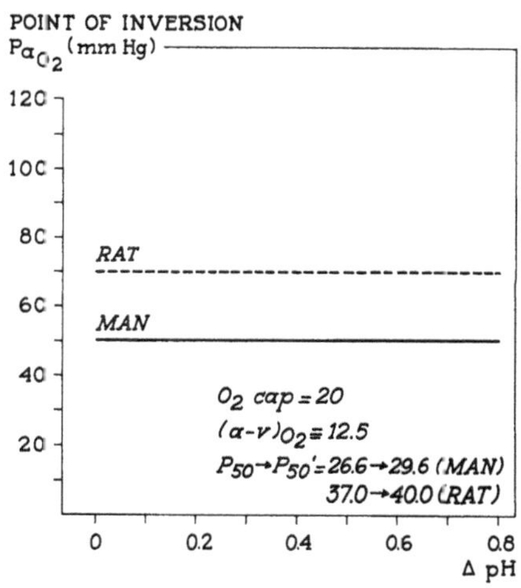

Fig.6. Absence of any significant effect of a shift of the dissociation curve to the right during the passage through the heart due to an increase of the arterio-venous pH difference. The arterial dissociation curve is shifted to the right by 3 mm Hg.

(P_{O_2} = 0) at the end of the cylinder, i.e. in the area where P_{O_2} already was quite low. A detailed discussion of this phenomenon and its possible clinical implication is beyond the scope of this paper.

As might be expected, the P_{O_2} at the point of inversion also depends on the extent of the right shift; a greater shift to the right also increases the P_{O_2} at the point of inversion (Fig. 5).

It is necessary to carefully distinguish between a shift of the DC due to factors operating in the whole body and changing oxygen affinity already in the arterial blood, i.e. before it reaches the heart (changes of acid-base equilibrium, temperature, 2,3-DPG, etc.), and a shift due to a decrease of oxygen affinity during the passage of the blood through the heart (e.g. because of a higher production of H^+ ions). Our whole preceding analysis refers to a shift of the DC already before the organ only. The P_{O_2} of the point of inversion is practically independent of a shift of the DC that occurs later during the passage through the organ (Fig. 6). The shift of the DC to the right during the passage through the organ (Bohr effect) is a different process; here the arterial point does not change its position and only the venous point is shifted to the right. This always results, at the same arterio-venous O_2 difference, in a higher P_{O_2} at the venous (or any capillary) point as compared with the situation where no shift occurs during the passage.

REFERENCES

Adair, G.S.: J.biol.Chem. 63; 529, 1925.
Duvelleroy, M.A., Mehmel, H., Laver, M.B.: J.Appl.Physiol. 35; 480, 1973.
Kety, S.S.: Federation Proc. 16; 666, 1957.
Krogh, A.: The Anatomy and Physiology of Capillaries, New Haven, Yale University Press, 1922.
Rakušan, K.: Oxygen in the Heart Muscle, Springfield, Ill., C.C.Thomas, 1971.
Roughton, F.J.W., Severinghaus, J.W.: J.Appl.Physiol. 35; 861, 1973.
Rushmer, R.P.: Cardiovascular Dynamics, Philadelphia, Saunders, 1961.
Thews, G.: Pflügers Arch. ges. Phys. 271; 197, 1960.
Turek, Z., Kreuzer, F., Hoofd, L.J.C.: Pflügers Arch. 342; 185, 1973.

ACKNOWLEDGMENT

This work was supported in part by a grant from the Stiftung Volkswagenwerk.

TISSUE BLOOD FLOW AND OXYGENATION DURING LARGE VESSEL SURGERY

Edward A.Ernst, M.D., Dennis Nelson, Ph.D., and Ralph DePalma, M.D.
Departments of Anesthesiology, Biomedical Engineering, Surgery
Case Western Reserve University, Cleveland, Ohio, U.S.A.
Supported by NIH Grant Number GM 19599

Tissue PO_2 and blood flow through gastrocnemius muscle and overlying subcutis were continuously determined in patients undergoing major vascular surgery for abdominal aneurysm or arteriosclerotic occlusive disease. Polarographic oxygen detection using paired flow-dependent and independent electrodes in each tissue allowed on-line computation of blood flow during the intraoperative and immediate perioperative periods.

Flow-dependent properties of diffusion membranes and their potential use in the determination of tissue blood flow was presented at the first ISOTT in 1973.[1] In 1974, a mass balance model of gas transport was described[2] built upon models proposed by Stuck[3] and Perl[4] but also incorporating a term acknowledging and utilizing data derived from a thin membrane, flow-dependent probe.

$$\frac{dC_{tz}}{dt} = \frac{\dot{Q}_t}{V_t}(C_{az} - C_{tbz}) - \frac{\eta}{V_t} - \frac{\gamma P_{tz}}{V_t} + \mu_z$$

(1) (2) (3) (4) (5)

where: C_{tz} is the concentration of gas z in tissue about the probe.
Q_t is tissue perfusion expressed as volume flow rate.
V_t is the compartment volume about the probe.
C_{az} is the concentration of gas z in arterial blood.
C_{tbz} is the concentration of gas z in blood within the compartment.
P_{tz} is the partial pressure of gas z in the tissue.
n is the consumption of gas z within the compartment.
y is the depletion factor for the tissue probe.
u is the volume flow rate at which gas z enters from neighboring compartments.

Term n is negative for production of gas. Term C_{tbz} includes fat and water components as well as blood. Term 4 accounts for gas harvested by the detecting probes.

The thin membrane, flow-dependent probe harvests more O_2 than the flow independent one, and it has been shown that a depletion factor can be determined from a ratio[2] of flow-dependent and independent oxygen electrode readings.

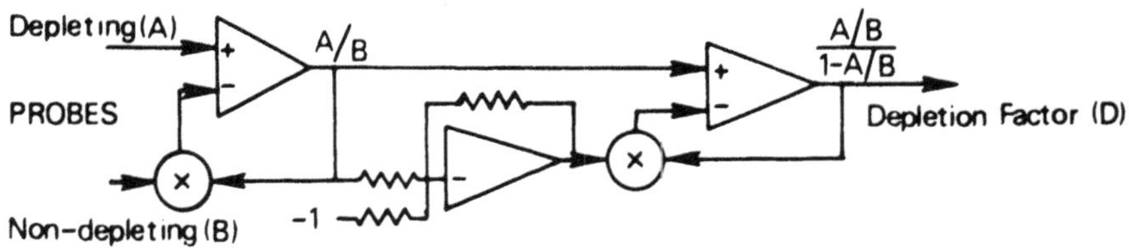

Block diagram of device for measuring tissue perfusion during steady-state conditions

This depletion factor (D) correlated well with dog hind leg blood flow measured with an electromagnetic flow meter.[2] The present investigation utilized this background information to study patients during surgery and provide the surgeon and anesthesiologist with real time lower extremity perfusion information.

Figure I shows measured PO_2 in subcutaneous and muscle tissue during successful abdominal aneurysmectomy. Subcutaneous PO_2 was always higher than muscle, and flow in both tissues prior to aorta cross-clamping was approximately equal. At cross-clamping, muscle PO_2 fell very rapidly and recovered much more slowly than subcutaneous tissue, a manifestation of its higher metabolic rate. When the cross-clamp was removed, flow through muscle greatly exceeded flow through subcutaneous tissue. This has been described by other investigators and can be interpreted as an autoregulatory mechanism in hypercarbic, hypoxic and acidotic tissue. Two step changes in flow occurred during each surgical procedure at aorta cross clamping and at subsequent clamp release, and time constants for both tissues are summarized in Figure II.

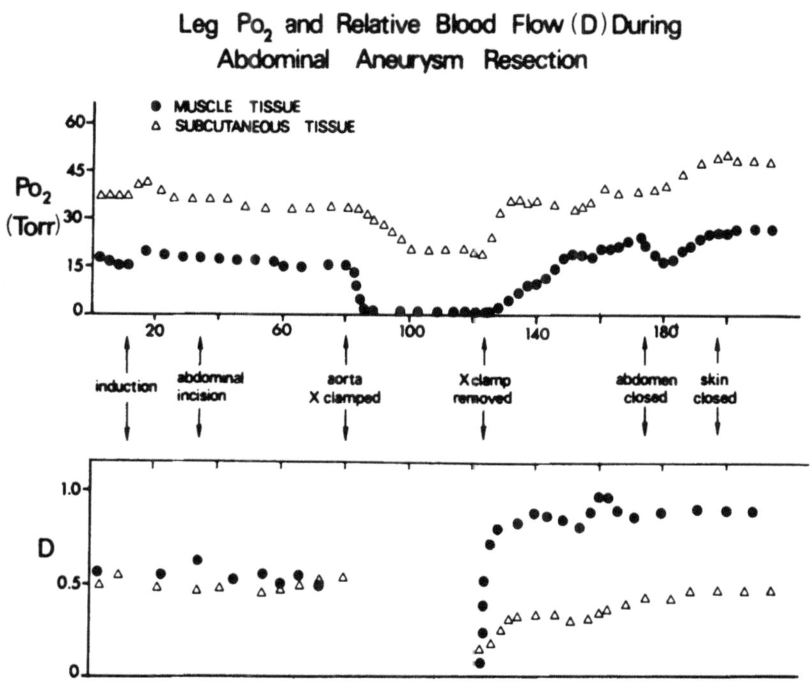

FIGURE I

63% PO_2 RESPONSE TIMES (τ) TO STEP CHANGE IN BLOOD FLOW INTO PATIENTS LEGS (Means and standard errors - n = 10)

	Muscle	Subcutis
τ_1 (min) aorta X clamped	2.65 ± 0.32	9.32 ± 1.00
τ_2 (min) clamp removed	10.16 ± 1.30	3.45 ± 0.47

FIGURE II

Objective measurements made in this study were compared with patients' clinical course. On two occasions, intraoperative measurements indicated that an embolus had probably occurred and the surgeon was able to extract it with a Fogarty Catheter while the patient was still on the operating table. On one occasion, measurements in the recovery room predicted postoperative atheromatous embolization before any clinical signs such as changes in peripheral pulse, temperature or limb cyanosis were clinically apparent.

In our study flow information from muscle tissue was much more predictively valuable than information from subcutaneous tissue when compared with the patients' actual clinical course.

References:
1. Nelson, et al.: Flow limited Properties of Diffusion Membranes. Advances in Medicine and Biology. Oxygen Transport to Tissue. Plenum Press, New York, 1973, 121-125.
2. Nelson, Ernst, et al.: Verification of Model for O_2 Delivery to Tissue. FASEB. April, 1974.
3. Stuck, et al.: Analysis of Oxygen Diffusion to a Measuring Probe in Animal Tissue. J. Theor. Biol. 31:509-532, 1971.
4. Perl, et al.: Intertissue Diffusion Effect for Inert Fat Soluble Gases. J. Appl. Physiol. 20:621-627, 1965.

MECHANISMS OF INCREASED TISSUE OXYGEN DELIVERY FOLLOWING RELEASE OF ARTERIAL OCCLUSION IN CANINE SKELETAL MUSCLE AND SKIN

H. I. Chen, A. H. Goodman, and H. J. Granger

Department of Physiology and Biophysics
University of Mississippi School of Medicine
Jackson, Mississippi 39216

INTRODUCTION

Tissue oxygen delivery is dependent on the local blood flow and the extent of oxygen extraction. Concerning the intrinsic microvascular control of tissue O_2 delivery, a recent system analysis (1) and experimental data (2) suggest that adequate tissue oxygenation is maintained over a wide range of metabolic stresses, the relative contribution of blood flow and O_2 extraction to the regulation of tissue O_2 delivery being determined by the prevailing venous oxygen level. The previous study (2) has shown that in skeletal muscle perfused with constant pressure, both reactive hyperemia and elevated arteriovenous (A-V) O_2 difference contribute to the O_2 debt repayment following arterial occlusion when the initial A-V O_2 difference is in the normal range. However, at low prevailing A-V O_2 difference, increased O_2 extraction is the major mechanism by which the tissue repays its O_2 debt and the contribution of blood flow is minimal. As the prevailing venous O_2 reserve is lowered, the contribution of O_2 extraction diminishes and reactive hyperemia becomes more important for the compensation. Thus, the immediate post-occlusion O_2 extraction is only slightly elevated or even transiently depressed.

In the present study, further experiments are carried out in order to investigate the contribution of O_2 extraction to the debt repayment following the release of arterial occlusion in 1) skeletal muscle perfused with constant flow to eliminate blood flow regulation, and 2) cutaneous circulation in which reactive hyperemia is weak or absent.

METHODS

The experiments were done on mongrel dogs anesthetized with pentobarbital. A tracheotomy was done and the animal ventilated with room air. In both hindlimb (mainly skeletal muscle) and hindpaw (mainly skin) preparations, the following parameters were monitored: arterial pressure, venous pressure, arterial blood flow and arteriovenous oxygen difference. The hindlimb preparation included isolation of femoral artery and vein and clamping of the paw. In the hindpaw preparation, the anterior tibial artery was isolated, cannulated and perfused by the femoral arterial blood. In addition, the saphenous vein was catheterized. For monitoring the arteriovenous O_2 difference, arterial blood was taken from the contralateral femoral artery and venous blood was taken from the femoral for the hindlimb experiments or from the saphenous vein in the paw experiments. In both preparations, all the collateral blood supply was tied off. To assure the absence of collateral flow, the femoral or anterior tibial artery was occluded for more than 1 minute until the arterial pressure reached a steady state close to the venous pressure.

A blood reservoir was connected to the arterial system via a carotid catheter. The height of the reservoir was adjusted to control the perfusion pressure. In order to perfuse the tissue with constant pressure and constant flow at different times, we connected a large two-way PE tubing between the proximal and distal end of femoral artery (hindlimb), or between femoral and anterior tibial artery (hindpaw). One path was for constant pressure perfusion, the other was connected to a pulsatile perfusion pump (constant flow perfusion). Constant pressure or constant flow perfusion was accomplished by alternately opening one circuit and closing the other.

To study the contribution of O_2 extraction to the O_2 debt repayment following release of arterial occlusion in muscle and hindpaw, we clamped the artery blood supply for 1 and 2 minutes, and compared the magnitude and duration of increased arteriovenous O_2 difference following the release of occlusion under the condition of constant pressure versus constant flow perfusion.

RESULTS

Table 1 summarizes the averaged changes of A-V O_2 difference and blood flow (with constant pressure perfusion) or perfusion pressure (with constant flow perfusion) in skeletal muscle following release of arterial occlusion. Figure 1 exemplifies the responses. Both blood flow (3.5 X control) and O_2 extraction (1.5 X) increased to repay the O_2 debt following 1 minute arterial occlusion. The magnitude and duration or reactive hyperemia were only slightly enhanced, but the A-V O_2 difference increased more (2.1 X) and lasted

Table 1. Post-occlusion changes in blood flow or perfusion pressure and A-V differences in skeletal muscle

Const Pres or Flow	No of Obs	Period of Occl (min)	Blood Flow (ml/min)			A-V O_2 Difference (vols%)				
			Cont	Peak	P/C (times)	Cont	Peak	P/C (times)	P-C	Dura (min)
Const Pres	12	1	76	266	3.5	3.8	5.8	1.5	2.0	0.8
110 mm Hg	12	2	75	274	3.7	4.0	8.2	2.1	4.2	1.4
			Perfusion Pressure (mm Hg)							
			Cont	MAX Red	MR/C (times)					
Const Flow	12	1	106	30	0.29	3.8	8.8	2.3	5.0	2.0
76 ml/min	12	2	108	28	0.26	317	10.9	3.0	7.2	2.8

P/C = peak/control
P - C = peak - control
Max Red = maximum reduction
MR/C = maximum reduction/control

longer when the period of occlusion was 2 minutes. As the reactive hyperemia was eliminated by constant flow perfusion, increased O_2 extraction became the only mechanism for O_2 debt repayment. In this condition, both the magnitude and duration of increased O_2 extraction was augmented. In some experiments the level of A-V O_2 difference returned to control and then was slightly above control for as long as 3-6 minutes.

In contrast to skeletal muscle in which vascular resistance was consistently depressed (0.25-0.3 X control) after arterial occlusion, the cutaneous circulation of the hindpaw exhibited variable responses. In the same animal, the immediate post-occlusion vascular resistance might increase, remain the same, or actually decrease. Figure 2 illustrates an example. Panel A shows a reduction of blood flow after 1 minute occlusion. Perfusion pressure increased at subsequent constant flow perfusion (panel C). Approximately 5 minutes later, the same arterial occlusion brought about a slight reduction of vascular resistance as was evidenced by increased blood flow at a constant pressure perfusion (panel B) and decreased perfusion pressure at constant flow perfusion (panel D). Table 2 summarizes the post-occlusion changes in blood flow (or perfusion pressure) and A-V O_2 difference in the cutaneous circulation for two types of responses: one with post-occlusion reduced flow, the other with normal flow or slight hyperemia. In group 1, when blood flow was reduced to 0.7 X control and gradually returned to control in 2-3 minutes, O_2 extraction increased 9-10 times and lasted 1.5-3.2 minutes.

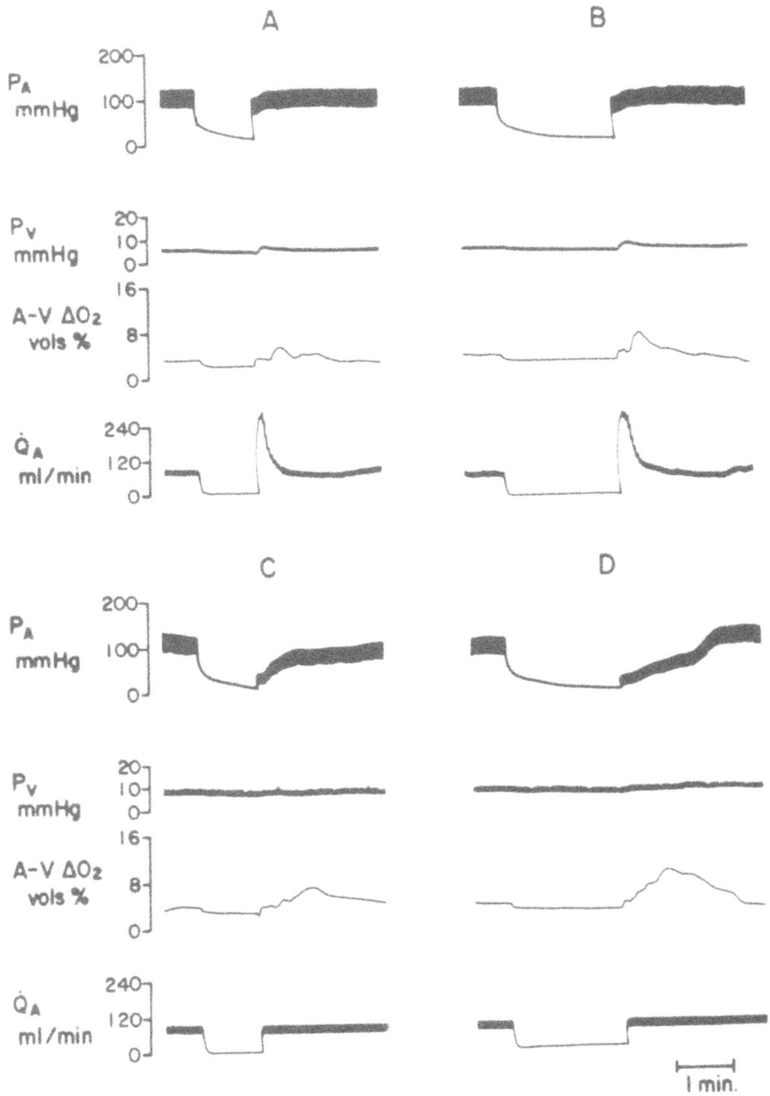

Figure 1. Effect of arterial occlusion on skeletal muscle circulation.

This elevation of O_2 extraction was very much greater and longer than that seen in skeletal muscle exhibiting reactive hyperemia. During subsequent constant flow perfusion of the paw, perfusion pressure increased to 1.7 X control immediately following release of occlusion. The magnitude and duration of elevated A-V O_2 difference were less than during constant pressure perfusion in which reduction of blood flow occurred.

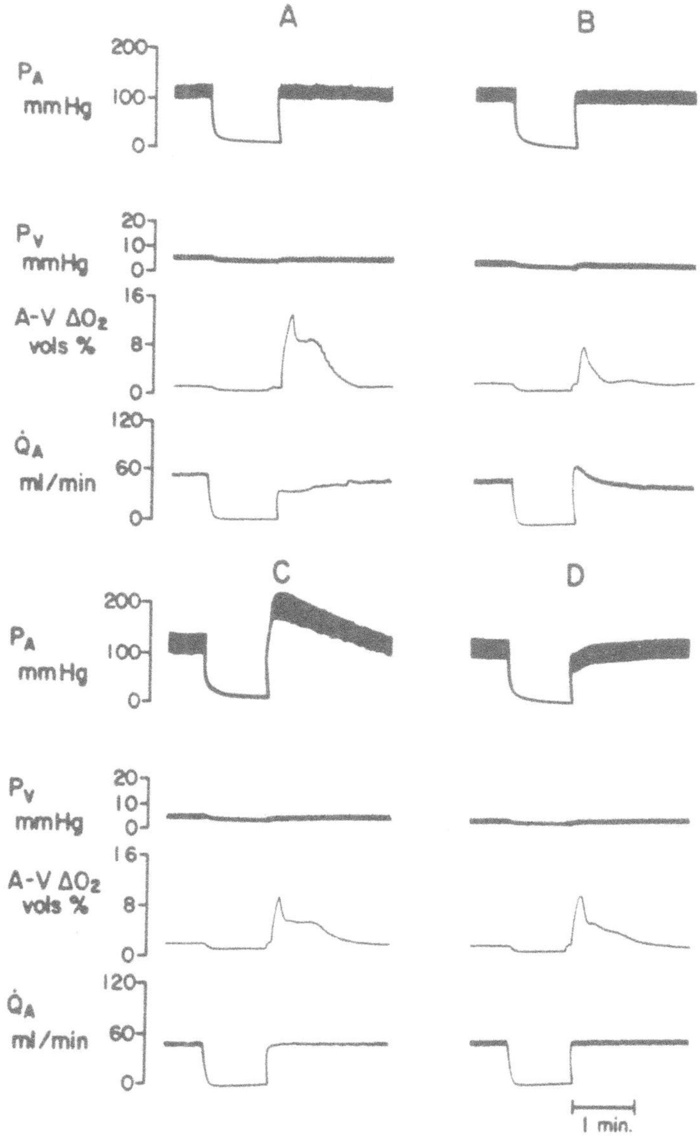

Figure 2. Effect of arterial occlusion on cutaneous circulation.

Table 2. Post-occlusion changes in blood flow or perfusion pressure and A-V O_2 difference in skin

Const Pres or Flow	No of Obs	Period of Occl (min)	Blood Flow (ml/min) Cont	Max Red	MR/C (times)	A-V O_2 Difference (vols%) Cont	Peak	P/C (times)	P-C	Dura (min)
Group 1: Reduction of blood flow following occlusion										
Const Pres 105 mm Hg	12	1	49	34	0.67	1.2	10.4	8.7	9.2	1.5
	12	2	47	32	0.67	1.3	12.5	9.6	11.2	3.2
			Perfusion Pressure (mm Hg) Cont	Max Inc	MI/C (times)					
Const Flow 48 ml/min	12	1	105	180	1.7	1.5	7.7	5.1	6.2	1.0
	12	2	105	184	1.7	1.3	8.8	6.7	7.5	1.4
Group 2: No change or increase of blood flow following occlusion										
			Blood Flow (ml/min) Cont	Max Inc	MI/C (times)					
Const Pres 105 mm Hg	12	1	46	51	1.1	1.4	6.8	4.8	5.4	1.1
	12	2	47	53	1.1	1.3	8.1	6.2	6.8	1.3
			Perfusion Pressure (mm Hg) Cont	Max Red	MR/C (times)					
Const Flow 48 ml/min	12	1	105	80	0.77	1.4	7.9	5.6	6.5	1.0
	12	2	105	80	0.77	1.4	9.1	6.5	7.7	1.2

Max Inc = Maximum Increase
MI/C = Maximum Increase/Control

In contrast, when normoremia or slight hyperemia was observed (Group 2), the increase in extraction of O_2 was less than in those paws showing reduced flow. In these preparations, A-V O_2 difference increased a little more when the slight hyperemia was prevented by constant flow perfusion.

DISCUSSION

It has been proposed that oxygen delivery to tissue cells is regulated by metabolic feedback to arterioles and precapillary sphincters (1, 2). The function of the arteriolar control system is to minimize changes in capillary PO_2 following alterations in the O_2 availability-to-demand ratio. This is achieved by feedback adjustment of blood flow in accordance with tissue oxygen requirement. On the other hand, precapillary sphincters maintain tissue oxygenation by modulating diffusion parameters through changes in effective capillary density, thereby altering O_2 extraction. In skeletal muscle, both mechanisms operate for the O_2 debt repayment following a period of arterial occlusion. However, their contributions depend on the initial blood flow and venous O_2 reserves. At higher prevailing levels of O_2 extraction (Figure 3B), the peak reactive hyperemia for a given period of arterial occlusion was higher than under normal conditions indicating an increased sensitivity of the arteriolar or flow control mechanisms at low tissue PO_2. Under this condition O_2 extraction even decreased below control level. These results suggest that the high reactivity of local flow control system at low tissue O_2 levels cause an over-comensation via the reactive hyperemia, thus extraction is transiently depressed. As the prevailing A-V O_2 difference is lowered, increased O_2 extraction became the major factor, and the reactivity of flow control mechanism is minimized. Furthermore, the present investigation shows that when the flow regulation mechanism is prevented by constant flow perfusion, the precapillary sphincter control system is more effective and the increase in O_2 extraction is greater and longer; under this condition extraction is of paramount importance for it is the only factor available for compensation. This elegant control and interaction of the flow and O_2 extraction mechanisms are further evident from the responses in the cutaneous circulation. Reactive hyperemia in the skin, if there is any, is weak, and O_2 extraction is the major mechanism by which the O_2 debt is repaid. In the skin, an unexpected phenomenon of post-occlusion hypoemia was commonly observed concomitant with very high increases in O_2 extraction. This particular finding may even imply that in the skin, the high reactivity of precapillary sphincter control mechanism to tissue hypoxia causes an over-compensation via the increased O_2 extraction; thus the arteriolar control system is depressed and the blood flow is reduced.

Supported by HL-11678 and a grant from the Mississippi Heart Association.

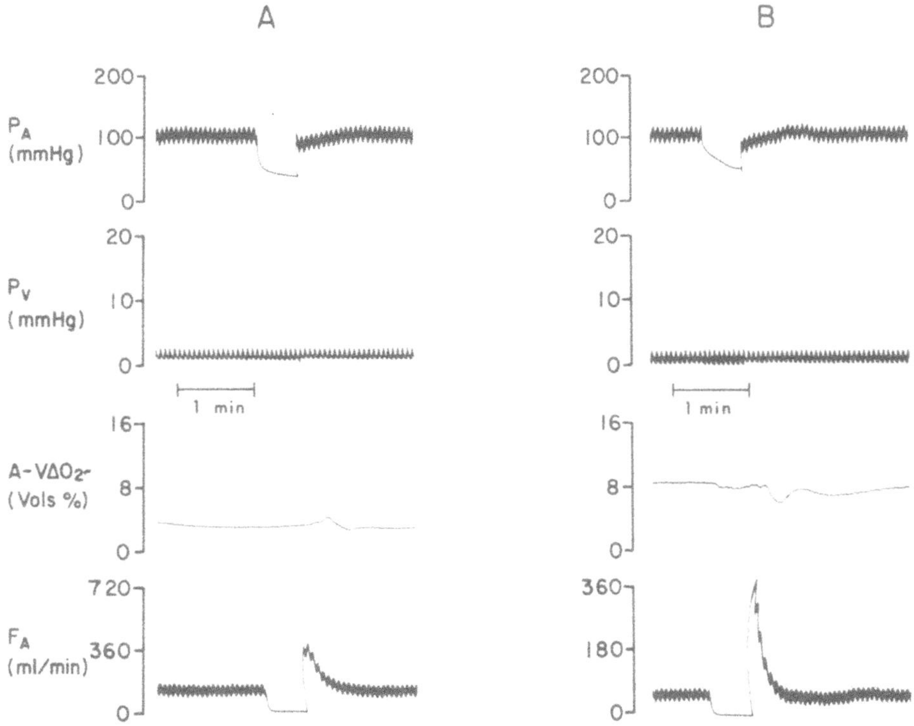

Figure 3. Reactive hyperemia and O_2 extraction at low and high A-VΔO_2

1. Granger, H. J., and A. P. Shepherd, Jr. Intrinsic microvascular control of tissue oxygen delivery. Microvas. Res. 5:49-72, 1973.

2. Granger, H. J., A. H. Goodman, and D. N. Granger. Intrinsic metabolic regulation of blood flow, O_2 extraction and tissue O_2 delivery in dog skeletal muscle. In: Oxygen Transport to Tissue, ed. by H. I. Bicher, and D. F. Bruley, Plenum Publishing Corporation, New York, 1974, pp. 451-456.

ACKNOWLEDGEMENTS:
The authors are indebted to Ms. Dianne Langford for excellent secretarial assistance.

MEAN MYOGLOBIN OXYGEN TENSION DURING EXERCISE AT MAXIMAL OXYGEN UPTAKE

R.F. Coburn and B.J. Clark

Department of Physiology, School of Medicine
University of Pennsylvania
Philadelphia, Pennsylvania 19174

We have applied the method of estimating intracellular oxygen in skeletal and cardiac muscle from binding of CO to myoglobin to intact man. This study has been published in detail elsewhere (1).

Figure 1 shows schematically the theory back of this method. The CO tension in tissue is determined by the P_{CO} in mean capillary blood. CO and O_2 compete for binding to myoglobin and under conditions of a constant tissue P_{CO} falls in intracellular PO_2 in proximity to myoglobin will result in an increase in binding of CO to myoglobin. It is possible to compute a "mean" myoglobin PO_2 in a muscle tissue from binding of CO to myoglobin at a given tissue P_{CO} assuming chemical equilibrium between CO and O_2 and myoglobin at every point in the tissue, as described previously (3,4). Calculations show that tissue P_{CO} is relatively fixed under a variety of conditions and suggest that changes in binding of CO to myoglobin reflect changes in mean myoglobin PO_2. The reaction of CO and myoglobin is used as a PO_2 indicator. Evidence that the binding of CO to myoglobin is a specific PO_2 indicator is summarized elsewhere (3). HbCO are at normal levels (1 to 2% sat.) in this study.

In previous experiments performed on anesthetized dogs, where CO binding to myoglobin was determined in biopsied hamstring muscle, it was found that mean myoglobin PO_2 under control conditions (PaO_2 80-120 mm Hg) was 4 to 6 mm Hg giving a normal oxymyoglobin % saturation of 60-70. CO binding to myoglobin remained constant as PaO_2 was varied from 300 to 400 mm Hg, giving calculated falls in mean myoglobin PO_2 of 1 to 1.5 mm Hg, but when PaO_2 fell below 40 mm Hg (by having the animal breathe hypoxic gas mixtures), large shifts of CO occurred, out of blood into skeletal and cardiac muscle and computed mean myoglobin PO_2 fell to values below 1 mm Hg.

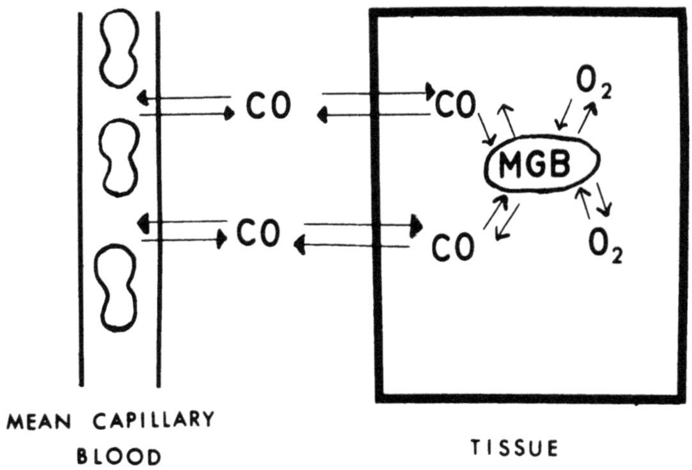

Figure 1. Competition of CO and O_2 for myoglobin.

There is evidence (3,4) that this shift of CO into heart or skeletal muscle occurred when intracellular PO_2 fell below the "critical PO_2" (by critical PO_2 we mean the PO_2 below which oxygen availability limits aerobic metabolism).

In applying this method to intact man we have determined shifts of CO in muscle from measured shifts of CO out of the vascular compartment under conditions where the body CO stores remain nearly constant. Best estimates of the makeup of the body CO stores indicate that over 95% of the stores are found either bound to hemoglobin or to myoglobin. This evidence includes: (a) muscle biopsy experiments referred to above showing that muscle CO can entirely explain the extravascular CO stores in dogs, within the measurement error; (b) low affinity constants for CO and cytochromes, including a_3 and P_{450}, compared to affinity constants for CO and myoglobin; (c) the finding that under conditions where CO shifted out of blood into muscle during hypoxic hypoxemia, loss from blood could be explained by increases in skeletal and cardiac muscle (3); (d) the inability to find extravascular CO stores in the dog liver, an organ with a high concentration of CO binding hemoproteins (unpublished data, R.F. Coburn). Therefore, increase of binding of CO to myoglobin will be mirrored by a fall in intravascular CO.

Figure 2 shows the CO shift out of blood which occurred with hypoxic hypoxemia in an anesthetized dog. In this experiment CO loss via the lungs was prevented by having the animal respire in a closed system.

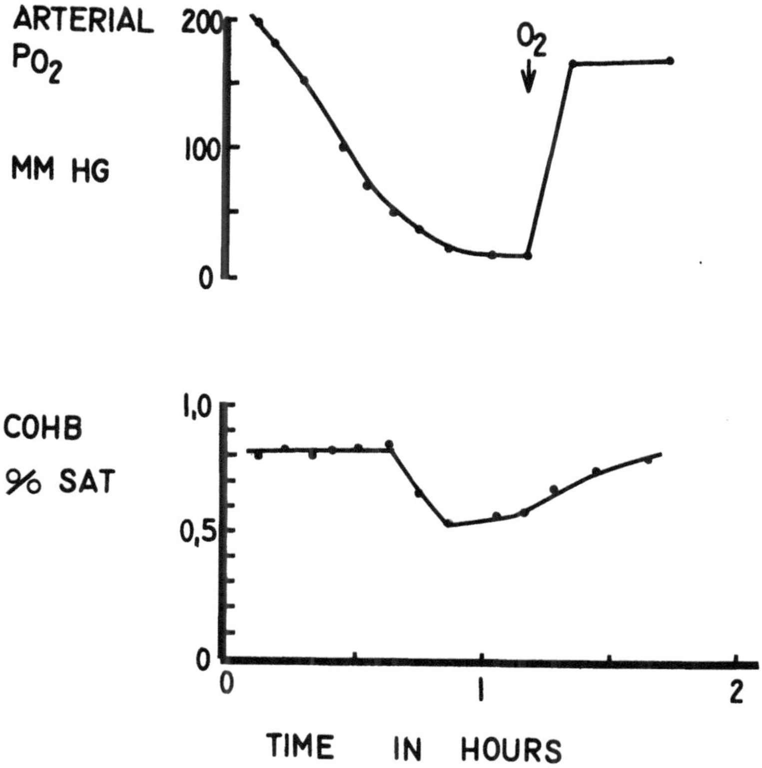

Figure 2. Experiments performed on a pentobarbital anesthetized dog breathing in a closed system. Inspired oxygen tension was allowed to fall progressively. HbCO was measured in mixed venous blood.

Note that blood HbCO% sat. remained constant as PaO_2 fell progressively to levels of 40 mm Hg. As PaO_2 fell below 40 mm Hg, blood HbCO decreased, indicating a shift of CO out of the vascular compartment. Muscle biopsies were performed and the loss of CO from the blood could be explained by increases in skeletal muscle, using assumed values for muscle mass.

In the present study we exercised human subjects at maximal oxygen uptake ($\dot{V}O_2$Max) and looked for a CO shift out of blood. We are asking the question, does intracellular PO_2 limit aerobic metabolism during exercise using the CO shift as an index of change in muscle intracellular PO_2.

Subjects exercised on a bicycle ergometer and breathed in a closed system which included a CO_2 absorber and pump. Oxygen was added to this rebreathing system and rate of oxygen uptake could be determined from the rate of oxygen delivery necessary to keep a constant gas PO_2 in the system. The closed system was used to prevent CO exchange across the lung during exercise. On the first day of each study we determined the work load - $\dot{V}O_2$ relationship. On the second day, venous catheters were inserted and the subject exercised at varying loads for time periods of 1½ to 8 minutes. The subjects rested for at least 40 minutes between "runs". Venous blood samples were taken just prior to and at the end of each run.

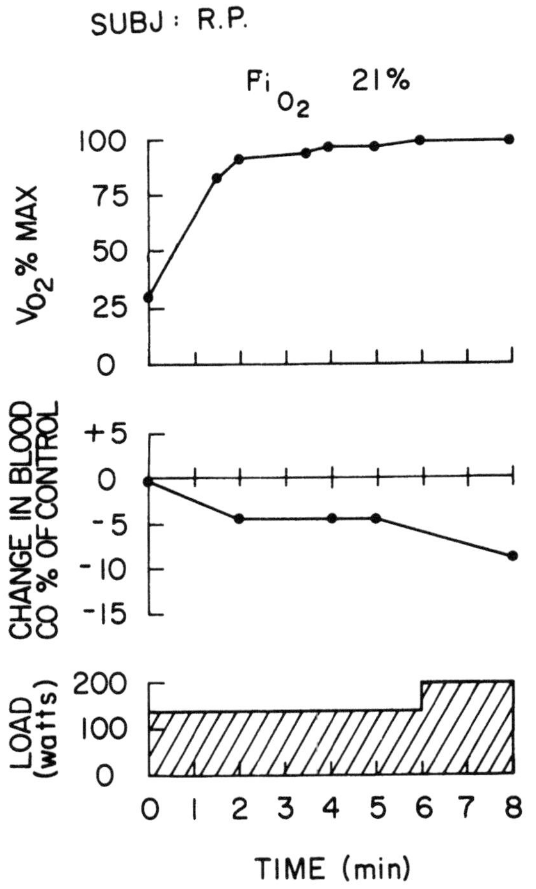

Figure 3. Exercise study in a normal male subject. Reproduced with the permission of the J. of Applied Physiology.

Figure 3 shows data; at the beginning of exercise where $\dot{V}O_2$Max was not reached, a small shift of CO out of blood is seen; later in the run where $\dot{V}O_2$Max was achieved, a larger shift out of blood occurred.

Fig. 4 shows data from several experiments where the effects of $\dot{V}O_2$Max exercise with the subject breathing 21% oxygen are compared with effects with the subject breathing 13-14% oxygen. $\dot{V}O_2$Max fell in all but one subject breathing 13-14% O_2. Likewise the shift of CO out of blood increased with $\dot{V}O_2$Max exercise breathing 13-14% O_2. (The one subject where the shift did not increase was the same subject where $\dot{V}O_2$Max did not decrease, breathing 13-14% O_2).

It is possible to compute increases in binding of CO to myoglobin, from shifts of CO out of blood, if the ratio of the relative sizes of total body hemoglobin and myoglobin stores in exercising muscle is known. We have computed increases in MbCO % sat. using a ratio of 9 which was computed in two different ways; from the relative sizes of the blood and extravascular CO space (2) and from published values of total body myoglobin and total body hemoglobin (5), both methods giving about the same value. We assume that the normal resting MbCO/HbCO is 1.0, as found in canine skeletal and cardiac muscle (3,4). CO binding to myoglobin is plotted in terms of the ratio of MbCO/HbCO (both given in % sat.). As indicated above, this ratio determines a value for mean myoglobin PO_2 (computed for a mean capillary PO_2 of 50 mm Hg), which is plotted on the X axis and the solid line shows the relationships of MbCO/HbCO to mean myoglobin PO_2. Average values of MbCO/HbCO and computed mean myoglobin PO_2 from previous animal experiments are shown for comparison with human data. Note that the increase in MbCO/HbCO at $\dot{V}O_2$Max exercise with the subject breathing 13-14% O_2 is practically identical to that found in canine hamstring muscle biopsies under conditions of severe hypoxic hypoxemia (PaO_2 less than 35 mm Hg) where there is evidence that the intracellular PO_2 was below the critical PO_2. There was increased CO binding with $\dot{V}O_2$Max exercise with the subject breathing 21% O_2 but less than expected if all exercising muscle fibers had falls in mean myoglobin PO_2 below the critical level, at least by comparison with our previous animal data.

Thirty % of the patients had very small shifts of CO out of blood during $\dot{V}O_2$Max breathing 21% O_2. Figure 6 illustrates such a subject. Data were collected over a three day period and results are consistent.

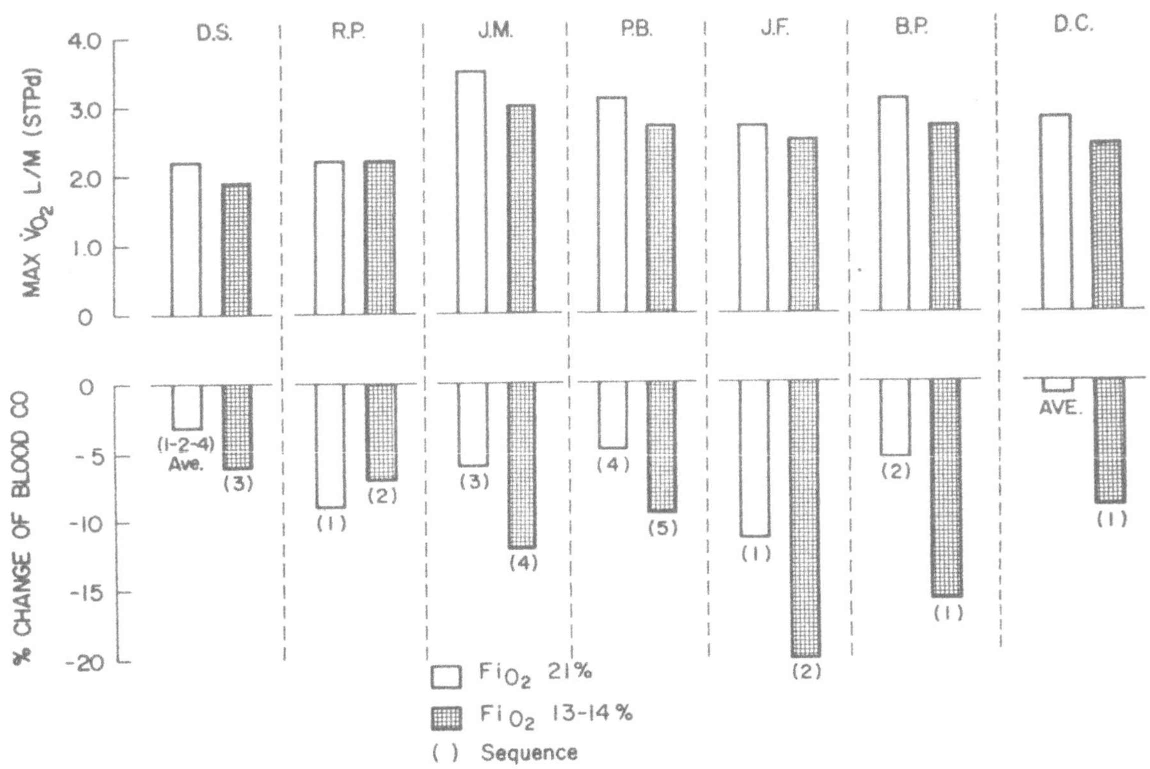

Figure 4. Exercise at maximal oxygen uptake breathing 21% and 13-14% O_2. Reproduced with the permission of the J. of Applied Physiology.

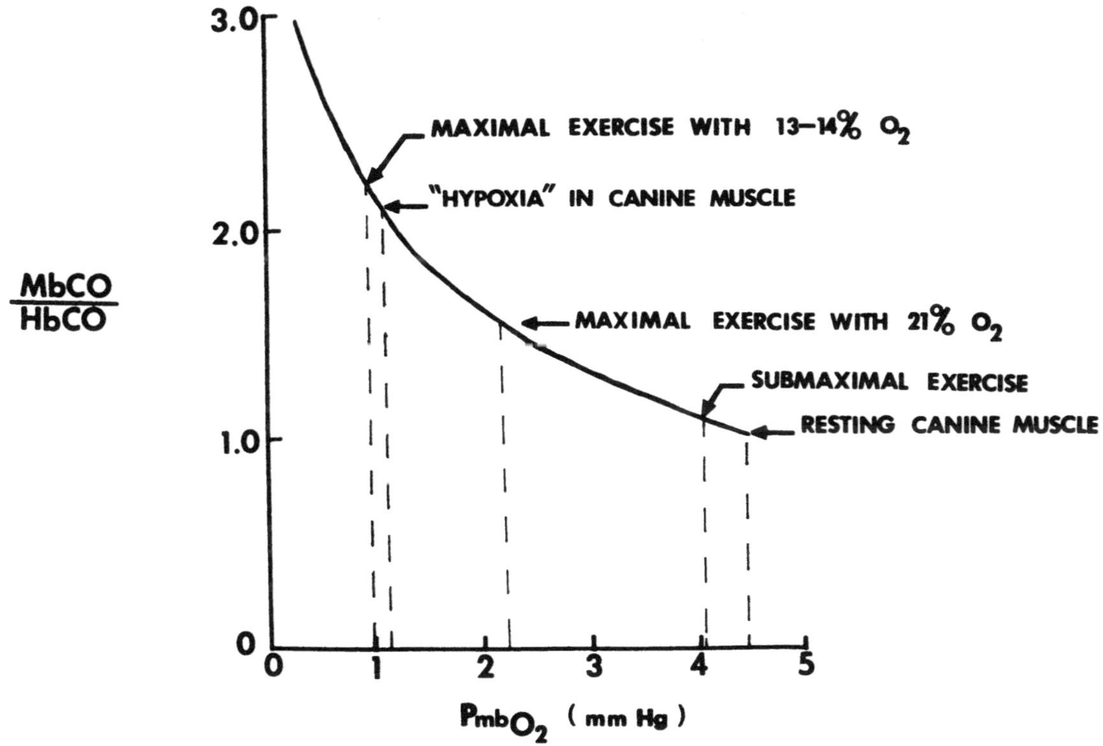

Figure 5. Average data obtained in exercise studies. Reproduced with the permission of the J. of Applied Physiology.

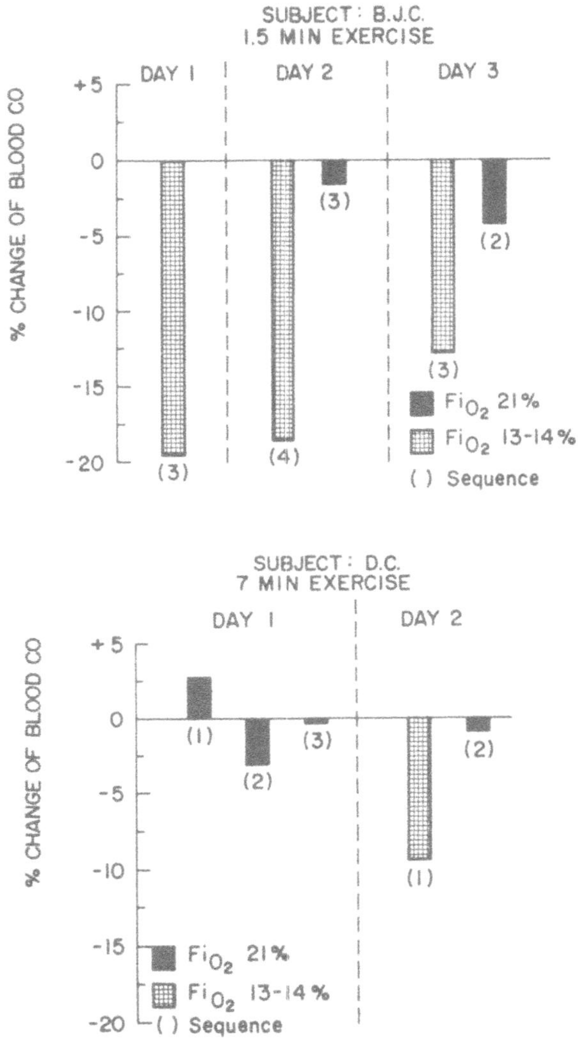

Figure 6. Data obtained on two subjects studied on several different days. These data illustrate the finding of a very small shift of CO at $\dot{V}O_2$Max exercise breathing 21% O_2 and a large "shift" with $\dot{V}O_2$Max exercise breathing 13-14% O_2.

In discussing these data, we have some evidence that we are nearly in steady state in that sequential blood sampling supports this (see Fig. 3); furthermore, studies of CO mixing in animals and in man show rapid mixing in the extravascular CO stores (6). We have performed experiments which suggest that changes in temperature or in capillary or intracellular pH of muscle cannot explain the CO shifts (1). Mean myoglobin PO_2 in this study represents a "mean" value for exercising muscle containing myoglobin.

In conclusion, our data suggest there is little or no fall in intracellular PO_2 with submax exercise, compared to the resting state. With exercise at $\dot{V}O_2Max$ with the subject breathing 21% O_2, on the whole, there is evidence of a fall in mean myoglobin PO_2 but not to levels which, by comparison with our previous animal studies, are expected if PO_2 is below the critical PO_2 in all exercising red muscle fibers. Mean myoglobin PO_2 does fall to these very low levels at $\dot{V}O_2Max$ exercising with the subject breathing 13-14% O_2. The surprising finding was, in a sizeable number of subjects, that $\dot{V}O_2Max$ was achieved without much of a fall in mean myoglobin PO_2, which suggests that oxygen availability is not limiting aerobic metabolism in these subjects. Our data are most consistent with several factors limiting maximal aerobic metabolism - one of these factors is O_2 availability, or delivery to sites of metabolism, the other factor or factors are unknown.

REFERENCES

1. Clark, B.J. and R.F. Coburn. Mean myoglobin oxygen tension during exercise of maximal oxygen uptake. J. Appl. Physiol. In press.
2. Coburn, R.F. The carbon monoxide body stores. Annals of the N.Y. Acad. of Sciences. 174:11-22, 1970.
3. Coburn, R.F. and L.B. Mayers. Myoglobin O_2 tension determined from measurements of carboxymyoglobin in skeletal muscle. Am. J. Physiol. 220:66-74, 1971.
4. Coburn, R.F., F. Ploegmakers, P. Gondrie and R. Abboud. Myocardial myoglobin oxygen tension. Am. J. Physiol. 224:870-876, 1973.
5. Drabkin, D.L. The distribution of the chromoproteins, hemoglobin, myoglobin and cytochrone c, in the tissue of different species and the relationship of the total content of each chromoprotein to body mass. J. Biol. Chem. 182:317-349, 1950.
6. Luomanmakki, K. and R.F. Coburn. Effects of metabolism and distribution of carbon monoxide on blood and body stores. Am. J. Physiol. 217:354-363, 1969.

Supported by Grant HL 10331 from the National Institutes of Health, Bethesda, Maryland

OXYGEN TRANSPORT IN SKELETAL MUSCLE: CAPILLARY GEOMETRY IN LONGITUDINAL SECTION

A.C. Groom, M. J. Plyley and G. Sutherland

Department of Biophysics, University of Western Ontario

London, Ontario N6A 5C1 Canada

For more than half a century researchers have recognised the need for quantitative measurements of the geometrical distribution of capillaries in the various organs of tissues of the body. Yet even today such information is very scarce in the literature, the reason, of course, being that spatial distribution of capillaries is a very complicated matter. Although it is easy to take pictures of the microcirculation it is not easy to reduce the information they contain to numerical form.

During the last 10 years or so, mathematical-modelling techniques that could be applied to the study of O_2 transport have become available but these cannot yet be used fully because the necessary input data needed for precise modelling is not available. Honig & Bordeau-Martini (1973) stated, with regard to the coronary circulation in particular:

"Nothing is presently known of the 3-dimensional arrangement of capillaries except that it is non-random. We are completely ignorant of the degree of order in alignment of arterial and venous ends of capillaries.... The extent of capillary branching is unknown, as is the orientation of the branches." They concluded "progress in O_2 transport is chiefly limited by lack of knowledge of parameters."

In our presentation at the Charleston meeting (Groom and Plyley, 1973) we discussed capillary geometry in transverse section and asked, "How many capillaries are needed around the perimeter of a muscle fibre to provide O_2 transport to the fibre?" In 18 different muscles from five mammalian species plus frog plus Japanese quail, we always found a mean value between 3 and 4, with an overall mean 3.6. This was independent of mean fibre diameter and seemed to provide a unifying concept underlying microvascular architecture in striated muscle. Put another way, we suggested that O_2 transport be looked at from the consumer's point of view (the individual fibre) and that we must consider diffusion from either a triangular or a square array of capillaries as seen in cross-section (this has been considered in more detail in a recent paper: Plyley and Groom, 1975). Grunewald (1973) presented a mathematical modelling study of the latter arrangement.

In this paper we want to discuss capillary geometry in longitudinal section. Because it is difficult to obtain sections which are cut precisely parallel to the fibres over distances of centimetres, we have used instead a thin, flat muscle which may be transilluminated. This is the sartorius of frog, about 0.7 mm thick. Frogs weighing 50 gm (approx.) were anesthetized by injection of urethane (3 to 4 mg/g) into the dorsal lymph sac. The abdominal aorta was cannulated and the blood in the hind limbs was washed out by infusing amphibian Ringer solution containing papaverine to induce maximal arteriolar vasodilation. Then a silicone elastomer (Microfil: Canton Biomedical Products, Inc.) of viscosity 20 cP was infused; it filled the capillary network and passed on into the venous outflow. After 15 - 20 minutes the material set and after one hour the hind quarters were cut off and fixed for several days in isotonic, buffered formalin. Later both sartorii were carefully dissected out and placed between glass microscope slides to keep them flat.

Each preparation was then placed on a micrometer stage under a light microscope and photographs of adjacent fields of view covering the whole muscle were taken. Then a large composite, such as shown in Fig. 1, was prepared. This picture, cut in two, for ease of presentation, shows the undersurface of the muscle; 'X' denotes the knee end (R. lateral aspect) and 'Y' the thigh end. Major vessels enter at the middle and at each end, then run across the muscle obliquely to the long axis. To determine which of the major vessels were arteries we infused additional sartorius muscles with Microfil whilst observing them under the dissecting microscope. When the elastomer just reached the arterial ends of the capillaries the infusion was stopped. Comparison of these muscles with these fully perfused enabled us to identify the arteries and veins. For ease of measurement magnified pictures of selected areas were prepared, such as that contained within the black frame on Fig. 1, as shown in Fig. 2. What we are seeing here is really the vessels in a layer of thickness equivalent to one fibre diameter. Vessels lying near the top of that layer are in clear focus whilst those near the bottom of the layer are fainter and less well focussed. In identifying the routes of vessels and branches on the composite picture we could check, where necessary, with the original muscle preparation, focussing up and down as necessary. In Fig. 2, vessels of the arterial inflow ('A')

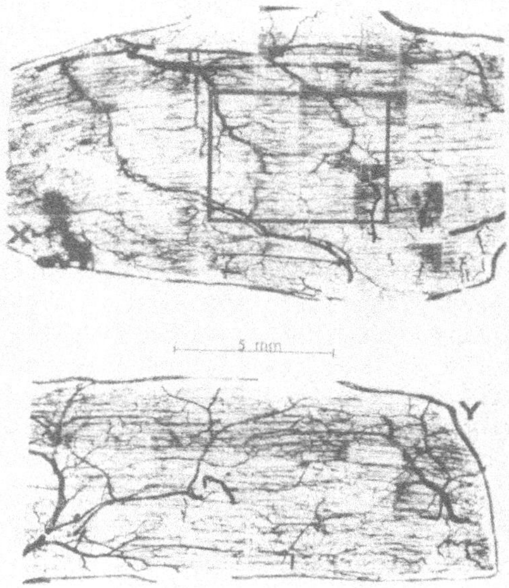

FIG. 1 - Composite photograph of microvasculature immediately beneath undersurface of frog sartorius muscle (see text).

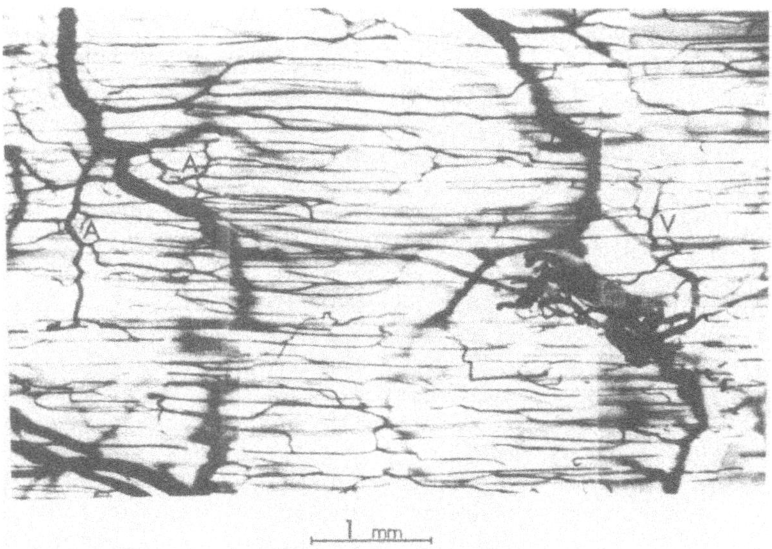

FIG. 2 - Magnified view of area of muscle shown bounded by the black rectangle in Fig. 1. Capillary paths running from arteriolar inflows 'A' to venular outflows 'V' were measured.

may be seen and a few mm to the right, the venules ('V') to which capillaries from ('A') run. One can thus follow along and measure a whole series of capillary paths between 'A' and 'V'. In amphibians the diameters of capillaries and fibres are larger than in mammals, and total capillary paths are longer; this makes our present task simpler.

From the arterioles at 'A' capillaries run both to the left and the right; similarly at the venules 'V' capillaries enter from both left and right. In between 'A' and 'V' the flow in adjacent capillaries is concurrent, as evidenced by observations of red cell flow in the living preparation and also by observations of branching angles in fixed preparations such as this. A very striking feature is the way the capillaries anastomose frequently, each vessel thus being divided into a number of segments. This has been noted previously in cat tenuissimus by Eriksson and Myrhage (1972).

In our studies we assign an identification number to each segment and measure its length. We list the various flow paths from A to V in terms of the segments involved and determine the total length of each path. We can also measure branching ratios and so forth. In this presentation we wish to concentrate on total path lengths (Fig. 3) and segmentation of capillaries (Figs. 4, 5, 6). It may be seen from Fig. 3 that the total path lengths varied from 1.5 to 7.5 mm with a mean of 3.70 ± 1.27 (S.D.). The frequency distribution was bell-shaped and near-normal, but slightly skewed toward longer paths. In contrast, segment lengths varied from 0.1 mm to 3.0 mm (approx.) and the distribution was decidedly exponential in character (Fig. 4). In fact a log-transformation yields a quite good Gaussian curve. The mean value was 0.88 mm and the variance 47% of the mean. In Fig. 5 the frequency distribution of the number of segments per path is shown for all the paths studied. The mean is 4.38 and the variance is large (79% of mean). This is not unlike a Poisson distribution. Subtracting ONE from the number of segments gives the number of branch points per path and this corresponds closely to a Poisson distribution, i.e. a set of randomly-distributed points along a capillary. One cannot really treat the data that way, however, since the path length was not constant. We can, however, study the variation of total path length with number of segments per path. A significant correlation ($p < .001$) exists between these two variables. In Fig. 6 is shown the relationship between mean path length and number of segments per path. The line shown is the least squares fit to the original data points (scattergraph); the numbers beneath each mean value indicate the number of separate observations involved.

From the point of view of constructing a suitable geometrical model for computations of O_2 diffusion to the fibres it is important to 'draw our data to scale' and we have chosen to

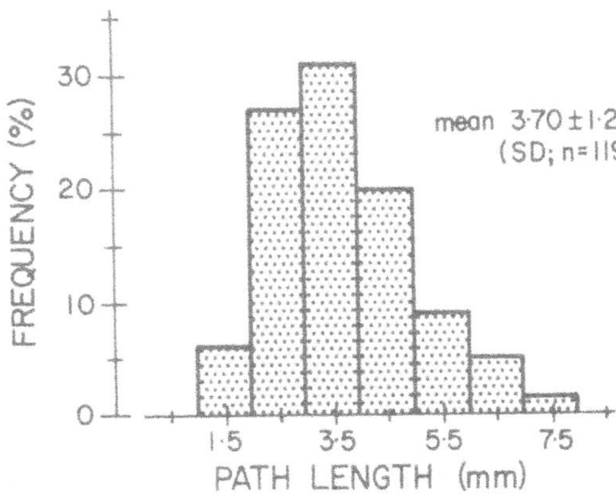

FIG. 3 - Frequency distribution of total path length for 119 capillary paths.

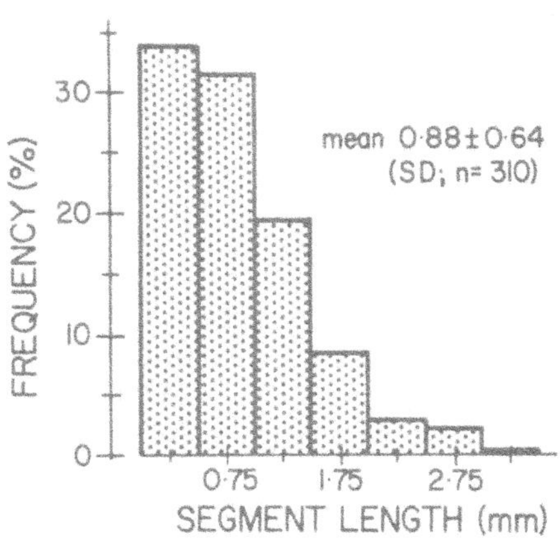

FIG. 4 - Frequency distribution of capillary segment lengths.

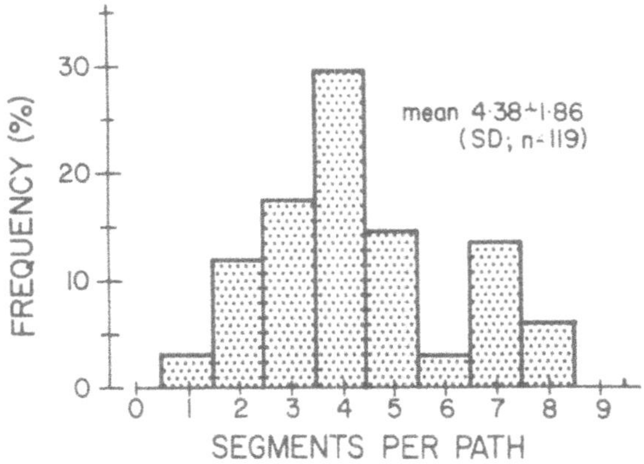

FIG. 5 - Frequency distribution of number of segments per total capillary path.

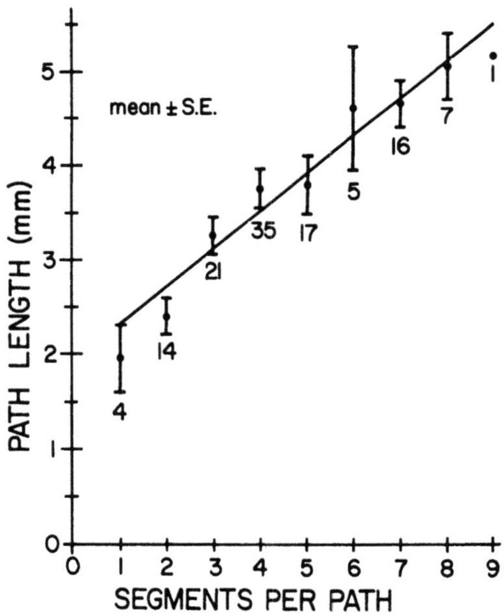

FIG. 6 - Mean total capillary path length versus number of segments per path.

express both segment and total path lengths as multiples of the mean fibre diameter. The mean segment length was 13 diameters (range 1.5 to 45) and total path length 55 diameters (range 22 to 110).

In summary, therefore, we have the following model for capillary distribution in discrete areas of frog sartorius muscle:

(i) arterial and venous ends of capillaries are aligned. The flow occurs in opposite directions in alternate regions as one scans from thigh to knee.

(ii) the flow is concurrent, at least in this layer of fibres nearest the undersurface of the muscle.

(iii) the mean capillary path length is 55 times the mean fibre diameter and three to four capillaries run alongside each muscle fibre. In transverse section these capillaries are seen as distributed around the perimeter of each fibre.

(iv) the capillaries anastomose with each other at approximately every 13 fibre diameters distance along their path, thereby forming a mean number of 4.4 capillary segments per path.

(v) approximately one-half of the branchings are divergent and one-half are convergent, thereby maintaining a mean of three to four capillaries around each fibre along its length.

These findings raise a very important and fundamental question that, to our knowledge, has not been previously considered: "What is the role or functional significance of the capillary anastomoses in skeletal muscle?" Clearly they can be thought of as a safety measure in the event of blockage of a vessel by a white blood cell or by a microthrombus. It seems to us, however,that the capillary anastomotic network is too highly developed for this to be its major role. An alternative possibility could be that the anastomoses play a basic role in maintaining or improving normal oxygenation of the tissue in working muscle. This is a very attractive possibility, but although it is our own 'prejudice' we have no experimental results to date that lend any support whatever to this view. We would certainly appreciate your critical discussion and any ideas about this intriguing question.

REFERENCES

Eriksson, E., and Myrhage, R. (1972). Microvascular dimensions and blood flow in skeletal muscle. Acta physiol. scand. 86, 211-222.

Groom, A.C. and Plyley, M.J. (1973). Oxygen transport in skeletal muscle: how many blood capillaries surround each fibre? in Oxygen Transport to Tissue: Ed. H. I. Bicher & D.F. Bruley. Adv. Exper. Med. Biol. Vol. 37B, 911-916.

Grunewald, W. (1973). Computer calculation for tissue oxygenation and the meaningful presentation of results. in: Oxygen Transport to Tissue: Ed. H. I. Bicher & D. F. Bruley. Adv. Exper. Med. Biol. Vol. 37B, 783-792.

Honig, C.R. and Bordeau-Martini, J. (1973). Oxygen and the number and arrangement of coronary capillaries: effect on calculated tissue P_{O_2}. in Oxygen Transport to Tissue: Ed. H. I. Bicher and D.F. Bruley. Adv. Exper. Med. Biol. Vol. 37A, 519-524, Plenum Press, N.Y.

Plyley, M.J. and Groom, A.C. (1975). Geometrical distribution of capillaries in mammalian striated muscle. Amer. J. Physiol. 228, (in press).

THE MEASUREMENT OF MYOCARDIAL MICROFLOW AND ITS REACTION TO HYPOXIA AND HYPERCAPNIA

K. Skolasinska, D. W. Lübbers, R. Wodick

Max-Planck-Institut fur Systemphysiologie
46 Dortmund, German Federal Republic

Determination of moycaridal microcirculation was performed using chemically generated hydrogen (Lübbers and Stosseck 1970). With this measurement a tissue area is involved which is smaller than the average capillary supply volume. Thus, the usual representation of flow as flow/volume cannot be strictly applied. As Wodick (1973) has shown this method measures the flow which penetrates a perpendicular plane, therefore the flow is expressed as flow/area. The radius of this plane is approximately 150 μm. Hydrogen coming from the generating "electrode" must pass through this theoretical plane, and the microflow is calculated as an intergrated value of flow velocity over the surface of this plane. To compare the flow/area with the flow/volume values we have to divide our value by the vessel lengths through which gas exchange can occur. Not being able to exactly determine the length of the vessels, we assume from a mean blood flow of 75 ml/100 g min a length of approximately 2.4 mm.

This method was used for calculating flow values quantitatively from single impulse H_2 desaturation curves as well as from the desaturation curves of continuously generated hydrogen. Changes of flow that occur during the continuous generation of H_2 can be expressed as quantitative values of flow, by means of a calibration curve.

Method. Experiments were performed on 20 rabbits, anesthetized with sodium pentobarbital (50 mg/kg). The animals were relaxed with Flaxedil and artificially ventilated with air. Respiratory CO_2 was measured and mean arterial blood pressure (MABP) from the dorsal aorta were recorded. The chest was opened at the midsternal line and the pericardial sac fixed to the thoracic wall to minimize the influence of respiratory movements. The flow probe consisting of a generating electrode (200 μm Ø) and a measuring electrode (100 μm Ø) with the distance between their centers being 315 μm. The probe was fixed to the heart with Histacryl blau (B. Braun, Co.). The site of fixation was between the left descendance coronary artery and the septal artery.

The following factors were taken into consideration to avoid the possibility of artifacts: 1.) The position of the probe should be longitudinal to the muscle fibers. 2.) The electrode should be placed in such a way to avoid large vessels and fatty tissue. 3.) The position of the reference electrode for eliminating, as such as possible, the influence of ECG. 4.) The fixation, in such a way, on the heart curvature that the contractile forces of the heart and the respiratory movements will not influence the course of the washout curve.

The single H_2 clearance curves were obtained by a current of 0.3 - 0.4 μA applied to the generating electrode for a period of 1 second. The signals from the measuring Pt wire were fed into a special amplifier which stored and amplified the signal according to the signal and time dependent function $p(t) \cdot t^{3/2}$ (for theoretical explanation see Wodick). The t_{max} of the curve was estimated by taking successive values for the geometrical mean of the curve according to the formula $\sqrt{t_1 \cdot t_2}$

where t_1, t_2 are coordinate pairs of time for which

$p(t_1) \cdot t_1^{3/2} = p(t_2) \cdot t_2^{3/2}$ (Fig. 1)

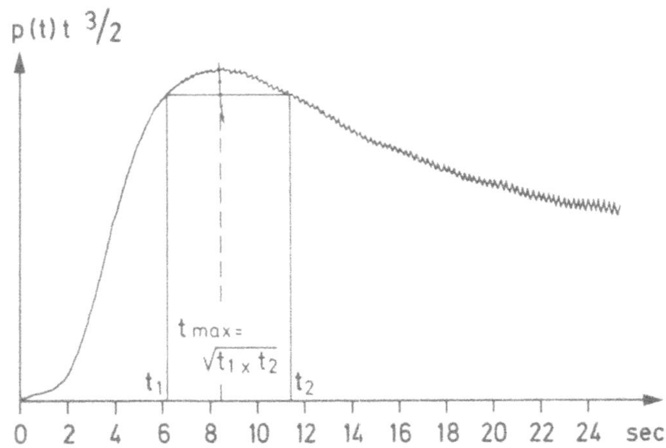

Figure 1

Estimation of t_{max} by the time dependent function curve

The mean flow velocity is given by the formula

$$\bar{v} = \frac{r}{\sqrt{t_1 \cdot t_2}}$$

where $\bar{v}$ is equal to flow per area, r is equal to the distance between the centers of the electrode wires.
The flow volume was expressed in $\frac{ml}{min \cdot 100\ g}$.

The continuous method for measuring flow was done by applying a continuous current of 0.31 - 0.53 μA to the generating electrode. Using the method described for the single pulses, it was possible to calculate the blood flow from the desaturation curve which is produced by switching off the continuous impulses. The calibration curve for the continuous method was obtained by plotting flow per area - $\bar{v}$ measured the desaturation curves against the values of π where π represents the height in millimeters of the continuous trace above base line, just before desaturation.

Experimental Procedure. To start each experiment several measurements of flow were made using the single impulse method in order to obtain average values of myocardial microflow. During periods (10 - 15 min) of continuously recording flow, the animals were ventilated with either a) 10 % O_2 in N_2 for 1 - 3 minutes, b) N_2 for 15 - 30 seconds, c) 9 % CO_2 in 21 % O_2 + balance N_2 for 1 - 3 minutes. For illustrating the dynamic changes of the epicardial microflow the following parameters were used: 1.) Response time for different stimuli. 2.) Time of maximal changes. 3.) Time of recovery to control values.

Results. From these experiments 170 single flow values were obtained. The flow velocity ranged from 0.012 - 0.067 mm/s and expressed in flow volume 32 - 170 ml/100 g . min. They were plotted against mean arterial blood pressure. The data points were fitted to a polynomial of the 8th order (see Fig. 2). A mean value for myocardial flow was calculated by averaging all values of flow for MABP between 35 - 80 mm Hg, this value was 68 $\pm$ 1.89. It should be noted that in the range from 35 - 80 mm Hg MABP the flow increase is not proportional to the increase of MABP. The flow values obtained from the desaturation curves of the continuously generated hydrogen agree very well with the values from single impulse hydrogen curves.

A 1 - 3 minute period of inhalation with 10 % O_2, while using the continuous method showed a 12 % increase in MABP above normal, and a quite variable increase in microflow. The increase in microflow +24 % above control precedes the increase in MABP by 6 - 8 s and remains at an elevated level for a longer period of time about 20 s (Fig. 3). Inhalation with 100 % N_2 for 10 - 30 s caused a

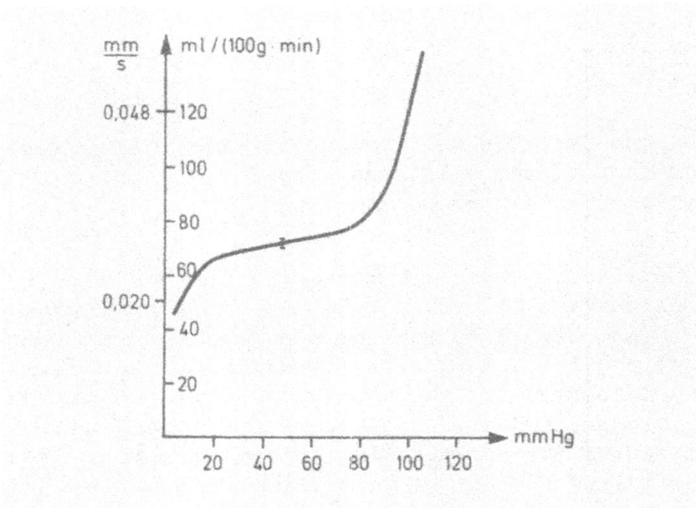

Figure 2
Relationship between flow units and mean arterial blood pressure

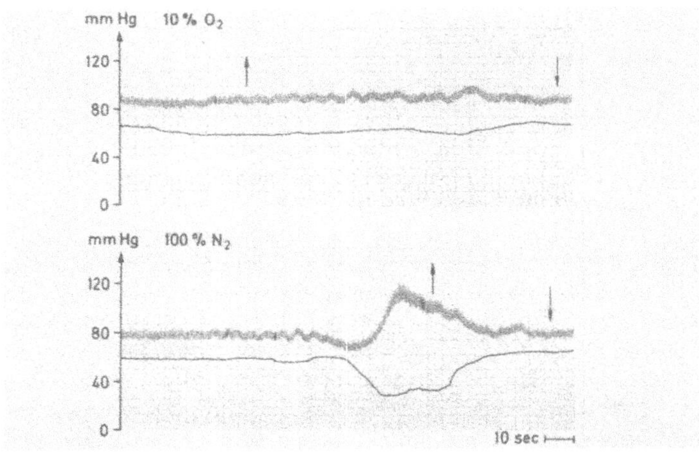

Figure 3
The effect of hypoxia and anoxia on the myocardial circulation. The lower curve represents flow from left to right

sharp 3-fold rise of the microflow (Fig. 4) usually simultaneously with increase of blood pressure to 45 % above control. This period of high increased flow was a short lasting on (15 - 20 s) and was followed by a long lasting (150 - 180 s) period of slight increased microflow independent from the arterial pressure which recovered earlier to the initial value. Significant changes in respiratory CO_2 were not observed.

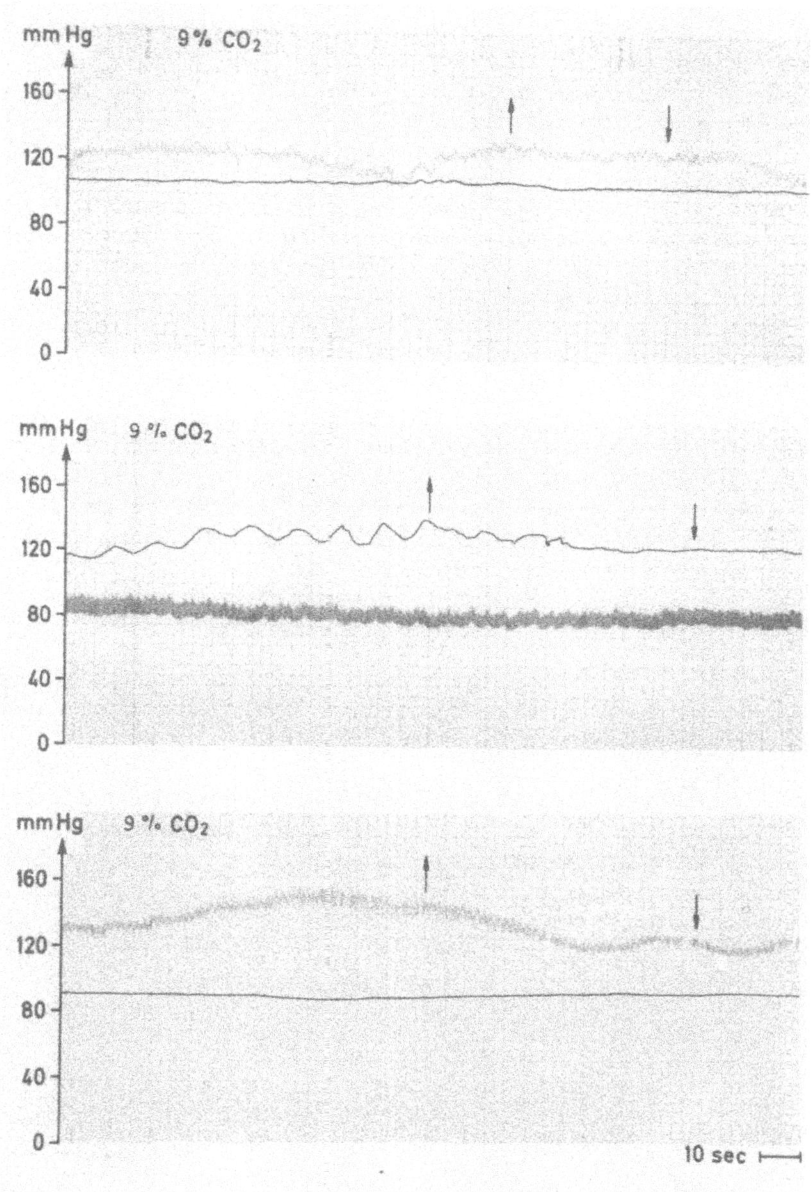

Figure 4
Different responses with 9 % CO_2 inhalation . Upper curves represent myocardial microflow, lower mean arterial blood pressure (from left to right)

Inhalation with 9 % CO_2 for 1 - 3 min caused in average a slight decrease of microflow (18 %). It must be noted that 3 types of responses were observed: decrease, increase and periodical changes of flow (Fig. 4). The effect of CO_2 was observed also after recovery to steady state for 140 - 180 s. The CO_2 level increase above 93 % of control.

Conclusion.

1) This method is useful for measuring the intergrated flow velocity in small areas. It should be possible in the future, with a multi-wire electrode to obtain more information about the myocardial microflow system.
2) The fact that we have been able to observe autoregulatory effects in the myocardial microflow system, indicates that with this method real physiological effects can be observed.
3) Myocardial microcirculation can reflect the blood flow changes of larger vessels, for example the flow increase in deep hypoxia. On the other hand a stimulus that has a given effect on the general circulation can produce diversified responses in the microcirculation such as the effect of increased CO_2 inhalation.

References

1. Lübbers D. W., Stosseck, K.: Quantitative Bestimmung der lokalen Durchblutung durch elektrochemisch im Gewebe erzeugten Wasserstoff. Naturwissensch. 57, 311 - 312 (1970)

2. Wodick, R.: Möglichkeiten und Grenzen der Bestimmung der Blutversorgung mit Hilfe der lokalen Wasserstoffclearance. Habilitationsschrift, Bochum 1973

SUMMARY OF DISCUSSION - SESSION XII:

OXYGEN SUPPLY OF MUSCLE TISSUE

Chairmen: C. R. Honig and K. Kunze

Paper of Dr. Honig

Dr. Kunze asked whether the intrinsic neurones participate in reflex reactions involving the central nervous system. Honig replied that the long post-ganglionic fibers from the sympathetic chain which mediate active sympathetic vasodilation appear to synapse on the non-adrenergic intrinsic neurones. (Fibers which mediate vasoconstriction do not synapse in the muscle). The significance of this is that the intrinsic neurones are a common anatomical element in active sympathetic vasodilation and post-contraction vasodilation.

Dr. Duhm asked how Honig's hypothesis applies to the heart, and what initiates activity in the intrinsic nerves. Honig replied that he has no information as to the possible role of intrinsic nerves in myocardium. In skeletal muscle it is likely that the stimulus to intrinsic nerves is deformation produced by contraction. Other non-myelinated C fibers are excellent low-threshold mechanoreceptors, and one might expect intrinsic nerves to behave similarly.

Dr. Groom asked about the extent of the ramification of an intrinsic neurone. Honig replied that processes of one neurone are probably confined to a single arteriole.

Paper of Dr. Kunze

There was considerable interest in the origin of the oscillations. Dr. Kreuzer suggested that respiratory changes in PaO_2 may appear in tissue PO_2. Dr. Goldstick raised the possibility that the oscillations are electrical artifacts from muscle fibers. Kunze replied that motor unit activity in the muscles was monitored continuously, and that results exclude this possibility. Moreover, the oscillations are best demonstrated in fully relaxed muscle. Dr. Honig commented that oscillation in intercapillary distance occurs in chronically denervated muscles, and should be accompanied by corresponding oscillation in tissue PO_2. This shows that local as well as systemic mechanisms can produce oscillation.

Paper of Drs. Whalen, et al.

Dr. Honig pointed out that the central point at tissue is whether areas of ischemia exist in muscles of small animals sufficient, in the aggregate, to account for the flow dependence of $\dot{V}O_2$.Whalen's older observations indicate that such areas exist, his new ones indicate that they do not. Dr. Honig reported that Dr. LaCelle, Univ., of Rochester, has found cells in mouse cremaster in which PO_2 is not distinguishable from zero. In these experiments care was taken to position the PO_2 probe at the venous end of capillaries, and to average PO_2 over small time intervals (about 10 sec). These procedures should increase the probability that hypoxic cells will be encountered. Dr. Honig also pointed out that measurements of $\dot{V}O_2$ and intercapillary distance in rat gracilis indicate that regions of zero PO_2 should exist in that muscle under normal circumstances.

Whalen replied that he did not think classical hypoxia could be the answer in cat muscle, because $\dot{V}O_2$ increased up to 5 fold with flow, whereas in only about 5% of locations was PO_2 below 5 mmHg. Whalen suggested that in vivo, with intact nerves, it may be different.

Dr. Jöbsis raised the possibility that there may be O_2-utilizing systems in the muscle not mediated by cytochrome A_3. He suggested that such mechanisms may contribute more importantly under certain circumstances than presently believed.

Dr. Siesjö pointed out that similar questions have raised with regard to brain, and asked whether biochemical studies have been done on muscle to support the notion that areas of anaerobiasis exist. Whalten replied that he has not made such measurements.

Dr. DiPrampero reported experiments on dog gracilis muscles perfused in situ. At rest, $\dot{V}O_2$ was independent of Q, but during isotonic tetani 0.2 - 1.2 sec. in duration, at rate of 20/min, $\dot{V}O_2$ became dependent on Q. there were no changes in lactic acid output, however, suggesting that no change in anaerobic metabolism occurred.

In summary, Whalen stated that at present it is not known whether classical hypoxia in small regions of the tissue or unorthodox biochemistry explains the flow dependence of $\dot{V}O_2$ in muscle.

Paper of Drs. Turek and Kreuzer

Dr. Thews noted that myocardial metabolism is not in a steady state, due to rhythmic fluctuation in Q and $\dot{V}O_2$, and asked what effect this might have on the dissociation curve. Turek replied that he had no data on which to base an opinion.

Dr. Versmold pointed out that a constant PaO_2 is assumed in Turek's calculations, and that in hypoxemia due to right-left shunt SaO_2 rather than PaO_2 should be nearly constant. In view of this, he suggested that the beneficial effect of a curve shift, (produced for example, by exchange transfusion in new-borns), would be diminished, but never reversed at low PaO_2. Turek replied that his colleague, Dr. Frans, had made calculations which supported Dr. Versmold's suggestion.

Dr. Duhm observed that Turek explored changes in mixed venous PO_2 at a given extraction, but did not consider the effect of a curve shift on O_2 extraction at a given mixed-venous PO_2. Turek answered that animals adapted to high altitude have the same $\dot{V}O_2$ as controls, that cardiac $\dot{V}O_2$ is not dependent on O_2 delivery, and that changes in O2 affinity change venous O_2 tension rather than $\dot{V}O_2$. Turek therefore considers change in venous PO_2 rather than change in unloading at constant venous PO_2 to be the more appropriate analysis.

Dr. Siesjö commented that brain blood flow increases about 5-fold in severe hypoxia, and that in this situation CaO_2 limits $\dot{V}O_2$. Under these conditions he believes a left-shift of the dissociation curve would be beneficial. Turek agreed that a left shift might be favorable in very severe arterial hypoxia.

Paper of Drs. Ernst, Nelson and DiPalma

Questions about the size, properties and location of the cathodes and reference electrodes were raised by several people, but were not resolved in discussion.

Paper of Drs. Skolazinska, Lübbers and Wodick

Dr. Forster was concerned about the extent to which the H_2 clearance method may be influenced by change in effective diffusion coefficient for H_2. Dr. Lübbers replied that the equation which describes the current at the measuring electrode includes 3 constants which depend on diffusion as well as convection. The ratio of two of these constants, however, depends only on convection. The flow per area is found from this ratio to be:

$$\bar{v} = r \frac{C}{A}$$

where r is the distance between the H_2 generating site and the detecting site. Thus v is dependent only on flow. For details consult Pflüger's Arch. 348: 225 - 238, 1974.

Dr. Siesjö asked whether venous pressure was considered in developing pressure-flow curves. Dr. Lübbers replied that venous pressure was not measured, but should not strongly influence the shape of the curves.

Paper of Drs. R. F. Coburn and B. J. Clark

Dr. Cerretelli remarked that the drop in $\dot{V}O_2$ max induced by 13 - 14% O_2 seemed low for the type of exercise used, and asked the consequences of such an underestimate for the conclusions drawn. Coburn replied that $\dot{V}O_2$-load curves were performed to define $\dot{V}O_2$ max in experiments in which blood samples were drawn. At apparent $\dot{V}O_2$ max no increase in $\dot{V}O_2$ was observed when load was increased for 1 min.

Paper of Drs. A. C. Groom and M. H. Plyley

Dr. Grunewald pointed out that segment lengths reported in this study are minimum values, attained only when all capillaries and anastomoses are open. In resting muscle, and in msucles doing submaximal work some anastomoses would be closed, and capillary segment lengths would be correspondingly longer. Dr. Grunewald than asked whether the frequency distribution of capillary segment lengths is significantly different in various muscles. Groom replied that other muscles have not yet been studied quantitatively, but that visual impression suggests the arrangement described is a common one.

Dr. Honig stated that comparable capillary branch patterns have been observed in living rat heart in situ. Dr. Honig asked wether capillaries which arise from one arteriole anastomose with those from another, for this would tend to minimize longitudinal O_2 gradients in capillaries. Groom replied that such anastomoses do exist, but most appear to occur among capillaries derived from a single arteriole.

Dr. Fletcher asked whether capillary segment length is the same before and after branching. Groom replied that no difference was observed.

Perinatal Oxygen Supply

OXYGEN UPTAKE OF THE GUINEA PIG AT DECREASED AND INCREASED MATERNAL PLACENTAL BLOOD FLOW

Waldemar Moll and Joachim Herberger

Institut für Physiologie

Universität Regensburg

The transfer of oxygen from the maternal organism to the fetal tissue is a complex mechanism: As indicated in fig. 1 oxygen is (1) transported to the placenta by maternal placental flow, (2) transferred to the fetal umbilical blood, (3) delivered via the fetal arteries to the fetal capillaries and finally (5) transferred by diffusion to the fetal mitochondria.

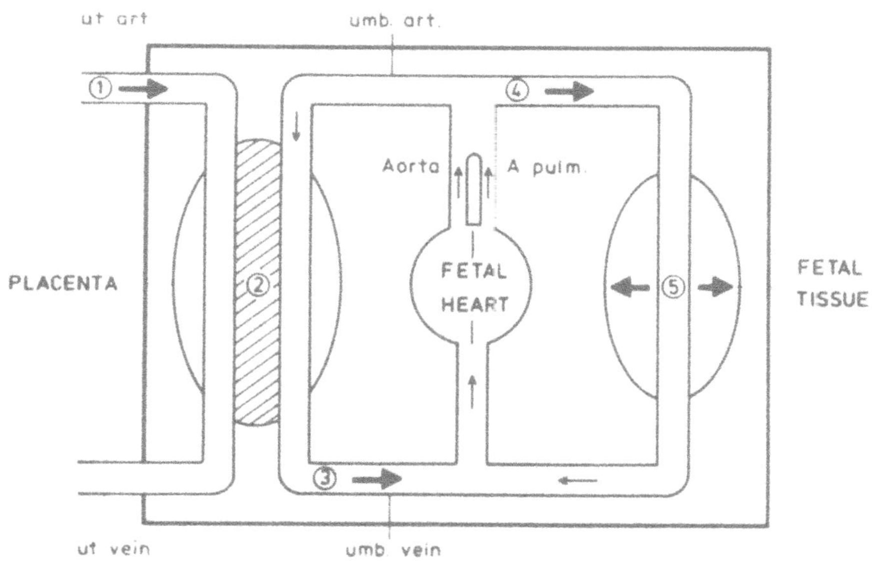

Fig. 1: A simple model of the fetoplacental unit (after MOLL, 1973b).

Thus, the oxygen tension inside the growing fetal tissue is a function of a series of parameters.Maternal placental flow of hemoglobin is one of the most important parameters; it is the maternal flow that is prone to various disturbances during birth and possibly even before.

In previous studies, we tried to obtain a quantitative understanding of the relation between maternal placental flow and fetal oxygen supply by studying mathematical models like in fig. 1 (MOLL, 1972; MOLL, 1973a) and by measuring placental oxygen transfer during spontaneous fall of placental blood flow (KÜNZEL and MOLL, 1972). It is the aim of the present paper to measure placental oxygen uptake after arbitrary changes of uterine blood flow in both directions, i.e. after an increase as well as after a decrease of maternal placental flow. In order to be able to increase as well as to decrease placental flow we shunted the aorta and the final part of a uteroplacental artery. To explain this procedure, we have to deal first with the location of the flow limiting resistance of the hemochorial placenta.

THE AORTO-SPIRAL-SHUNT AS A WAY TO EXPERIMENTALLY INCREASE MATERNAL PLACENTAL FLOW

The hemochorial placenta (the placenta of rodents, rabbits and primates including man) seems to be associated with a very peculiar type of uteroplacental arteries: The spiral arteries. These arteries progressively dilate when they approach to the placenta. In fig. 2 a cast of uteroplacental artery is shown. The vessel is narrow at its central part and wide at its peripheral part. This shape indicates that the flow limiting resistance of the uteroplacental vascular system is located in the central parts of the arteries, opposite of the situation in the conventional vascular beds where the resistance is located in the periphery. This view is substantiated by physiological measurements: Pressure measurements in the spiral arteries (MOLL and KÜNZEL, 1972, 1973) showed that more than 2/3 of the resistance to placental flow is located upstream of the spiral arteries. The central location of the vascular resistance to placental flow was confirmed by measuring the vascular resistance of the placenta. The vascular resistance of the guinea pig placenta was found to be too low (around 1 mm Hg min/ml) as to be an essential limitation of placental flow.

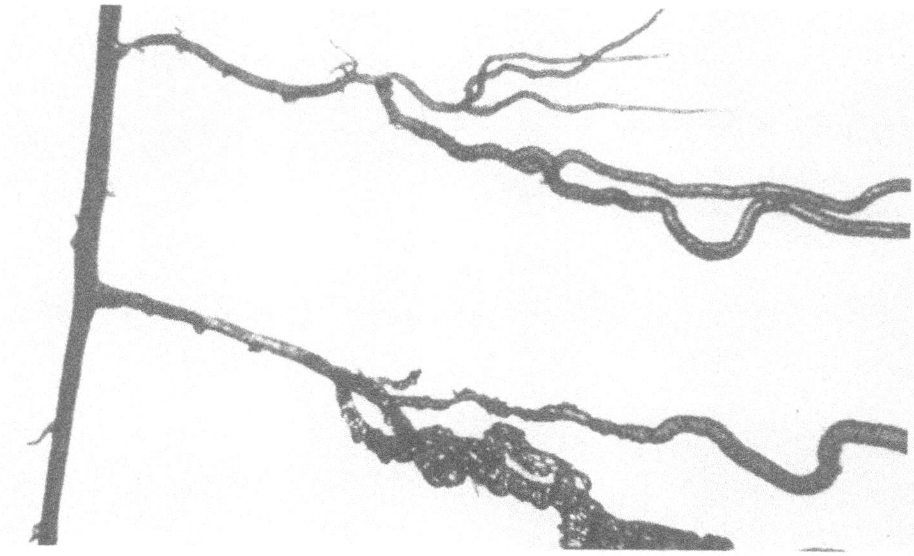

Fig. 2: Plastoid cast of the final part of a uteroplacental artery. Note the peripheral dilation.

We took advantage of the central location of the vascular resistance to get data on placental oxygen uptake at increased placental flow rate. As indicated in fig. 3, we connected the aorta through the carotid artery with the spiral artery in order to circumvent the flow limiting central portions of the uteroplacental arteries. The preparation yielded higher rates of placental blood flow (up to 30 ml/min) than measured ever before. Using a clamp placental blood flow could be decreased. In other words: The preparation allows to vary placental flow in a wide range around the value found in anaesthetized guinea pigs.

EXPERIMENTAL DETAILS

Preparation. The guinea pigs were anaesthetized with Ketamin (50 mg/kg) and Diacepam (2 ml). The uterus was exposed. Its surface was covered by plastic sheets. The temperature of the uterine surface was controlled by heating lamps. The animals were given heparin (200 IE). To set up the aorto-spiral shunt the carotid artery and the spiral artery were canulated with 1 mm wide polyethylene tubings, which were connected with a 3 mm wide silastic tubing. The shunted blood was adjusted to body temperature by a thermostatted water jacket.

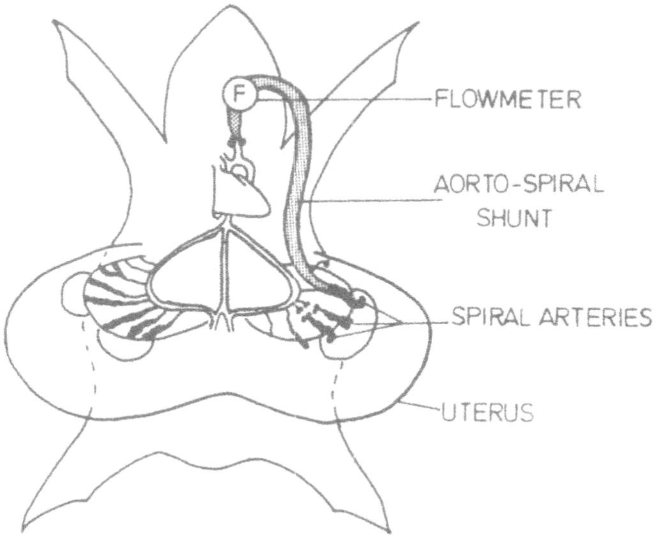

Fig. 3: The aorto-spiral shunt.

<u>Measurements</u>. The oxygen concentration was determined by a coulometric method (Lex-O_2-Con). The placental flow was monitored by an electromagnetic flowmeter. The fetal heart rate was determined with an ultrasonic device. Hemoglobin concentration was measured spectrophotometrically. Placental oxygen transfer was calculated from placental flow and AVD_{O2}.

PLACENTAL O_2 UPTAKE AT DECREASED PLACENTAL FLOW RATE

In fig 3, the measured placental oxygen uptake (●) at decreased placental flow rate is plotted against the flow of hemoglobin across the maternal placenta, i.e. the product of blood flow and hemoglobin concentration. It can be seen that oxygen uptake is nearly proportionate to the placental flow of hemoglobin. This is to be expected on the basis of a most simple model of the fetoplacental unit (KÜNZEL and MOLL, 1972). The values are in good agreement with previous data (O). This agreement is surprising as the approach and the methods used were quite different in the 2 studies. In the present study, placental oxygen uptake was measured after arbitrary changes of blood flow in an artificially perfused placenta. In the previous study oxygen transfer was measured during spontaneous changes of placental blood flow the placenta being perfused via the uterine arteries.

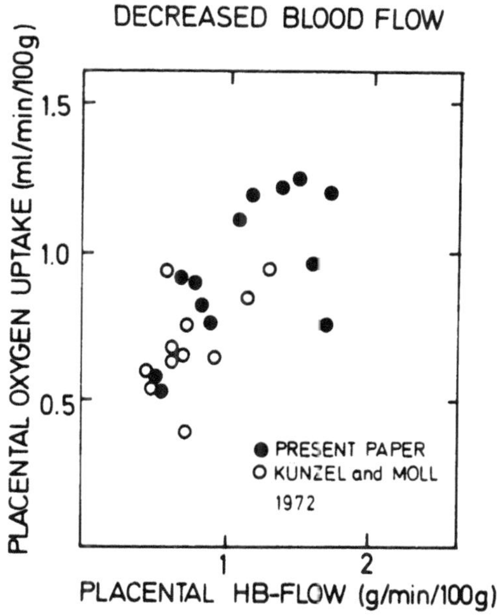

Fig. 4: Placental O_2 transfer at decreased flow of Hb.

PLACENTAL OXYGEN UPTAKE AT INCREASED PLACENTAL FLOW

In 6 animals placental hemoglobin flow was increased above the value determined in anaesthetized animals (hemoglobin flow in anaesthetized animals is around 2.2 g/min per 100 g of fetal weight according to the maternal hemoglobin concentration, the blood pressure and the vascular conductance of the placenta). In fig. 5, placental oxygen uptake is related to placental hemoglobin flow over the whole range of flow. The results were quite unexspected: It can be seen that placental oxygen uptake still rises when placental hemoglobin flow surpasses 2.2 g/min/100g. The slope of the curve, however, is much less than in the range of decreased flow. At flow rates above 3 g/min/100g placenta oxygen uptake seems to level off. The increase of placental oxygen uptake was correlated with an increase of fetal heart rate (fig. 6). At fetal oxygen uptake of 1.1 ml/min per 100 g of fetal weight fetal heart rate was found to be 220 beats per minute. Both values were found previously in nonanaesthetized animals (MOLL et al., 1970). Fetal heart rate, however, exceeded 250 beats per minute when fetal oxygen uptake rose to more than 1.5 ml/min/100g.

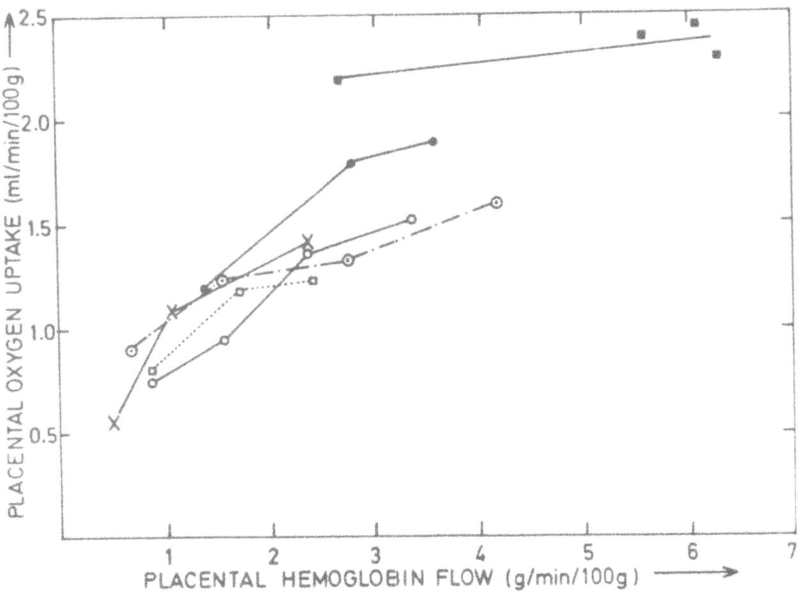

Fig. 5: Placental oxygen transfer at decreased and increased placental flow of hemoglobin.

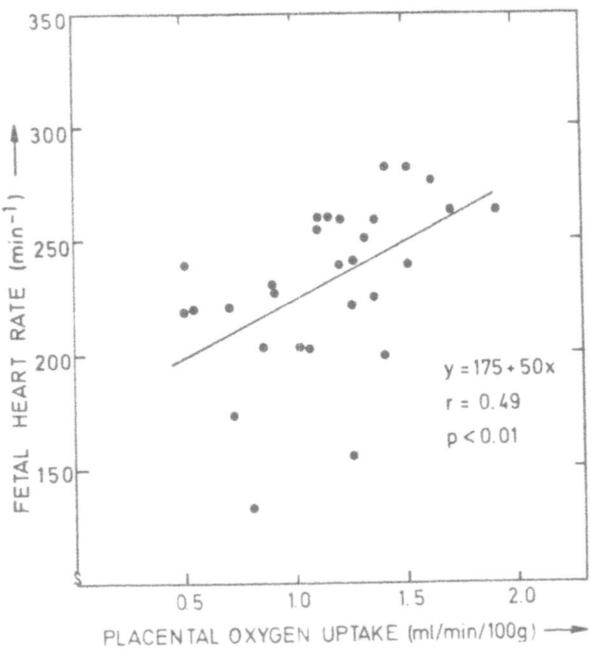

Fig. 6: Fetal heart rate related to placental oxygen uptake.

The present results indicate that placental oxygen transfer is not at its maximum at the probably normal placental flow of 2.2 g/min/100 g; variations of placental flow result in variations of oxygen uptake. The observations on the fetal heart rate indicate that the action of the fetal heart is limited by the oxygen supply.

It may be speculated that the observed variations of placental oxygen transfer represent variations of growth intensity and that placental flow limits fetal growth. It has been found in rabbits by BRUCE and ABDUL-KARIM (1973) that variations of growth rate are associated with variations of placental flow rate. In this laboratory (MOLL and PFOERRINGER, unpublished results) we found that bigger fetuses are supplied by more spiral arteries than smaller ones. All these findings indicate that maternal placental flow limits fetal growth. The variations of fetal growth may be reflected by variations of fetal oxygen uptake found in this study.

CONCLUSIONS

As the flow limiting resistance of the uteroplacental vascular system is located in the central parts of the arterial system, blood flow can be varied in a wide range around the normal value found in anaesthetized guinea pigs when an aorto-spiral shunt is set up; placental oxygen transfer can be observed at decreased and increased placental flow under these conditions.

At decreased placental flow, placental oxygen uptake is almost proportionate to the placental flow of hemoglobin. This observation is in accordance with conclusions made on the basis of simple models of the feto-placental unit.

At increased placental flow, placental oxygen uptake is increased above the value found in unanaesthetized animals. The results indicate that normal variations of placental flow result in variations of fetal oxygen uptake. The conclusions are in agreement with the view that placental blood flow is a limiting factor of fetal growth.

REFERENCES

BRUCE, N.W. and R.W. ABDUL-KARIM: Relationship between fetal weight, placental weight and maternal placental circulation in the rabbit at different stages of gestation. J. Reprod. Fertil., 32, 15-24 (1973)

KÜNZEL, W. and W. MOLL: Uterine O_2 consumption and blood flow of the pregnant uterus. Z. Geburtsh. Perinat., 178, 108-117 (1973)

MOLL, W.: Gas exchange in concurrent, countercurrent and crosscurrent flow systems. The concept of the fetoplacental unit. In: Longo, L.D. and H. Bartels (ed.): Respiratory gas exchange and blood flow in the placenta. U.S. Department of health, education and welfare, Bethesda, Maryland, 1972

MOLL, W.: Placental function and oxygenation in the fetus. In: Bruley, D.F. and H.I. Bicher (ed.): Oxygen transport to tissue, advances in experimental medicine and biology. Vol. 37B, Plenum Press, New York, London, 1973a

MOLL, W.: Oxygen supply of the human fetus. Bull. Physio-path. resp., 9, 1345-1364 (1973b)

MOLL, W. and W. KÜNZEL: The blood pressure in arteries entering the placentae of guinea pigs, rats, rabbits and sheep. Pflügers Arch., 338, 125-131 (1973)

MOLL, W., W. KÜNZEL and H.G. ROSS: Gas exchange of the pregnant uterus of anaesthetized and unanaesthetized guinea pigs. Respir. Physiol., 8, 303-310 (1970)

DEVELOPMENT AND ADAPTATION OF HEART MITOCHONDRIAL RESPIRATORY CHAIN FUNCTION IN FETUS AND IN NEWBORN

C. W. Goodwin, L. Mela, C. Deutsch, R. E. Forster,
L. D. Miller, and M. Delivcria-Papadopoulos

Departments of Physiology, Pediatrics and Surgery,
University of Pennsylvania, Philadelphia, Pennsylvania

The ability of mitochondria to undergo alterations in response to changes in oxygen availability is suggested by the data from animals studied at high altitude (1,2). During the transition from intrauterine to extrauterine life, the animal experiences a marked change in oxygen environment which might affect mitochondrial function. In order to investigate the roles of development and adaptation, freshly isolated cardiac mitochondria from lambs and puppies were studied. The development of mitochondrial respiratory function was examined in fetal lambs. The changes in respiratory capacity, cytochrome concentration, and calcium transport subsequent to the increase in oxygen environment following birth were determined in newborn lambs and puppies.

METHODS

Fetal lambs near term were delivered by Caesarean section after the ewe had been anesthetized by a high epidural block. Determination of fetal age was based on the known length of the pregnancy and on an assumed gestational period of 150 days. Fetal puppies were delivered after maternal anesthesia was induced with sodium pentobarbital (30 mg/kg). Newborn lambs and puppies were studied at various ages up to two weeks. Fetal puppies at term, which had not breathed, served as controls for the canine postnatal studies. The newborn animals were anesthetized by intracisternal injection of lidocaine (10 mg.).

Immediately following anesthesia, the chest was entered through a sternotomy incision, and ascending aortic blood was sampled anaerobically. P_{O2}, P_{CO2} and pH were determined with standard calibrated electrodes. After collection of blood samples, the ventricular portion of the heart was excised, placed in ice-cold buffer, and minced with sharp scissors. The tissue was then gently homogenized. The mitochondria were isolated in a medium composed of 0.225 M mannitol, 0.075 M sucrose and 100μM EDTA at $0^{\circ}C$ as previously described (3). However, no bacterial proteinase (Nagarse) was used in animals less than ten days of age.

Mitochondrial respiratory activity was determined by a Clark electrode, using 10mM glutamate plus 10mM malate, or 10mM succinate in presence of 10μM rotenone, as substrates and ADP as the phosphate acceptor. Cytochrome concentrations were determined in a Chance dual-wavelength spectrophotometer. Cytochrome c and cytochrome oxidase ($a+a_3$) were measured at 550-540 nm and 445-460 nm respectively, and their extinction coefficients of 19 mM^{-1} and 160 mM^{-1} were used for calculations (4).

Mitochondrial calcium transport activity was measured in the same spectrophotometer using murexide as the calcium indicator at 540-507 nm according to the method of Mela and Chance (5). Protein concentrations were determined by the Biuret method.

RESULTS

Mitochondria display maximal respiratory activity in the presence of ADP (State 3), and the changes in this active state were followed during the animals' development (6). All preparations exhibited tight coupling, as reflected by respiratory control ratios (RCR) greater than 10. As seen in Figure 1, State 3 respiratory capacity of fetal lamb cardiac mitochondria rose from around 75 nmoles O_2 utilized /min/mg mitochondrial protein at 30 days preterm to 140 nmoles/min/mg protein at term. Presumably, the oxygen tension in the fetal tissues is relatively constant (and low). Following birth of the lambs, State 3 oxygen uptake dropped markedly from 140 to 60 nmoles/min/mg protein by postnatal day four. In Figure 2, the same pattern of postnatal respiratory activities is seen in newborn puppies. Cardiac mitochondria from fetal tissue at term obtained before breathing exhibited a respiratory rate of about 70 nmoles/min/mg. protein. This level fell to 20 nmoles/min/mg protein by postnatal day four and then began to climb more slowly toward adult levels.

In the fetal puppy the oxygen tension in the ascending aorta is quite low and varies between 8 and 15 torr (mean 12.0). Following birth there is a rapid and quite linear climb to around 70 torr by the fourth postnatal day, after which oxygen tension rises more slowly toward adult levels. As seen in Figure 3, there appears to be a direct relation between arterial oxygen tension and mitochondrial respiratory capacity.

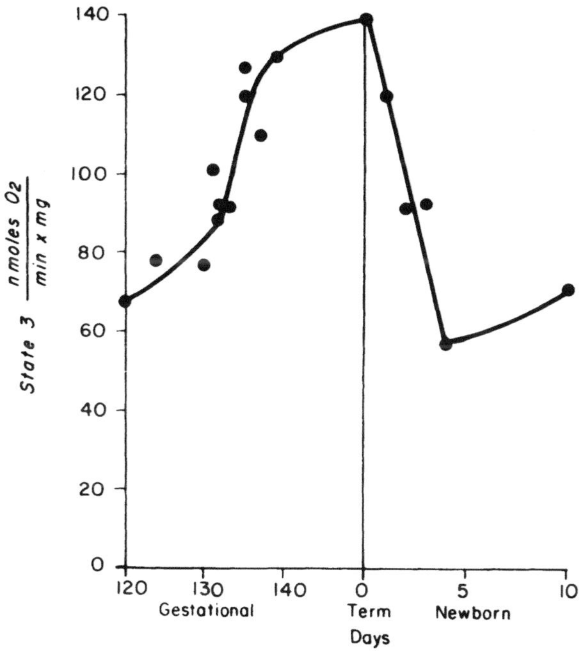

Figure 1. State 3 respiratory capacity in heart mitochondria of lambs as a function of age, expressed in nmoles/min/mg protein. Each point represents one animal.

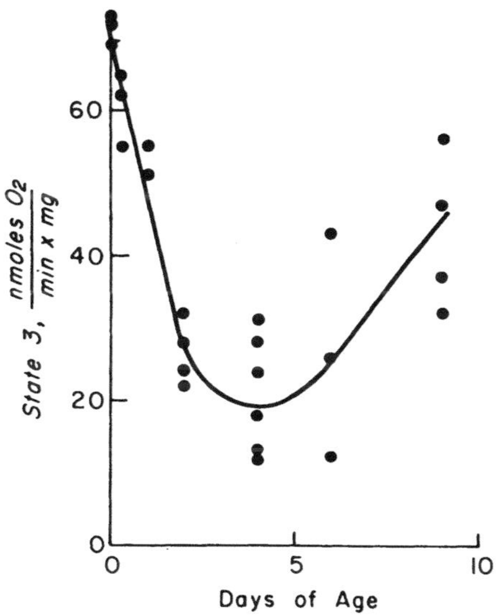

Figure 2. State 3 respiratory capacity in puppy heart mitochondria as a function of postnatal age. Each point represents one animal.

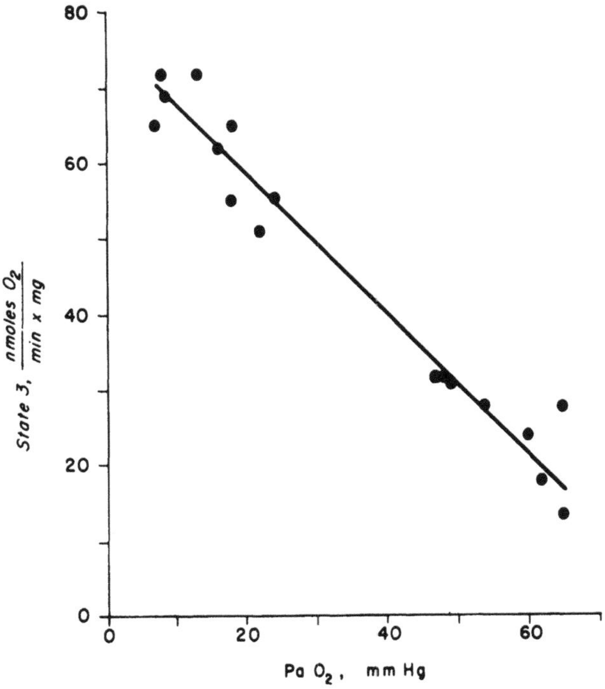

Figure 3. Changes in State 3 respiratory capacity as a function of arterial oxygen tension in puppies. Each point represents one animal.

Cytochrome c in the puppy heart increased from 30% at term to nearly 100% of the adult level (0.25 nmole/mg protein to 0.65 nmoles/mg protein respectively) by 48 hours postnatally. As seen in Figure 4, cytochrome oxidase ($a+a_3$) increased more slowly, increasing from 27% at term to only 60% of the adult value by the end of the first postnatal week (from 0.06 nmoles/mg protein to 0.14 nmoles/mg protein respectively).

If respiratory capacity is related to cytochrome concentration, oxygen utilization is seen to drop from 1100 moles O_2/min/mole of cytochrome $a+a_3$ at birth to 200 moles O_2/mm/mole $a+a_3$ at 4 to 7 days after birth.

Calcium transport capacity, as shown in Figure 5, dropped from around 100 nmoles Ca^{++}/min/mg protein (1000 moles Ca^{++} accumulated min/mole $a+a_3$) to undetectable levels by day seven.

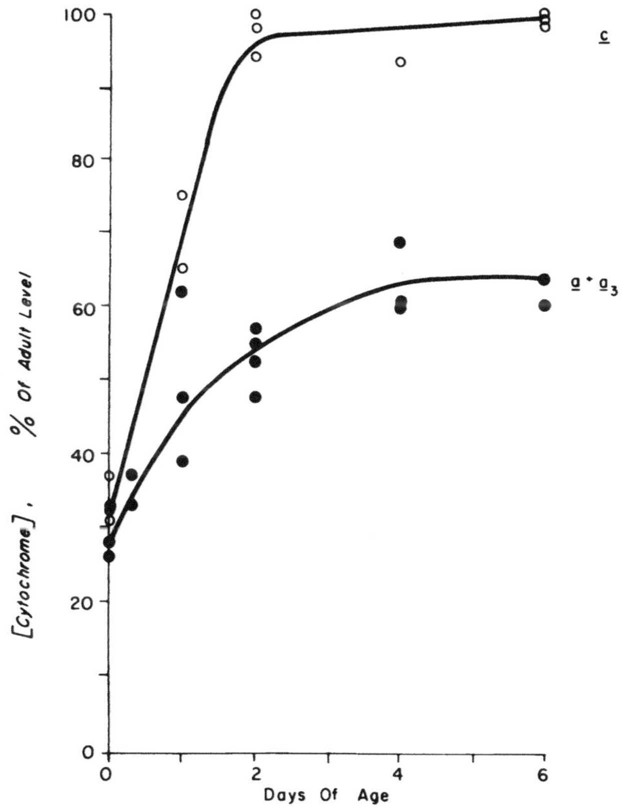

Figure 4. Concentrations of canine heart cytochrome c (o) and cytochrome $a+a_3$ (•) as a percentage of adult level. Each point represents one animal.

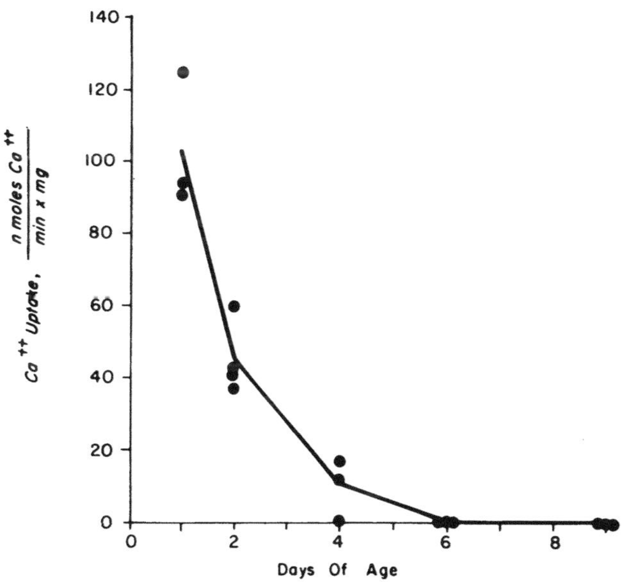

Figure 5. Calcium accumulation in the absence of added phosphate as a function of age in the puppy. Each point represents one animal.

DISCUSSION

The data presented here indicate that heart mitochondria respond to oxygen availability in vivo by adaptive changes in their functional states. That these changes are not seen in isolated mitochondria from normoxic animals suggests that these alterations are the results of interactions within the entire cell. In earlier work, we demonstrated an overall increase in State 3 respiratory capacity in adult dogs made chronically hypoxic by a vascular shunting procedure (3). Months later, when these animals were reoxygenated, the pattern was reversed, with respiratory capacity decreasing in a pattern similar to the present data (7). In addition, cardiac mitochondria from patients with congenital cyanotic heart disease exhibited the same decrease when normoxic conditions were established by cardiopulmonary bypass. The perinatal changes in cytochromes in rats have been shown to follow a course like those of the puppies and lambs, and the expected postnatal increase in cytochromes could be inhibited if the rats were kept in a hypoxic environment following birth (8).

The postnatal increase in mitochondrial enzymes found in the present study probably reflects a continuation of fetal development, which is subject to modulation by oxygen availability. Respiratory capacity, on the other hand, seems to depend more directly on oxygen regulation. At this time we can only speculate as to the control mechanism for this decreased cytochrome enzymatic turnover, but carrier-mediated mechanisms are obvious choices to be investigated.

ACKNOWLEDGEMENT

This work was supported by GM 01540, GM 19867, and HD 07135 from the National Institutes of Health.

REFERENCES

1. Ou, L.C. and S.M. Tenney. Properties of mitochondria from hearts of cattle acclimatized to high altitude. Resp. Physiol. 8:151-159, 1970.

2. Shertzer, H.G. and J. Cascarano. Mitochondrial alterations in heart, liver, and kidney of altitude-acclimated rats. Am. J. Physiol. 223:632-636, 1972.

3. Park, C.D., L. Mela, R. Wharton, J. Reilly, P. Fishbein, and E. Aberdeen. Cardiac mitochondrial activity and chronic cyanosis. J. Surg. Res. 14:139-146, 1973

4. Chance B. and B. Hagihara. Direct spectroscopic measurements of interaction of components of the respiratory chain with ATP, ADP, phosphate and uncoupling agents. In Proceedings of the Fifth International Congress of Biochemistry, Oxford. Elmsford, New York, Pergamon Press, 1963, page 3

5. Mela, L. and B. Chance. Spectrophotometric measurements of the kinetics of Ca^{2+} and Mn^{2+} accumulation in mitochondria. Biochemistry 7:4059-4063, 1968.

6. Chance, B. and G. R. Williams. The respiratory chain and oxidative phosphorylation. Advan. Enzym. 17:65-134, 1956.

7. Goodwin, C.W., L. Mela, C.D. Park, J. Campbell. Adaptation to oxygen by cardiac mitochondria in newborn and chronically hypoxic adult dogs. Surg. Forum 25:185-187, 1974.

8. Hallman, M. Changes in mitochondrial respiratory chain proteins during perinatal development. Evidence for the importance of environmental oxygen tension. Biochim. Biophys. Acta. 253:360-372, 1972.

EXPERIMENTAL AND THEORETICAL ANALYSIS OF OXYGEN TRANSPORT IN FETAL BRAIN

Eric J. Guilbeau and Daniel D. Reneau

Department of Biomedical Engineering
Louisiana Tech University
Ruston, Louisiana 71270

The purpose of this investigation was to experimentally and theoretically determine the transient response of the fetal brain PO_2 to dynamic changes in maternal arterial PO_2. In the experimental analysis transient changes in maternal arterial PO_2 of two specific types were studied; 1) the transient change from a condition of maternal hyperoxia to maternal normoxia, 2) a transient change from a condition of maternal hyperoxia to maternal hypoxia followed by a return to hyperoxia. In the theoretical analysis the response of fetal brain PO_2 during the transition from a condition of maternal hyperoxia to maternal normoxia was simulated mathematically by solving equations which represent the placental exchange system, fetal circulatory system, and fetal brain.

Past theoretical studies describing oxygen transfer in the placental-fetus system (6, 9, 10, 16) showed that the response of fetal brain PO_2 to transient changes in maternal arterial PO_2 was a slower process than the response of adult brain PO_2. This may be primarily contributed to the increased circulation time (maternal blood from lung to placenta; fetal blood from placenta to fetal brain) and the placental transport processes. One specific purpose of the present study was to measure the pure transport delay associated with fetal brain oxygenation and to estimate the total time required for the fetal brain PO_2 to reach a new equilibrium value following a transient change in maternal arterial PO_2.

It has been shown that the fetus increases flow to the brain during periods of hypoxia (3, 11, 12). A second specific purpose of this study was to determine if an overshoot phenomena can be observed in the response of fetal cortical PO_2 to brief periods of maternal hypoxia, and hence, if the fetus has a control mechanism for compensation following hypoxia as has been demonstrated in the adult (4, 14, 15).

EXPERIMENTAL PROCEDURE

Ten experiments were performed on Spanish brush goats in their nineteenth to twentieth week of gestation, with the exception of one nanny which was in her fifteenth week, under chlorolose anesthesia.

Two types of response were evoked in each experiment. First, with the nanny in a stable condition breathing a mixture of oxygen and air via a T-shaped tracheal cannula the oxygen was removed and the response of fetal brain PO_2 was measured using oxygen microelectrodes (1μ tip). Blood samples were collected from the maternal femoral artery and analyzed via a radiometer blood gas analyzer for oxygen PO_2 just prior to oxygen removal, after the nanny had stabilized on air, and after the animal was returned to the oxygen-air gas mixture. Second, with the nanny initially breathing a mixture of oxygen and air, nitrogen was administered via an anesthesia apparatus connected to a T-shaped tracheal cannula. Maternal carotid artery blood pressure, maternal femoral artery PO_2 and fetal brain PO_2 responses were measured. Nitrogen administration was continued until one of the following three conditions were satisfied: 1) survival of the nanny appeared to be in jeopardy, 2) survival of the fetus appeared to be in jeopardy, or 3) fetal brain PO_2 appeared to have reached a constant value. In most experiments nitrogen administration was discontinued to insure survival of the nanny. After each period of nitrogen administration the nanny was returned to the air-oxygen gas mixture and allowed to stabilize. Fetal brain PO_2 was measured using microelectrodes of the type developed by Silver (17).

THEORETICAL ANALYSIS

In previous mathematical analyses of oxygen transport, distributed, lumped-distributed, and lumped parameter analyses have been used to study the response of the microscopic exchange unit of the placenta (6, 8, 9, 10, 16). Initially the placenta was represented by two microscopic exchange units, one in which maternal and fetal blood flow was in a concurrent manner and the other in which flow was countercurrent. Later development included the fetus in the analysis so that the effects of maternal placental flow changes on fetal oxygenation could be investigated (9). Cameron (6) described a basic framework for the feto-placental unit and presented a mathematical model based on this system which described oxygen transport in 1) the major fetal blood vessels, 2) the placenta, and 3) the fetal organs. This analysis followed closely the techniques of Bischoff (5) who modeled drug administration in the adult circulation.

The present analysis uses the system shown in Figure 1. The placenta was represented by two exchange units, one in which maternal and fetal bloods flow in a concurrent manner and another in which flow is countercurrent. These exchange units were represented by dividing them into a series of compartments (i.e., the system was finite differenced). Oxygen transfer in the compartmentalized exchange units was then represented by a set of non-linear ordinary differential equations. The following equations resulted from this type analysis.

Concurrent Exchange Unit:

Maternal Equation,

$$\frac{d\lambda'_{mn}}{dt} = \frac{1}{2}\,\frac{Q_m}{V_m}\left(\lambda'_{mn-1} - \lambda'_{mn+}\right) - \frac{H'_n}{V_m N_m}$$

Fetal Equation,

$$\frac{d\lambda'_{fn}}{dt} = \frac{1}{2}\,\frac{Q_f}{V_f}\left(\lambda'_{fn-1} - \lambda'_{fn+1}\right) + \frac{H'_n}{V_f N_f}$$

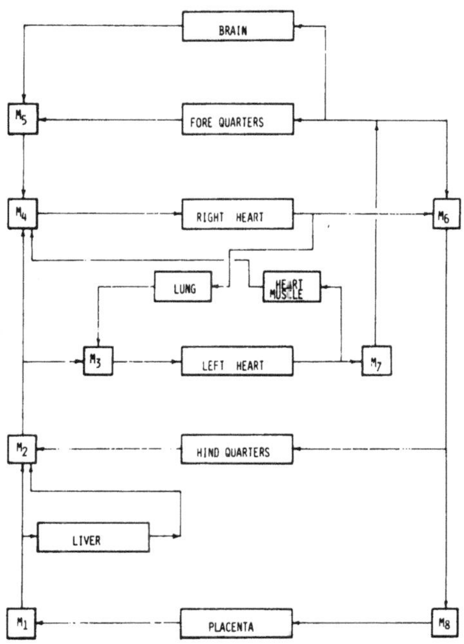

Figure 1. System for Mathematical Analysis

Countercurrent Exchange Units:

Maternal Equation,

$$\frac{d\lambda''_{mn}}{dt} = \frac{1}{2}\frac{Q_m}{V_m}\left(\lambda''_{mn-1} \quad \lambda''_{mn+1}\right) - \frac{H''_n}{V_m N_m}$$

Fetal Equation,

$$\frac{d\lambda''_{fn}}{dt} = \frac{1}{2}\frac{Q_f}{V_f}\left(\lambda''_{fn+1} - \lambda''_{fn-1}\right) + \frac{H''_n}{V_f N_f}$$

Where,

$$H''_n = KA_s\left(P''_{mn} - P''_{fn}\right)$$

The fetal brain was treated in a similar manner by dividing the fetal brain capillary and surrounding tissue into a set of compartments. The following equations apply:

Capillary:

$$\frac{d\lambda_{bn}}{dt} = \frac{1}{2}\frac{Q_b}{V_{bc}}\left(\lambda_{bn-1} - \lambda_{bn+1}\right) - \frac{H_{bn}}{V_{bc}N_f}$$

Tissue:

$$\frac{dP_{tn}}{dt} = \frac{H_{bn}}{\alpha_n V_{bt}} - \frac{A_n}{\alpha_n V_{bt}}$$

Where,

$$H_{bn} = K_b A_{sb}\ (P_{bn} - P_{tn})$$

The other fetal organs and the arterial and venous circulating blood compartments (m_1-m_8) were represented by single ordinary differential equations of the following form:

$$\frac{d\lambda_o}{dt} = \frac{1}{V_o}\left(\sum_{j=1}^{m} Q_{ij}\lambda_{ij} - Q_o\lambda_o\right) - \frac{A_o}{N_f V_o}$$

with the input term $\sum_{i=1}^{m} Q_{ij}\lambda_{ij}$ varying with each particular organ.

The relationship between PO_2 and fractional saturation of hemoglobin (blood) and myoglobin (heart muscle) was represented quantitatively by the Hill equation. The model equations were arranged in a continuous manner with all organs interconnected. The resulting continuous, unsteady-state model was solved to yield transient changes in the PO_2 of the various organs in the fetal circulation. The model also yielded axial PO_2 profiles in the placental and in the fetal brain capillary and tissue. Solutions were obtained using variable step Runge Kutta numerical intergration via IBM CSMP III on an IBM 370 computer.

RESULTS

The results obtained in this study will be divided into two sections, hyperoxia results and hypoxia results.

Hyperoxia

In ten experiments the nanny was allowed to reach equilibrium conditions while spontaneously breathing a mixture of 100% O_2 and air. This resulted in increased maternal arterial blood PO_2 values which ranged between 176 and 372 mm Hg. After equilibration with the O_2 rich gas, the mixture was removed and the animal was allowed to spontanesouly breathe air. Records of the fetal brain PO_2 response were obtained. A typical record is shown in Figure 2. In this experiment the nanny had been maintained on a mixture of 100% oxygen and air for thirty minutes. A stable fetal brain PO_2 of 24.5 mm Hg was established and was maintained within relatively close limits. Reading the record from left to right the first mark represents the drawing of a blood sample from the maternal femoral artery. Analysis of this sample showed a corresponding maternal arterial blood PO_2 of 241 mm Hg. At the second mark the nanny was removed from the oxygen rich gas mixture and allowed to spontaneously breathe air. Following a 24 second period, fetal brain PO_2 began to decrease and continued to decrease for 6.2 minutes. At the third and fourth mark maternal arterial blood samples were collected and analyzed. The maternal arterial blood PO_2 had decreased to 81.0 mm Hg. A PO_2 of 12.0 mm was established to represent the new equilibrium condition in fetal brain.

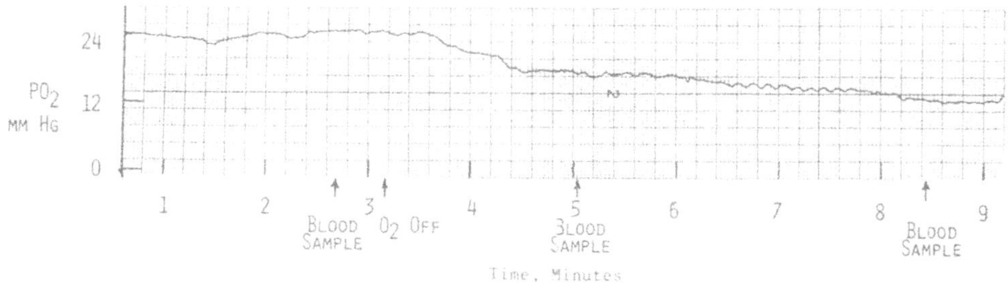

Figure 2. Fetal Brain Oxygen Tension Response to Removal of 100% Oxygen.

In this record the time delay before any significant decrease in fetal brain PO_2 was observed represents the pure transport delay associated with the fetal and maternal circulation and the placental transport process. The subsequent decrease in fetal brain PO_2 following this initial delay corresponds to the gradual decrease in maternal arterial PO_2 and subsequent decrease in fetal arterial PO_2 following placental exchange.

Behrman (2) has shown in the monkey that increasing maternal arterial PO_2 by 137% resulted in a 36% increase in umbilical vein PO_2 and a 24% increase in umbilical artery PO_2. Our results indicate that these increased fetal umbilical PO_2 levels result in increased fetal brain PO_2 levels.

Other investigators (1, 2) who have studied the effects of maternal hyperoxia on the fetus have shown that unless maternal arterial PO_2 approaches hyperbaric conditions (3 atm) no significant increase or decrease in umbilical or uterine flow or fetal O_2 consumption rate occurs. This fact permits mathermatical simulation of hyperoxia without the necessity of having detailed flow and consumption rate data as a function of PO_2. Using the previously described mathematical analysis the model was solved by placing a step change on maternal arterial PO_2 (240 mm Hg to 80 mm Hg) so that the experimentally obtained response could be simulated theoretically. The results of this simulation are shown in Figure 3. The upper curve shows the experimental response of Figure 1 redrawn as the fractional decrease in fetal brain PO_2 versus time. The lower curve shows the response of the mathematical model following the step change (initiated at time = 0) on maternal arterial PO_2. Note that the shape of the curves corresponds well, a time delay is

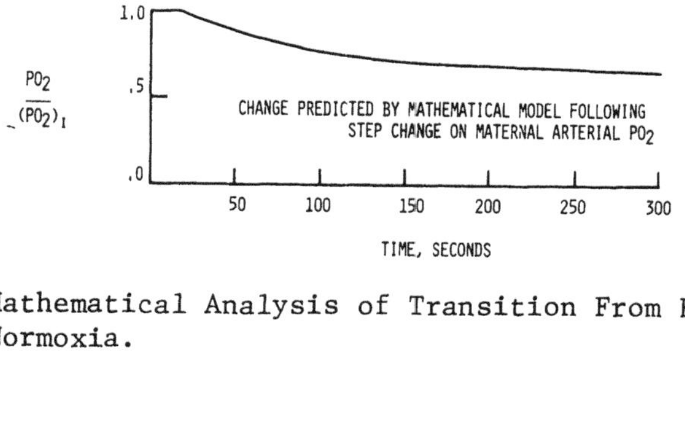

Figure 3. Mathematical Analysis of Transition From Hyperoxia to Normoxia.

present in both, and the fractional change is essentially the same in both and requires the same total time to occur.

In other experiments the decrease in fetal brain PO_2 was not so significant as in this record. In several animals no decrease was observed. The magnitude of the decrease in fetal brain PO_2 following removal of the oxygen appeared to be related to the magnitude of the equilibrium PO_2 value measured during oxygen inhalation. The higher the initial fetal brain PO_2 the larger the subsequent decrease in PO_2 following oxygen removal and vice versa. The mathematical analysis verified these experimental findings. Larger changes were predicted at the arterial end of the fetal brain capillary than at the venous end.

Hypoxia

Immediately following the oxygen responses in each of the experiments, the animal was allowed to stabilize while spontaneously breathing a mixture of 100% pure oxygen and air. When a stable record of fetal brain PO_2 was established the oxygen rich gas mixture was removed and the animal was allowed to spontaneously breathe 100% nitrogen. Following each period of nitrogen inhalation the nanny was returned to the original oxygen-air gas mixture.

A typical fetal brain PO_2 response to maternal hypoxia is shown in Figure 4. This record shows that with the nanny breathing the oxygen-air gas misture, fetal brain PO_2 was stable at 6.5 mm Hg. At the moment the nanny was allowed to spontaneously breathe 100% nitrogen (indicated by the first arrow) the fetal brain PO_2 trace was slightly off scale, a scale change was made (calibration corresponds to the trace following the scale change). Approximately 67 seconds after nitrogen administration fetal brain PO_2 began a gradual decrease to a minimum value slightly greater than two mm Hg over a time period of approximately 3.5 minutes. The nanny was then switched from nitrogen to the oxygen-air gas mixture as indicated by the second arrow, and the fetal PO_2 began a very gradual increase to 5.5 mm Hg then increased more rapidly to 9.5 mm Hg followed by a decrease to a new equilibrium value of 6.0 mm Hg. Maternal arterial blood PO_2 in the femoral artery was measured to be 197 mm Hg prior to nitrogen administration, decreased to a minimum value of 11.3 mm Hg during nitrogen administration, and returned to a value of 197 mm Hg immediately following return to the oxygen-air gas mixture. Since quantitative information regarding the redistribution of flows in the fetal circulation during hypoxia is not available mathematical simulation of this response was not attempted. In all of the experiments the observation was made that the fetal brain PO_2 values seemed considerably lower than those which have been measured in adult brain. This agrees with the results of Erdmann (7).

The hyperoxia studies, Figures 2 and 3, as well as the hypoxia

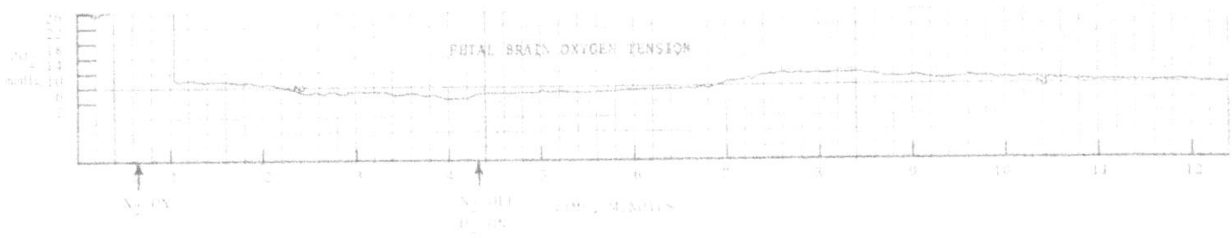

Figure 4. Fetal Brain Oxygen Tension Response to Maternal Hypoxia

studies, Figure 4, also indicate that the time required for the fetal brain PO_2 to respond to a transient change in maternal arterial PO_2 is considerably longer than the time required for the PO_2 in adult brain to respond to similar changes in arterial PO_2.

The hypoxia responses also indicate that the fetus like the adult has some control mechanism available to protect the microenvironment of fetal brain during maternal hypoxia. This is indicated by the fact that the fetal brain PO_2 overshoots the initial value following a brief period of maternal hypoxia. The results of this investigation do not permit postulation of the mechanism of this control other than to say it is most likely flow related.

CONCLUSIONS

Based on the results obtained in this study and the results of others it seems safe to conclude the following:

1) Fetal brain PO_2 values are considerably lower than those found in adult brain.
2) Administration of 100% oxygen to the mother can (but not always) significantly raise the PO_2 at a specific point in the fetal cortex.
3) The response of fetal brain PO_2 to changes in maternal arterial PO_2 is delayed by a finite quantity of time of the order of magnitude of 38 seconds.
4) The time required for the fetal brain PO_2 to reach a minimum following a decrease in the PO_2 of maternal arterial blood coincides closely with the time required for the maternal arterial PO_2 to reach its minimum plus the pure transport delay time (38 seconds).
5) The fetus has available a control mechanism which acts to compensate for periods of reduced PO_2 in the microenvironment of the fetal cortex.

ACKNOWLEDGEMENTS

This study was supported by a grant from the Frost Foundation, Shreveport, Louisiana.

Special appreciation is afforded to Dr. Ian Silver of Bristol University, Bristol, England, and Dr. Marian Silver, Cambridge University, Cambridge, England, for their aid in electrode development techniques and fetal surgical techniques.

NOMENCLATURE

A	metabolic rate of fetal tissue, $cm^3 O_2$/sec.
A_s	surface area, cm^2
K	mass transfer coefficient, $cm^3 O_2/cm^2$-second- mm Hg.
N	oxygen capacity blood, $cm^3 O_2/cm^3$blood.
P	oxygen partial pressue, mm Hg.
Q	volumetric flow rate, cm^3blood/second.
t	time, seconds.
V	volume, cm^3.
λ	fractional saturation.
b	brain value.
f	fetal value.
i	inlet value.
m	maternal value.
n	refers to nth compartment.
o	organ values.

REFERENCES

1. Assali, N. S., T. H. Kirschbaum, and P. V. Dilts, Jr. Circulation Res. 22:573-588, 1968.
2. Berhmann, R. E., E. N. Peterson, and C. W. deLannog. Resp. Physiol. 6:271-283, 1969.
3. Berhmann, R. E., M. H. Lees, E. N. Peterson, C. W. deLannog, and A. E. Seeds. Amer. J. Obstet. Gynec. 108:956-69, 1970.
4. Bicher, H. I., D. D. Reneau, D. F. Bruley, and M. H. Knisely. Amer. J. Phys. 224:274-82, 1973.
5. Bischoff, K. B., and R. G. Brown, Chemical Engineering in Medicine, Chemical Engineering Progress Symposium Series, AICHE, N.Y. 62:32-45 (1965).
6. Cameron, J. M., D. D. Reneau, and E. J. Guilbeau. Proceedings of the Summer Computer Simulation Conference, Houston, TX, 1974.
7. Erdmann, E. Respiratory Gas Exchange and Blood Flow in the Placenta, ed. by L. D. Longo and H. Bartels, H.E.W. Pub. 459, 1972.

8. Guilbeau, E. J., D. D. Reneau, and M. H. Knisely. Advances in Chemistry Series No. 118, Chemical Engineering in Medicine, American Chemical Society, 1973.

9. Guilbeau, E. J., and D. D. Reneau. Oxygen Transport to Tissue, Pharmacology, Mathematical Studies, and Neonatology, ed. by D. F. Bruley and H. I. Bicher, Plenum, 1973.

10. Hill, E. P., G. G. Power, and L. D. Longo. J. of Applied Physiol. 222:721-29 (1972).

11. Mann, L. I. Clin. Gynecology 13:638-50, 1970.

12. Purves, M. J., and I. M. James. Cir. Res. 25:651-67, 1969.

13. Reneau, D. D., D. F. Bruley, and M. H. Knisely. A.I.Ch.E. J. 15:916-925, 1969.

14. Reneau, D. D., H. I. Bicher, D. F. Bruley, and M. H. Knisely. Blood Oxygenation ed. by Daniel Hershey, Plenum Press, New York, 1970.

15. Reneau, D. D., H. I. Bicher, D. F. Bruley, W. C. Reardon, and M. H. Knisely. Biomedical Engineering Computer Simulation, Preprint 10f 69th National Meeting of A.I.Ch.E., Cincinnati, May, 1971.

16. Reneau, D. D., E. J. Guilbeau, and J. M. Cameron. Microvascular Research 8:346-361, 1974.

17. Silver, I. A., Med. Electron. Biol. Eng. 3:377-387, 1965.

FETAL AND PLACENTAL O_2 CONSUMPTION AND THE UPTAKE OF DIFFERENT METABOLITES IN THE RUMINANT AND HORSE DURING LATE GESTATION

Marian Silver & R. S. Comline

Physiological Laboratory

University of Cambridge, Cambridge, CB2 3EG

The use of conscious pregnant animals with indwelling catheters in both fetal and maternal circulations has enabled a variety of measurements to be made on a long-term basis. In the sheep, changes in uterine and umbilical blood flows have been followed during the latter part of gestation (for references see Comline & Silver 1974) and such measurements coupled with analyses of arterio-venous differences in oxygen and other metabolites allow the calculation of fetal and utero-placental oxygen consumption and metabolite uptake (Battaglia & Meschia 1973). The picture which has emerged is that the rates of both uterine and umbilical blood flow keep pace with the growth of the fetus so that its oxygen uptake per unit weight remains relatively constant. However, in their calculations of the energy balance of the sheep fetus Battaglia & Meschia (1973) noticed that the amount of oxygen used by the fetus was greater than could be explained by the uptake and metabolism of glucose, amino acids and other possible metabolic fuels; at least 20-25% of the total oxygen consumption remained unaccounted for. It seemed possible that some of this apparent energy deficit might be supplied by volatile fatty acids since these play an important role in the metabolism of the adult ruminant.

In a re-examination of this problem we have compared the ruminant fetus (cow) with a non-ruminant of comparable size (horse). Determinations of the oxygen consumption of the uterus as well as the fetus have been made in conscious animals, and the uptakes of glucose, acetate and other possible metabolic fuels have been assessed for their role in fetal metabolism. Some of these findings have already been published (Comline & Silver 1975a; Silver & Comline 1975).

METHODS

Nine pregnant cows and four pony mares in late gestation were used. In the mother catheters were inserted into a maternal artery and peripheral vein and into the main uterine vein; in the fetus the umbilical artery and vein were catheterised. Details of the techniques used are given elsewhere (Comline, Hall, Lavelle, Nathanielsz & Silver, 1974; Comline & Silver, 1975b). All measurements were begun after a 3-4 day recovery period. Uterine and umbilical blood flows were determined by the diffusion equilibrium method (Huckabee, Metcalfe, Prystowsky & Barron, 1961; Crenshaw, Huckabee, Curet, Mann & Barron, 1968), with antipyrine as test substance. At the same time arterio-venous differences in oxygen content and in glucose, acetate and free fatty acid (F.F.A.) concentrations were measured; in some animals artery-to-artery plasma urea differences were also determined. Blood flow measurements were made at 3-7 day intervals, while blood gas tensions, pH and metabolite concentrations were monitored daily until delivery. Live births were obtained in all the cows but in the mares still-born fetuses were delivered 5 - 40 days after operation.

RESULTS & CONCLUSIONS

Uterine and umbilical blood flows, expressed per unit weight, did not appear to change during the last few weeks of gestation i.e. the absolute rates of blood flow to the uterus and the umbilical circulation increased with fetal weight. Since, in ruminants at least, fetal growth rate is highest and placental enlargement is minimal during late gestation, the rate of blood flow per g of tissue must therefore increase considerably on both fetal and maternal sides of the placenta.

The mean values for umbilical and uterine blood flow obtained in the cows (Table 1) were essentially similar to those reported previously for sheep (Huckabee et al 1961; Crenshaw et al 1968): uterine blood flows in the mare were also in the same range.

Table 1. Mean umbilical and uterine blood flows (± S.E.M.) in conscious mares and cows in late gestation

Species	No. of animals	Blood Flow (ml/kg/min)	
		Uterine*	Umbilical**
Mare	4	315 ± 14	171 ± 21
Cow	9	329 ± 21	230 ± 11

*Per kg uterus & tissues contents including fetus. **Per kg fetus

However, mean umbilical blood flow in the foal was low compared with values for ruminants. This may well be due to the high vascular resistance to umbilical flow in the foal since the ductus venosus is absent in this species.

Umbilical and uterine arterio-venous differences in oxygen content were inversely related to blood flow rates, so that although rates of flow showed considerable individual variation, the actual uptake of oxygen by both uterus and fetus remained within a relatively narrow range; the mean values obtained for both cow and mare are given in Table 2. Utero-placental oxygen consumption was estimated using a weight ratio of utero-placental tissue: fetus of 4:6 (obtained from acute experiments performed in late pregnancy). Utero-placental oxygen consumption was much higher than that of the fetus, and since 85-90% of the total uterine blood flow supplies the placental areas (see Comline & Silver 1974) the oxygen utilization of this tissue is likely to be even higher while endometrial and myometrial uptakes will be correspondingly low.

Of the possible metabolic fuels used by the fetus, glucose is by far the most important in most species (Battaglia & Meschia 1973). In both cow and mare an uptake of glucose by the fetus was found but it was much lower than that of the uterus as a whole (Table 2). Thus, a major part of the total uterine consumption appeared to be due to utero-placental usage. Setchel, Bassett, Hinks and Graham (1972) calculated that 70% of the total glucose metabolism of the pregnant sheep may be accounted for by uterine uptake. Obviously much of this must be due to placental utilization for the placenta is not just an organ for exchange - it is an endocrine gland of considerable importance and a high rate of metabolism is not unexpected. The conversion of glucose to fructose also occurs in the placenta, but there is little or no evidence for a significant utilization of fructose by the fetus in any of the fructogenic species. In the present experiments the arterio-venous differences in fructose across the umbilical circulation were negligible in both foal and calf.

Measurement of acetic acid concentration differences across the uterine and umbilical circulations in the cow showed a consistent uterine uptake of this volatile fatty acid and a small but significant uptake by the fetus (Table 2). The amount removed by the fetus appeared to be dependent on the maternal concentration; thus in poorly fed animals little or no acetate uptake by the fetus occurred.

In neither the mare nor the cow was there a detectable F.F.A. difference across the umbilical circulation although the absolute plasma concentrations were much higher in the foal than in the

Table 2. Mean values (± S.E.M.) for O_2, glucose and acetate uptakes by the uterus and fetus (U), fetus alone (F) and the utero-placental tissue (UPT)* in 9 cows and 4 mares in late gestation.

Species	O_2 (ml/kg/min)			Glucose (mg/kg/min)			Acetate (mg/kg/min)		
	U	F	UPT	U	F	UPT	U	F	UPT
Cow	8.5 (± 0.7)	6.8 (± 0.2)	11	9.1 (± 0.6)	5.0 (± 0.3)	15	5.0 (± 0.6)	1.7 (± 0.7) n=5	10
Mare	8.5 (± 0.3)	7.4 (± 0.3)	10	11.9 (± 1.1)	6.8 (± 0.6)	17			

*Estimated using the weight ratio of 6:4 for fetus: UPT

calf fetus. Battaglia & Meschia (1973) failed to detect any F.F.A. uptake by the sheep fetus nor any usage of β.OH butyrate (Morris, Boyd, Makowski, Meschia & Battaglia, 1974). No uterine uptake of F.F.A. was seen in the cow while the uterine A-V differences in the mare were inconsistent. Thus the extent of uterine and fetal F.F.A. uptake in these species remains equivocal.

Measurements of fetal urea clearance for quantitative estimates of amino acid breakdown were not made in the present experiments. However, artery-to-artery urea concentration differences were lower than those previously reported for the sheep (Battaglia & Meschia 1973). This suggests that amino acid catabolism contributes less to fetal energy metabolism in these species than in the sheep.

The relative roles of glucose and acetate in the metabolism of the calf fetus are given by calculation of the glucose/oxygen quotient (0.55) and the acetate/oxygen quotient (0.17). These show that 55% of the total fetal oxygen consumption may be used for the aerobic metabolism of glucose and about 17% for acetate breakdown. If a further 15-20% is used for amino acid catabolism, then most of the oxygen consumption of the calf fetus can be accounted for in terms of known metabolic fuels. In the fetal foal glucose probably plays a more important role since the glucose/oxygen quotient is 0.7 in this species. However, there may be small contributions to the total energy balance of the foal from amino acids, acetate, F.F.A. and even fructose, although the precise contribution made by each has yet to be assessed quantitatively.

This work was supported by grants from the Milk Marketing Board and the Horserace Betting Levy Board. We are grateful to many members of the Assistant Staff of the Laboratory for their help with experiments and care of the animals.

References

Battaglia, F. C. & Meschia, G. (1973) in Foetal & Neonatal Physiology pp. 382-397. Eds. R. S. Comline, K. W. Cross, G. S. Dawes, & P. W. Nathanielsz. Cambridge University Press.

Comline, R. S. & Silver, M. (1974) in Recent Advances in Physiology pp. 406-454. Ed. R. J. Linden. Churchill, London.

Comline, R. S. & Silver, M. (1975a) J. Physiol. Lond. **245**, 75-76P.

Comline, R. S. & Silver, M. (1975b) J. Reprod. Fert. Suppl. 23 in press.

Comline, R. S., Hall, L. W., Lavelle, R. B., Nathanielsz, P. W. & Silver, M. (1974) J. Endocr. **63**, 451-472.

Crenshaw, C., Huckabee, W. E., Curet, L. B., Mann, L. & Barron, D. H. (1968) Q. J. exp. Physiol. **53**, 65-75.

Huckabee, W. E., Metcalfe, J., Prystowsky, H. & Barron, D. H. (1961) Am. J. Physiol. **200**, 274-278.

Morris, F. H., Boyd, R. D. H., Makowski, E. L., Meschia, G. & Battaglia, F. C. (1974) Proc. Soc. exp. Biol. Med. **145**, 879-883.

Setchell, B. P., Bassett, J. M., Hinks, N. T. & Graham, N. M. (1972) Q. J. exp. Physiol. **57**, 257-266.

Silver, M. & Comline, R. S. (1975) J. Reprod. Fert. Suppl. 23 in press.

CONTINUOUS PO_2 AND HEART RATE RECORDING IN THE HUMAN NEWBORN

Albert Huch, Dietrich W. Lübbers and Renate Huch

Department of Obstetrics and Gynaecology
University of Marburg, Marburg/Germany and
Max-Planck-Institut für Systemphysiologie
Dortmund/Germany

In numerous obstetrical and pediatric departments caring for healthy and sick newborns, continuous heart rate monitoring is used as an indirect reflection of oxygenation. This is based on the theory that a sudden fall in arterial Po_2 or chronic hypoxaemia is reflected in a change in heart rate and thus, alert the physician to a possible hypoxaemic state.

With the transcutaneous Po_2 method (1,2,3,4,5,6), which allows continuous monitoring of arterial Po_2 as previously presented to this society in 1971 and 1973, simultaneous heart rate and Po_2 monitoring is possible in sick and healthy newborns. Also, with this method, it has become possible to monitor the fetus prenatally with increased success (7). This simultaneous and continuous monitoring of heart rate and arterial Po_2 values has enabled us to observe heart rate behaviour during normal and pathological arterial oxygenation. We should like to first present our observations of healthy newborns in our clinic and then those of sick infants transferred from our clinic to pediatric centers and those observed in intensive care units elsewhere.

In each child we monitored

1. heart rate, (beat to beat); (HR)
2. the relative local perfusion (electrical current required to keep the preset temperature of the heated electrode constant); (rel. loc. perfusion)
3. the transcutaneous Po_2; ($tcPo_2$)

4. the transthoracic impedance
5. the respiratory rate (integrated); (resp. rate)

It is well known that heart rate varies with a child's degree of activity. We have observed a similar relationship between arterial Po_2 and activity. As an example, Fig. 1 shows considerable variation of both heart rate and arterial Po_2 in an active child. Note, that the heart rate is recorded beat to beat without integration.

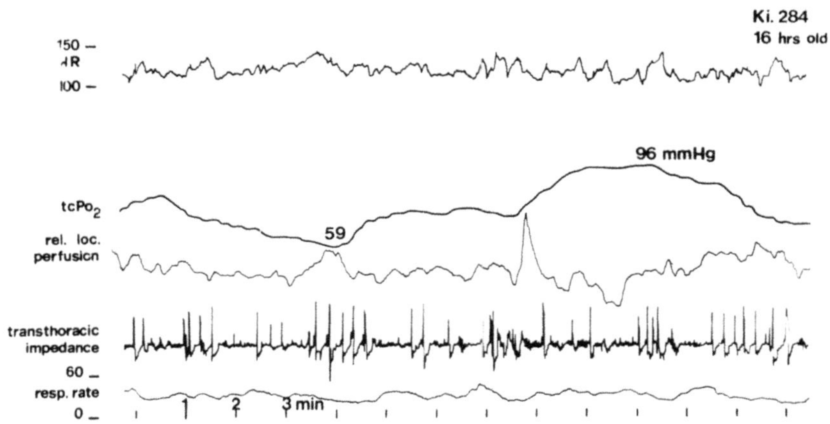

Fig. 1: Part of a continuous registration of transcutaneous Po_2 together with beat to beat recording of heart rate, with relative local perfusion, transthoracic impedance and respiratory rate. In this healthy, unquiet infant all parameters show rather great changes.

In Fig. 2 this observation is even more dramatically illustrated as we awoke a child from deep sleep. Note all parameters studied displayed a monotonous tracing during the time that the child was in a state of deep sleep and great variability during the aroused state. Because of the observed marked variability in all parameters in the aroused child, for our comparative studies, we selected periods of sleep or quiet.

Fig. 3 illustrates the collected data for infants during the first 24 hours of life. We studied 259 newborns, monitoring for at least one hour each. This group was divided into three sub-groups according to age. Transcutaneous Po_2 was transformed to arterial Po_2 utilizing the mean conversion factor (c = 0,89) determined from paired values (4). We observed

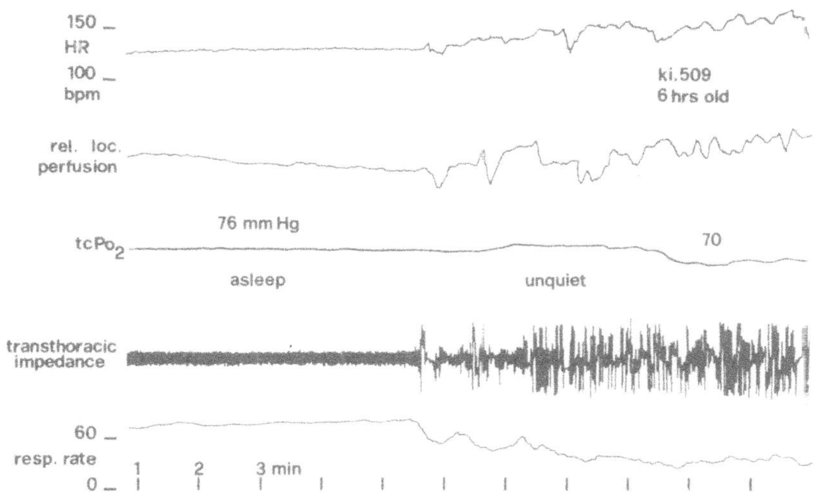

Fig. 2: Part of a continuous registration of $tcPo_2$ together with beat to beat heart rate recording, with relative local perfusion, transthoracic impedance and respiratory rate. All recorded parameters change their performance when the child is woken up.

that heart rate was highest immediately post partum and declines continuously throughout the first day of life from 130 to 108 beat per minute. It is interesting that we found no difference in the mean arterial Po_2 values throughout the first three hours of life. Our observations of heart rate behaviour are in agreement with those reported by others who studied only the heart rate behaviour (8, 9, 10). However, our additional monitoring of arterial Po_2 failed to support the proposed relationship between tachycardia and hypoxaemia. The statistical analysis failed to show any relationship between heart rate and arterial Po_2 in the normal Po_2 range. It is important to understand that we were monitoring a group of apparently healthy infants and therefore seldom measured in an extrem hypoxic range. One of the exceptions is illustrated in Fig. 4. It is a record of a spontaneous apnoeic episode which occured in an otherwise asymptomatic, normal appearing infant. Here, a relationship between arterial Po_2 and heart rate was noted; however, the degree of change in heart rate is small compared to the dramatic Po_2 fall. In addition, it is important to note that, of the 259 infants studied, 16 infants displayed heart rates

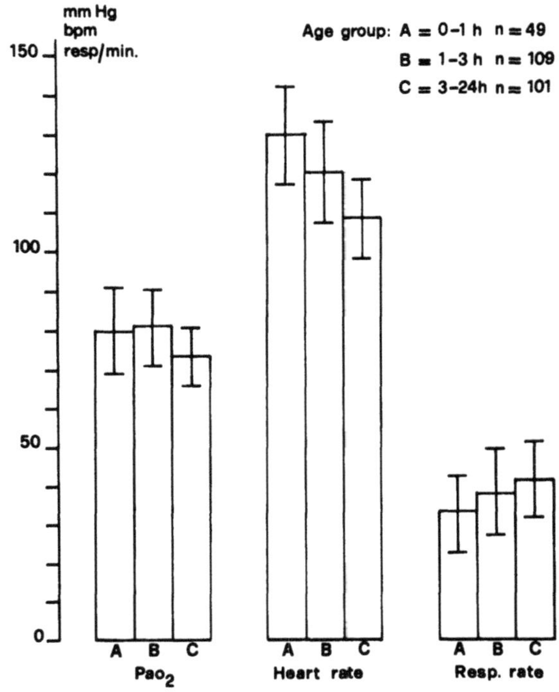

Fig. 3: Representation of mean values and standard deviations of Po_2, heart rate and respiratory rate in 259 healthy, calm newborn infants.

between 80 - 95 beat per minute with normal Po_2 in the course of deep sleep.

Fig. 5 presents the data from a group of 21 sick infants we studied. The left columns illustrate a mean heart rate of 143 bpm with the corresponding mean arterial Po_2 of 30 mm Hg, values obviously different from those just described from healthy infants. A big surprise was the heart rate values observed in the same children when respiratory therapy brought their arterial Po_2 values into normal range. Despite improvement of Po_2 values, the heart rates remain abnormal and not significantly different from those recorded from the infants while hypoxic.

Particular impressive to us were the following individual examples where we observed a striking lack of relation between heart rate and Po_2. Despite the 5 minute period of hypoxaemia in this premature (1800 g), there is no noticable change in heart

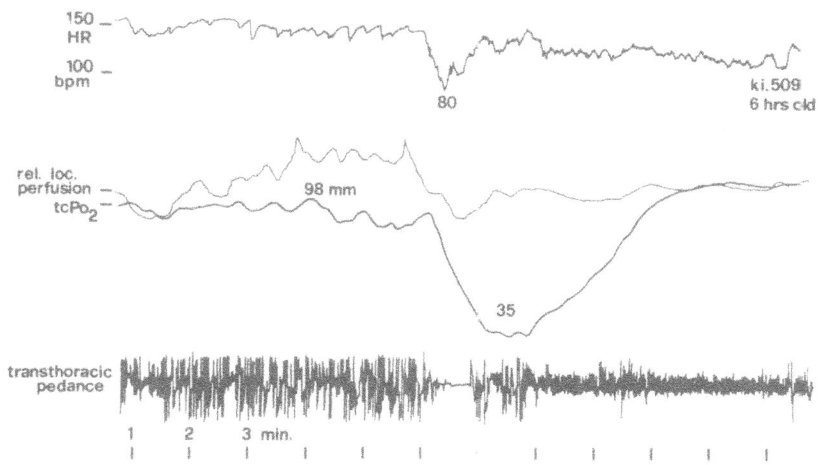

Fig. 4: Part of a continuous registration of $tcPo_2$ together with beat to beat recording of heart rate, with relative local perfusion, transthoracic impedance and respiratory rate. An apnoeic phase of about 35 sec. leads to a parallel drop in heart rate and Po_2.

rate (Fig. 6).

During an unavoidable disconnection from the respirator this child (Fig. 7) was monitored. Here, again, we note no significant change in heart rate desplite marked hypoxaemie. Because of the constance of the perfusion tracing, we are certain that the fall in arterial Po_2 is real. We note even a slight increase in the local perfusion which probably reflects a slight increase in blood pressure.

In addition we have investigated the fluctuation of heart rate and its relationship to Po_2. In order to study heart rate fluctuations and resulting patterns, a beat to beat recording device is required. Various obstetrical groups (11, 12) have identified repetitive patterns which were considered suggestive of fetal hypoxaemia and distress. One of these is the silence, type zero-oscillation, in which there is less than 5 bpm fluctuation. Unfortunately, we have only integrated heart rate recordings in our data from sick infants from other clinics. Therefore we have only been able to review fluctuation patterns from the tracings taken in our clinic. These are mostly healthy newborns and we thus have only few hypoxic tracings. From our many tracings, we selected all those with silent heart rate oscillations and all those with low Po_2 recordings (n = 24) and compared these selected charts with a number of random tracings

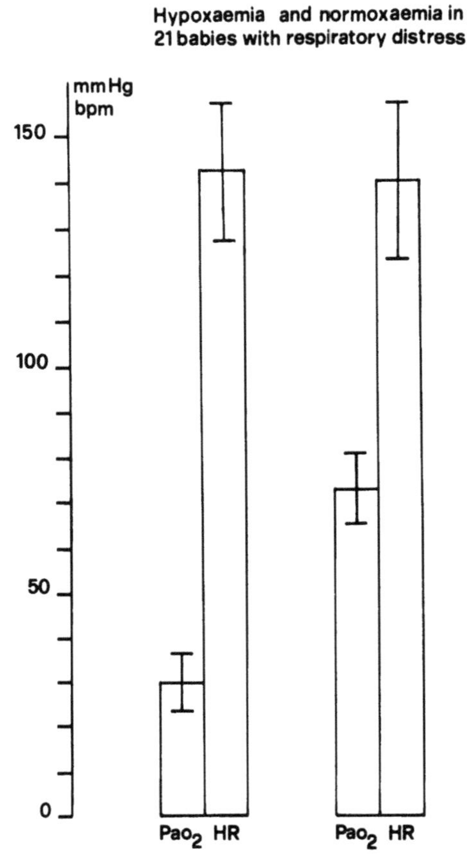

Fig. 5: Representation of mean values and standard deviations of Po_2 and heart rate an 21 sick infants. Left: hypoxaemia. Right: normoxaemia after treatment.

(n = 76; Fig. 8). It is worth noting that all of the low Po_2 values we recorded were accompagnied by a silent heart rate oscillation. However, it must also be noticed that many silent heart rate oscillations were observed together with a normal Po_2 value.

So let us review and summarize our results:

1. The decline in heart rate level seen throughout the first day of age is independent of the Po_2 level.
2. Also, within each age group we could demonstrate no relationship between heart rate and Po_2 values.

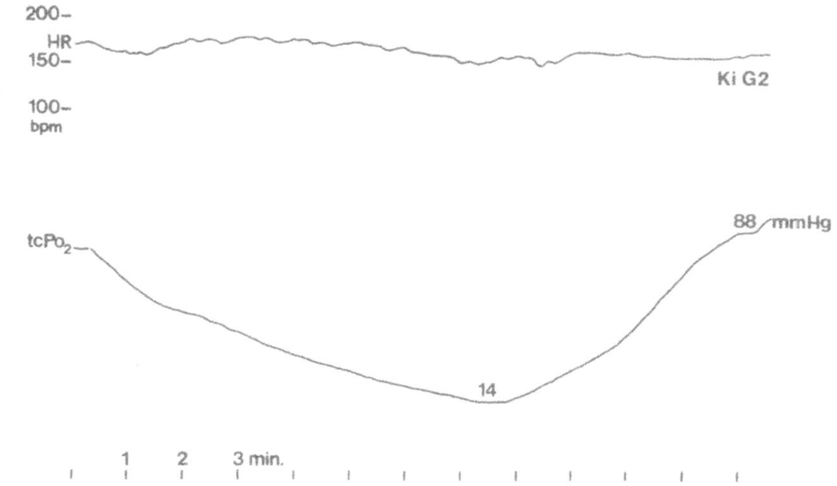

Fig. 6: Part of a continuous registration of $tcPo_2$ and integrated heart rate in a premature. Hypoxaemia over several minutes does not change the heart rate level markedly.

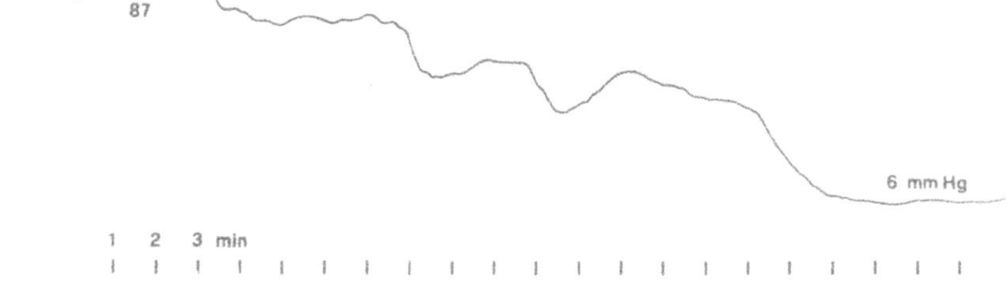

Fig. 7: Simultaneous recording of integrated heart rate, relative local perfusion and $tcPo_2$ in a ventilated infant during uravoidable disconnection from the respirator.
Note the unchanged level in heart rate.

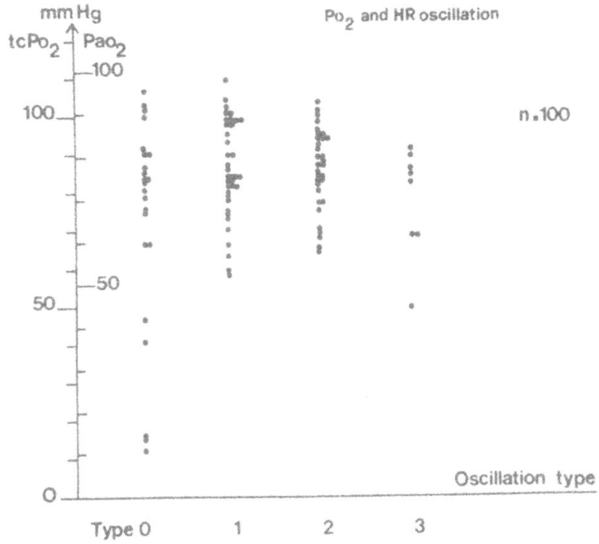

Fig. 8: Relation between Po_2 and heart rate oscillations

3. A spontaneous prolonged apnoeic episode, in an otherwise clinically normal infant, only demonstrated a 10 second depression of heart rate.

4. We have shown that the heart rate level in sick infants with hypoxia, mean Po_2 of 30 mm Hg, is significantly higher than the heart rate of healthy infants. However, this abnormally elevated heart rate persists even when ventilatory support improves the Po_2 values to normal range.

5. According to our numerous individual observations of respiratorily depressed infants, acute or chronic hypoxaemia is not always accompanied by the same dramatic changes in heart rate.

6. From our first comparative observations of Po_2 and beat to beat heart rate recordings we suggest that the patterns and not the absolute rate may provide a screening method for the detection of hypoxaemia.

These results, particularly the poor correlation of heart rate and Po_2 values in sick infants lead us to suggest a very cautious interpretation when only integrated heart rate is monitored. Also, we advise against false security when heart rate is normal, since hypoxaemia may still be present.

References

1. HUCH, A., HUCH, R., MEINZER, K., LÜBBERS, D.W.: Medizin-Technik 16.5.1972 in Stuttgart

2. HUCH, R., LÜBBERS, D.W., HUCH, A.: J. Perinat. Med. 1, 183, 1973

3. HUCH, A., HUCH, R., ARNER, B., ROOTH, G.: Scand. J. Clin. Lab. Invest. 31, 3, 1973

4. HUCH, R., LÜBBERS, D.W., HUCH, A.: Archives of Disease in Childhood 49, 213, 1974

5. HUCH, R., LÜBBERS, D.W., HUCH, A.: in Bicher/Bruley: Oxygen Transport to Tissue, Plenum Publishing Corporation, New York 1973, 1121

6. HUCH, R., LÜBBERS, D.W., HUCH, A.: A Symposium on Current Status of Oxygen Measurement in Biology and Medicine, 27.-28.6.1974 in Marlow-on-Thames

7. HUCH, A., HUCH, R., BUCHHOLZ, R., LÜBBERS, D.W.: Geburtsh. u. Frauenheilkunde 33, 856, 1973

8. CORDERO, JR., L.: Biol. Neonate 20, 270, 1972

9. KLÖCK, F.K., CLOOS, H.P., LAMBERTI, G., SCHWENZEL, W.: Z. Geburtsh. Perinat. 176, 266, 1972

10. RÜTTGERS, H., LORENZ, U., HALLER, H.U., FOEISCH, H., KUBLI, F.: Perinatale Medizin, Band IV, hrsg. von Dudenhausen u. Saling, Georg-Thieme-Verlag 1973, page 468

11. HAMMACHER, K.: Gynäkologie u. Geburtshilfe, Bd. II, hrsg. von O. Käser, V. Friedberg, G.Ober, K. Thomsen, J. Zander, Stuttgart 1967

12. HON, E.H.: Harty Press. Inc., New Haven, Connecticut 1968

A COMPARISON OF TRANSCUTANEOUS AND ARTERIAL PO_2 IN SICK NEONATES

Linda P. Soutter and Dawood Parker

Department of Medical Physics

University College Hospital, London

We have investigated the reliability of a transcutaneous PO_2 sensor - the Hoffmann la Roche Oxygen Monitor 5300 - for the continuous assessment of the arterial PO_2 of sick infants over periods of several hours. The PO_2 transducer - developed by Eberhard and his colleagues[1] - uses a large cathode 4 mm in diameter in conjunction with a membrane of low oxygen permeability to prevent alteration of the oxygen profile in the tissue by the oxygen consumption of the sensor. The transducer is heated to produce local hyperemisation of the skin - most of our measurements were made with the sensor at 42°, more recently some were made with the temperature increased to 43°. 22 premature babies in the Neonatal Unit at University College Hospital were monitored. All were undergoing oxygen therapy during treatment for respiratory disease. 13 of the subjects, aged 4 to 101 hours, had an umbilical artery catheter with a built in PO_2 transducer, providing a means of continuous comparison of arterial with skin PO_2 (the catheter-tip transducer has been used in more than 50 infants at U.C.H. and has been shown to give a linear response to P_aO_2[2,3]). The other 9 infants, aged 7 to 32 days had no arterial catheter and comparisons were made by analysis of blood samples obtained by arterial puncture with a Radiometer Type E5046 PO_2 electrode which was also used to check the calibration of the catheter-tip transducer.

After preparation of the membrane, the skin PO_2 sensor was allowed to stabilize overnight then calibrated using the electronic zero and air PO_2. The infant's skin was cleaned, wiped with alcohol and dried and the sensor attached using an adhesive tape ring. The upper part of the chest was used for most measurements both because this has been recommended by other authors[1,4] and

Table 1

Case	Birthweight (g)	Diagnosis	No. of Sensor Applications	Total Monitoring Time (hr)	Sensor Temp. 42° Skin PO_2 / P_aO_2 % Mean (range)	Sensor Temp. 43° Skin PO_2 / P_aO_2 % Mean (range)
1	1786	HMD	1	6	88(83-92)	
2	1790	HMD	2	8	62(31-88)	
3	1940	Hydrops foetalis	4	21	39(26-85)	
4	1641	HMD	1	6	83(78-104)	
5	1878	HMD	2	7	50(21-83)	
6	883	Lung liquid retention	1	12	92(72-126)	
7	1250	Pneumonia & septicaemia	3	16	60(39-89)	
8	1445	Hydrops foetalis	2	10	80(59-93)	
9	1175	HMD	4	24	66(25-100)	
10	2114	Hydrops foetalis	2	10	93(75-107)	
11	2930	Pulmonary haemorrhage	6	36	72(21-115)	119(60-200)
12	995	HMD	3	14	92(70-106)	121(76-135)
13	2383	Pneumonia	3	13	95(85-104)	145(109-162)

HMD = hyaline membrane disease

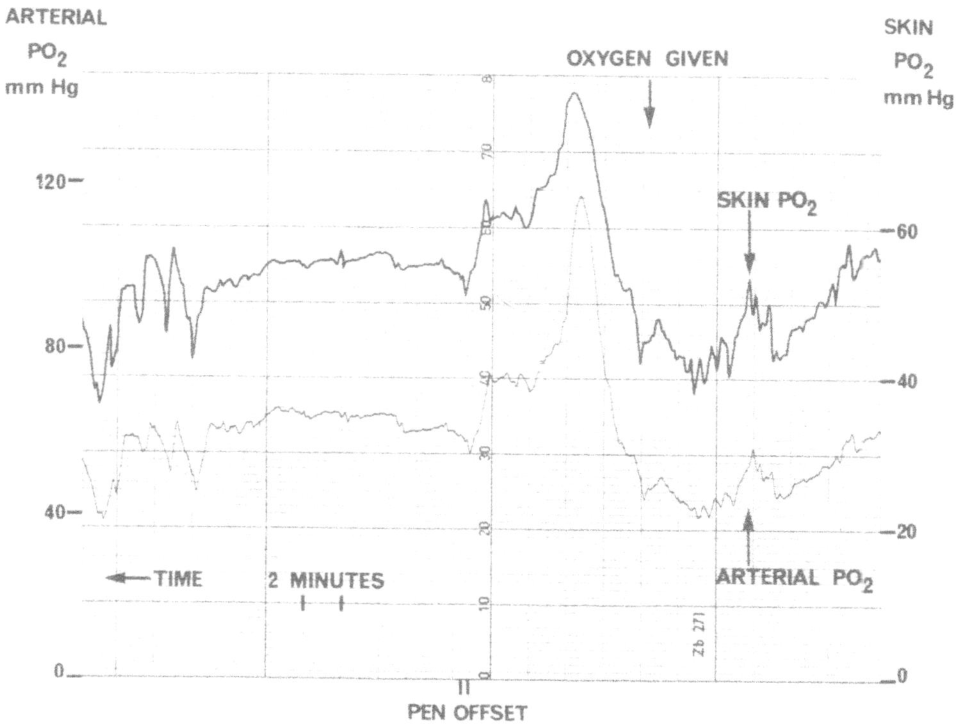

Fig. 1 shows good correlation between skin and arterial PO_2 but the skin response is damped at higher PO_2s. The subject was a 12 hour old baby (birthweight 883 g) breathing air with intermittent oxygen via a face mask.
(N.B. pen offset - arterial trace in advance of skin trace.)

because it was often the only flat area on very small babies. The sensor output was allowed to stabilize for twenty minutes before measurements were started. Readings for comparison with catheter-tip transducer PO_2 were taken every 24 minutes. In the older babies arterial puncture samples were taken when clinically necessary. After periods of 3 to 12 hours the sensor was removed from the skin and its calibration checked.

The 22 subjects were monitored for a total of 228 hours with 43 applications of the sensor. The mean air PO_2 calibration of the sensor on removal from the skin was 99% (range 89%-104%) of the original calibration. Table 1 summarises the results obtained by

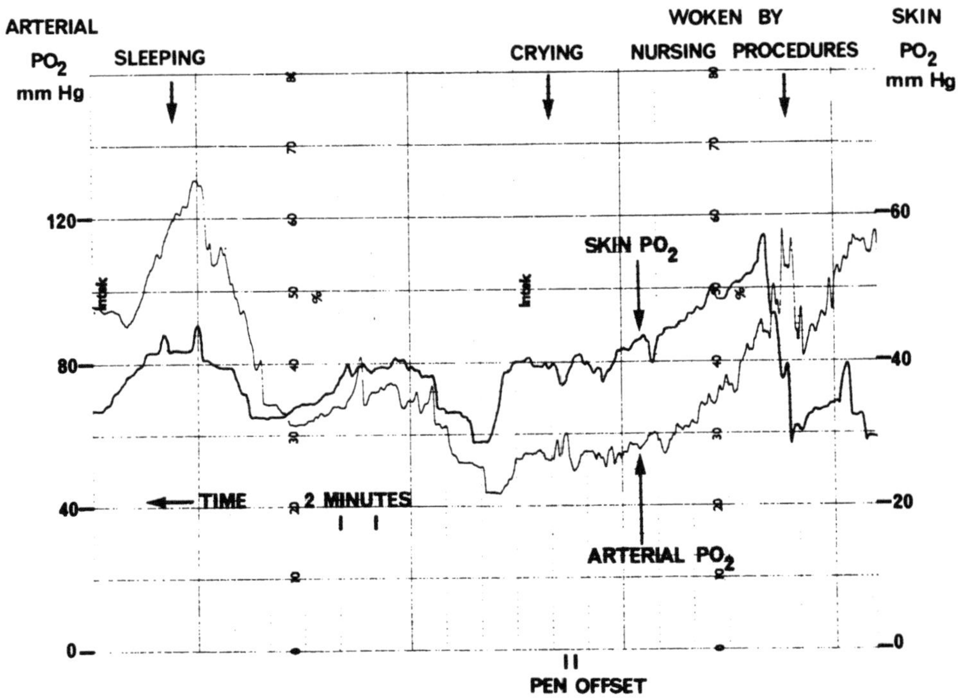

Fig. 2 shows a lack of correlation between skin and arterial PO_2 while the baby slept. When he woke and cried the skin PO_2 reading increased. The subject was aged 70 hours (birthweight 2930 g) breathing spontaneously (F_1O_2 44%) while recovering from a pulmonary haemorrhage.
(N.B. pen offset - arterial trace in advance of skin trace.)

comparison of arterial catheter PO_2 transducer output with skin PO_2. The most obvious feature of the comparison is the wide variation in degree of correlation, that is skin PO_2 expressed as a percentage of P_aO_2, between the two measurements. In 3 cases (subjects 1, 4 and 6) skin PO_2 followed the general trends of P_aO_2 throughout the periods of comparison as shown in fig. 1, giving a good correlation with P_aO_2 (mean 88%) although correlation was better at lower PO_2s - below 50 mm Hg PO_2 the mean correlation was 101% and above 70 mm Hg it was 79%. In the other 10 subjects the degree of correlation between the two measurements varied during the course of each comparison. In 2 subjects (cases 2 and 5) this variation took the

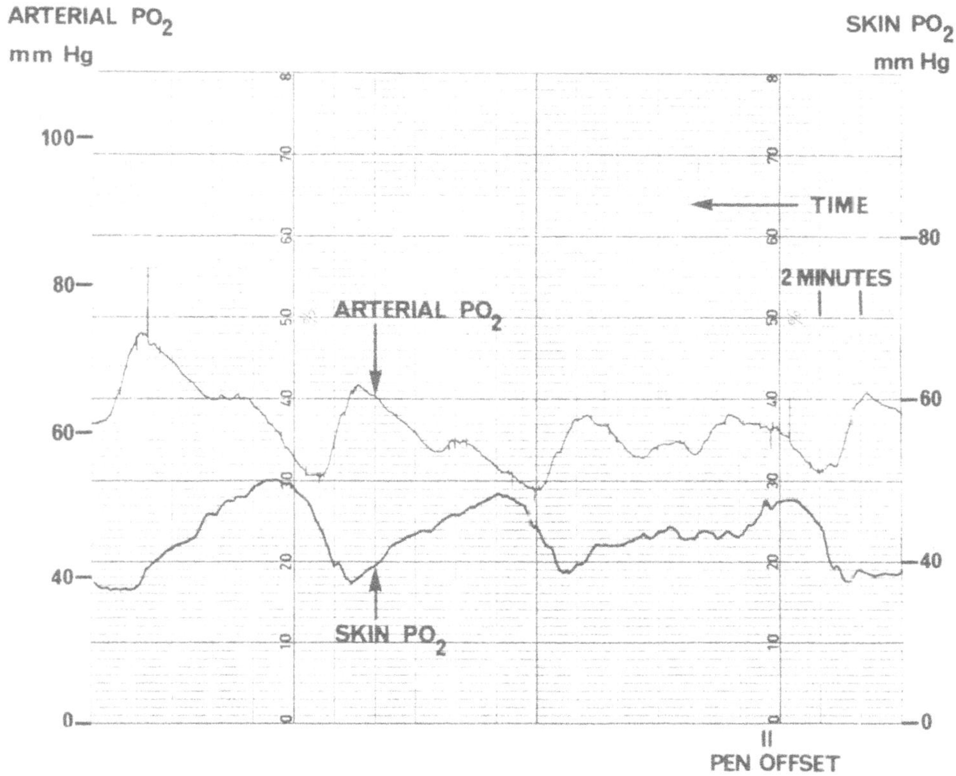

Fig. 3 shows inverse correlation between skin and arterial PO_2. The subject was a 28 hour old Rhesus affected Hydrops foetalis (birthweight 1940 g) undergoing mechanical ventilation (F_1O_2 65%). 24 hours after this recording the baby went into irreversible shock. (N.B. pen offset - arterial trace in advance of skin trace.)

form of an apparent gradual decrease in sensitivity of the skin PO_2 sensor although at the end of the period of measurement the calibration of the sensor was normal. The skin immediately beneath the sensor in these cases was pale and puffy in appearance, unlike the normal red of hyperemised skin. In the remaining subjects there was intermittent loss of correlation between the two measurements, skin PO_2 almost always being lower than arterial PO_2. The loss of correlation occurred more frequently in the infants with the most severe clinical symptoms (cases 3, 7, 9 and 11) - examples of this are shown in figures 2 and 3. Recently a modification has been made to the Oxygen Monitor to enable the sensor to be used at a higher temperature. Preliminary results with the sensor at 43°

have shown an increase in the overall level of the skin PO_2 reading but in 2 out of 3 trials variations in correlation still occurred. Use of the sensor on one baby at 44° for only 2 hours produced a dark red mark still visible 2 days later so we did not think it wise to use this temperature routinely.

20 comparisons of skin PO_2 with the PO_2 of arterial puncture samples in the 9 older infants gave a mean value of skin PO_2 of 82% of P_aO_2 (range 66-111). All samples were in the PO_2 range 40 to 100 mm Hg.

In this investigation skin PO_2 did not provide a consistently reliable monitor of arterial PO_2 for 10 of the 22 subjects and gave the most variable correlation with P_aO_2 for the 4 most severely distressed infants. In 2 cases the infants' skin appeared to react unfavourably to the presence of the sensor. The variations in correlation are presumably due to fluctuation in perfusion of the skin beneath the sensor, therefore a means of measuring this perfusion is necessary for the safe use of the transcutaneous method in this situation.

References

1. P. Eberhard, W. Mindt, F. Jann and K. Hammacher. "Oxygen monitoring of newborns by skin electrodes. Correlation between arterial and cutaneously determined PO_2." Advances in Experimental Medicine and Biology 37B 1097 (1973).

2. D. Parker and L.P. Soutter. "In vivo monitoring of blood PO_2 in newborn infants." Proc. symposium on Current Status of Oxygen Measurements in Biology and Medicine, Marlow, June 1974. Butterworths (in press).

3. M. Conway, G.M. Durbin, D. Parker, E.O.R. Reynolds and L.P. Soutter. "Continuous measurement of arterial oxygen tension using a new-catheter-tip polarographic electrode". Proc. N.I.H. Conference on Perinatal Intensive Care, Bethesda (1974) edit J. Dancis (in press).

4. R. Huch, A. Huch and D.W. Lubbers. "Transcutaneous measurement of blood PO_2 - Method and application in perinatal medicine". J. Perinat. Med. 1 183 (1973).

EFFECT OF UMBILICAL ARTERY CATHETERS ON OXYGEN SUPPLY TO EXTREMITIES

Anthony V. Beran, Robert F. Huxtable, Kenneth G. Proctor and Donald R. Sperling.

University of California, Irvine, College of Medicine
Department of Pediatrics, Irvine, California, U.S.A.

Umbilical artery catheters are routinely used in patient management. Reported complications of this procedure include thrombosis, infection, vessel perforation, extremity blanching, and visceral necrosis (1,2). A catheter placed in an artery produces a partial acute mechanical obstruction equivalent to coarctation of the aorta.

Theoretical consideration used as a rationale for this study are given in the following equation for streamline flow of a Newtonian fluid through an annular system:

$$\dot{Q} = \frac{\pi(\Delta P)}{L(8\lambda)}\left[R_2^4 - R_1^4 - \frac{(R_2^2 - R_1^2)^2}{\ln \frac{R_2}{R_1}}\right];$$

where $\dot{Q}$=flow, ΔP=pressure drop, L=tube length, λ=viscosity, R_2= radius of outer tube (aorta) and R_1=radius of inner tube (catheter). $\dot{Q}$ is primarily effected by ΔR which is a fourth power variable. Although an *in vivo* situation differs from the ideal *in vitro* situation (Non-Newtonian characteristics of blood, pulsatile rather than steady flow, elasticity of the outer vessel wall, etc.), we speculated that because of the anomalous viscosity of blood, and the turbulent rather than laminar flow along the inner tube, the flow would be decreased even further than predicted. The purpose of this study was to evaluate the effect of "R" (3.5 and 5.0F umbilical artery catheter) on blood flow and oxygen supply to the extremities.

METHODS

Experimental Procedure

Male New Zealand rabbits (1.6 to 3.5 kg) were anesthetized with intravenous sodium pentobarbital (25 mg/kg) and placed on a heating blanket (Gorman-Rupp) maintained at 39°C. In 10 animals, the right common iliac artery was exposed intraperitoneally, and a blood flow probe was secured around the vessel. A needle thermistor was placed subcutaneously in the foot distal to the flow probe. An oxygen electrode was implanted in the right gracilis muscle, distal to the flow probe and proximal to the thermistor. An arterial catheter (3.5F or 5F) was then inserted in the left femoral artery, 3 cm from the bifurcation of the abdominal aorta. Control data for the physiologic variables described below were obtained at this point in time. The catheter was advanced 15-20 cm and left in place for 10-30 min. If the 3.5F produced a significant obstruction as manifested by decrease in blood flow or tissue oxygen availability, the 5F catheter was not used. Zero tissue oxygen availability and blood flow levels were obtained by periodic occlusion of the vessel or at death. In 10 additional animals (.55 to 2.6 kg) the above procedure was repeated, without placement of the blood flow probe, in order to eliminate possible vascular constriction by the probe.

Physiologic Variables

Arterial blood pressure (BP) was continuously monitored by a pressure transducer (Statham P23DB). Temperature (T) was measured by thermistor (Yellow Springs, Tele-thermometer). Blood flow (BF) was continuously monitored by electromagnetic blood flow meter (IVM EMF 101). Muscle tissue oxygen availability (O_2a) was continuously monitored polarographically (3) using commercially available electrodes (International Biophysics Corp. Irvine, California). All dynamic variables were recorded on a chart recorder.

RESULTS

Mean and standard deviation for BP, BF, O_2a and T produced by insertion of 3.5F and 5F catheters advanced 15-20 cm are presented in Table 1. Values obtained at "o" time represent control values prior to catheter advance, while values obtained at 5 and 10 min. represent values after the advance.

The 3.5F catheters produced a slight increase in BP and a decrease in O_2a and BF to 66 ± 48% and 72 ± 39% respectively. T decreased from 37.1 ± 2.4°C to 36.7 ± 2.6°C. Out of 16 determinations obtained with this catheter, 5 showed a decrease in BF, O_2a and T, while the remaining did not change. The 5.0F catheter produced a

Table 1

Changes in Physiologic Variables Produced by 15-20 cm Insertion of 3.5 and 5.0F Arterial Catheters

CATHETER SIZE		3.5 F			5.0 F	
Time (min)	0	5	10	0	5	10
BP (mm Hg)	104±16 / 76±11	108±18 / 79±13	108±18 / 79±13	120±17 / 80±10	124±19 / 81±9	123±19 / 83±11
O_2a (%)	100	68±40	66±48	100	30±33	23±31
BF (%)	100	73±35	72±39	100	42±38	35±38
T (°C)	37.1±2.4	36.5±2.9	36.7±2.6	37.7±1.1	36.8±1.4	36.3±1.7

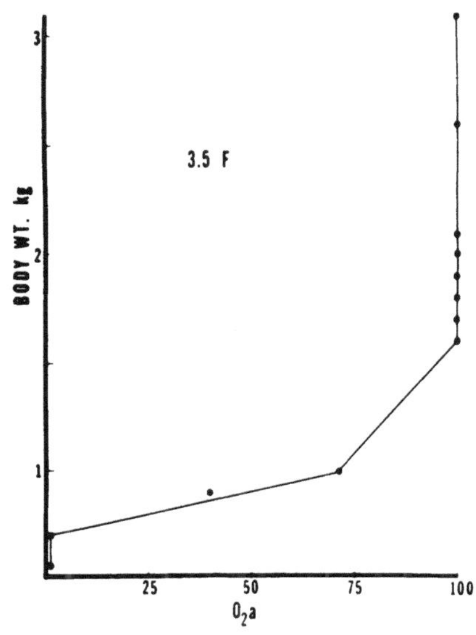

Fig. 1: Changes in O_2a as a function of body weight produced by 3.5 F catheters.

moderately greater increase in BP and a decrease in O_2a and BF to 23 ± 31% and 35 ± 38%, respectively. T decreased from 37.7 ± 1.1°C to 36.3 ± 1.7°C. Of 14 determinations obtained with 5.0F, all showed a decrease in BF, O_2a and T.

O_2a changes as a function of body weight produced by insertion of 3.5F catheters in a group of animals in which the blood flow probe was not implanted, are shown in Fig. 1. Insertion of this catheter in animals weighing more than 1.6 kg did not produce any change in O_2a. In those weighing less than 1.6 kg but more than .7 kg, the gradual decrease was proportional to body weight, while in those weighing less than .7 kg, O_2a was 100% decreased.

DISCUSSION

Effects of 3.5F and 5.0F catheters on blood flow and oxygenation of lower extremities were evaluated in animals weighing .55 - 3.5 kg. Our results indicate that reduction in BF, O_2a, and T is related to the relative dimensions of the vessel and the catheter (Δr). 3.5F catheters decreased BF, T and O_2a in animals weighing less than 1.6 kg, while 5.0F catheters produced similar decreases in animals weighing less than 2.1 kg. Although the radius of the 3.5F catheter is 70% of that of the 5.0F, the obstructing cross sectional area of the latter is doubled, accounting for the impressive difference in flows through the annular space, and resulting in a significant reduction in oxygen supply to the extremities. This suggests that only 3.5F (or smaller) catheters should be used in small newborns. Clinically, various sites have been suggested for catheter placement such as: abdominal aorta distal to the renal and inferior mesenteric arteries, and proximal to the aortic bifurcation (4); thoracic aorta, distal to the ductus arteriosus (4); and iliac artery or just above the aortic bifurcation (5). Our data indicate that there is no change in oxygen supply to the opposite extremity when the catheter is placed below the aortic bifurcation suggesting this as a preferred site. This concurs with recent reports by others (6,7). These factors should be considered during clinical application of umbilical artery catheters. Undesirable changes could be detected by continuous monitoring of extremity O_2a or differential core and extremity T.

REFERENCES

1. Kitterman JA, Phibbs RH and Tooley WH. Catheterization of umbilical vessels in newborn infants. Pediat Clin N Amer 17:895-912, 1970.

2. Lackey DA and Taber P. An unusual complication of umbilical artery catheterization. Pediatrics 49:281-283, 1972.

3. Beran AV, Strauss J, Sperling DR, Norton AC, Garwood VP and Yamazaki J. Effect of Thalidomide on brain oxygenation. Pediat Res 5:199-205, 1971.

4. James LS. Complications arising from catheterization of the umbilical vessels. In Problems of Neonatal Intensive Care Units (Report of the Fifty-Ninth Ross Conference on Pediatric Research Stowe, Vt., 1969).

5. Vidyasagar D, Downes JJ and Boggs TR. Respiratory Distress Syndrome of Newborn Infants II. Technic of catheterization of umbilical artery and clinical results of treatment of 124 patients. Clin Pediat 9:332-337, 1970.

6. Book LS, Herbst JJ and Atherton S. Gluteal Necrosis and gastrointestinal bleeding: complications of Ca gluconate infusion through umbilical artery catheterization. Clin Res 23:157, 1975.

7. Powers WF and Swyer PR. Limb blood flow following umbilical arterial catheterization. Pediatrics 55:248-256, 1975.

TISSUE OXYGEN AVAILABLE (O_2a) AS A CRITERION FOR THE EFFECTIVENESS OF CONTINUOUS POSITIVE PRESSURE BREATHING (CPPB)

Anthony V. Beran, Donald R. Sperling, Kenneth G. Proctor, and Robert F. Huxtable

University of California, Irvine, College of Medicine
Department of Pediatrics, Irvine, California, U.S.A.

Since Gregory's report (1) on the effectiveness of Continuous Positive Airway Pressure for treatment of infants with the Idiopathic Respiratory Distress Syndrome (IRDS), the method has been widely accepted throughout the world. This method provides increased proximal airway pressure (Ppa) sufficient to prevent alveolar collapse at the end of expiration, while the subject is breathing spontaneously. In the normal lung, as little as 3-5 cm H_2O Ppa may reduce cardiac output ($\dot{Q}$). Contrary to this, it is postulated that in IRDS, decreased pulmonary compliance (SC_L) acts as a barrier and minimizes this effect. Pulmonary compliance varies widely between normal subjects and those with IRDS of varying severity. Therefore, a wide range of Ppa is required to provide optimal oxygenation without reducing $\dot{Q}$. Since $\dot{Q}$ is not routinely measured, a reduction in $\dot{Q}$ could follow an excessive increase in Ppa; in addition, excessive reduction in $\dot{Q}$ could accompany regression of the disease while Ppa is unchanged.

This study was undertaken to determine whether O_2a could be used to detect changes in perfusion when excessive Ppa is applied during CPPB.

METHODS

Thirteen adult male New Zealand rabbits (1.8-2.6 kg) were divided into two groups. The control group (N) consisted of 5 normal animals and the experimental group (E) consisted of 8 animals with lungs damaged by exposure to high oxygen concentrations for 36-48 hours.

Animal model

Individual animals in the experimental group were placed in a chamber with adequate food and water supply and normobaric 100% O_2 circulating at 6 l/min. After 36-48 hours, the animals were removed from the chamber and exposed to room air for 1-3 hours before the initiation of any experimental procedure.

Experimental procedure

Animals were anesthetized with intravenous sodium pentobarbital (25 mg/kg) and placed on a heating pad (Gorman Rupp K-1) maintained at 39°C. A tracheostomy tube was inserted and secured. A 5F arterial catheter, containing a monopolar oxygen sensor (International Biophysics Corp., Irvine, Calif--IBC), was advanced from the femoral artery to a point distal to the aortic bifurcation for monitoring of blood pressures (BP), arterial partial oxygen pressure (PaO_2) and for blood sample collection. A venous catheter was advanced from the femoral vein into the right atrium for pressure measurement (Pra) and blood sample collection. $\dot{Q}$ was determined by the Fick principle. A balloon secured to PE 260 tubing was inserted orally to the cardiac sphincter and then withdrawn to the lower 1/3 of the esophagus for measurement of esophageal pressure (Pes). A monopolar oxygen electrode (IBC) was implanted in the right triceps muscle for measurement of O_2a (2). Reference electrodes were secured to the skin and connected to the monitoring systems. The treacheostomy tube was connected to a pneumotachograph in series with a CPPB system similar to one described by Gregory (1). A humidified airflow of 12 l/min was circulated through the system. Control values for all physiologic variables measured were obtained at this point. Ppa was then increased from .5-15 cm H_2O in 3 cm increments at 10 min intervals. At 12 cm H_2O, the fraction of inspired O_2 (FiO_2) was increased from ambient to 50% and 100%. During these procedures animals were breathing spontaneously and regulating their own respiratory rates and tidal volumes.

Static lung compliance (SC_L) and histologic evaluations were performed in six normal and six oxygen treated animals not exposed to CPPB in order to verify the validity of the experimental model. In addition, SC was measured immediately after death in all animals following CPPB application. To permit comparison of lungs of different sizes, volume was expressed as ml of gas per gram of lung tissue (3).

RESULTS

Representative static pressure volume curves from the control (normal lung) and experimental (oxygen damaged lung) groups are presented in Fig. 1. The minimum pressure required to initiate inflation was 12 cm H_2O in the normal lung, and 16 cm H_2O in the oxygen damaged lung. At the maximally applied pressure of 25 cm H_2O the normal lung appeared fully inflated, while the damaged lung demonstrated multiple lobulation surrounded by uninflated segments of tissue. In addition, at this pressure, the normal lung contained almost twice as much gas per gram of tissue as the damaged lung. Furthermore, the slope of the pressure volume curve over the entire range was reduced in the damaged lung. Histologic evaluation of damaged lungs showed pulmonary hemorrhage, atelectasis, and edema but no evidence of cellular atypia or hyaline membrane formation. SC_L at the peak inflation pressure at 25 cm H_2O was 9.5±1.8 cc/g of tissue in the control group, and 5.5±1.4 cc/g of tissue in the experimental group.

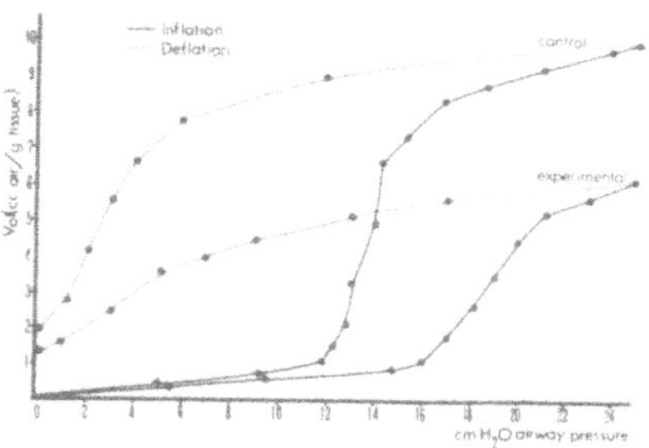

Fig. 1. Representative pressure-volume curves.

Mean Pra in the control group increased with each increment in Ppa. In contrast to this, in the experimental group, this increase in Pra did not occur until a Ppa of greater than 6 cm H_2O was reached. At 6 cm H_2O, the difference between the two groups was statistically significant ($t=9.58$, $p<.005$). At the maximum Ppa of 15 cm H_2O, mean Pra for control and experimental groups was 10.0±1.8 cm H_2O (240% of control) and 5.9±1.8 cm H_2O (140% of control), respectively. $\dot{Q}$ in the control group decreased with each increment in Ppa. At 9 cm H_2O it had decreased to 60%, reaching 22% of control at 15 cm H_2O Ppa. In the experimental group, $\dot{Q}$ remained essentially unchanged until 9 cm H_2O Ppa, subsequently it decreased, and at 15 cm H_2O Ppa it was 57% of control.

Mean and standard deviation changes for PaO_2 and O_2a obtained at .5,3,6,9 and 12 cm H_2O Ppa and at an FiO_2 of 20.9%, 50% and 100% at 12 cm H_2O Ppa are presented in Table 1. In normal animals PaO_2 decreased from 96 to 88 mm Hg when Ppa was increased from .5 to 12 cm H_2O. O_2a decreased with each increment in Ppa, reaching 22% of control at 12 cm H_2O Ppa. In experimental animals, changes in PaO_2 were similar to those observed in normal animals. However, in contrast to normals, O_2a initially increased, then fell below the control levels at 9 cm H_2O Ppa, reaching a 36% of control at 12 cm H_2O Ppa. The difference between normal and experimental animals at this pressure was statistically significant.

TABLE 1

Effect of increased Ppa on PaO_2 and O_2a in Normal(N) and Pulmonary Damaged(E) animals.

Ppa cm H_2O		.5	3	6	9	12	12	12
FiO_2%		20.9	20.9	20.9	20.9	20.9	50	100
PaO_2mm Hg	N	96±7	96±6	98±5	94±3	88±10	197±23	408±32
	E	56±9	56±9	55±11	46±9	39±8	154±55	316±80
O_2a%	N	100	92±10	72±11	55±10	22±11	40±13	45±18
	E	100	107±12	100±21	78±20	36±17	146±144	201±192

DISCUSSION

CPPB at 3-15 cm H_2O Ppa was evaluated in animals with normal and low lung compliance. Animals with normal compliance could not tolerate any increase in Ppa. This was manifested by an immediate increase in Pes and Pra and a decrease in $\dot{Q}$ and O_2a when as little as 3 cm H_2O Ppa was applied. Contrary to this, animals with low compliance lungs exhibited the protective "barrier effect", tolerating much higher pressures. Pes and Pra increased and $\dot{Q}$ and O_2a decreased only at 6-9 cm H_2O Ppa. Furthermore, at 12 cm H_2O Ppa these changes were less magnitude in animals with low compliance lungs. This manifests that changes in $\dot{Q}$ are accompanied with changes in the muscle O_2a.

PaO_2 in both groups was decreased only when a Ppa of 12 cm H_2O was reached. Administration of 100% O_2 at this pressure increased PaO_2 as high as 408 mm Hg while O_2a in control and experimental group was 45% and 201% of control respectively. This exemplifies that PaO_2 can be at normal or hyperoxic levels while O_2a is markedly decreased suggesting a reduction in perfusion. The reduction in perfusion was of greater magnitude in animals with normal compliance lungs. Our data indicate that the mechanism of the reduction in perfusion is by means of pressure transmission across the alveolar wall, which in turn produces an increase in Pes, followed by increase in Pra and a decrease in pulmonary venous return, $\dot{Q}$ and O_2a, and that this mechanism is compliance dependent. This suggest the importance of measuring variables which reflect changes in perfusion in addition to changes in systemic oxygenation.

Because changes in O_2a occur concurrently with changes in Pes, Pra and $\dot{Q}$, we stress that a reduction in O_2a would accurately reflect excessive Ppa. Since changes in $\dot{Q}$ during CPPB are compliance dependent and since O_2a is $\dot{Q}$ dependent, O_2a could provide a means of selecting optimal Ppa during CPPB.

REFERENCES

1. Gregory GA, Kitterman JA, Phibbs RH, Tooley WH and Hamilton WK. Treatment of the idiopathic respiratory distress syndrome with continuous positive airway pressure. New Eng J Med 284:1333, 1971.
2. Beran AV, Strauss J, Sperling DR, Norton AC, Garwood VP, and Yamazaki J. Effect of Thalidomide on brain oxygenation. Pediat Res 5:199, 1971.
3. Gribetz I, Frank NR and Avery ME. Static volume pressure relations of excised lungs of infants with hyaline membrane disease, newborn and stillborn infants. J Clin Invest 38:2168, 1959.

SUMMARY OF DISCUSSION - SESSION XIII:

PERINATAL OXYGEN SUPPLY

Chairmen: M. Silver, M. Mochizuki, and W. Moll

The first, third and fourth papers of this session concerned different aspects of fetal oxygenation. Dr. Moll showed that an increase in placental blood flow in the guinea pig resulted in increased placental oxygen uptake and a rise in fetal heart rate. In answer to two questions from Dr. Silver, he said that predominantly placental rather than uterine blood flow and oxygen uptake were measured because the arterial supply to the uterine muscle had been ligated. He discussed the possibility that the oxygen supply to the guinea pig fetus may be limited, so that an artificial increase in this supply led to better fetal oxygenation and an increase in its heart rate although the mechanism for the latter was not known.

Dr. Guilbeau showed, experimentally and mathematically, the changes in fetal brain (cortical) PO_2 which occurred during maternal hypoxia and hyperoxia in the goat. Dr. Bicher commented that these changes might be considered as autoregulatory as he had suggested for the adult animal. However, the authors felt that although both "delay" and "over shoot" phenomena were seen in the fetal brain PO_2 changes, the underlying mechanisms for these were not yet fully understood. The delayed response in the fetus could be accounted for by the sequential transport changes in the maternal circulation, placenta and fetal circulation. The PO_2 overshoot seen on reoxygenation might be due to a number of factors e.g., local or general hyperemia. Dr. Moll asked whether the oxygen saturation difference between fetal arterial blood to the head and that in the lower aorta was taken into account in the mathematical model used, because this could be an important factor in cerebral oxygen supply. He was assured that this was being incorporated into a new, more complex model of the fetal circulation in which output to different organs and the degree of cardiac mixing varies with fetal oxygenation.

In measurements of fetal oxygen and metabolite uptake in conscious cows and horses, Dr. Silver showed that more oxygen was used by the fetus than could be accounted for by uptake of known metabolic fuels. Dr. Siesjo wondered if the "missing substrate" might be β-OH-butyrate or aceto-acetate but was assured that these are not used by sheep fetuses (according to Meschia and colleagues). He asked if R.Q's had been measured because if the values were close to 1.0 then carbohydrates, perhaps from the glycogen stores in the placenta, were implicated as the main source of energy. Dr. Silver thought that the very high placental glucose uptake might result in the formation of some other metabolic fuel for fetal use; fructose would be an obvious substrate but unfortunately no fetal utilization of this sugar could be detected. Fetal R.Q.'s were not measured in these experiments but in sheep the value is just under 1.0. Dr. Moll pointed out that in sheep there is a very low fetal glucose level and that, unlike the cow, fetal glucose uptake is dependent on maternal concentration (according to Battaglia and Meschia); he asked about fetal and maternal glucose levels in cows. Dr. Silver replied that bovine fetal values were higher than in fetal lambs; concentrations ranged between 20 and 30 mg/100 ml over a maternal range of 65-85 mg/100 ml, and under these conditions the fetal glucose uptake appeared to be independent of maternal concentrations.

In the second paper of the session Dr. Goodwin showed some of the respiratory enzyme changes which occur in heart mitochondria during the perinatal period in puppies and lambs. Drs. Versmold and Longmuir were concerned that the respiratory rate had been related only to mitochondrial protein. Dr. Longmuir thought it should be related to the DNA content since protein losses might occur, while Dr. Versmold suggested relating the measurements to tissue weight. He also wondered if the known increase in number of mitochondria per cell during the perinatal period might be relevant. Dr. Goodwin said that the standard method of relating all measurements to mitochondrial protein seemed the most reliable and that it should eliminate variables such as changes in number of mitochondria. However, the authors were examining tissue mitochondrial changes in E.M. pictures taken during the perinatal period. In reply to a question from Dr. Dora, the speaker said that Ca^{++} transport had not been measured after the sixth postnatal day. Dr. Netter asked whether the decreased turnover of O_2 after birth indicated the induction of a new cytochrome with a low O_2 turnover number during the post natal period. Dr. Goodwin thought this unlikely since a number of factors, such as variations in both substrate and enzyme concentrations can produce changes in the O_2 turnover number.

The last three papers of the session dealt with various clinical applications of transcutaneous (T.C.) and catheter PO_2 electrodes. Dr. Huch demonstrated how their T.C. PO_2 electrode could be used to estimate arterial PO_2 in the fetus during labour and in the neonate and showed that changes in neonatal PaO_2 bore little if any relation to alterations in heart rate. Dr. Beran congratulated the authors on the very close correlation between T.C. PO_2 and PaO_2 even when large PO_2 gradients across the dermis were present. He and Dr. Dora asked if the close relationship still existed at low arterial pressure, and whether blood pressure had been monitored. Dr. Huch replied that the babies were normal cases and it was not permissible to monitor blood pressure. However, she and Dr. Lubbers emphasized that provided stringent control of the conditions (particularly the temperature) at the measuring site were observed then T.C. PO_2 is virtually independent of flow. The local hyperemia is maintained by careful control of the heating current and under these conditions general blood flow to the area may be reduced by 2/3 without affecting T.C. PO_2. However, if the blood pressure falls very low then the local flow might become insufficient. In reply to a question by Dr. Kreuzer, Dr. Huch explained that T.C. PO_2 is about 11% higher than PaO_2, the full data for correcting T.C. to arterial PO_2 being available in Arch. Dis. Child. 49, 1974. Dr. Huch thought that it was very difficult to know why there was no correlation between PaO_2 and heart rate but pointed out that systematic experimental investigations could not be made on human babies. Dr. Versmold emphasised that in some babies heart rate does drop during hypoxemia, but in those cases where no changes are found with decreased PaO_2 very careful monitoring is necessary.

In contrast to the previous paper Dr. Soutter found little correlation between T.C. PO_2 and PaO_2 in neonates; a La Roche T.C. electrode was used in this study. Dr. Bicher thought that commercially available electrodes should always be tested thoroughly before clinical use since manufacturers' claims were not always reliable. Dr. Lubbers pointed out that the type of electrode used in this study was known to have a poor correlation with PaO_2 because of a number of constructional features. In some simultaneous tests with the Huch/Lubbers electrode, the latter invariably gave a good correlation with PaO_2 while the La Roche electrode gave variable results; that is shown in the Figure on the next page. Dr. Soutter replied that they had used the La Roche electrode in good faith, had followed the makers instructions and that she merely wanted to show the results which they had obtained.

In the last paper of the session Dr. Beran showed how different sizes of intra-arterial catheters inserted into one iliac artery in rabbits may affect the blood pressure, and the blood flow, O_2 availability and skin temperature in the contralateral limb. Dr. Strauss was very glad that such inherent dangers of arterial catheterization had been brought to our notice and thought that the results should make everyone think a little more carefully and test more thoroughly any equipment to be used clinically, whether on new born infants or adults.

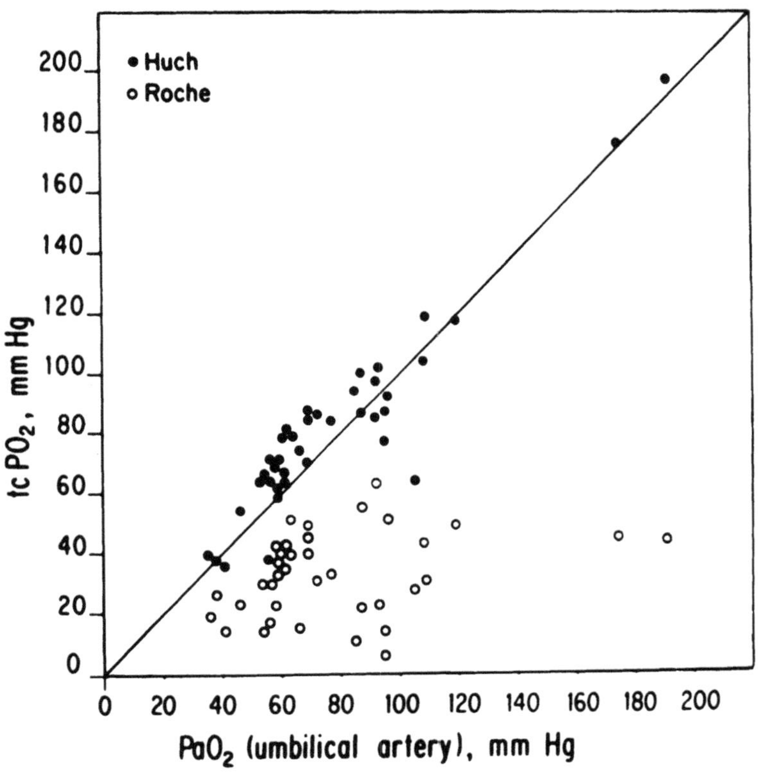

Arterial PO_2 (PaO_2) and transcutaneous PO_2 ($tcPO_2$) values in ventilated children of the Pediatric Intensive Care Unit in Zürich. Different correlations obtained during simultaneous measurements on the same children with the percutaneous instrument of Hofmann-LaRoche (o) and the transcutaneous electrode according to Huch, Lübbers, Huch (•). (From a study performed by G. Duc, Zürich.)

CONTRIBUTORS

Dr. H. Acker
Max-Planck-Institut für Systemphysiologie,
Dortmund, Fed. Rep. Germany

Dr. D. R. Antonenko
Department of Surgery, Royal Alexandra Hospital,
Edmonton, Alberta, Canada

Dr. A. von Ardenne
Forschungsinstitut Manfred von Ardenne,
Dresden, GDR

Dr. M. von Ardenne
Forschungsinstitut Manfred von Ardenne,
Dresden, GDR

Dr. W. Barnikol
Institute of Physiology, University of Mainz,
Mainz, Fed. Rep. Germany

Dr. R. E. Barr
Department of Ophthalmology, University of Missouri,
Columbia, Missouri, USA

Dr. A. V. Beran
Department of Pediatrics, University of California,
Irvine, California, USA

Dr. H. I. Bicher
Department of Pharmacology, University of Arkansas,
Little Rock, Arkansas, USA

Dr. D. F. Bruley
Chemical Engineering Department, School of Engineering,
Tulane University, New Orleans, Louisiana, USA

Dr. S. M. Cain
Department of Medicine, Pulmonary Division, University of Alabama, Birmingham, Alabama, USA

Dr. P. Cerretelli
Department of Physiology III, University of Milano, Milano, Italy

Dr. R. F. Coburn
Department of Physiology, University of Pennsylvania, Philadelphia, Pennsylvania, USA

Dr. T. B. Constable
MRC Cyclotron Unit, Hammersmith Hospital, London, England

Dr. J. Ditzel
Department of Medicine, Section of Endocrinology and Metabolism, Aalborg Regional Hospital, Aalborg Denmark

Dr. E. Dóra
Experimental Research Department, Medical University of Budapest, Budapest, Hungary

Dr. W. J. Dorson
Engineering Center, Ariczona State University, Tempe, Arizona, USA

Dr. J. Duhm
Institute of Physiology, University of Munich, Munich, Fed. Rep. Germany

Dr. E. A. Ernst
Department of Anesthesiology, University Hospital, Case Western Reserve University, Cleveland, Ohio, USA

Dr. N. T. S. Evans
MRC Cyclotron Unit, Hammersmith Hospital, London, England

Dr. J. E. Fletcher
Division of Computer Research and Technology, National Institute of Health, Bethesda, Maryland, USA

Dr. R. W. Flower
Applied Physics Laboratory, Johns Hopkins University and Hospital, Silver Spring, Maryland, USA

Dr. R. E. Forster
Department of Physiology, University of Pennsylvania, Philadelphia, Pennsylvania, USA

Dr. W. J. Gibson
Department of Surgery, Royal Alexandra Hospital, Edmonton, Alberta, Canada

Dr. T. K. Goldstick
Chemical Engineering Department, Northwestern University, Evanston, Illinois, USA

Dr. C. A. Goresky
University Medical Clinic, Montreal General Hospital, Montreal, Quebec, Canada

Dr. M. Gosalvez
Bioquimica Experimental, Clinica Puerta de Hierro, Madrid, Spain

Dr. A. C. Groom
Department of Biophysics, University of Western Ontario, London, Ontario, Canada

Dr. J. Grote
Institute of Physiology, University of Mainz, Mainz, Fed. Rep. Germany

Dr. W. Grunewald
Institute of Physiology, University of Regensburg, Regensburg, Fed. Rep. Germany

Dr. E. J. Guilbeau
Department of Biomedical Engineering, Louisiana Tech University, Ruston, Louisiana, USA

Dr. P. M. Gullino
Laboratory of Pathophysiology, National Cancer Institute, National Institute of Health, Bethesda, Maryland, USA

Dr. C. R. Honig
Department of Physiology, University of Rochester, Rochester, New York, USA

Dr. L. J. C. Hoofd
Department of Physiology, University of Nijmegen, Nijmegen, Netherlands

Dr. A. Huch
Department of Obstetrics and Gynecology, University of Marburg, Marburg, Fed. Rep. Germany

Dr. R. Huch
Department of Obstetrics and Gynecology, University of Marburg, Marburg, Fed. Rep. Germany

Dr. P. Hunt
Department of Pharmacology, University of Arkansas, Little Rock, Arkansas, USA

Dr. H. Hutten
Institute of Physiology, University of Mainz, Mainz, Fed. Rep. Germany

Dr. C. Ikrényi
Experimental Research Department, Medical University of Budapest, Budapest, Hungary

Dr. F. Jesch
Institute for Surgical Research, University of Munich, Munich, Fed. Rep. Germany

Dr. F. F. Jöbsis
Department of Physiology, Duke University
Durham, North Carolina, USA

Dr. T. Kawashiro
Max-Planck-Institut für Experimentelle Medizin, Abteilung Physiologie, Göttingen, Fed. Rep. Germany

Dr. H. P. Kimmich
Department of Physiology, University of Nijmegen, Nijmegen, Netherlands

Dr. H. Kiwull-Schöne
Institute of Physiology, University of Bochum, Bochum, Fed. Rep. Germany

Dr. A. G. B. Kovách
Experimental Research Department, Medical University of Budapest, Budapest, Hungary

Dr. F. Kreuzer
Department of Physiology, University of Nijmegen, Nijmegen, Netherlands

Dr. K. Kunze
Department of Clinical Neurophysiology,
University of Giessen,
Giessen, Fed. Rep. Germany

Dr. A. Lehmkühler
Institute of Physiology,
University of Münster,
Münster, Fed. Rep. Germany

Dr. E. Leniger-Follert
Max-Planck-Institut für Systemphysiologie,
Dortmund, Fed. Rep. Germany

Dr. I. S. Longmuir
Department of Biochemistry,
North Carolina State University,
Raleigh, North Carolina, USA

Dr. D. W. Lübbers
Max-Planck-Institut für Systemphysiologie,
Dortmund, Fed. Rep. Germany

Dr. A. Mayevsky
Department of Life Sciences, Bar-Ilan University,
Ramat-Gan, Israel

Dr. J. H. Meldon
Department of Physiology, University of Odense,
Odense, Denmark

Dr. M. Mochizuki
Department of Physiology, Yamagata University,
Yamagata, Japan

Dr. W. Moll
Institute of Physiology, University of Regensburg,
Regensburg, Fed. Rep. Germany

Dr. R. W. Ogilvie
Department of Pathology,
Medical University of South Carolina,
Charleston, South Carolina, USA

Dr. J. M. M. Oomens
Department of Mechanical Engineering,
University of Technology Eindhoven,
Netherlands

Dr. W. Pawlik
Institute of Physiology, Medical Academy of Krakow, Krakow, Poland

Dr. J. Piiper
Max-Planck-Institut für Experimentelle Medizin, Abteilung Physiologie, Göttingen, Fed. Rep. Germany

Dr. H. W. Puffer
Department of Pathology, University of Southern California, Los Angeles, California, USA

Dr. P. E. di Prampero
Centro Studi Fisiologia del Lavoro Muscolare (CNR), Milano, Italy

Dr. D. D. Reneau
Department of Biomedical Engineering, Louisiana Tech University Ruston, Louisiana, USA

Dr. E. L. Roetman
Department of Mathematics, University of Missouri, Columbia, Missouri, USA

Dr. E. Seidl
Max-Planck-Institut für Systemphysiologie, Dortmund, Fed. Rep. Germany

Dr. K. Skolasinska
Max-Planck-Institut für Systemphysiologie, Dortmund, Fed. Rep. Germany

Dr. G. Schneiderman
Chemical Engineering Department, Northwestern University, Evanston, Illinois, USA

Dr. V. S. Shapot
Department of Biochemistry, Institute of Experimental and Clinical Oncology, Moscow, USSR

Dr. B. K. Siesjö
Research Department 4, E-Blocket, University Hospital, Lund, Sweden

Dr. I. A. Silver
Department of Pathology, University of Bristol, Bristol, England

Dr. M. Silver
Physiological Laboratory, University of Cambridge, Cambridge, England

Dr. E. Sinagowitz
Urologische Universitätsklinik Freiburg, Freiburg, Fed. Rep. Germany

Dr. L. P. Soutter
Department of Medical Physics, University College Hospital, London, England

Dr. J. A. E. Spaan
Department of Mechanical Engineering, University of Technology Eindhoven, Eindhoven, Netherlands

Dr. E. Standl
Diabetes Research Unit, City Hospital Schwabing, Munich, Fed. Rep. Germany

Dr. J. Strauss
Department of Pediatrics, University of Miami, Miami, Florida, USA

Dr. P. Stroeve
Department of Physiology, University of Nijmegen, Nijmegen, Netherlands

Dr. I. Tannock
Department of Medicine, Toronto General Hospital, Toronto, Ontario, Canada

Dr. G. Thews
Institute of Physiology, University of Mainz, Mainz, Fed. Rep. Germany

Dr. M. Tsacopoulos
Department of Ophthalmology, University of Geneva, Geneva, Switzerland

Dr. Z. Turek
Department of Physiology, University of Nijmegen, Nijmegen, Netherlands

Dr. P. Vaupel
Institute of Physiology, University of Mainz, Mainz, Fed. Rep. Germany

Dr. H. Versmold
Kinderklinik der Universität München, Munich, Fed. Rep. Germany

Dr. H. Weigelt
Max-Planck-Institut für Systemphysiologie,
Dortmund, Fed. Rep. Germany

Dr. Ch. Weiss
Institute of Physiology, University of Kiel,
Kiel, Fed. Rep. Germany

Dr. W. J. Whalen
St. Vincent Charity Hospital, Cleveland, Ohio, USA

Dr. D. F. Wilson
Johnson Research Foundation, Department of Biophysics
and Physical Biochemistry, University of Pennsylvania,
Pennsylvania, USA

Dr. R. Wodick
Max-Planck-Institut für Systemphysiologie,
Dortmund, Fed. Rep. Germany

Dr. W. Wrabetz
Max-Planck-Institut für Systemphysiologie,
Dortmund, Fed. Rep. Germany

Dr. R. Zander
Institute of Physiology, University of Mainz,
Mainz, Fed. Rep. Germany

Dr. W. Erdmann
Department of Anestesiology,
Birmingham, Alabama, USA

INDEX

GPSR Compliance
The European Union's (EU) General Product Safety Regulation (GPSR) is a set of rules that requires consumer products to be safe and our obligations to ensure this.

If you have any concerns about our products, ycu can contact us on

ProductSafety@springernature.com

In case Publisher is established outside the EU, the EU authorized representative is:

Springer Nature Customer Service Center GmbH
Europaplatz 3
69115 Heidelberg, Germany

www.ingramcontent.com/pod-product-compliance
Ingram Content Group UK Ltd.
Pitfield, Milton Keynes, MK11 3LW, UK
UKHW051240300926
15471UKWH00015B/1126

* 9 7 8 1 4 6 8 4 3 2 7 4 9 *